Sleep in Childhood Neurological Disorders

Sleep in Childhood Neurological Disorders

Sanjeev V. Kothare, MD
Associate Professor of Neurology
Harvard Medical School

Attending Pediatric Neurologist and Sleep Specialist
Department of Neurology
Associate Director (Neurology)
Center for Pediatric Sleep Disorders
Children's Hospital
Boston, Massachusetts

Suresh Kotagal, MD
Professor of Neurology
Division of Child Neurology
Mayo Clinic
Professor of Neurology
Mayo Clinic Center for Sleep Medicine
Rochester, Minnesota

demosMEDICAL
New York

Acquisitions Editor: Beth Barry
Cover Design: Joe Tenerelli
Compositor: S4Carlisle Publishing Services
Printer: Hamilton Printing

Visit our Website at www.demosmedpub.com

Medicine is an ever-changing science. Research and clinical experience are continually expanding our knowledge, in particular, our understanding of proper treatment and drug therapy. The authors, editors, and publisher have made every effort to ensure that all information in this book are in accordance with the state of knowledge at the time of production of the book. Nevertheless, the authors, editors, and publisher are not responsible for any errors or omissions or for any consequences from application of the information in this book and make no warranty, express or implied, with respect to the contents of the publication. Every reader should examine carefully the package inserts accompanying each drug and should carefully check whether the dosage schedules mentioned therein or the contraindications stated by the manufacturer differ from the statements made in this book. Such examination is particularly important with drugs that are either rarely used or have been newly released on the market.

Library of Congress Cataloging-in-Publication Data

Sleep in childhood neurological disorders / [edited by] Sanjeev V. Kothare, Suresh Kotagal.
p. ; cm.
Includes bibliographical references and index.
ISBN 978-1-933864-96-9
1. Sleep disorders in children. 2. Nervous system—Diseases—Complications. 3. Child psychiatry. I. Kothare, Sanjeev V. II. Kotagal, Suresh.
[DNLM: 1. Sleep Disorders—complications. 2. Adolescent. 3. Child. 4. Mental Disorders—complications. 5. Nervous System Diseases—complications. WL 108]
RJ506.S55S575 2011
618.92'8498—dc22

2010046352

Special discounts on bulk quantities of Demos Medical Publishing books are available to corporations, professional associations, pharmaceutical companies, health care organizations, and other qualifying groups. For details, please contact:

Special Sales Department
Demos Medical Publishing
11 W. 42nd Street, 15th Floor
New York, NY 10036
Phone: 800-532-8663 or 212-683-0072
Fax: 212-941-7842
E-mail: rsantana@demosmedpub.com

Made in the United States of America
11 12 13 14 15 5 4 3 2 1

This book is dedicated to our patients and their families and our own families

Contents

Preface ix
Contributors xi

1. The Science of Sleep: Ontogeny, Phylogeny, and More 1
Kiran Prasad Maski, Suresh Kotagal, and Sanjeev V. Kothare

2. The Clinical and Laboratory Assessment of Childhood Sleep–Wake Problems 27
Suresh Kotagal

3. Sleep and ADHD: Daytime and Nighttime Phenotypes 41
Karen Spruyt and David Gozal

4. Restless Legs Syndrome 57
Daniel L. Picchietti and Matthew A. Picchietti

5. Sleep and Epilepsy 71
Joseph Kaleyias and Sanjeev V. Kothare

6. Sleep-Potentiated Spike-Wave Discharges and Electrical Status Epilepticus of Slow-Wave Sleep 97
Tobias Loddenkemper and Prakash Kotagal

7. Childhood Parasomnias 113
Radhika Dhamija and Suresh Kotagal

8. Smith–Magenis Syndrome 123
Gabor P. Szuhay and Andrea L. Gropman

9. Autism and Other Neurodevelopmental Disorders 143
Suzanne E. Goldman and Beth A. Malow

10. Psychiatric Disorders and Sleep 153
Oliviero Bruni, Luana Novelli, Valeria Savoja, and Raffaele Ferri

11. Sleep and Wakefulness in Children With Brain Tumors 173
Gerald Rosen and Audrey Schor

12. Narcolepsy 189
Marcin Zarowski, Suresh Kotagal, and Sanjeev V. Kothare

13. Circadian Rhythm Disorders 219
Tifenn Raffray, Eliza Van Reen, Leila Tarokh, and Mary A. Carskadon

14. Sleep and Circadian Dysfunction in Children With Mental Retardation or Cerebral Palsy 235
Jonathan Lipton

15. Sleep-Related Breathing Disorders in Children With Miscellaneous Neurological Disorders 245
Madeleine Grigg-Damberger and Jeffrey J. Stanley

16. Management of Sleep-Disordered Breathing in Children With Neuromuscular Disease 275
Eliot S. Katz and Carolyn M. D'Ambrosio

17. Congenital Central Hypoventilation Syndrome 295
Debra E. Weese-Mayer, Pallavi P. Patwari, Michael S. Carroll, and Casey M. Rand

18. Assessment of Sleep Fragmentation 313
Shalini Paruthi and Ronald D. Chervin

19. Imaging Modalities in Pediatric Sleep Medicine 325
Robert Joseph Thomas

20. Pediatric Sleep Pharmacology 345
Rafael Pelayo and Kin Yuen

21. Sleep and Headaches 367
Martina Vendrame and Sanjeev V. Kothare

22. Sleep in Traumatic Brain Injury in Children 381
Stephen H. Sheldon

23. Craniofacial Disorders and Sleep 387
Tarig Ali-Dinar and Nalton F. Ferraro

24. Multidisciplinary Team Approach for the Evaluation of Children With Sleep Disorders 399
Umakanth A. Khatwa, Rachel Rosen, Eric Chiou, and Greg R. Licameli

25. Drug Development for Pediatric Sleep Disorders: Opportunities and Challenges 417
O'Neill D'Cruz and Virinder Nohria

Index 425

Preface

The sleep–wake problems of infants, children, and adolescents with neurological disorders have thus far been discussed in print through scattered review articles in textbooks and journals. *Pediatric neurosomnology* is an emerging, multidisciplinary field in need of a firm foundation. This state-of-the-art compilation of reviews by leading authorities is intended to help solidify the base of this important discipline that contributes so much to enhancing the quality-of-life of children with neurological problems. We have tried to minimize overlap between the chapters, but some repetition is unavoidable given the multidimensional nature of sleep disruption in childhood neurological disorders. It is our hope that this book will be a trusted resource and practical guide for pediatricians and family care physicians, neurologists, sleep specialists, and others who are involved in the care of children with neurologically based sleep problems.

The editors are deeply indebted to all the authors for their hard work, adherence to deadlines, and flexibility in modifying their manuscripts when requested. We would like to thank Beth Barry at Demos Publishing for her assistance in launching this project and Tom Hastings for his marketing advice and cover design management.

Sanjeev V. Kothare, MD
Suresh Kotagal, MD

Contributors

Tarig Ali-Dinar, MD
Assistant Professor of Clinical Pediatrics
Department of Pediatrics
Miller School of Medicine
University of Miami
Miami, Florida

Oliviero Bruni, MD
Associate Professor
Department of Developmental Neurology and Psychiatry
Center for Pediatric Sleep Disorders
Sapienza University
Rome, Italy

Michael S. Carroll, PhD
Computational Neuroscientist
Center for Autonomic Medicine in Pediatrics
Children's Memorial Hospital
Chicago, Illinois

Mary A. Carskadon, PhD
Professor, Psychiatry and Human Behavior
Brown University
Director
E.P. Bradley Sleep Research Laboratory
Providence, Rhode Island

Ronald D. Chervin, MD, MS
Professor of Neurology
Michael S. Aldrich Collegiate Professor of Sleep Medicine
Director, Sleep Disorders Center
Department of Neurology
University of Michigan
Ann Arbor, Michigan

Eric H. Chiou, MD
Clinical Fellow
Division of Pediatric Gastroenterology
Children's Hospital Boston
Boston, Massachusetts

Carolyn M. D'Ambrosio, MD
Associate Professor
Division of Pulmonary Diseases
Tufts-New England Medical Center
Boston, Massachusetts

O'Neill D'Cruz, MD, MBA
Medical Director
Department of Neurology
UCB Pharma
Raleigh, North Carolina

Radhika Dhamija, MBBS
Resident
Department of Neurology
Mayo Clinic
Mayo Clinic Center for Sleep Medicine
Rochester, Minnesota

Nalton F. Ferraro, MD
Oral and Maxillofacial Surgery
Division of Plastic and Faciomaxillary surgery
Children's Hospital Boston
Harvard Medical School
Boston, Massachusetts

Raffaele Ferri, MD
Head, Department of Neurology
Sleep Research Centre
Oasi Institute for Research on Mental Retardation and Brain Aging (IRCCS)
Troina, Italy

Suzanne E. Goldman, PhD
Assistant Professor
Department of Neurology
Sleep Disorders Program
Vanderbilt University Medical Center
Nashville, Tennessee

David Gozal, MD
The Herbert T. Abelson Professor and Chair
Department of Pediatrics
University of Chicago
Chicago, Illinois

Madeline Grigg-Damberger, MD
Professor of Neurology
University of New Mexico School of Medicine
Medical Director, Pediatric Sleep Medicine Services
University Hospital Sleep Disorders Center
University of New Mexico Medical Center
Albuquerque, New Mexico

Andrea L. Gropman, MD
Associate Professor
Department of Neurology
Children's National Medical Center
George Washington University of the Health Sciences
Washington, District of Columbia

Joseph Kaleyias, MD, PhD
Director of Child Neurology
Division of Child Neurology
Department of Pediatrics
University Hospital of Patras
Patras, Greece

Eliot S. Katz, MD
Instructor in Pediatrics
Division of Respiratory Diseases
Children's Hospital Boston
Boston, Massachusetts

Umakanth A. Khatwa, MD
Codirector
Pulmonary Program of Center for Aerodigestive Disorders
Department of Medicine
Division of Respiratory Diseases
Children's Hospital Boston
Harvard Medical School
Center for Pediatric Sleep Disorders
Boston, Massachusetts

Prakash Kotagal, MD
Head, Pediatric Epilepsy Section
Neurological Institute
The Cleveland Clinic Foundation
Cleveland, Ohio

Suresh Kotagal, MD
Professor of Neurology
Division of Child Neurology
Mayo Clinic
Professor of Neurology
Mayo Clinic Center for Sleep Medicine
Rochester, Minnesota

Sanjeev V. Kothare, MD
Associate Professor of Neurology
Harvard Medical School
Attending Pediatric Neurologist and Sleep Specialist
Department of Neurology
Associate Director (Neurology)
Center for Pediatric Sleep Disorders
Children's Hospital
Boston, Massachusetts

Greg R. Licameli, MD, FACS
Associate in Otolaryngology
Department of Otolaryngology and Communication Enhancement
Assistant Professor
Children's Hospital Boston
Boston, Massachusetts

Jonathan Lipton, MD, PhD
Instructor in Neurology
Department of Neurology
Children's Hospital Boston
Faculty Member
Division of Sleep Medicine
Harvard Medical School
Boston, Massachusetts

Tobias Loddenkemper, MD
Assistant Professor of Neurology
Department of Neurology
Harvard Medical School
Children's Hospital Boston
Boston, Massachusetts

Beth A. Malow, MD, MS
Professor/Medical Director
Department of Neurology
Sleep Disorders Program
Vanderbilt University Medical Center
Nashville, Tennessee

Kiran Prasad Maski, MD
Instructor
Department of Neurology and Sleep Medicine
Children's Hospital Boston
Boston, Massachusetts

Virinder Nohria
Executive Vice President
Chief Medical Officer
Alaven Pharmaceuticals, LLC
Marietta, Georgia

Luana Novelli, PhD
Research Assistant
Department of Developmental Neurology
and Psychiatry
Center for Pediatric Sleep Disorders
Sapienza University
Rome, Italy

Shalini Paruthi, MD
Assistant Professor
Department of Pediatrics
Saint Louis University
St. Louis, Missouri

Pallavi P. Patwari, MD
Assistant Professor of Pediatrics
Feinberg School of Medicine
Northwestern University
Center for Autonomic Medicine in Pediatrics
Children's Memorial Hospital
Chicago, Illinois

Rafael Pelayo, MD
Associate Professor
Department of Psychiatry
and Behavioral Science
Stanford Sleep Disorders Center
Stanford University School of Medicine
Stanford, California

Daniel L. Picchietti, MD
Department of Pediatrics
Carle Foundation Hospital
University of Illinois School of Medicine
Urbana, Illinois

Matthew A. Picchietti, BA
Department of Psychology
Southern Illinois University, Carbondale
Carbondale, Illinois

Tifenn Raffray, MD, MS
Research Fellow
Department of Psychiatry and Human Behavior
Brown University
Providence, Rhode Island
Chief of Clinic
Department of Adult Psychiatry
University Hospital
Lausanne, Switzerland

Casey M. Rand, BS
Research Coordinator
Center for Autonomic Medicine in Pediatrics
Children's Memorial Hospital
Chicago, Illinois

Eliza Van Reen, PhD
Instructor
Department of Psychiatry and Human Behavior
Warren Alpert Medical School
of Brown University
Research Associate
Sleep and Chronobiology Lab
E.P. Bradley Hospital
Providence, Rhode Island

Gerald Rosen, MA, MPh
Director of Sleep Center
Children's Hospital of Minnesota
St. Paul, Minnesota
Associate Professor
Department of Pediatrics
University of Minnesota School of Medicine
Minneapolis, Minnesota

Rachel Rosen, MD, MPH
Assistant Professor of Pediatrics
Department of Gastroenterology
Children's Hospital Boston
Boston, Massachusetts

Valeria Savoja, MD
Research Assistant
Department of Neurosciences, Mental
Health, and Sensory Functions
Sapienza University
Unit of Psychiatry
Sant'Andrea Hospital
Rome, Italy

Audrey Schor, PhD
Assistant Professor
Department of Biology
Saint Leo University
Saint Leo, Florida

Stephen H. Sheldon, DO, FAAP
Professor of Pediatrics
Feinberg School of Medicine
Northwestern University
Director
Sleep Medicine Center
Children's Memorial Hospital
Chicago, Illinois

Karen Spruyt, PhD
Assistant Professor
Department of Pediatrics
University of Chicago
Chicago, Illinois

Jeffrey J. Stanley, MD
Assistant Professor
Department of Otolaryngology-Head
and Neck Surgery
Michael Aldrich Sleep Disorders Center
University of Michigan Health System
Ann Arbor, Michigan

Gabor P. Szuhay, MD
Assistant Professor
Department of Neurology
Children's National Medical Center
George Washington University
of the Health Sciences
Washington, District of Columbia

Leila Tarokh, PhD
Instructor (Research)
Department of Psychiatry and Human
Behavior
Warren Alpert Medical School
of Brown University
Providence, Rhode Island
Academic Guest
Institute of Pharmacology and Toxicology
University of Zurich
Zurich, Switzerland

Robert Joseph Thomas, MD, MMSc.
Assistant Professor of Medicine
Division of Pulmonary
Critical Care and Sleep Medicine
Beth Israel Deaconess Medical Center
Boston, Massachusetts

Martina Vendrame, MD, PhD
Assistant Professor
Department of Neurology
Boston University Medical School
Boston, Massachusetts

Debra E. Weese-Mayer, MD
Professor of Pediatrics
Feinberg School of Medicine
Northwestern University
Director
Center for Autonomic Medicine in Pediatrics
Children's Memorial Hospital
Chicago, Illinois

Kin Yuen, MD, MS
Stanford Sleep Disorders Center
Stanford University School of Medicine
Stanford, California

Marcin Zarowski, MD, PhD
Division of Epilepsy and Clinical Neurophysiology
Center for Pediatric Sleep Disorders
Department of Neurology
Children's Hospital Boston
Harvard Medical School
Boston, Massachusetts
Polysomnography and Sleep Research Unit
Department of Developmental Neurology
Poznan University of Medical Sciences
Poznan, Poland

CHAPTER 1

The Science of Sleep: Ontogeny, Phylogeny, and More

Kiran Prasad Maski, Suresh Kotagal, and Sanjeev V. Kothare

Phylogeny of Sleep

Many mysteries still remain about the function of sleep. "If sleep does not serve an absolutely vital function, then it is the biggest mistake the evolutionary process has ever made," Allan Rechtschaffen, a sleep pioneer, wrote in 1971. Indeed, sleep is a highly conserved behavior found in mammals and nonmammal species alike. To discuss sleep across species, a definition for sleep must be established. Major criteria defining behavioral sleep states include (1) behavioral quiescence when motor activity may be reduced; (2) adoption of specific postures; (3) elevated arousal thresholds during which time a higher intensity stimulus is required to elicit a response compared with wake state; (4) rapid spontaneous reversibility, which distinguishes sleep from coma or anesthetic-induced state; and (5) homeostatic regulation, which drives species to sleep in response to sleep deprivation and are (6) partially governed by circadian or ultradian biorhythms [1–3]. Behaviorally defined sleep states have been characterized in the fruit fly (*Drosophila melanogaster*), zebra fish (*Danio rerio*), and most recently nematodes (*Caenorhabditis elegans*) [4–6]. Among mammals, there is more diversity in the behavior defined as sleep with sleeping patterns varying with diet, metabolic rate, gestational periods, and brain weight [7]. Certainly, the presence of sleep states in such a diverse array of creatures raises the question of whether sleep evolved independently in each organism or whether sleep was present in a common ancestor. Genetic analysis and molecular mechanisms linked to sleep control of model organisms such as *Drosophila* reveal remarkable conservation in the underlying mechanisms controlling sleep behavior, suggesting a common ancestor of all bilaterally symmetric organisms more than 600 million years ago [8].

Reptiles and amphibians exhibit clear sleep behavior but do not have the more sophisticated physiologic signatures of sleep seen in birds and mammals. Reptiles may show subcortical electrical signs on electroencephalogram (EEG) suggestive of non-rapid eye movement (NREM) sleep [9], but reptiles and amphibians do not have convincing neuronal activity suggestive of rapid eye movement (REM) sleep [10]. In mammals and birds, REM and NREM sleep can be distinguished on EEG, electrooculogram (EOG), and electromyelogram (EMG) data—These states may have evolved with endothermy (the maintenance of high, constant body temperature) [1]. The exception to this rule is in the primitive egg-laying mammals, echidnae, *Tachyglossus aculeatus*, where REM/NREM mixed state has been described [11]. Notably, birds have a smaller difference in their EEG spectrum between wakefulness and NREM sleep than mammals. Mammalian sleep is unique in the ability to generate sleep spindles and slow waves on EEG monitoring during NREM sleep [3,12].

Birds are believed to have a lower percentage of REM sleep, the occurrence of REM sleep in clusters, and a much briefer REM periods compared with mammals [1]. The amount of

REM sleep in mammals seems to correlate with species lifestyle, risk of predation, and degree of exposure of the sleeping environment [13]. Some birds and marine mammals also have brief or absent REM sleep and unihemispheric NREM sleep. This pattern of sleep may be developed by ecological pressures for migrating birds to keep moving or marine mammals to breathe air while diving [14]. The period length of each REM-NREM epoch increases with brain size across species [7]. In altricial mammalian species (those born immature such as the cat, dog, and human), REM sleep percentage is higher initially and declines to some degree with maturity whereas REM sleep stays at low values throughout life in precocial mammalian species (those born fairly mature such as the guinea pig and sheep) [15]. Although the quality and quantity of NREM/REM sleep vary considerably by species and within species, the conservation of these sleep states over time despite ecological pressures suggests that they do indeed serve some compelling vital function.

Function of Sleep

The ability to feed, mate, and protect oneself is lost during sleep. Research still has not yielded any conclusive data on the function of sleep, though several theories exist. Sleep deprivation in rodents and flies can cause death more quickly than food deprivation [16]. In rats, total sleep deprivation after 2 to 3 weeks leads animals to become hyperphagic but lose weight, become hyperthermic and then hypothermic, and debilitated before death [17,18]. In contrast, findings in marine mammals such as the killer whale (*Ornicus orca*) have been noted to have near absence of sleep behavior in neonates and postpartum mothers without deleterious effects or need for catch-up sleep [19]. Voluntary sleep deprivation in humans reveals impaired cognition and labile mood before sleep intrudes into waking states as micro-sleep [20]. Chronic and partial sleep deprivation in humans has been associated with abnormalities in immune function and host defense mechanisms, alterations in metabolism, nitrogen balance, protein catabolism, psychological disturbances, learning and memory, as well as quality-of-life measures [21].

Restorative Theory

The earliest theory about the function of sleep is the restorative theory of sleep, which proposes that sleep serves to reverse and restore biochemical and physiologic processes that are progressively degraded during prior wakefulness and thereby restore normal daytime functioning [22]. Indirect evidence supports this hypothesis [23]: (1) increased growth hormone secretion follows sleep onset in humans and baboons [24]; (2) increased amounts and intensity (as measured by slow-wave density and increased arousal threshold of sleep) during a period of sleep recovery after 24 hours of sleep deprivation in humans and most terrestrial mammals [25]; (3) the release of endogenous anabolic steroids (prolactin, testosterone, and luteinizing hormone) during specific sleep stages [26,27], and nadir of catabolic steroids during the first few hours of sleep [28]; (4) increased mitosis of lymphocytes and increased rate of bone growth during sleep [29]. Studies on the effects of exercise on sleep argue against the restorative theory of sleep. Increased sleep following the elevated catabolic state produced by physical exertion showed no evidence of increased postexercise sleep [30]. Studies did show an increase in NREM sleep postexercise, but this was thought to be the result of increased body temperature produced by exercise [31]. In addition, there is substantial evidence that circadian rhythms affect various somatic functions arguing against the restorative effects of sleep in itself. For instance, day-night variations in both the mitotic index and DNA synthesis were found in oral mucosa [32], corneal epithelium [33], and bone marrow [34], suggesting regulation by an endogenous circadian rhythm.

Most tantalizing to the neurologist are findings that sleep provides restorative function to the central nervous system (CNS). Microarray strategies that allow measurements of tens of thousands of transcripts simultaneously have provided comprehensive assessments of molecular changes in the brain during sleep and wakings. Research studying molecular changes in the brain during the sleep-wake cycle and after sleep deprivation using cerebral cortex and cerebellar gene expression in rats has shown that more than 15,000 transcripts were expressed, and a similar number of transcripts (5%) were affected by behavioral states and by time of day [35]. The study confirmed that the involvement of immediate-early shock genes as well as genes involved in synaptic plasticity and memory acquisition, energy metabolism, synaptic excitatory neurotransmission, and response to cellular stress are upregulated during waking. In sleep, genes involved in brain protein synthesis, lipid metabolism, myelin formation, synaptic vesicle turnover, and membrane trafficking and maintenance are upregulated [35]. Similarly, in the mouse cerebral cortex and to a lesser extent in the hypothalamus, other microarray studies have found upregulation of genes involved in enzyme production for cholesterol synthesis and synthesis of proteins for lipid transport and energy-regulating pathways [36]. The consequences of sleep deprivation were also analyzed using similar molecular technology. Rats were sleep deprived for 8 hours to 1 week, and the expression of more than 24,000 transcripts in the cerebral cortex was analyzed [37]. Long-term sleep deprivation induced overexpression of genes involved in many inflammatory processes and stress response genes mainly in glial cells, suggesting a trend toward generalized brain pathology. Such molecular research seems to support the view that synthesis of proteins and other macromolecules is a key function of sleep and that it is transcriptionally regulated.

Energy Conservation Theory

Another popular theory about sleep function is that sleep allows for an adaptive state during which energy is conserved across a 24-hour day. Findings that endothermic mammals reduce their metabolic rate and body temperature during periods of rest possibly to support the waking energy demands may support this theory [7]. Certainly, it is for endothermic mammals to reduce energy expenditure when food supply is scarce to ensure survival. When endothermic mammals fall asleep, thermoregulation continues through NREM sleep at functional levels below those of wakefulness. Their metabolic rates decrease as mediated by the preoptic nucleus of the hypothalamus and about 10% of heat is dissipated from their bodies through peripheral vasodilation [38,39]. However, it is widely held that this reduction in metabolism is minimal and the energy savings may not be sufficient to explain the natural selection of NREM/REM sleep in endothermic mammals during the course of evolution [14]. Further arguing against this hypothesis is that REM sleep, a state where temperature is partially unregulated, is associated with increased whole-body oxygen consumption [40]. Lastly, sleep is distinct from hibernation, a state selected to save energy. Animals emerging from hibernation, experience a sleep rebound as in sleep deprivation [41].

Learning and Memory Theory

In humans, the effects of sleep deprivation on higher cortical functions such as cognition, attention, and memory are immediate and seemingly unavoidable [14]. This observation has led to the theory that sleep is needed for brain plasticity, specifically in the process of learning and memory. There is a mounting wealth of data using neuroimaging, behavioral studies, electrophysiological studies, and cellular and molecular techniques that describe sleep-dependent brain plasticity in animals and humans [42–44]. Behavioral studies have shown that learning and memory are improved by subsequent sleep without repetition of the task, suggesting offline information processing and long-term memory consolidation and enhancement in sleep. Declarative memories benefit particularly from slow-wave sleep (SWS), whereas procedural memories benefit from REM sleep [45–47].

Neuroimaging techniques have shown that patterns of brain activity elicited during initial task training are replayed during subsequent sleep. Activation patterns on positron emission tomography (PET) during practice of motor skill tasks before sleep reappear during subsequent REM sleep episodes [48]. Furthermore, subjects' retest performances postsleep had improved relative to their initial training performances. The extent of sleep-dependent performance improvement was found to have a direct relationship with the subsequent reactivation during REM sleep [49]. Likewise, use of functional magnetic resonance imaging in conjunction with a procedural visuomotor pursuit task has also shown sleep-dependent plasticity [50]. Subjects allowed normal sleep showed significantly enhanced behavioral performance and selective increase in activation of the superior temporal gyrus at retest compared with subjects who were deprived of sleep.

REM and NREM contain numerous and unique electrophysiological phenomena implicated in the process of plasticity by potentiation or depression of synaptic connectivity [51]. After declarative learning tasks, the density of sleep spindles seen during stage 2 NREM sleep is significantly higher than that with a nonlearning control task and is greatest within the first 90 minutes of sleep [52]. It has been proposed that sleep spindles can provide depolarizing inputs to targets in the cortex that may be similar to the process of long-term potentiation (LTP), the process of enhanced synaptic stability in the hippocampus [53–55]. Similarly, theta waves seen in the hippocampus during REM sleep in humans and animals are also thought to greatly facilitate the induction of hippocampal LTP [56,57].

A form of sleep-dependent plasticity at the cellular level has been demonstrated during early postnatal development in the visual system of cats. Under normal circumstances, brief periods of monocular deprivation during critical periods of development lead to remodeling of synaptic connectivity, with the deprived eye's inputs to cortical neurons being functionally weakened [58]. Monocular deprivation plus a period of sleep was found to double the size of the monocularity shift [59]. It was concluded that sleep could contribute to the developmental changes seen in synaptic connectivity, as do visual experiences by enhancing changes occurring during a prior period of monocular deprivation. Contrary to this work, other cellular data have shown that the transcript expression at higher levels during sleep are involved in synaptic depression and depotentiation, whereas wakefulness leads to upregulation of activity-dependent processes of synaptic potentiation [35,60]. This suggests that sleep is necessary to renormalize synapses to a baseline level that leaves only the most robust synapses intact. Synaptic downscaling would also strengthen connectivity to improve performance as well as accelerate memory transfer from the hippocampus to the cortex [61].

Although the behavioral, neuroimaging, and cellular data pointing to an offline role of sleep in learning and memory are intriguing, the theory suggests that the benefit of sleep is corticocentric and does not account for the need for sleep in the development of sleep in animals without a telencephalon [62].

Sleep Architecture and Cycling

Normal sleep is a highly structured process involving cycling of REM and NREM sleep through the night [63] (Figure 1.1). In adults, a night of sleep begins with about 80 minutes of NREM sleep followed by 10 minutes of REM sleep. The approximate 90-minute NREM-REM cycle is then repeated about 3 to 6 times during the night. In successive cycles of the night, the amounts of stage 3 NREM sleep decrease and the proportion of REM sleep tends to increase. Wakefulness in sleep usually accounts for less than 5% of the night.

Criteria for sleep stages have been largely set by Rechtschaffen and Kales in 1968 [64] and modified over time [65]. NREM is conventionally divided into 3 stages based on the EEG findings and described as synchronous, with characteristic waveforms. Overall, NREM sleep is associated with preserved ability to move the body and active regulating brain and varying arousal thresholds depending on the stage of NREM sleep. The first sleep cycle in the normal young adult begins with stage 1 sleep, which is characterized by a decrease in alpha activity, mostly low-voltage, mixed-frequency activity ranging 3 to 7 Hz. Slow rolling eye movements on EOG may appear, and tone measured by EMG activity is moderate to low. Vertex waves and high-amplitude (up to 250 μV) and negative polarity waveforms that last less than 200 milliseconds can also be seen during stage 1 and stage 2 sleep. Stage 2 sleep consists of low-voltage and mixed theta and delta activity and is characterized by bursts of distinct 12- to 14-Hz sinusoidal waves called sleep spindles on EEG. Sleep spindles are believed to arise from generators located in the reticular nucleus of the thalamus and are believed to represent the electrical signature of cerebral deafferentation that occurs when the primary sensory pathways are gated [66]. Eye movements are rare and EMG tone is again low to moderate. K-complexes are characterized by a sharp negative wave followed by a slower positive wave, last at least 0.5 seconds, and are often followed by sleep spindles. Both vertex and K-complexes tend to occur in short spontaneous bursts but can appear in response to sensory stimuli. Stage 3 sleep (formerly known as stage 3 and 4 sleep) is characterized by high-amplitude (>75 mV), delta frequency activity, termed slow

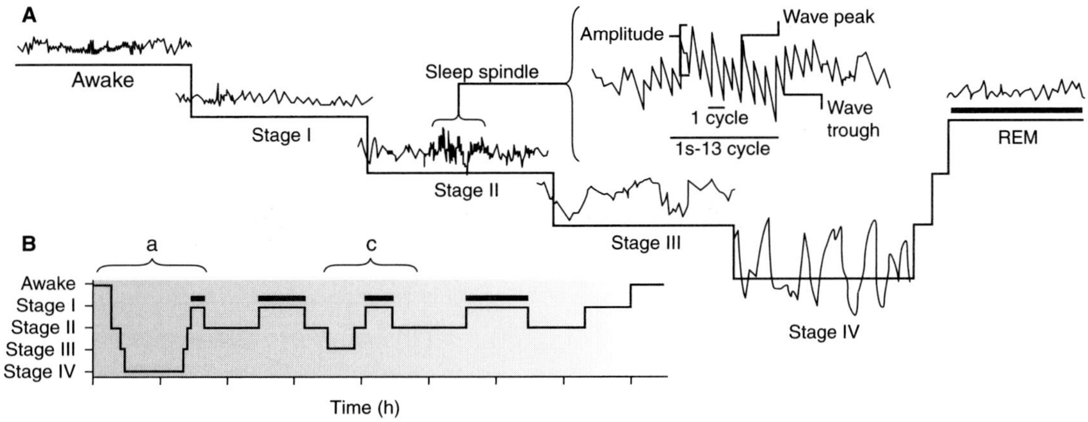

Figure 1.1 Sleep architecture and cycle basics. In mammals, NREM and REM sleep states exist and are defined in part by characteristic features on EEG (panel A). NREM sleep is divided into distinct stages, which correspond to the depth of sleep. Stage 1 NREM sleep is defined by a decrease in alpha activity and presence of mostly low-voltage, mixed-frequency activity ranging 3 to 7 Hz and vertex waves. Stage 2 NREM sleep is characterized by bursts of fast-frequency waveforms termed sleep spindles as well as K-complex waveforms. Stage 3 NREM sleep (formerly known as stage 3 and 4 NREM sleep) is associated with high-voltage, lower frequency, and synchronous slow (0.5–2 Hz) waveforms. REM sleep is characterized by wake-like, high-frequency, low-amplitude, and desynchronized activity on the EEG. NREM and REM sleep alternate in each of the 4 to 5 cycles that occur every night during sleep (panel B). Early in the night (a), NREM sleep is deeper and longer and becomes shallower later in the night. REM sleep (bar) is short in the first sleep cycle and increases in late sleep cycles (c). Adapted with permission from Ref. [204].

waves. Cortical cells governed by cells in the dorsal thalamus and connected by various thalamocortical projections generate these waves. The stages of NREM sleep correspond with the depth of sleep with stage 1 having the lowest arousal threshold and stage 4 the highest [63].

REM sleep is a state with electrical appearance and cerebral metabolic rate similar to wakefulness. In REM sleep, the EEG reverts to a low-voltage, high-frequency pattern with irregular activity. Another characteristic of REM sleep on EEG is the presence of sawtooth waves that have a frequency of 2 to 5 Hz, range 20 to 100 μV, and occur in a cluster of 3 or more waves. In addition, subcortical spike waves that arise in the pons and transmitted to lateral geniculate nucleus and visual cortex called PGO (ponto-geniculo-occipital waves) have been recorded in cats and more recently with deep brain electrodes in humans [67,68]. REM stage is characterized by episodic bursts of REM or saccades of quick conjugate eye movements on EOG. The background EMG is virtually absent representing muscle atonia with intermittent muscle twitching. REM sleep is generally not divided into stages, but there are tonic and phasic aspects of REM sleep. Phasic REM sleep events are intermittent with REMs and muscle twitches generally of the fingers, toes, and face, and tonic REM sleep events are persistent with desynchronized EEG and muscle inhibition [63]. Arousal threshold is lighter in REM sleep with increased neuronal activity compared with wakefulness and sometimes even greater than wakefulness reflecting a highly active mental state. Accordingly, dreaming is reported more frequently on awakenings from REM than NREM [69]. In REM sleep, there is suspended thermoregulation and predominance of sympathetic activity. Brain temperature increases as does cerebral blood flow (CBF) [70]. Heart rate, respiratory rate, and blood pressure are more variable during REM than during NREM. Lastly, penile erections occur during REM periods but rarely in NREM sleep [71].

Maturation of Sleep

Sleep is a maturational process with sleep architecture and cycling changing over the course of infancy and childhood [72]. Sleep can be distinguished from wakefulness on the basis of EEG and behavioral observation by 26 to 28 weeks postconceptional age (PCA). By 30 to 32 weeks, there is clear differentiation of sleep into quiet sleep (NREM) and active (REM) sleep. At this age, active sleep constitutes about 80% of total sleep, with quiet sleep being the remaining 20%. The EEG of quiet (NREM) sleep shows bursts of symmetric high-voltage slow waves lasting 4 to 5 seconds alternating with periods of low-amplitude activity of a similar duration (tracé alternans). During active sleep, the EEG is composed of irregular, mixed-frequency 4- to 8-Hz activity of less than 50 μV representing rudimentary REM sleep. By full term or 40 weeks PCA, the proportion of active sleep declines to about 50% of total sleep time, along with a corresponding increase in quiet sleep. Sleep generally begins with active sleep in the newborn. The ultradian rhythms (recurrent periods or cycles in a 24-hour period) of quiet/active sleep at birth have a period length of 50 to 60 minutes. By age 5 years, a 90-minute sleep cycle is established, which persists into adulthood.

At about 3 months of postnatal age, more defined waking stages are evident with emergence of a posterior dominant background rhythm. A clear circadian pattern develops at this age as sleep starts to move into longer portions during the night compared with the day. Quiet sleep develops features of more definite NREM sleep as sleep spindles start to appear between 3 and 6 months, but these spindles may still be asymmetrical till 12 to 18 months of age. By 6 months of age, stages of NREM sleep can be differentiated as vertex and K-complexes become identifiable. All stages of sleep are easily discernable by middle childhood and become very similar to adult sleep stages, though amplitude may be higher. SWS is maximal in young children and decreases with age (Figure 1.2). By the second decade of life, SWS decreases by nearly 40% by 75 years of age, SWS may be completely absent [63].

Active sleep may exceed 50% of sleep time in the newborn [72]. The need for the high levels of active sleep in the newborn period is not clear but may be important for the maturation of the brain and synaptic plasticity discussed earlier. By the end of the first year of life, the percentage of REM sleep decreases to about 30% of total sleep time and to 25% by age 3 to 5 years. REM sleep as a percentage is maintained well into healthy old age [63]. The EEG during REM sleep also undergoes significant changes with slight increase in mixed frequencies and decrease in amplitude and development of sawtooth waves between 3 and 12 months of age. The saccadic eye movements of sleep do not require retinal development or conscious fixation but do require development of the vestibular system [73]. An increase in phasic movements during sleep may persist till 18 months of age and reflects the maturation of the brain stem [74].

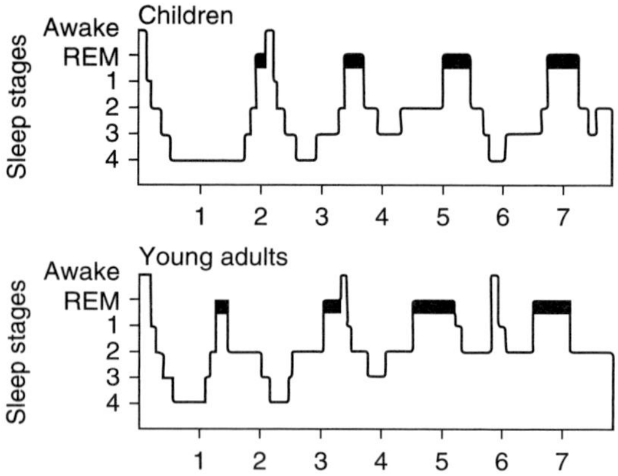

Figure 1.2 Sleep maturation from childhood to the adult period. Slow-wave sleep is maximal in childhood and decreases with age. REM sleep gradually decreases from childhood to adulthood.

Lastly, the arousal threshold decreases with age [75]. Extended wake episodes of which the individual is aware of and can report as well, as brief and unremembered arousals, increase with aging.

Wake and Sleep Anatomy and Physiology

Wakefulness

In 1949, Moruzzi and Magoun identified the ascending reticular activating system "whose direct stimulation activates or desynchronizes the EEG, replacing high-voltage slow waves with low-voltage fast activity" [76]. Based on their findings, wakefulness has been attributed to pathways of this diffuse "reticular activating system" involving glutamate concentrating neurons and connections to neurons of the thalamus and cerebral cortex. It is now known that the ascending pathways originate in well-defined cell groups in the brainstem and the basal forebrain (BF) and involve specific neurotransmitters and connections [77] (Figure 1.3). The wake pathway has 2 distinct branches. The dorsal branch ascends to the thalamus to activate the reticular nucleus and the relay nuclei, which are critical for thalamocortical transmission. The major sources of input to these thalamic nuclei are 2 cholinergic cell groups in the mesopontine tegmentum—the laterodorsal tegmental (LDT) and pedunculopontine tegmental (PPT) nuclei but modulating input is also received from the locus coeruleus (LC) and dorsal and median raphe nucleus (DR/MR) [79]. Cholinergic projections to the thalamus allow flow of sensory information and play a critical gatekeeper like role for thalamocortical transmission [77].

The ventral branch of the ascending arousal system bypasses the thalamus and activates neurons in the lateral hypothalamic area (located

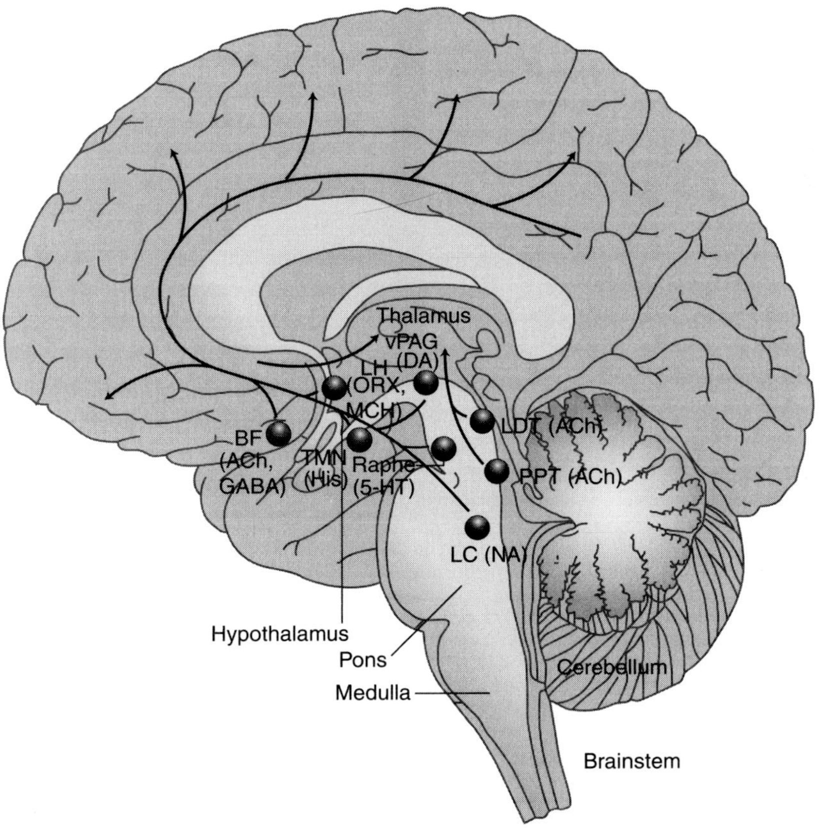

Figure 1.3 Arousal mechanisms. A major input to the relay and reticular nuclei of the thalamus originates from cholinergic (ACh) cell groups in the upper pons, the pedunculopontine (PPT), and laterodorsal tegmental (LDT) nuclei. These inputs facilitate thalamocortical transmission. A second pathway activates the cerebral cortex to facilitate the processing of inputs from the thalamus. This arises from neurons in the monoaminergic cell groups, including the tuberomammillary nucleus (TMN) containing histamine (His), the ventral periaquaductal gray matter (vPAG) containing dopamine (DA), the dorsal and median raphe nuclei containing serotonin (5-HT), and the locus coeruleus (LC) containing noradrenaline (NA). This pathway also receives contributions from peptidergic neurons in the lateral hypothalamus (LHA) containing orexin (ORX) or melanin-concentrating hormone (MCH), and from basal forebrain (BF) neurons that contain γ-aminobutyric acid (GABA) or ACh. Adapted with permission from Ref. [80].

in the posterior hypothalamus), BF, and diffuse areas of the cerebral cortex [80]. The inputs arise from the upper brainstem (noreadrenergic LC, dopaminergic ventral periaquaductal gray matter, serotonergic DR/MR) and caudal hypothalamus [histaminergic tuberomammillary neurons (TMN)] [81–84]. They ascend through the lateral hypothalamus (LHA) and terminate on neurons in the BF including nucleus basalis, magnocellular neurons in the substantia innominata, medial septum nucleus, and nucleus of the diagonal band of Broca [85], regions that project to cortical targets. Lesions of the cholinergic neurons of the BF produce slowing of cortical activity and loss of vigilance, which may explain characteristic findings of Alzheimer disease [86].

These brainstem inputs are joined by 2 distinct populations of neurons in the LHA that contribute to the regulation of wakefulness. LHA neurons contain a neuropeptide called orexin (otherwise known as hypocretin) in the perifornical area lateral hypothalamic nuclei as well as the melanin-concentrating hormone (MHC) [87–89]. These inputs join the cholinergic and γ-aminobutyric acidergic (GABAergic) BF neurons in providing direct input to the cerebral cortex [90,91]. Orexin neurons also project to the LC, TMN, and DR/MR, the ventral tegmentum, and the brainstem cholinergic nuclei and have an important role in modulating or strengthening the arousal systems [92]. The functional importance of this orexin system in the arousal system is highlighted in narcolepsy, a condition associated with low or absent orexin levels and intrusions of REM sleep into wake states. Clearly coordinated activity of thalamocortical, hypothalamocortical, and basalocortical systems is required for full arousal and cortical activation, but the interconnections help ensure that waking is still possible if there is injury to one of these systems.

REM Sleep

REM sleep has been described as "paradoxical sleep" or "active sleep" as the cortical EEG closely resembles that of the waking state [93]. Indeed, there is marked overlap between the neurobiology of REM sleep and waking states. REM sleep is thought to originate from the mesopontine junction with firing of the "REM on" cholinergic neurons located in LDT/PPT [66,94,95]. Electrolytic lesions of these cells permanently destroy REM sleep in cats [96]. These neurons increase discharge rate often above waking levels to activate the thalamus and produce cortical desynchrony during REM sleep [66,97,98]. Proportional destruction of these "REM on" cholinergic neurons results in loss of REM sleep (including loss of PGO waves and atonia) [99]. During wakefulness and NREM sleep, these REM-on neurons are turned off by norepinephrine, serotonin, and histamine, which are found in the brainstem nuclei [100]. "REM-off" neurons have been localized to the mesopontine tegmentum and include the ventrolateral periaquaductal gray matter (vLPAG), laterodorsal pontine tegmentum (LPT), dopaminergic neurons of the ventral PAG, DR nucleus, and LC [101]. Notably, specific lesions of the vLPAG and LPT in freely moving box turtles doubled REM sleep and increased both the number and duration of bouts of REM sleep [102].

The discharge rates of these REM-off neurons decline during the transition to sleep from wakefulness, due in part to active inhibition from GABAergic interneurons [103]. In contrast, the pontine aminergic system is tonically active and inhibits the pontine cholinergic system during wake. The neurochemicals involved in REM-on/off switches explain REM state changes with the use of certain medications. For instance, acetylcholine agonist medications are found to increase REM sleep but medications such as selective serotonin reuptake inhibitors and tricyclic antidepressants decrease REM sleep.

Different groups of neurons in the pontine reticular formation are instrumental in the various manifestations of REM sleep (Figure 1.4). The pontine reticular formation contains the neural generator for the production of both REMs and PGO waves. REMs are the result of phasic firing by the reticular and vestibular cells, which stimulate the motor layers of the superior colliculus, which in turn acts on the paramedian pontine reticular formation to produce saccadic eye movements [104]. PGO waves, the phasic potentials recorded in the pons, thalamic lateral geniculate body, and occipital cortex of the cat, are the result of tonic disinhibition and phasic excitation of burst cells in the lateral pontomesencephalic tegmentum [66]. Another characteristic finding of REM sleep is the finding on hippocampal EEG of irregular rhythms to a regular theta rhythm

REM sleep

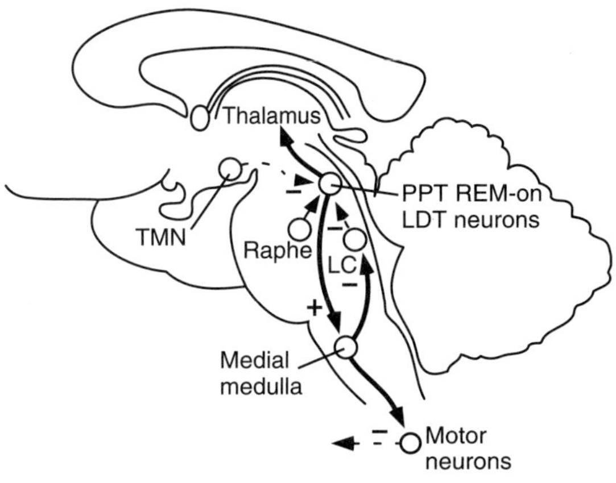

Figure 1.4 REM sleep. REM-on neurons in the laterodorsal tegmental (LDT)/pedunculopontine tegmental (PPT) nuclei are disinhibited as the aminergic neurons fall silent. These cholinergic neurons produce atonia of REM sleep by activating the medial medulla, which releases glycine and inhibits spinal and brainstem motor neurons. The medial medulla then reduces excitatory signals from the locus coeruleus (LC) that normally increases motor tone as well as synapses. The LDT/PPT neurons release ACh to activate the thalamus and produce cortical desynchrony. Adapted with permission from Ref. [141].

influenced by the brainstem and mediated by the medial septal nucleus of the BF [105]. These theta waves are mostly described in nonprimate mammals and postulated to have an important function in learning [106].

In REM sleep, there is up to 35% increase in heart rate, but use of beta-blockers tends to reduce heart rate, suggesting that REM sleep surges are primarily mediated by cardiac sympathetic activity [107]. Similarly, cardiac decelerations during REM sleep precede eye movement burst and may be mediated by cardiac vagus nerve efferent fiber burst activity [107,108]. Ventilatory responses to chemical stimuli such as hypercarbia and respiratory reflexes are inhibited in REM sleep, especially phasic REM. The irregular respiratory pattern during REM sleep does not depend on chemoreceptor or vagal nerve activity, but is secondary to brainstem neuronal activity [109].

Lastly, atonia is a fundamental characteristic of REM sleep, where only the diaphragm, ocular muscles, and muscles of the middle ear are spared [93]. Atonia is thought to originate by activity in the dorsal pontine reticular formation and exerts its effects on the ventrolateral medulla and the gamma motor neurons of the spinal cord through the reticulospinal tract. Specifically, neurons of the LDT/PPT and adjacent areas use ACh, glutamate, and probably other neurotransmitters to activate atonia-producing neurons in the medial medulla. The medullary cells release glycine onto the spinal and brainstem motor neurons during REM sleep, leading to hyperpolarization and inhibition. The medial medulla also inhibits motor neurons by reducing excitatory signals from the red nucleus and LC [110]. Thus, atonia results from a direct inhibition as well as loss of excitation of motor neurons at the level of the medulla. Disconnection of the medulla from the pons eliminates atonia, but leaves PGO spikes and REMs intact during REM sleep, though the timing of these later events may be altered [111].

Why Do We Dream?

Undoubtedly, dreaming is one of the most fascinating aspects of REM sleep, but there has been little scientific evidence about the mechanism, purpose, and effects of dreams. Although the exact timing of the emergence of adult-type dreaming is debated, it is not observed before the age of 5 years and may be seen as late as 8 years [112]. Although the distinctive features of dreams are maximally correlated with REM sleep, they are also found in NREM sleep (mostly in stage I, sleep onset, and stage II sleep) [113]. REM sleep dreams are associated with an increase in bizarre, hyperassociative elements, emotions, and episodic memory loss [114,115]. It is widely believed that the ascending cholinergic activation and lack of aminergic control during REM sleep provides the best physical substrate for distinctive formal features of dreaming. Recent PET neuroimaging studies have shown that there is relative deactivation of the dorsolateral prefrontal cortex, a region involved in working memory and reasoning, compared to waking [116]. In contrast, increased activity in the medial limbic structures, which includes the anterior cingulate, medial frontal cortexes, and amygdala, are activated to levels at or above waking levels during REM sleep [117,118]. The selective activation of these areas may be supportive of the synthesis of instinctual drive, emotional feelings, and associative cognition in dreaming [115]. Activation of limbic structures such as amygdale and anterior cingulate gyrus, which mediates anxiety, may augment dream emotional content.

Others have suggested that the lack of episodic memory in REM sleep dreams reflects the inaccessibility of stored information in the hippocampus [106]. The flow of information from the hippocampus to the cortex is suppressed during waking and REM sleep because of elevated levels of ACh, but this flow might be particularly restricted in the absence of aminergic neuromodulation during REM sleep [119]. As mentioned earlier, PGO waves originating in the mesopontine brainstem indirectly activate the visual cortex in the cat. Similar waves may occur in humans and have been hypothesized to stimulate the visual association areas to develop the complex visual imagery reported in REM sleep dreams [120].

The function of dreams still remains elusive, though many from the disciplines of philosophy, neuroscience, psychology, and psychiatry have contributed to this discourse, which is outside the realm of this chapter. From a neurocognitive standpoint, perhaps the function of dreaming is entwined with the framework of offline memory processing during sleep [121]. In this way, dreaming may reflect the neuronal activity, and specifically the activity of the brain that includes reactivation of memories and emotions from earlier experiences. Dreaming then becomes the conscious experience of activated and edited neural networks for the purposes of off-line learning and memory consolidation that occur during sleep.

NREM Sleep

Neurons that are involved in promoting NREM sleep are concentrated in the midline brainstem, dorsolateral medullary reticular formation, anterior hypothalamus and preoptic area, ventrolateral preoptic area, and the BF (including substantia innominata and diagonal band nuclei) [122]. Dampening of the brainstem, hypothalamus, and BF activating systems leads to disfacilitation and hyperpolarization of the thalamus, which shifts their mode from fast, tonic discharges to slow bursting discharges that are reflected as spindles and slow-wave activity on EEG. Specifically, neurons in the monoaminergic systems, cholinergic neurons in PPT/LDT, and orexin neurons in the LHA, which are discharging rapidly during wake, will slow their discharge during NREM sleep.

Promotion of NREM sleep involves a few key neurochemicals. γ-Aminobutyric acid (GABA) transmission from the hypothalamus and cortex is fundamentally involved in the induction and maintenance of N3 sleep or SWS by inhibiting activating systems [123]. Furthermore, GABAergic neurons from the thalamic reticular centers initiate, pace, and sustain thalamocortical burst discharges that underlie spindling and slow-wave activity [124]. Adenosine is present in the extracellular space as a byproduct of adenosine triphosphate and increases with progressive waking and decreases with sleep. Adenosine may promote sleep by inhibition of the cholinergic neurons of the brainstem and BF [125]. In the thalamus and cortex, adenosine hyperpolarizes projection neurons and facilitates the burst discharges of slow-wave activity during SWS [126]. The physiologic effects of 5-HT on sleep and wake states are controversial with conflicting reports that 5-HT promotes sleep and induces wakefulness [127]. Other molecules such as somatostatin, opioid peptides, galanin, growth hormone-releasing factor, interleukins, prostaglandin D_2, and cortistatin also have sleep-promoting effects [122].

The sleep-inducing neurons overlap with autonomic, particularly parasympathetic regulating systems. Neurons in the anterior hypothalamus project directly to the solitary nucleus and adjacent region in the medulla, which constitutes the parasympathetic control centers, thus promoting decrease in blood pressure and heart rate and causes pupillary miosis [122]. Sleep-inducing neurons may be promoted by environmental factors that reduce sensory input and increase somatic and visceral sensory input such as warmth and satiation [92].

Sleep/Wake Transitions

The orchestration of wake and the ultradian rhythm of NREM/REM sleep has been the focus of much of sleep research in the last 20 years. As already discussed, the state of wakefulness is maintained by specific neural groups in the brainstem reticuloactivating system, which in turn excites neurons in the thalamocortical projections, posterior hypothalamus, and BF. These thalamocortical, hypothalamocortical, and basalocortical projections serve to activate the cerebral cortex in a global and long-lasting fashion. During NREM sleep, there is a shift from sympathetic to parasympathetic systems and there is reduced firing of the reticuloactivating system. The clear transition from wake to sleep suggests a switch mechanism that is actively inhibited [77]. Retrograde transport experiments identified a set of neurons within a small cluster in the anterior hypothalamus called the ventrolateral preoptic nucleus (VLPO), which primarily contains the inhibitory neurotransmitters galanin and GABA and innervates all the major brainstem components of the ascending arousal system (Figure 1.5) [128,129]. These preoptic neurons seem to be active during sleep, especially deep NREM sleep [130,131], but REM sleep is also affected [132]. In contrast, the neurons in the VLPO were also found to be inhibited by noradrenergic afferents, which mainly originate from the ventrolateral medulla and serotonergic inputs from the dorsal raphe nucleus thus promoting wakefulness [133,134]. VLPO neurons also respond to the GABA, galanin, and endomorphin originating from TMN, all of which are inhibitory projections [135–137]. Somnogens such as adenosine increase activity in VLPO, in turn promoting sleep to further modulate control of VLPO [138].

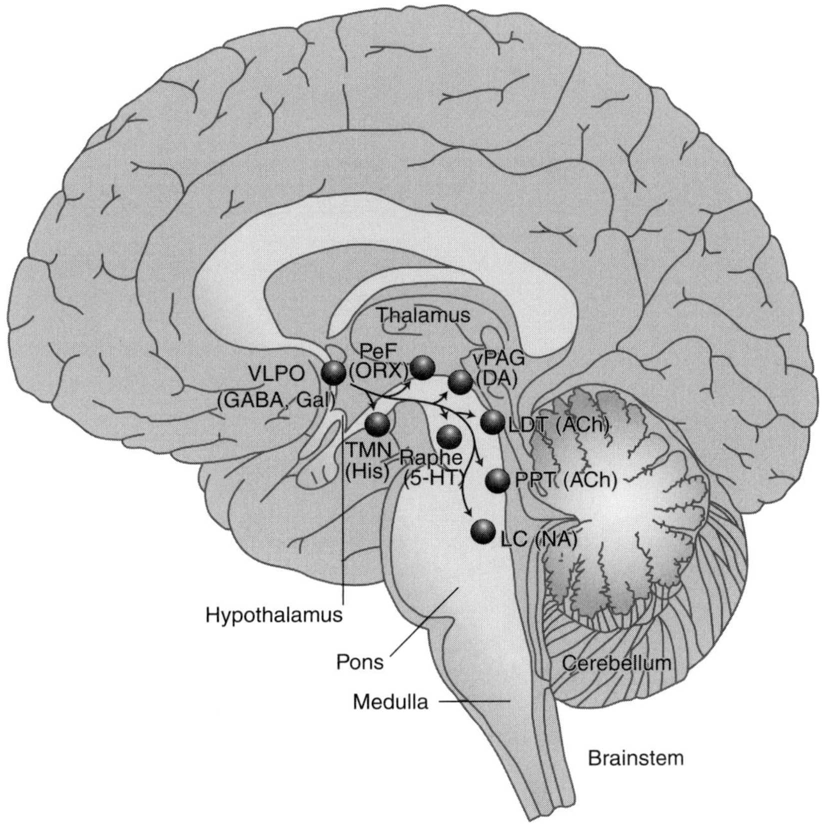

Figure 1.5 Targets of ventrolateral preoptic nucleus. The GABAergic ventrolateral preoptic nucleus (VLPO) neurons to specified targets fire faster as sleep deepens. Targets of the VLPO include the monoaminergic cell groups such as the tuberomammillary nucleus (TMN), the raphe cell groups, and the locus coeruleus (LC). It also innervates neurons in the lateral hypothalamus (LHA), including the perifornical (PeF) orexin (ORX) neurons, and interneurons in the cholinergic (ACh) cell groups, the pedunculopontine (PPT), and laterodorsal tegmental (LDT) nuclei. 5-HT, serotonin; GABA, γ-aminobutyric acid; Gal, Galanin; NA, noradrenaline; His, histamine. Adapted with permission from Ref. [80].

The mutually inhibitory interaction between the VLPO and the components of the arousal system produces a circuit similar to what electrical engineers call a "flip-flop switch" (Figure 1.6) [77]. If either side gains the advantage, it shuts off the other and disinhibits its own firing of the system. In this way, wake and NREM sleep states are transitioned quickly and completely. In fact, both humans and animals spend only a small part of each day (<1%−2%) in transitional states [80]. Such a switch has obvious advantages for the animal so as to prevent moving when not fully alert and increasing risk of predation. Behavioral states become less stable with loss of neurons on either side of the "switch" so that unwanted state transitions between wake and sleep can occur [134]. The animals with VLPO lesions have normal circadian patterns of sleep

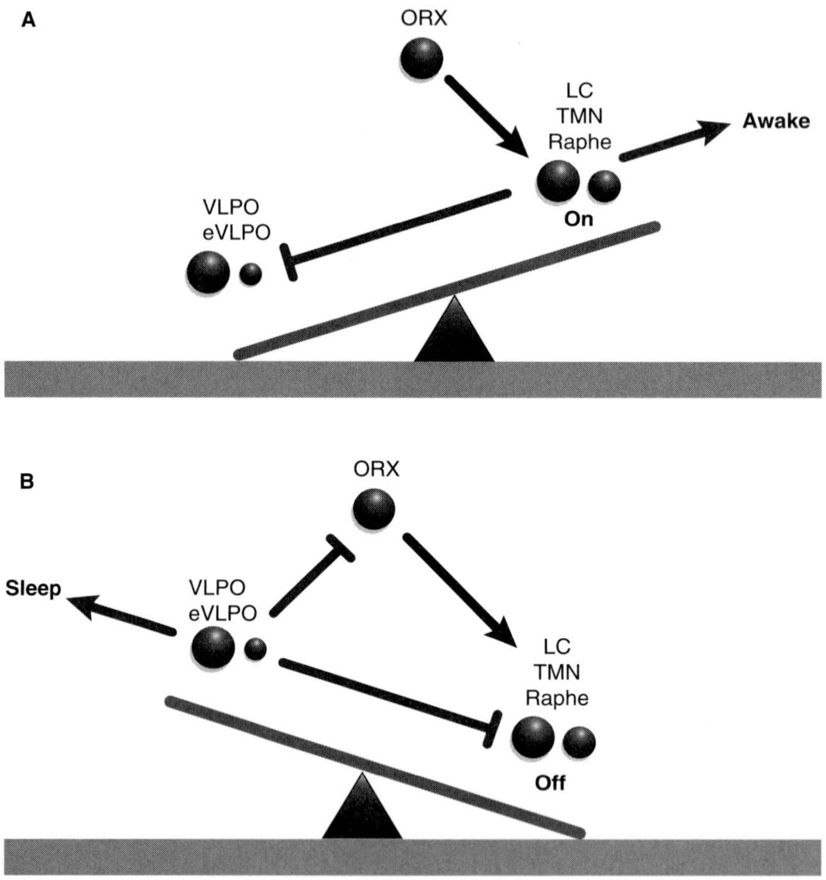

Figure 1.6 Flip-flop switch. During wakefulness A, the monoaminergic nuclei inhibit the ventrolateral preoptic nucleus (VLPO), thereby relieving the inhibition of the monoaminergic cells, and that of the orexin (ORX) neurons, and the cholinergic pedunculopontine (PPT) and laterodorsal tegmental (LDT) nuclei. Because the VLPO neurons do not have orexin receptors, the orexin neurons serve primarily to reinforce the monoaminergic tone, rather than directly inhibiting the VLPO on their own. During sleep B, the firing of the VLPO neurons inhibits the monoaminergic cell groups, thereby relieving their own inhibition. This also allows it to inhibit the orexin neurons, further preventing monoaminergic activation that might interrupt sleep. The direct mutual inhibition between the VLPO and the monoaminergic cell groups forms a classic flip-flop switch, which produces sharp transitions in state, but is relatively unstable. The addition of the orexin neurons stabilizes the switch. 5-HT, serotonin; ACh, cholinergic; eVLPO, extended ventrolateral preoptic nucleus; GABA, γ-aminobutyric acid; gal, galanin; LC, locus coeruleus; NA, noradrenaline; PeF, perifornical; REM, rapid eye movement; TMN, tuberomammillary nucleus. Adapted with permission from Ref. [80].

Table 1.1 State-specific firing rates of brainstem and cortical neuronal groups

Site	Neurotransmitters	Wakefulness	NREM	REM
Basal forebrain	Acetylcholine	++++	+	++++
Laterodorsal tegmentum/ pedunculopontine tegmentum	Acetylcholine	++++	+++ → 0	++++
Dorsal and median raphe	Serotonin	++++	++	0
Locus coeruleus	Norepinephrine	++++	++	0
Tuberomammillary nucleus	Histamine	++++	++	0
Posterior/lateral hypothalamus	Hypocretin/orexin	++++	+	+
Ventrolateral preoptic area	GABA	+	+++	++++

GABA, γ-aminobutyric acid; NREM, non-rapid eye movement; REM, rapid eye movement
Adapted with permission from Ref. [142]

but have a 50% to 60% reduction in REM and NREM sleep time, wake more often during their sleep cycle, and fall asleep more often during a wake cycle [139]. Lesions of the VLPO are rare in clinical practice but sedating drugs such as benzodiazepines and barbiturates may promote sleep by enhancing the GABA signaling in the descending pathways from VLPO [140,141]. Once sleep onset occurs, firing rates of VLPO neurons increase and get progressively faster as sleep deepens [142]. This firing increases further inhibition of arousal centers that allow for more uninterrupted and deeper sleep. A transition to REM occurs during NREM sleep when GABAergic neurons disinhibit REM-on neurons located in LDT/PPT. Acetylcholine is then released to the thalamus producing cortical dysynchrony as the aminergic neurons of TMN, raphe, and LC are silenced by afferent signals produced by the VLPO (Table 1.1) [141].

The orexin neurons located in the lateral and posterior hypothalamus play an essential role in stabilizing the wake-sleep states. Orexin neurons innervate the LC, TMN, median raphe nuclei, and mesopontine reticular formation, similar to the brainstem arousal system targets as the VLPO [143], yet the VLPO neurons do not have orexin receptors [144]. The orexin neurons stabilize the flip-flop switch into the "wake" position primarily through upregulation of the monoaminergic arousal tone [77]. These orexin neurons are less active during NREM sleep, but it is not clear if they are active during REM sleep [145]. In turn, the VLPO neurons inhibit the orexin neurons, creating a negative feedback loop to promote sleep [134]. Observation in animals that lack the gene for orexin or its receptor leads to narcolepsy and highlights the importance of orexin on the flip-flop switch, as these animals have many more state transitions both during wake and sleep but do not exhibit increased total sleep time [146,147].

Two-Process Model of Sleep

An influential model proposed by Borbely and Tobler posits that human and animal sleep depends on 2 major factors: the circadian regulator that defines the diurnal rhythm and the homeostatic regulator that defines the relationship between wake and sleep timings [148]. The homeostatic component, named Process S (sleep), is believed to derive from a substrate or protein that registers the homeostatic "need to sleep" during periods of extended wakefulness that is subsequently relieved by sleep. As NREM sleep appears to take precedence over REM sleep following acute sleep loss, it is probable that the homeostatic mechanisms for the 2 sleep states differ [128]. The second component of the sleep-wake regulatory mechanism was termed by Borbely as Process C, which involves circadian influences and is independent of sleep and waking. Dijk and Czeisler confirmed the role of this circadian pacemaker in the timings of the sleep-wake cycle and regulation of internal sleep structure during a forced desynchrony protocol on men who lived in an environment free of time cues [149]. Process C ensures continued sleep despite decreased homeostatic need for it toward the end of the sleep cycle; on the other hand, circadian waking drive builds up and is maximal just before sleep onset (Figure 1.7).

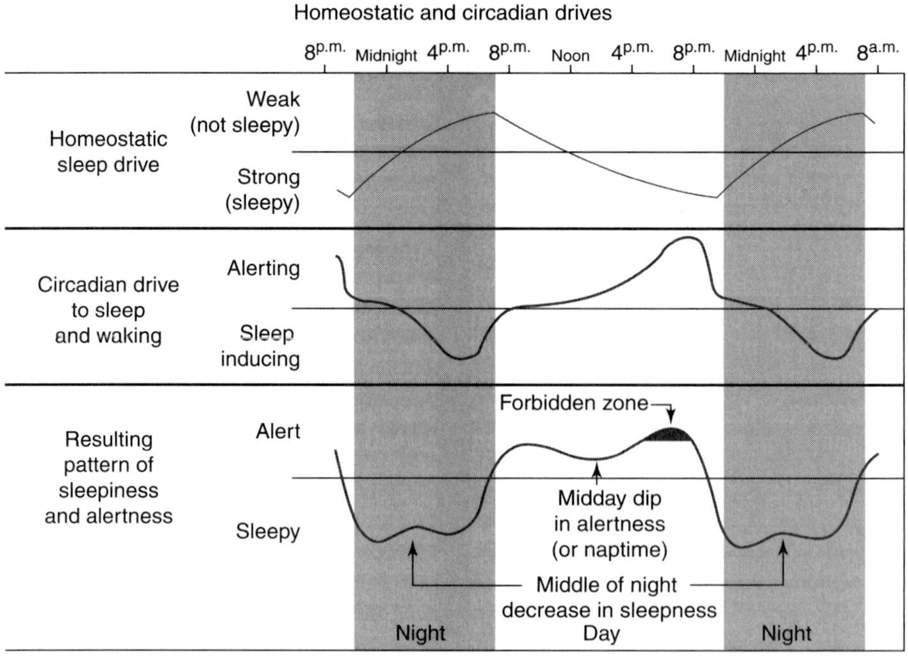

Figure 1.7 Two-process model of sleep and wake. Homeostatic process (Process S) accumulates during wake and dissipates in sleep, whereas the circadian process (Process C) oscillates with a 24-h periodicity. The forbidden zone is the period during which Process S and Process C are maximal and is a poor time to expect a child to sleep. Adapted with permission from Ref. [205].

Homeostatic Regulation of Sleep

Unlike other homeostatic mechanisms that seek to recover a set point when perturbed, sleep deprivation is followed by extra recovery sleep that is proportional to the sleep loss [80]. The purpose of this additional sleep is unknown, but may serve a restorative function in the brain as discussed earlier in this chapter. The mechanism for this homeostatic sleep drive is yet unclear. McCarley has shown that adenosine acting in the BF is a key mediator of homeostatic control [150]. Extracellular stores of adenosine may build up and accumulate near the BF as brain glycogen stores are broken down into adenosine during sustained wakefulness [151]. Injection of adenosine or adenosine A1 receptor agonists into the BF of cats or A2a receptor agonists near the VLPO in rats promotes sleep by inhibiting multiple wake-promoting regions of the brain or exciting sleep-promoting cell groups [152]. In addition, adenosine might disinhibit VLPO via adenosine A1 receptors by reducing inhibitory GABAergic inputs [153]. In sum, adenosine may act as a homeostatic regulator of sleep need by local inhibition of the BF arousal system and triggering VLPO nucleus. Future research may identify other mediators of homeostatic sleep drive.

Circadian Sleep Regulation

Circadian timing in which the neurons fire in a near-24-hour cycle is organized in a hierarchy of tissue-specific structures located throughout the body. These tissue-specific rhythms are coordinated by the suprachiasmatic nucleus (SCN) of the hypothalamus, which acts as a "master clock." This clock is synchronized by light input from the environment and endogenous melatonin secreted during the dark cycles [154,155]. The light signal is received from a specialized set of retinal ganglion cells that contain the photopigment melanopsin, which increases the firing of the SCN [156]. Melatonin is secreted by the highly vascularized pineal gland located in the posterodorsal aspect of the third ventricle into the cerebral sinuses in response to photic information received by the eyes (dark). Melatonin is inhibited by light cues received by the SCN via the sympathetic intermediolateral cell column in the thoracic spinal cord, which has a negative feedback loop with the pineal gland [157].

The SCN has the bulk of its output to the adjacent subparaventricular zone (SPZ) and the dorsomedial nucleus of the hypothalamus (DMH); in contrast, there is little transmission to the VLPO or orexin neurons [87,128, 158]. The SPZ appears to be a complex region involved in sleep and temperature rhythms. Lesions of the ventral SPZ have been shown to disrupt measures of the circadian index of sleep by 90% but had little effect on body temperature; in contrast, lesions of the dorsal SPZ resulted in lowered circadian rhythms of temperature by 75% but had little effect on sleep [159]. The major purpose of the SPZ serves to link the SCN to the DMH to amplify circadian responses [80].

The DMH is particularly important for delivering signal from the SCN to the sleep regulatory system. Lesions of DMH have been shown to reduce circadian rhythms of wakefulness, feeding, locomotor activity, and serum corticosteroid secretion [160]. The DMH is one of the largest sources of input to the VLPO and orexin neurons [134] and is crucial for conveying SCN influence to the wake-sleep regulatory system. DMH sends GABAergic projections to the VLPO nucleus to promote wakefulness by inhibiting sleep as well as glutamate-related thyrotropin-releasing hormone to excite LHA, orexin, and MHC neurons for waking and feeding [160]. Thus, the DMH plays a major role in regulation of circadian sleep behavior by integrating information received from the SCN and SPZ with feeding, temperature, and social cues.

One rational for the complexity of this 3-stage pathway for circadian control of sleep and other behaviors may be that it gives animals the flexibility to adapt their behaviors and physiologic cycles to environmental cues to maximize their chances for survival [80]. Whereas the SCN seems to stay locked in the set light-dark cycle, there seems to be a shift of activation in the DMH. For example, when rats are given access to food only during the light cycle (when they normally are asleep), they invert their daily cycles of feeding, wake-sleep, and locomotor activity and corticosteroid secretion [161]. This behavior persists even if food is withheld for 2 days, thus underlying the point that circadian pattern is not dependent on external cues. More recently, clock genes including *Clock*, *Bmal1*, *Per*, and *Cry*, which form a complex transcriptional-translational network, have been found to be associated with SCN function [162]. The products of these genes bind to sequences in the promotors of effector genes to establish a central clock.

Sleep and Effect on Target Organs

Sleep provides dynamic physiologic effects on many body organs, some of great clinical significance. Evaluation of disease process and treatment response should include consideration of variations of organ functioning in sleep. These changes to the CNS, as well as to the cardiovascular, respiratory, gastrointestinal, and endocrine systems, are further discussed.

Brain Physiology and Sleep

Animal experiments have revealed that there are variations in CBF during sleep with different areas of the brain exhibiting different magnitudes of alteration. There is a marked increased CBF during REM sleep at an estimated 8% over baseline [70]. During REM sleep, there is an increase in blood flow to the entorhinal cortex, anterior cingulate, amygdala, thalamus, dorsal mesencephalon, and pontine tegmentum, whereas blood flow decreases to these structures during NREM sleep [163]. Likewise, cerebral metabolic rate for glucose and oxygen consumption increases in REM sleep. Spinal cord blood flow also increases during REM sleep. In contrast, there is a consistent decrease in CBF during NREM sleep with an overall average of 10% during SWS [70]. The decrease in CBF to the pons, mesencephalon, thalamus, hypothalamus, and BF during NREM [164] may point to an energy-saving value of both the bursting discharge mode of the brain stem and the synchronizing activity of the thalamocortical circuits seen during NREM sleep [165]. In NREM sleep, a slight hypercapnia develops (2–3 mm Hg) which counteracts the effects of decreased metabolic rate and may account for the small increase in CBF in some species [166]. Intrinsic changes in CBF are altered by the chemical environment, specifically arterial carbon dioxide tension ($PaCO_2$), which can become an important determinant of CBF in pathological conditions such as sleep apnea [167]. In contrast, alterations in arterial oxygen tension (PaO_2) within physiologic range do not significantly affect CBF or cerebral metabolic rate [168]. If PaO_2 is lowered below 50 mm Hg, CBF increases precipitously in response to hypoxia [169].

Intracranial pressure (ICP) may also vary by sleep state. Although there is little variation of ICP from wake to NREM sleep, large ICP waves occur in REM sleep that almost double the steady-state pressure [170]. In most individuals, these ICP waves have no clinical significance but in patients with little ICP reserve, small increases may affect cerebral functioning.

Cardiovascular Changes in Sleep

Heart rate varies during NREM and REM sleep. When compared with quiet wake, heart rate decreases by 4 to 8 beats per minute in NREM sleep [171] and there is typically a normal sinus arrhythmia produced by normal respiratory activity coupled with cardiorespiratory activity [172]. In this state, heart rate acceleration accompanies inspiration as there is an increase in venous return resulting in increased cardiac output. In expiration, a progressive slowing of heart rate occurs. Normal sinus variability may be attributed to the increased vagal nerve activity in NREM states and is a sign of cardiac health. Systemic blood pressure may fall during NREM sleep, which could lead to significant limitations of cardiac perfusion in those with stenotic cardiac vessels, precipitating cardiac ischemia.

In REM sleep, the heart rate becomes increasingly variable with episodes of tachycardia and bradycardia [173]. During phasic REM periods, there can be a transient 35% increase in heart rate [174]. In animal models, these phasic REM state heart rate surges are linked to CNS activation as reflected by concomitant increase in hippocampal theta activity, PGO activity, and eye movements [107]. The heart surges seen in REM are accompanied by a rise in mean arterial blood pressure. Clinically, the surges in sympathetic activity in REM sleep and increased heart rate increase the risk of ventricular arrhythmias in REM sleep [175]. Furthermore, cardiac vulnerability [176] is present during phasic REM sleep when episodic surges in coronary blood flow correspond with decrease in vascular resistance. In coronary artery stenosis, there are phasic decreases in blood flow during REM sleep, rather than increases, coincident with heart rate surges [177]. Sympathovagal imbalances present in sleep may shift to increased sympathetic activity in patients with sleep apnea [178]. Such autonomic factors may be conducive to cardiac ischemia or myocardial infarction during sleep.

Respiratory Physiology in Sleep

Respiratory rate tends to be slower and more regular in NREM and increases and becomes more irregular in REM sleep [176,179]. In NREM sleep, upper airway resistance increases, tidal volume increases, minute ventilation decreases, and end tidal CO_2 increases [180]. In REM sleep, tidal volume and minute ventilation decreases and there is a decrease in responses to chemical stimuli such as hypoxia and hypercarbia [181]. These normal irregular respirations in REM may result in central apneas or hypopneas secondary to brainstem neuronal activity [176]. Furthermore, many upper airway muscles are atonic or hypotonic, and laryngeal and diaphragmatic response to occlusion is inconsistent and variable. Such physiology in REM sleep promotes worsening of obstructive sleep-disordered breathing in REM sleep, with longer obstructive events and more severe oxygen desaturations.

Gastrointestinal Physiology in Sleep

The sleep-driven changes in the gastrointestinal system vary depending on the organ studied, but are driven by a combination of CNS activity, subserosal neural plexus activity, autonomic activity, and circadian rhythm factors. Whereas there is minimal basal gastric acid secretion in waking that increases with meal intake, there is a peak between 10 PM and 2 AM, suggesting an internal circadian rhythm to basal acid secretion [182]. In healthy individuals, this increase in gastric secretion does not result in gastroesophageal reflux disease (GERD). However, in those who do suffer from GERD in sleep, there is a decrease in acid clearance possibly because of delay in conscious response to the presence of acid and decline of swallowing [183,184] and salivation in sleep [185]. There are conflicting data regarding the gastric motor function during sleep with some research suggesting a decline in peristaltic movement in sleep [186], an increase in gastric motility in sleep [187], and variations in motility based on NREM versus REM sleep stage [188,189]. There seems to be a clear inhibition of the colonic motility index in sleep and an increase in motility on awakening [190]. Sudden awakenings from sleep result in segmental colonic contractions without propagation [191]. Lastly, the decrease in anal canal resting pressure during sleep may create risk for fecal incontinence but this is prevented by retrograde rectal propulsions [192,193].

Endocrine Function in Sleep

There is a predictable pattern of hormonal secretion during sleep that is driven by circadian and ultradian rhythms. Plasma growth hormone in prepubertal children is generally secreted in maximal concentrations in SWS (stage N3), and peaks at 90 minutes after sleep onset [194]. During adolescence and adulthood, the pattern of GH secretion is modified with age, with older adults having a less significant correlation between growth hormone secretion and sleep [195]. Interestingly, GH surges seem independent of circadian rhythmicity [24]. A 180-degree reversal of sleep phase results in a 180-degree shift in the peak of GH secretion. In contrast, cortisol secretion peaks between 4 and 8 AM, demonstrating clear circadian influence [196]. Prolactin concentrations begin to increase 1 hour after sleep onset and are maximal between 5 and 7 AM [197]. On awakening, prolactin concentrations reach their nadir. Thyroid-stimulating hormone (TSH) secretion also follows a circadian pattern with peak levels at night and low levels at daytime. TSH secretion reaches its peak before the onset of sleep and then declines across the sleep phase [198].

Leutenizing hormone (LH) and follicle-stimulating hormone (FSH) increase during sleep during puberty in boys and girls [199]. In boys, LH surges are followed by elevations in testosterone levels that induce changes in

Sleep Pearls

1. Sleep is a behavioral state highly conserved across species.
2. The function of sleep is unclear, though theories about its role in functional restoration, energy conservation, and synaptic plasticity exist.
3. In adults, a night of sleep begins with about 80 minutes of non-rapid eye movement (NREM) sleep followed by 10 minutes of rapid eye movement (REM) sleep. The approximate 90-minute NREM-REM cycle is then repeated about 3 to 6 times during the night. In children, these cycles may be 60 minutes in duration.
4. Sleep is a maturational process. REM sleep is at maximal amount in the newborn period and declines to near-adult levels by age 5 years. Slow-wave sleep is maximal in young children and decreases with age.
5. The wake state is maintained by multiple coordinated activities of thalamocortical, hypothalamocortical, and basalocortical systems originating in the pontine and midbrain tegmentum, but interconnections help ensure that waking is still possible if there is injury to one of these systems.
6. REM sleep is associated with saccadic eye movements, muscle atonia (with exception to eye muscles, diaphragm, and middle ear muscles), and electroencephalogram features similar to alert waking.
7. During NREM sleep, there is a shift from sympathetic to parasympathetic systems and reduced firing of the reticular activating system. The switch from wake to sleep is mediated by the ventrolateral preoptic nucleus.
8. A two-process model exists to control sleep and wakefulness. The homeostatic process (Process S) accumulates during wakefulness and declines during sleep whereas the circadian process (Process C) is independent of sleep and waking.
9. Sleep provides dynamic physiologic effects on different body organs, which must be considered in disease processes and treatment regimens.

secondary sexual characteristics [200]. Pubertal girls show sleep-coupled release of FSH and LH during sleep, but estrodiol levels do not increase until 10 to 14 hours later [201]. Although there is no established relationship between the secretion of leptin and ghrelin in sleep [202], these metabolic hormones secreted by adipose cells may influence circadian rhythms. Leptin and ghrelin may enter the hypothalamus and be relayed to the ventromedial nucleus and arcuate nucleus, respectively, and project input to the SPZ and dorsomedial nucleus to influence sleep timings (Figure 1.8) [92]. Furthermore, it has been reported that people with shorter

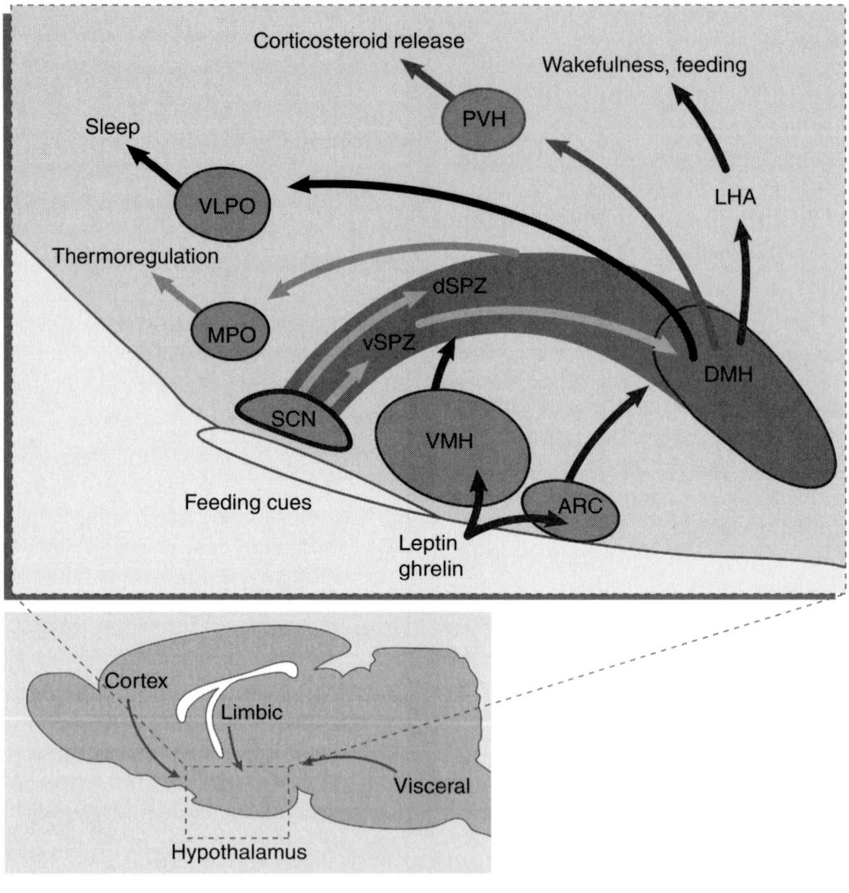

Figure 1.8 Circadian integrator pathway of the brain. The suprachiasmatic nucleus (SCN) serves as a biological clock, but has few outputs to sleep regulatory systems. Most of its output goes to ventral (vSPZ) and dorsal (dSPZ) subparaventricular zone, and the dorsomedial nucleus of the hypothalamus (DMH). Neurons in the vSPZ relay information necessary for organizing daily cycles of wake-sleep, whereas dSPZ neurons are crucial for rhythms of body temperature. Outputs from the SPZ are integrated in the DMH with other inputs, and DMH neurons drive circadian cycles of sleep, activity, feeding, and corticosteroid secretion. Cycles of body temperature are maintained by dSPZ projections back to the medial preoptic area (MPO), whereas the DMN is the origin of projections to the ventrolateral preoptic nucleus for sleep cycles, to the corticotropin-releasing hormone (CRH) neurons of the paraventricular nucleus (PVH) for corticosteroid cycles, and to the lateral hypothalamic (LHA) orexin and melanin-concentrating hormone neurons for wakefulness and feeding cycles. The integrative steps in the SPZ and DMH allow circadian rhythms to adapt to environmental stimuli, such as food availability (eg, leptin and ghrelin action via the ventromedial [VMH] and arcuate [ARC] nuclei), as well as visceral sensory inputs, cognitive influences from the prefrontal cortex, and emotional inputs from the limbic system (inset). Adapted with permission from Ref. [80].

sleep times have increased circulating ghrelin and decreased leptin, a hormonal pattern consistent with decreased energy expenditure and increased appetite and obesity [203].

Conclusion

Although many mysteries about sleep linger, it is clear that sleep is not simply a passive state and may serve some evolutionary purpose. Sleep may provide an opportunity for functional restoration, energy conservation, and/or enhancement of learning and memory, though these theories are debatable. Specific circuitry and neurotransmitters have been identified that smoothly transit mammals from wakefulness, NREM sleep, and REM sleep. Likewise, multiorgan changes in sleep are now known, that have clinical importance to health. The basic understanding of the anatomy and physiology involved in mammalian sleep discussed in this chapter will help the clinician understand unique disease and health conditions that occur during sleep further discussed in this book.

References

1. Zepelin H, Siegel J, Tobler I. Mammalian sleep. In: Kryger MH, Roth T, Dement WC, eds. *Principles and Practice of Sleep Medicine*. Philadelphia, PA: Elsevier/Saunders; 2005:91–100.
2. Siegel JM. Do all animals sleep? *Trends Neurosci.* 2008;31(4):208–213.
3. Siegel JM. Clues to the functions of mammalian sleep. *Nature.* 2005;437(7063):1264–1271.
4. Hall JC. Genetics and molecular biology of rhythms in Drosophila and other insects. *Adv Genet.* 2003; 48:1–280.
5. Zhdanova IV. Sleep in zebrafish. *Zebrafish.* 2006; 3(2):215–226.
6. Raizen DM, Zimmerman JE, Maycock MH, et al. Lethargus is a Caenorhabditis elegans sleep-like state. *Nature.* 2008;451(7178):569–572.
7. Zepelin H, Rechtschaffen A. Mammalian sleep, longevity, and energy metabolism. *Brain Behav Evol.* 1974;10(6):425–470.
8. Allada R, Siegel JM. Unearthing the phylogenetic roots of sleep. *Curr Biol.* 2008;18(15):R670–R679.
9. De Vera L, Gonzalez JR, Rial RV. Reptilian waking EEG: slow waves, spindles and evoked potentials. *Electroencephalogr Clin Neurophysiol.* 1994;90(4): 298–303.
10. Eiland MM, Lyamin OI, Siegel JM. State-related discharge of neurons in the brainstem of freely moving box turtles, Terrapene carolina major. *Arch Ital Biol.* 2001;139(1–2):23–36.
11. Siegel JM, Manger PR, Nienhuis R, Fahringer HM, Pettigrew JD. The echidna Tachyglossus aculeatus combines REM and non-REM aspects in a single sleep state: implications for the evolution of sleep. *J Neurosci.* 1996;16(10):3500–3506.
12. Ursin R. The two stages of slow wave sleep in the cat and their relation to REM sleep. *Brain Res.* 1968;11(2):347–356.
13. Allison T, Cicchetti DV. Sleep in mammals: ecological and constitutional correlates. *Science.* 1976; 194(4266):732–734.
14. Tobler I. Phylogeny of sleep regulation. In: Kryger MH, Roth T, Dement WC, eds. *Principles and Practice of Sleep Medicine.* Philadelphia, PA: Saunders; 2005:77–90.
15. Jouvet-Mounier D, Astic L, Lacote D. Ontogenesis of the states of sleep in rat, cat, and guinea pig during the first postnatal month. *Dev Psychobiol.* 1970;2(4):216–239.
16. Rechtschaffen A. Current perspectives on the function of sleep. *Perspect Biol Med.* 1998;41(3): 359–390.
17. Everson CA, Bergmann BM, Rechtschaffen A. Sleep deprivation in the rat: III. Total sleep deprivation. *Sleep.* 1989;12(1):13–21.
18. Rechtschaffen A, Bergmann BM, Everson CA, Kushida CA, Gilliland MA. Sleep deprivation in the rat: X. Integration and discussion of the findings. 1989. *Sleep.* 2002;25(1):68–87.
19. Lyamin O, Pryaslova J, Lance V, Siegel J. Animal behaviour: continuous activity in cetaceans after birth. *Nature.* 2005;435(7046):1177.
20. Banks S, Dinges DF. Behavioral and physiological consequences of sleep restriction. *J Clin Sleep Med.* 2007;3(5):519–528.
21. Dinges DF, Rogers NL, Baynard MD. Chronic sleep deprivation. In: Kryger MH, Roth T, Dement WC., eds. *Principles and Practice of Sleep Medicine.* Philadelphia, PA: Saunders/Elsevier; 2005:67–76.
22. Sherington CS. *Man on His Nature.* Cambridge, MA: Cambridge University Press; 1946:413.
23. Sheldon SH. Introduction to pediatric sleep medicine. In: Sheldon SH, Ferber R, Kryger MH, eds. *Principles and Practices of Pediatric Sleep Medicine.* Philadelphia, PA: Elsevier Saunders; 2005:1.
24. Sassin JF, Parker DC, Mace JW, Gotlin RW, Johnson LC, Rossman LG. Human growth hormone release: relation to slow-wave sleep and sleep-walking cycles. *Science.* 1969;165(892): 513–515.
25. Berger RJ, Oswald I. Effects of sleep deprivation on behaviour, subsequent sleep, and dreaming. *J Ment Sci.* 1962;108:457–465.
26. Sassin JF, Frantz AG, Kapen S, Weitzman ED. The nocturnal rise of human prolactin is dependent on sleep. *J Clin Endocrinol Metab.* 1973;37(3):436–440.
27. Boyar RM, Rosenfeld RS, Kapen S, et al. Human puberty. Simultaneous augmented secretion of luteinizing hormone and testosterone during sleep. *J Clin Invest.* 1974;54(3):609–618.

28. Weitzman ED, Hellman L. Temporal organization of the 24 hour pattern of the hypothalamic-pituatary axis. In: M. Ferin, F. Halberg, R.M. Richart and R.L. Vande Wiele. Biorhythms and Human reproduction. John Wiley and Sons, New York 1974.
29. Valk I, Van der Bosch JSG. Intra-daily variation of the human ulnar length and short term growt-a longitudinal study in eleven boys. *Growth.* 1974;42:107.
30. Horne JA. The effects of exercise upon sleep: a critical review. *Biol Psychol.* 1981;12(4):241–290.
31. Atkinson G, Davenne D. Relationships between sleep, physical activity and human health. *Physiol Behav.* 2007;90(2–3):229–235.
32. Bjarnason GA, Jordan RCK. Circadian variation of cell proliferation and cell cycle protein expression in man: clinical implications. In: Meijer S, Guidet S, Philipe M, eds. *Progress in Cell Cycle Research.* New York, NY: Plenum Press; 2000:193–206.
33. Scheving LE, Pauly JE, von Mayersbach H, Dunn JD. The effect of continuous light or darkness on the rhythm of the mitotic index in the corneal epithelium of the rat. *Acta Anat (Basel).* 1974; 88(3):411–423.
34. Smaaland R. Circadian rhythm of cell division. *Prog Cell Cycle Res.* 1996;2:241–266.
35. Cirelli C, Gutierrez CM, Tononi G. Extensive and divergent effects of sleep and wakefulness on brain gene expression. *Neuron.* 2004;41(1):35–43.
36. Mackiewicz M, Shockley KR, Romer MA, et al. Macromolecule biosynthesis: a key function of sleep. *Physiol Genomics.* 2007;31(3):441–457.
37. Cirelli C. Cellular consequences of sleep deprivation in the brain. *Sleep Med Rev.* 2006;10(5):307–321.
38. Carpenter AC, Timiras PS. Sleep organization in hypo- and hyperthyroid rats. *Neuroendocrinology.* 1982;34(6):438–443.
39. Eastman CI, Rechtschaffen A. Effect of thyroxine on sleep in the rat. *Sleep.* 1979;2(2):215–232.
40. Parmeggiani PL. Thermoregulation and sleep. *Front Biosci.* 2003;8:s557–s567.
41. Heller HC, Ruby NF. Sleep and circadian rhythms in mammalian torpor. *Annu Rev Physiol.* 2004;66: 275–289.
42. Walker MP, Stickgold R. Sleep-dependent learning and memory consolidation. *Neuron.* 2004; 44(1):121–133.
43. Yoo SS, Hu PT, Gujar N, Jolesz FA, Walker MP. A deficit in the ability to form new human memories without sleep. *Nat Neurosci.* 2007;10(3): 385–292.
44. Walker MP, Stickgold R, Alsop D, Gaab N, Schlaug G. Sleep-dependent motor memory plasticity in the human brain. *Neuroscience.* 2005;133(4):911–917.
45. Peigneux P, Laureys S, Fuchs S, et al. Are spatial memories strengthened in the human hippocampus during slow wave sleep? *Neuron.* 2004;44(3): 535–545.
46. Plihal W, Weaver S, Mölle M, Fehm HL, Born J. Sensory processing during early and late nocturnal sleep. *Electroencephalogr Clin Neurophysiol.* 1996;99(3):247–256.
47. Marshall L, Born J. The contribution of sleep to hippocampus-dependent memory consolidation. *Trends Cogn Sci.* 2007;11(10):442–450.
48. Maquet P, Laureys S, Peigneux P, et al. Experience-dependent changes in cerebral activation during human REM sleep. *Nat Neurosci.* 2000;3(8): 831–836.
49. Peigneux P, Laureys S, Fuchs S, et al. Learned material content and acquisition level modulate cerebral reactivation during posttraining rapid-eye-movements sleep. *Neuroimage.* 2003;20(1): 125–134.
50. Maquet P, Peigneux P, Laureys S, et al. Memory processing during human sleep as assessed by functional neuroimaging. *Rev Neurol (Paris).* 2003; 159(suppl 11):6S27–6S29.
51. Benington JH, Frank MG. Cellular and molecular connections between sleep and synaptic plasticity. *Prog Neurobiol.* 2003;69(2):71–101.
52. Walker MP, Liston C, Hobson JA, Stickgold R. Cognitive flexibility across the sleep-wake cycle: REM-sleep enhancement of anagram problem solving. *Brain Res Cogn Brain Res.* 2002;14(3): 317–324.
53. Sejnowski TJ, Destexhe A. Why do we sleep? *Brain Res.* 2000;886(1–2):208–223.
54. Contreras D, Destexhe A, Steriade M. Spindle oscillations during cortical spreading depression in naturally sleeping cats. *Neuroscience.* 1997;77(4):933–936.
55. Contreras D, Destexhe A, Sejnowski TJ, Steriade M. Spatiotemporal patterns of spindle oscillations in cortex and thalamus. *J Neurosci.* 1997;17(3): 1179–1196.
56. Cantero JL, Atienza M, Stickgold R, Kahana MJ, Madsen JR, Kocsis B. Sleep-dependent theta oscillations in the human hippocampus and neocortex. *J Neurosci.* 2003;23(34):10897–10903.
57. Poe GR, Nitz DA, McNaughton BL, Barnes CA. Experience-dependent phase-reversal of hippocampal neuron firing during REM sleep. *Brain Res.* 2000;855(1):176–180.
58. Shaffery JP, Oksenberg A, Marks GA, Speciale SG, Mihailoff G, Roffwarg HP. REM sleep deprivation in monocularly occluded kittens reduces the size of cells in LGN monocular segment. *Sleep.* 1998;21(8):837–845.
59. Frank MG, Issa NP, Stryker MP. Sleep enhances plasticity in the developing visual cortex. *Neuron.* 2001;30(1):275–287.
60. Tononi G, Cirelli C. Sleep function and synaptic homeostasis. *Sleep Med Rev.* 2006;10(1):49–62.
61. Euston DR, Tatsuno M, McNaughton BL. Fast-forward playback of recent memory sequences in prefrontal cortex during sleep. *Science.* 2007;318(5853):1147–1150.
62. Mignot E. Why we sleep: the temporal organization of recovery. *PLoS Biol.* 2008;6(4):e106.
63. Carskadon M, Dement WC. Normal human sleep: an overview. In: Kryger MH, Roth T, Dement WC, eds. *Principles and Practice of Sleep Medicine.* Philadelphia, PA: Saunders; 2005: 13–23.

64. Rechtschaffen A, Kales A. *A Manual of Standardized Terminology, Techniques and Scoring System for Sleep Stages of Human Subjects*. Los Angeles: UCLA Brain Information Service/Brain Research Institute; 1968.
65. Iber C, Ancoli-Israel S, Chesson A and Quan SF for the American Academy of Sleep Medicine. *The AASM Manual for the Scoring of Sleep and Associated Events, Rules, Terminology and Technical Specification*. Westchester, IL: American Academy of Sleep Medicine; 2007.
66. Steriade M, Datta S, Paré D, Oakson G, Curró Dossi RC. Neuronal activities in brain-stem cholinergic nuclei related to tonic activation processes in thalamocortical systems. *J Neurosci*. 1990;10(8):2541–2559.
67. Callaway CW, Lydic R, Baghdoyan HA, Hobson JA. Pontogeniculooccipital waves: spontaneous visual system activity during rapid eye movement sleep. *Cell Mol Neurobiol*. 1987;7(2):105–149.
68. Fernandez-Mendoza J, Lozano B, Seijo F, et al. Evidence of subthalamic PGO-like waves during REM sleep in humans: a deep brain polysomnographic study. *Sleep*. 2009;32(9):1117–1126.
69. Middelkoop HA, Smilde-van den Doel DA, Neven AK, Kamphuisen HA, Springer CP. Subjective sleep characteristics of 1,485 males and females aged 50–93: effects of sex and age, and factors related to self-evaluated quality of sleep. *J Gerontol A Biol Sci Med Sci*. 1996;51(3):M108–M115.
70. Townsend RE, Prinz PN, Obrist WD. Human cerebral blood flow during sleep and waking. *J Appl Physiol*. 1973;35(5):620–625.
71. Sheldon SH. Polysomnography in infants and children. In: Sheldon SH, Ferber R, Kryger MH, eds. *Principles and Practices of Pediatric Sleep Medicine*. Philadelphia, PA: Elsevier Saunders; 2005:49–71.
72. Sheldon SH. Polysomnography in infants and children. In: Ferber R, Kryger MH, eds. *Principles and Practice of Sleep Medicine in the Child*. Philadelphia, PA: Elsevier Saunders; 2005:49–71.
73. Becker PT, Thoman EB. Rapid eye movement storms in infants: rate of occurrence at 6 months predicts mental development at 1 year. *Science*. 1981;212(4501):1415–1416.
74. Fukumoto M, Mochizuki N, Takeishi M, Nomura Y, Segawa M. Studies of body movements during night sleep in infancy. *Brain Dev*. 1981;3(1):37–43.
75. Carskadon MA, Brown ED, Dement WC. Sleep fragmentation in the elderly: relationship to daytime sleep tendency. *Neurobiol Aging*. 1982;3(4):321–327.
76. Moruzzi G, Magoun HW. Brain stem reticular formation and activation of the EEG. *Electroencephalogr Clin Neurophysiol*. 1949;1(4):455–473.
77. Saper CB, Chou TC, Scammell TE. The sleep switch: hypothalamic control of sleep and wakefulness. *Trends Neurosci*. 2001;24(12):726–731.
78. Aalto J, Kiianmaa K. Role of brain monoaminergic systems in the increased ethanol drinking caused by REM-sleep deprivation. *Alcohol Alcohol Suppl*. 1987;1:313–317.
79. Stenberg D. Neuroanatomy and neurochemistry of sleep. *Cell Mol Life Sci*. 2007;64(10):1187–1204.
80. Saper CB, Scammell TE, Lu J. Hypothalamic regulation of sleep and circadian rhythms. *Nature*. 2005;437(7063):1257–1263.
81. Tork I. Anatomy of the serotonergic system. *Ann N Y Acad Sci*. 1990;600:9–34, discussion 34–35.
82. Koella WP. Serotonin and sleep. *Exp Med Surg*. 1969;27(1–2):157–168.
83. Schonrock B, Busselberg D, Haas HL. Properties of tuberomammillary histamine neurones and their response to galanin. *Agents Actions*. 1991;33(1–2): 135–137.
84. Yang QZ, Hatton GI. Electrophysiology of excitatory and inhibitory afferents to rat histaminergic tuberomammillary nucleus neurons from hypothalamic and forebrain sites. *Brain Res*. 1997;773 (1–2):162–172.
85. Jasper H. Diffuse projection systems: the integrative action of the thalamic reticular system. *Electroencephalogr Clin Neurophysiol*. 1949;1(4):405–419; discussion 419–420.
86. Lo Conte G, Casamenti F, Bigl V, Milaneschi E, Pepeu G. Effect of magnocellular forebrain nuclei lesions on acetylcholine output from the cerebral cortex, electrocorticogram and behaviour. *Arch Ital Biol*. 1982;120(1–3):176–188.
87. Sakurai T, Nagata R, Yamanaka A, et al. Input of orexin/hypocretin neurons revealed by a genetically encoded tracer in mice. *Neuron*. 2005;46(2):297–308.
88. Bittencourt JC, Presse F, Arias C, et al. The melanin-concentrating hormone system of the rat brain: an immuno- and hybridization histochemical characterization. *J Comp Neurol*. 1992;319(2):218–245.
89. De Lecea L, Kilduff TS, Peyron C, et al. The hypocretins: hypothalamus-specific peptides with neuroexcitatory activity. *Proc Natl Acad Sci U S A*. 1998;95(1):322–327.
90. Rye DB, Wainer BH, Mesulam MM, Mufson EJ, Saper CB. Cortical projections arising from the basal forebrain: a study of cholinergic and noncholinergic components employing combined retrograde tracing and immunohistochemical localization of choline acetyltransferase. *Neuroscience*. 1984;13(3):627–643.
91. Gritti I, Mainville L, Mancia M, Jones BE. GABAergic and other noncholinergic basal forebrain neurons, together with cholinergic neurons, project to the mesocortex and isocortex in the rat. *J Comp Neurol*. 1997;383(2):163–177.
92. Saper CB. Staying awake for dinner: hypothalamic integration of sleep, feeding, and circadian rhythms. *Prog Brain Res*. 2006;153:243–252.
93. Siegel J. REM sleep. In: Kryger MH, Roth T, Dement WC, eds. *Principles and Practice of Sleep Medicine*. Philadelphia, PA: Elsevier/Saunders; 2005:120–135.
94. Greene RW, Gerber U, McCarley RW. Cholinergic activation of medial pontine reticular formation neurons in vitro. *Brain Res*. 1989;476(1):154–159.
95. Carli G, Armengol V, Zanchetti A. Brain stem-limbic connections, and the electrographic

aspects of deep sleep in the cat. *Arch Ital Biol.* 1965;103(4):725–750.
96. Jouvet M. The role of monoamines and acetylcholine-containing neurons in the regulation of the sleep-waking cycle. *Ergeb Physiol.* 1972;64:166–307.
97. Jasper HH, Tessier J. Acetylcholine liberation from cerebral cortex during paradoxical (REM) sleep. *Science.* 1971;172(983):601–602.
98. el Mansari M, Sakai K, Jouvet M. Unitary characteristics of presumptive cholinergic tegmental neurons during the sleep-waking cycle in freely moving cats. *Exp Brain Res.* 1989;76(3):519–529.
99. Webster HH, Jones BE. Neurotoxic lesions of the dorsolateral pontomesencephalic tegmentum-cholinergic cell area in the cat. II. Effects upon sleep-waking states. *Brain Res.* 1988;458(2):285–302.
100. Crochet S, Sakai K. Effects of microdialysis application of monoamines on the EEG and behavioural states in the cat mesopontine tegmentum. *Eur J Neurosci.* 1999;11(10):3738–3752.
101. Fuller PM, Saper CB, Lu J. The pontine REM switch: past and present. *J Physiol.* 2007;584(pt 3): 735–741.
102. Lu J, Sherman D, Devor M, Saper CB. A putative flip-flop switch for control of REM sleep. *Nature.* 2006;441(7093):589–594.
103. Xi MC, Morales FR, Chase MH. Evidence that wakefulness and REM sleep are controlled by a GABAergic pontine mechanism. *J Neurophysiol.* 1999;82(4):2015–2019.
104. Maciewicz RJ, Kaneko CR, Highstein SM, Eagen K. Vestibular and medullary brain stem afferents to the abducens nucleus in the cat. *Brain Res.* 1977;123(2):229–240.
105. Vertes RP, Albo Z, Viana Di Prisco G. Theta-rhythmically firing neurons in the anterior thalamus: implications for mnemonic functions of Papez's circuit. *Neuroscience.* 2001;104(3):619–625.
106. Stickgold R, Hobson JA, Fosse R, Fosse M. Sleep, learning, and dreams: off-line memory reprocessing. *Science.* 2001;294(5544):1052–1057.
107. Rowe K, Moreno R, Lau TR, et al. Heart rate surges during REM sleep are associated with theta rhythm and PGO activity in cats. *Am J Physiol.* 1999;277(3, pt 2):R843–R849.
108. Taylor WB, Moldofsky H, Furedy JJ. Heart rate deceleration in REM sleep: an orienting reaction interpretation. *Psychophysiology.* 1985;22(1): 110–115.
109. Orem J, Montplaisir J, Dement WC. Changes in the activity of respiratory neurons during sleep. *Brain Res.* 1974;82(2):309–315.
110. Mileykovskiy BY, Kiyashchenko LI, Siegel JM. Cessation of activity in red nucleus neurons during stimulation of the medial medulla in decerebrate rats. *J Physiol.* 2002;545(pt 3):997–1006.
111. Morrison AR. Paradoxical sleep without atonia. *Arch Ital Biol.* 1988;126(4):275–89.
112. Foulkes D. *Children's dreams: longitudinal studies.* New York, NY: Wiley; xi, 1982:477.
113. Foulkes WD. Dream reports from different stages of sleep. *J Abnorm Soc Psychol.* 1962;65:14–25.
114. Baylor GW, Cavallero C. Memory sources associated with REM and NREM dream reports throughout the night: a new look at the data. *Sleep.* 2001;24(2):165–170.
115. Hobson JA, Pace-Schott EF, Stickgold R. Dreaming and the brain: toward a cognitive neuroscience of conscious states. *Behav Brain Sci.* 2000;23(6): 793–842, discussion 904–1121.
116. Braun AR, Balkin TJ, Wesenten NJ, et al. Regional cerebral blood flow throughout the sleep-wake cycle. An H2(15)O PET study. *Brain.* 1997;120(pt 7): 1173–1197.
117. Maquet P, Lejeune H, Pouthas V, et al. Brain activation induced by estimation of duration: a PET study. *Neuroimage.* 1996;3(2):119–126.
118. Hobson JA, Stickgold R, Pace-Schott EF. The neuropsychology of REM sleep dreaming. *Neuroreport.* 1998;9(3):R1–R14.
119. Hasselmo ME. Neuromodulation and the hippocampus: memory function and dysfunction in a network simulation. *Prog Brain Res.* 1999;121:3–18.
120. Peigneux P, Laureys S, Fuchs S, et al. Generation of rapid eye movements during paradoxical sleep in humans. *Neuroimage.* 2001;14(3):701–708.
121. Stickgold R. Why we dream. In: Kryger MH, Roth T, Dement WC, eds. *Principles and Practice of Sleep Medicine.* Philadelphia, PA: Saunders/ Elsevier; 2005:579–588.
122. Jones BE. Basic mechanisms of sleep-wake states. In: Kryger MH, Roth T, Dement WC, eds. *Principles and Practice of Sleep Medicine.* Philadelphia, PA: Elsevier/Saunders; 2005:136–153.
123. Gritti I, Mainville L, Jones BE. Codistribution of GABA- with acetylcholine-synthesizing neurons in the basal forebrain of the rat. *J Comp Neurol.* 1993;329(4):438–457.
124. Steriade M, Deschenes M. The thalamus as a neuronal oscillator. *Brain Res.* 1984;320(1):1–63.
125. Rainnie DG, Grunze HC, McCarley RW, Greene RW. Adenosine inhibition of mesopontine cholinergic neurons: implications for EEG arousal. *Science.* 1994;263(5147):689–692.
126. Benington JH, Heller HC. Restoration of brain energy metabolism as the function of sleep. *Prog Neurobiol.* 1995;45(4):347–360.
127. Jouvet M. Sleep and serotonin: an unfinished story. *Neuropsychopharmacology.* 1999;21(suppl 2): 24S–27S.
128. Saper CB, Lu J, Chou TC, Gooley J. The hypothalamic integrator for circadian rhythms. *Trends Neurosci.* 2005;28(3):152–157.
129. Sherin JE, Shiromani PJ, McCarley RW, Saper CB. Activation of ventrolateral preoptic neurons during sleep. *Science.* 1996;271(5246):216–219.
130. Szymusiak R, Alam N, Steininger TL, McGinty D. Sleep-waking discharge patterns of ventrolateral preoptic/anterior hypothalamic neurons in rats. *Brain Res.* 1998;803(1–2):178–188.
131. Sherin JE, Elmquist JK, Torrealba F, Saper CB. Innervation of histaminergic tuberomammillary neurons by GABAergic and galaninergic neurons in the ventrolateral preoptic nucleus of the rat. *J Neurosci.* 1998;18(12):4705–4721.

132. Lu J, Bjorkum AA, Xu M, Gaus SE, Shiromani PJ, Saper CB. Selective activation of the extended ventrolateral preoptic nucleus during rapid eye movement sleep. *J Neurosci.* 2002;22(11):4568–4576.
133. Gallopin T, Fort P, Eggermann E. Identification of sleep-promoting neurons in vitro. *Nature.* 2000;404(6781):992–995.
134. Chou TC, Bjorkum AA, Gaus SE, Lu J, Scammell TE, Saper CB. Afferents to the ventrolateral preoptic nucleus. *J Neurosci.* 2002;22(3):977–990.
135. Vincent SR, Hokfelt T, Wu JY. GABA neuron systems in hypothalamus and the pituitary gland. Immunohistochemical demonstration using antibodies against glutamate decarboxylase. *Neuroendocrinology.* 1982;34(2):117–125.
136. Kohler C, Ericson H, Watanabe T, et al. Galanin immunoreactivity in hypothalamic neurons: further evidence for multiple chemical messengers in the tuberomammillary nucleus. *J Comp Neurol.* 1986;250(1):58–64.
137. Ericson H, Kohler C, Blomqvist A. GABA-like immunoreactivity in the tuberomammillary nucleus: an electron microscopic study in the rat. *J Comp Neurol.* 1991;305(3):462–429.
138. Porkka-Heiskanen T, Strecker RE, McCarley RW. Brain site-specificity of extracellular adenosine concentration changes during sleep deprivation and spontaneous sleep: an in vivo microdialysis study. *Neuroscience.* 2000;99(3):507–517.
139. Lu J, Greco MA, Shiromani P, Saper CB. Effect of lesions of the ventrolateral preoptic nucleus on NREM and REM sleep. *J Neurosci.* 2000;20(10):3830–3842.
140. Sallanon M, Denoyer M, Kitahama K, Aubert C, Gay N, Jouvet M. Long-lasting insomnia induced by preoptic neuron lesions and its transient reversal by muscimol injection into the posterior hypothalamus in the cat. *Neuroscience.* 1989;32(3):669–683.
141. Espana RA, Scammell TE. Sleep neurobiology for the clinician. *Sleep.* 2004;27(4):811–820.
142. Swick TJ. The neurology of sleep. *Neurol Clin.* 2005;23(4):967–989, v.
143. Peyron C, Tighe DK, van den Pol AN, et al. Neurons containing hypocretin (orexin) project to multiple neuronal systems. *J Neurosci.* 1998;18(23):9996–10015.
144. Marcus JN, Aschkenasi CJ, Lee CE, et al. Differential expression of orexin receptors 1 and 2 in the rat brain. *J Comp Neurol.* 2001;435(1):6–25.
145. Kiyashchenko LI, Mileykovskiy BY, Maidment N, et al. Release of hypocretin (orexin) during waking and sleep states. *J Neurosci.* 2002;22(13):5282–5286.
146. Lin L, Faraco J, Li R, et al. The sleep disorder canine narcolepsy is caused by a mutation in the hypocretin (orexin) receptor 2 gene. *Cell.* 1999;98(3):365–376.
147. Mochizuki T, Crocker A, McCormack S, Yanagisawa M, Sakurai T, Scammell TE. Behavioral state instability in orexin knock-out mice. *J Neurosci.* 2004;24(28):6291–6300.
148. Borbely AA, Tobler I. In McGinty DJ, Colin RD, Morrison A, and Parmeggiani PL. ed. *Brain Mechanisms of Sleep.* New York, NY: Raven Press; 1985:35–44.
149. Dijk DJ, Czeisler CA. Contribution of the circadian pacemaker and the sleep homeostat to sleep propensity, sleep structure, electroencephalographic slow waves, and sleep spindle activity in humans. *J Neurosci.* 1995;15(5, pt 1):3526–3538.
150. McCarley RW. Neurobiology of REM and NREM sleep. *Sleep Med.* 2007;8(4):302–330.
151. Kong J, Shepel PN, Holden CP, Mackiewicz M, Pack AI, Geiger JD. Brain glycogen decreases with increased periods of wakefulness: implications for homeostatic drive to sleep. *J Neurosci.* 2002;22(13):5581–5587.
152. Scammell TE, Gerashchenko DY, Mochizuki T, et al. An adenosine A2a agonist increases sleep and induces Fos in ventrolateral preoptic neurons. *Neuroscience.* 2001;107(4):653–663.
153. Chamberlin NL, Arrigoni E, Chou TC, Scammell TE, Greene RW, Saper CB. Effects of adenosine on gabaergic synaptic inputs to identified ventrolateral preoptic neurons. *Neuroscience.* 2003;119(4):913–918.
154. Johnson RF, Moore RY, Morin LP. Loss of entrainment and anatomical plasticity after lesions of the hamster retinohypothalamic tract. *Brain Res.* 1988;460(2):297–313.
155. Cassone VM, Chesworth MJ, Armstrong SM. Entrainment of rat circadian rhythms by daily injection of melatonin depends upon the hypothalamic suprachiasmatic nuclei. *Physiol Behav.* 1986;36(6):1111–1121.
156. Gooley J, Lu J, Saper CB. A broad role for melanopsin in nonvisual photoreception. *J. Neurosci.* 2003;23:7093–7106.
157. Provencio I, Rollag MD, Castrucci AM. Photoreceptive net in the mammalian retina. This mesh of cells may explain how some blind mice can still tell day from night. *Nature.* 2002;415(6871):493.
158. Yoshida K, McCormack S, España RA, Crocker A, Scammell TE. Afferents to the orexin neurons of the rat brain. *J Comp Neurol.* 2006;494(5):845–861.
159. Lu J, Zhang YH, Chou TC, et al. Contrasting effects of ibotenate lesions of the paraventricular nucleus and subparaventricular zone on sleep-wake cycle and temperature regulation. *J Neurosci.* 2001;21(13):4864–4874.
160. Chou TC, Scammell TE, Gooley JJ, Gaus SE, Saper CB, Lu J. Critical role of dorsomedial hypothalamic nucleus in a wide range of behavioral circadian rhythms. *J Neurosci.* 2003;23(33):10691–10702.
161. Stephan FK. The "other" circadian system: food as a Zeitgeber. *J Biol Rhythms.* 2002;17(4):284–292.
162. Dunlap JC. Molecular bases for circadian clocks. *Cell.* 1999;96(2):271–290.
163. Maquet P, Péters J, Aerts J, et al. Functional neuroanatomy of human rapid-eye-movement sleep and dreaming. *Nature.* 1996;383(6596):163–166.

164. Maquet P, Degueldre C, Delfiore G, et al. Functional neuroanatomy of human slow wave sleep. *J Neurosci.* 1997;17(8):2807–2812.
165. Zoccoli G, Walker AM, Lenzi P, Franzini C. The cerebral circulation during sleep: regulation mechanisms and functional implications. *Sleep Med Rev.* 2002;6(6):443–455.
166. Santiago TV, Guerra E, Neubauer JA, Edelman NH. Correlation between ventilation and brain blood flow during sleep. *J Clin Invest.* 1984;73(2): 497–506.
167. Hajak G, Klingelhöfer J, Schulz-Varszegi M, Sander D, Rüther E. Sleep apnea syndrome and cerebral hemodynamics. *Chest.* 1996;110(3): 670–679.
168. Greenberg JH. Sleep and the cerebral circulation. In: Orem J, ed. *Physiology in Sleep.* New York, NY; Academic Press; 1980:57–95.
169. Kogure K, Scheinberg P, Reinmuth OM, Fujishima M, Busto R. Mechanisms of cerebral vasodilatation in hypoxia. *J Appl Physiol.* 1970;29(2):223–229.
170. Gucer G, Viernstein LJ. Intracranial pressure in the normal monkey while awake and asleep. *J Neurosurg.* 1979;51(2):206–210.
171. Mancia G, Baccelli G, Adams DB, Zanchetti A. Vasomotor regulation during sleep in the cat. *Am J Physiol.* 1971;220(4):1086–1093.
172. Verrier RL, Harper RM, Hobson JA. Cardiovascular physiology: central and autonomic regulation. In: Kryger MH, Roth T, Dement WC, eds. *Principles and Practice of Sleep Medicine.* Philadelphia, PA: Saunders; 2000:192–202.
173. Dickerson LW, Huang AH, Nearing BD, Verrier RL. Primary coronary vasodilation associated with pauses in heart rhythm during sleep. *Am J Physiol.* 1993;264(1, pt 2):R186–R196.
174. Gassel MM, Ghelarducci B, Marchiafava Pl, Pompeiano O. Phasic Changes in Blood Pressure and Heart Rate during the Rapid Eye Movement Episodes of Desynchronized Sleep in Unrestrained Cats. *Arch Ital Biol.* 1964;102:530–544.
175. Lown B, Temte JV, Reich P, Gaughan C, Regestein Q, Hal H. Basis for recurring ventricular fibrillation in the absence of coronary heart disease and its management. *N Engl J Med.* 1976;294(12):623–629.
176. Orem J. Neuronal mechanisms of respiration in REM sleep. *Sleep.* 1980;3(3–4):251–267.
177. Kirby DA, Verrier RL. Differential effects of sleep stage on coronary hemodynamic function during stenosis. *Physiol Behav.* 1989;45(5):1017–1020.
178. Baharav A, Kotagal S, Rubin BK, Pratt J, Akselrod S. Autonomic cardiovascular control in children with obstructive sleep apnea. *Clin Auton Res.* 1999;9(6):345–351.
179. Orem J, Netick A, Dement WC. Breathing during sleep and wakefulness in the cat. *Respir Physiol.* 1977;30(3):265–289.
180. Orem J, Kubin L. Respiratory physiology: central and neural control. In: Kryger MH, Roth T, Dement WC, eds. *Principles and Practice of Sleep Medicine.* Philadelphia, PA: Saunders; 1989:213–222.
181. Phillipson EA. Control of breathing during sleep. *Am Rev Respir Dis.* 1978;118(5):909–939.
182. Moore JG, Englert E Jr. Circadian rhythm of gastric acid secretion in man. *Nature.* 1970;226(5252):1261–1262.
183. Orr WC, Johnson LF, Robinson MG. Effect of sleep on swallowing, esophageal peristalsis, and acid clearance. *Gastroenterology.* 1984;86(5, pt 1): 814–819.
184. Lichter I, Muir RC. The pattern of swallowing during sleep. *Electroencephalogr Clin Neurophysiol.* 1975;38(4):427–432.
185. Helm JH, Dodds WJ, Hogan W. Flow and acid neutralization capacity of human saliva. *Gastroenterology.* 1980;78:1181.
186. Orr WC, Dubois A, Stahl ML. Gastric Function during Sleep. *Sleep Res.* 1978;7:72.
187. Bloom PB, Filion RD, Stunkard AJ, Fox S, Stellar E. Gastric and duodenal motility, food intake and hunger measured in man during a 24-hr period. *Am J Dig Dis.* 1970;15(8):719–725.
188. Baust W, Rohrwasser W. [Gastric motility and pH during natural human sleep]. *Pflugers Arch.* 1969;305(3):229–240.
189. Yaryura-Tobias JA, Hutcheson JS, White L. Relationship between stages of sleep and gastric motility. *Behav Neuropsychiatry.* 1970;2(7):22–24.
190. Narducci F, Bassotti G, Gaburri M, Morelli A. Twenty four hour manometric recording of colonic motor activity in healthy man. *Gut.* 1987; 28(1):17–25.
191. Bassotti G, Bucaneve G, Betti C. Sudden awakenings from sleep: effects on proximal and distal colonic contractile activity in humans. *Eur J Gastroenterol Hepatol.* 1990;2:6.
192. Ronholt C, Rasmussen OO, Christiansen J. Ambulatory manometric recording of anorectal activity. *Dis Colon Rectum.* 1999;42(12): 1551–1559.
193. Rao SS, Welcher K. Periodic rectal motor activity: the intrinsic colonic gatekeeper? *Am J Gastroenterol.* 1996;91(5):890–897.
194. Parker DC, Sassin JF, Mace JW, et al. Human growth hormone release during sleep: electroencephalographic correlation. *J Clin Endocrinol Metab.* 1969;29(6):871–874.
195. Van Cauter E, Kerkhofs M, Caufriez A, et al. A quantitative estimation of growth hormone secretion in normal man: reproducibility and relation to sleep and time of day. *J Clin Endocrinol Metab.* 1992;74(6):1441–1450.
196. Weitzman ED, Fukushima D, Nogeire C, Roffwarg H, Gallagher TF, Hellman L. Twenty-four hour pattern of the episodic secretion of cortisol in normal subjects. *J Clin Endocrinol Metab.* 1971;33(1):14–22.
197. Sassin JF, Frantz AG, Weitzman ED, Kapen S. Human prolactin: 24-hour pattern with increased release during sleep. *Science.* 1972;177(55):1205–1207.
198. Lucke C, Hehrmann R, von Mayersbach K, von zur Mühlen A. Studies on circadian variations of plasma TSH, thyroxine and triiodothyronine in man. *Acta Endocrinol (Copenh).* 1977;86(1):81–88.
199. Fevre M, Segel T, Marks JF, Boyar RM. LH and melatonin secretion patterns in pubertal boys. *J Clin Endocrinol Metab.* 1978;47(6):1383–1386.

200. Judd HL, Parker DC, Siler TM, Yen SS. The nocturnal rise of plasma testosterone in pubertal boys. *J Clin Endocrinol Metab.* 1974;38(4):710–713.
201. Van Cauter E. Endocrine physiology. In: Kryger MH, Roth T, Dement WC, eds. *Principles and Practice of Sleep Medicine.* Philadelphia PA: Saunders; 2005:273.
202. Bodosi B, Gardi J, Hajdu I, Szentirmai E, Obal F Jr, Krueger JM. Rhythms of ghrelin, leptin, and sleep in rats: effects of the normal diurnal cycle, restricted feeding, and sleep deprivation. *Am J Physiol Regul Integr Comp Physiol.* 2004; 287(5):R1071–R1079.
203. Taheri S, Lin L, Austin D, Young T, Mignot E. Short sleep duration is associated with reduced leptin, elevated ghrelin, and increased body mass index. *PLoS Med.* 2004;1(3):e62.
204. Pace-Schott EF, Hobson JA. The neurobiology of sleep: Genetics, cellular physiology and subcortical networks. *Nat Rev Neurosci.* 2002;3(8):591–605.
205. Lipton J, Becker RE, Kothare SV. Insomnia of childhood. *Curr Opin Pediatr.* 2008;20(6):641–649.

CHAPTER 2

The Clinical and Laboratory Assessment of Childhood Sleep–Wake Problems

Suresh Kotagal

Introduction

The pervasive nature of sleep-wake problems in children with neurodevelopmental disabilities, their significant impact on quality of life, and the amenability in general to treatment underscore how important it is for health professionals to integrate the assessment of sleep-wake function into their comprehensive management plan. The sleep-wake assessment consists of a sleep history and clinical examination that are followed when necessary by diagnostic procedures that are specifically tailored to the needs of the patient. There are continuous changes in the organization of sleep-wake states and respiration from infancy through adolescence; thus, one needs to be familiar with age-related normal values for various physiologic parameters [1]. Specialized studies such as cerebrospinal fluid hypocretin analysis for the diagnosis of narcolepsy are discussed in their relevant chapters in the book.

History

The style of eliciting the sleep history may vary. This author finds it useful to guide the parent or patient through events and activities from the time of awakening in the morning into the afternoon, evening, then on to bedtime, and through the night's sleep. Conversely, one may also start inquiry with events around bedtime, through the night's sleep, morning, and then the day. A sample questionnaire that is completed by the family before consultation visit at the author's institution is shown in Figure 2.1. The design of such questionnaires varies from one institution to another. Despite the best of efforts, it may sometimes be difficult to sort out sleepiness from physical tiredness [2].

Daytime History

How the child feels on awakening is a key question from the standpoint of existence of an underlying sleep disorder—disturbed night sleep is frequently associated with feeling unrefreshed on awakening in the morning, regardless of the length of night sleep. The morning awakening time may be delayed to 10:00 or 11:00 hours or beyond in patients with delayed sleep-phase syndrome. Patients with major depressive disorders may have difficulty awakening and daytime sleepiness [3]. Sleepiness may also occur when children are dropped off at day care centers relatively early in the morning or when teenagers have to contend with early school start times [4]. Infants with obstructive sleep apnea (OSA) show problems with sucking or swallowing and choking on the feeds. Prior respiratory syncytial virus infection may be a risk factor for OSA in infancy [5]. The disturbed night sleep of preschool-aged children can be associated with daytime hyperactivity and inattentiveness [6]. One should inquire about daytime

Confidential
Pediatric Ages 3–17 Years
Not part of Medical Record. Discard after use.

Your physician has requested that your child have a consultation at the Center for Sleep Medicine. This questionnaire asks questions not only about your child's habits and behavior during sleep, but also about other factors that may influence the patterns of sleep and wakefulness. Please answer each question to the best of your ability. Mark questions that you cannot answer with a question mark.

Please bring the completed questionnaire to the Center for Sleep Medicine when you come for your consultation. if you have any questions about this questionnaire or your consultation, please call the Center for Sleep Medicine at 507-266-7456.

General Patient Information

Patient Name *(child)*			Mayo Clinic Number	Birth Date *(Month DD. YYYY)*
Name of Person Completing Questionnaire			Legal Authority *(if other than parent)*	
Address - Street			Home Phone *(including area code)*	
City	State	ZIP	Work Phone *(including area code)*	

Concerns

What are your main concerns about your child's sleep or level of alertness?

Sleep History

What time does your child enter bed at night to go to sleep? *(hh:mm)*

On school nights ______ : ______ On weekends and holidays ______ : ______

Where does the child lie down to sleep?

☐ In the child's own bed, in the child's own room

If the child sleeps in his or her own room, is the room shared with anyone else? ☐ Yes ☐ No

Do you have to be present in the room in order for the child to fall asleep? ☐ Yes ☐ No

☐ In the child's own bed, in the parents' bedroom

☐ In a parent's lap in an armchair

☐ Family room couch

☐ Some other place *(describe)*:

What does the child like to do in the 2 hours before bedtime?

Approximately how long does it take for the child to fall asleep? *(hh:mm)* ______ : ______

Does your child experience feelings of restlessness or the urge to move their legs (this may described as owwies, tickles, tingles, boo-boos, static, bugs, spiders, ants or a lot of energy in their legs)? ☐ Yes ☐ No

Do these sensations begin or become worse in the evening or at bedtime? ☐ Yes ☐ No

Do these sensations begin or become worse when the child is sitting or lying down? ☐ Yes ☐ No

Are these sensations relieved by moving the legs or walking about? ☐ Yes ☐ No

Does the child need any of the following to fall asleep? *(check all that apply)*

☐ Blanket ☐ Night light ☐ Stuffed animal ☐ Other toy ☐ Radio ☐ Television ☐ Pacifier

☐ Bedtime story ☐ Rocking ☐ Snack ☐ Car ride ☐ Patting ☐ Other *(describe)*: ____________

Does the child snore?

☐ Never ☐ Occasionally ☐ Frequently ☐ Always

Is the snoring heard when the child is:

☐ Sleeping on the back ☐ Sleeping on the side

☐ Sleeping face down ☐ in all body positions

Is the snoring interrupted by silent pauses and snorting sounds?

☐ Yes ☐ No

Does the child: *(Chech all that apply)*

☐ Have a tendency to sleep with the mouth open?

☐ Cry or act confused at night?

☐ Wake up at night with a dry mouth?

☐ Talk in sleep?

☐ Have bed wetting?

☐ Walk in sleep?

☐ Have any other unusual behavior at night? If yes, describe:

Figure 2.1 Center for Sleep Medicine Questionnaire.

napping—it is physiologic for toddlers to take one nap per day; thus, it is difficult to label them as having excessive daytime sleepiness unless it is of an extreme degree. Napping generally stops in all children by the age of 3 to 5 years [7]. In a school-age child, therefore, a tendency to habitually fall asleep in the classroom, while being driven in an automobile, on

***Steep History** Continued*

How many times does your child wake up at night?	What is the final morning wake up time? *(hh:mm)* On school days ______ : ______ On weekends and holidays ______ : ______
What does the child do after waking up during the night?	Upon awakening, the child feels: ☐ Tired ☐ Somewhat refreshed ☐ Refreshed Does he/she feel sleepy during the daytime? ☐ Yes ☐ No
What do you do to help the child fall back to sleep?	The child takes ______ naps per day, with each nap lasting approximately ______ minutes. The naps are: ☐ Refreshing ☐ Not refreshing

Pediatric Daytime Sleepiness Scale (PDSS)

Drake C, Nickel C, Burduvall E at al. The pediatric daytime sleepiness scale (PDSS): sleep habits and school outcomes in middleschool children. SLEEP 2003;26(4):455-458 used with permission granted by the Associated Professional Sleep Societies In October 2008

Please answer the following questions as honestly as you can by circling one answer only:

1. How often do you fall asleep or get drowsy during class periods?	Always	Frequently	Sometimes	Seldom	Never
2. How often do you get sleepy or drowsy while doing your home work?	Always	Frequently	Sometimes	Seldom	Never
3. Are you usually alert most of the day?	Always	Frequently	Sometimes	Seldom	Never
4. How often are you ever tired and grumpy during the day?	Always	Frequently	Sometimes	Seldom	Never
5. How often do you have trouble getting out of bed in the morning?	Always	Frequently	Sometimes	Seldom	Never
6. How often do you fall back to sleep after being awakened in the morning?	Very often	often	Sometimes	Seldom	Never
7. How often do you need someone to awaken you in the morning?	Always	Frequently	Sometimes	Seldom	Never
8. How often do you think you need more sleep?	Very often	often	Sometimes	Seldom	Never

Check the following if present: a tendency for the child's legs to become weak or rubbery whenever he/she becomes: ☐ Excited ☐ Emotionally upset ☐ Starts laughing The child sees vivid or scary dreams at the time of falling asleep? ☐ Yes ☐ No or upon waking up from sleep? ☐ Yes ☐ No There is a tendency for the child's body to get momentarily paralyzed as he/she is falling asleep? ☐ Yes ☐ No or upon waking up? ☐ Yes ☐ No	Are your child's sleep problems affecting school performance, self image or social activities: Other health problems that might be affecting sleep *(in your opinion)*:
Please provide any other information that you feel might be useful in your child's Sleep Center evaluation:	List medications:

Family History

Is there a family history of restless legs syndrome? ☐ Yes ☐ No ☐ Don't know If Yes, who has this condition?______
Is there a family history of sleep apnea? ☐ Yes ☐ No ☐ Don't know If Yes, who has this condition?______
Is there a family history of any other sleep disorder, and who has the condition?

Signature

Parent Signature (or legal authority)	Legal Authority (if not parent) ☐ Legal Guardian ☐ Surrogate ☐ Health Care Agent ☐ Conservator (Health Care Power of Attorney)	Signature Date (Month *DD.YYYY*)

Figure 2.1 ***(Continued)***

returning home from school, at the dinner table, while watching television, or while reading clearly suggests hypersomnolence. The excessively sleepy child is sometimes labeled as being "lazy" or lacking motivation [8]. The naps of children with narcolepsy may be associated with seeing vivid dreams at sleep onset (hypnagogic hallucinations) or a momentary inability to move (sleep paralysis). Cataplexy accompanies 60% to 70% of children with narcolepsy. It is characterized by abrupt loss of tone in the skeletal muscles in response to emotional stimuli such as laughter, fright, or surprise [9,10]. The antigravity muscles are most often affected, leading to head drops, the jaw dropping open, or partial or complete fall to the floor after becoming limp. Consciousness remains intact. Cataplexy may be relatively subtle in early childhood and may be easily overlooked unless inquired about specifically. Because sleepiness disrupts inhibitory functions of the prefrontal cortex, behavioral release phenomena such as mood swings and inattentiveness are common accompaniments, though they may also suggest coexistence of depression. Sleepy teens can manifest declining grades, chronic absence from school, and vulnerability to accidents/near-miss accidents. The degree of sleepiness can be quantified in 9- to 12-year-olds using scales such as the Pediatric Daytime Sleepiness Scale [11] or the modified Epworth Sleepiness Scale (ESS) [12] (Table 2.1). There may also be increased consumption of caffeinated beverages or nicotine in sleepy adolescents. Teenagers who show periods of hypersomnia lasting 10 to 14 days in conjunction with hyperphagia and hypersexual behavior alternating with intervening weeks of normal alertness may have periodic hypersomnia (Kleine-Levin syndrome). Inadequate sleep hygiene, substance abuse, and drug-seeking behavior may mimic a primary disorder of vigilance such as narcolepsy or idiopathic hypersomnia. Medication history for prescription drugs, over-the-counter agents, and street drugs is critical. Low self-esteem, feelings of sadness, and social withdrawal may suggest underlying depression. It is also important to inquire about whether daytime sleepiness is affecting quality-of-life measures such as attendance at school and social gatherings. One also needs to inquire about the level of participation in countermeasures for sleepiness such as physical activity and exercise. Excessive weight gain over the preceding year may be associated with OSA-hypopnea syndrome and narcolepsy-cataplexy [13,14].

Nighttime History

The bed onset time and sleep onset time (on school nights and nonschool nights) should be documented. Children with separation anxiety or behavioral insomnia of childhood may have become habituated to sleeping in the parents' bedroom. Elaborate rituals such as rocking the child to sleep or having the child fall asleep on the lap of the parent, which are actually counterproductive to the development of independent sleeping habits, may be seen in some children with autistic spectrum disorder. Restless legs syndrome (RLS) may be accompanied by an urge to move the limbs and a creeping or crawling feeling in the legs. This appears in the evenings or at night. This sensory disturbance is worsened by keeping the limbs still and is relived partially by stretching or moving the limb. Akathisia, a feeling of restlessness that is present throughout the day, is in contrast. Teens with inadequate sleep hygiene may use caffeinated beverages, tobacco, or alcohol before bedtime or watch television to "relax" and also use cell phones or surf the Internet till late at night. The history should also assess events at the sleep-wake transition such as hypnic starts, head rolling, and body rocking.

Patients with OSA may exhibit noisy snoring—the classic pattern is one of snoring that is interrupted by silent pauses, which terminate with snorting sounds; inspiratory stridor may also be encountered [1]. There is no correlation of the loudness of snoring with severity of OSA because infants and children with weak chest walls may not have forceful inspiration despite existence of a narrow upper airway. A tendency for dry mouth and keeping the mouth partially open (suggestive of nasal obstruction), restless sleep, excessive sweating, gastroesophageal reflux, and bed-wetting are other common manifestations of OSA. Periodic limb movements in sleep occur in approximately 80% of patients with RLS and appear as episodes of intermittent flexion at the hips, knees, and ankles at an interval of 4 to 90 seconds. Confusional arousals, sleep walking, and sleep terrors are non-rapid eye movement (NREM) parasomnias that typically occur 2 to 3 hours after initial onset. These events may last 15 to 20 minutes. Typically, the child has no recollection of the events on awakening the following morning. NREM parasomnias may be triggered by sleep instability because of OSA, RLS, or gastroesophageal reflux. Frontal lobe seizures are characterized by hypermotor, thrashing movements, or dystonic posturing of the limbs lasting 20 to 60 seconds [15] that occur randomly

Table 2.1 Scales for assessing sleepiness

Scale	Stanford Sleepiness Scale (SSS) [30]	Epworth Sleepiness Scale (ESS)	Pediatric Daytime Sleepiness Scale (PDSS)
Description	SSS asks patients to rate their degree of sleepiness at a single moment in time using a range of scores from 1 to 7.	Participants rate how likely they are to doze off or fall asleep in 8 different situations commonly encountered in daily life on a 4-point scale; 0 = no chance of dozing, 1 = slight chance of dozing, 2 = moderate chance of dozing, 3 = high chance of dozing.	The PDSS is an 8-item questionnaire developed to measure excessive sleepiness in younger school-age populations; responses are rated as: never (score 0), seldom (score 1), sometimes (score 2), frequently (score 3), and always (score 4). Reverse score item #3.
Items	Feeling active, vital, alert, or wide awake [1] Functioning at high levels, but not at peak, able to concentrate [1] Awake but relaxed; responsive but not fully alert [2] Somewhat foggy, let down [3] Foggy, losing interest in remaining awake Slowed down [4] Sleepy, woozy, fighting sleep; prefer to lie down [5] No longer fighting sleep, sleep onset soon, having dreamlike thoughts [6] Asleep (7)	Sitting and reading Watching TV Sitting inactive in a public place (eg, movie theater or a meeting) As a passenger in a car for an hour without break Lying down to rest in the afternoon when circumstances permit Sitting and talking to someone Sitting quietly after lunch In a car, while stopping for a few minutes in traffic	1. How often do you fall asleep or get drowsy during class periods? 2. How often do you get sleepy or drowsy while doing your homework? 3. Are you usually alert most of the day? 4. How often are you ever tired and grumpy during the day? 5. How often do you have trouble getting out of bed in the morning? 6. How often do you fall back to sleep after being awakened in the morning? 7. How often do you need someone to awaken you in the morning? 8. How often do you think that you need more sleep?
Score	No reference values and it is not validated with physiologic measures.	ESS total score >10 indicates need to determine excessive daytime sleepiness (EDS) cause.	Maximum score = 32; the 50th, 75th, and 90th percentiles for sleepiness scores are 16, 20, and 23, respectively.

Reproduced with permission from Ref. [2].

through the night. The seizures of benign rolandic epilepsy of childhood are accompanied by perioral and facial muscle twitching, preserved consciousness, and ictal aphasia.

Owens and Dalzell [16] have developed the mnemonics SIFT (Situation Impairment Frequency Tools) and BEARS (Bedtime Problems, Excessive daytime sleepiness, Awakening at night, Regularity and duration of sleep) that can facilitate elicitation of the sleep history in the office setting (Table 2.2).

The Sleep-Related Examination

Certain components of the general physical examination and that of respiratory and cardiovascular systems, nose, throat, craniofacial features, and the neurological assessment are used. Anthropometrics such as height, weight, body mass index, occipitofrontal head circumference, and blood pressure are important. OSA may be associated with poor weight gain during infancy and with obesity in older children [1]. The patient should be evaluated for craniofacial abnormalities such as micrognathia, dental malocclusion, enlarged tongue size, high arched palate, and mid-face hypoplasia. Deviated nasal septum, swollen inferior turbinates, tonsillar hypertrophy, and mouth breathing can be encountered in children with OSA. Consultation with an otolaryngologist may be required for excluding adenoidal hypertrophy. Brainstem anomalies such as Chiari types I and II malformation can be associated with snoring, hoarseness of the voice, decreased gag reflex, and an altitudinal abnormality in tendon reflexes [17]. Neuromuscular disorders such as myotonic dystrophy, congenital muscular dystrophy, congenital nonprogressive myopathies, spinal muscular atrophy, and myasthenia gravis show chronic obstructive hypoventilation because of a combination of pharyngeal muscle weakness that predisposes to upper airway collapse and chest and abdominal wall weakness [18]. The kyphoscoliosis that commonly accompanies neuromuscular disorders can further restrict chest and abdominal movement and exacerbate hypoventilation, which is manifested clinically as hypercarbia, with consequent early morning headache and daytime fatigue [19]. Goldstein et al have developed a clinical assessment scale for the evaluation of sleep-disordered breathing that is based on the history and clinical examination [20]. In situations where diagnostic tests such as nocturnal polysomnography (NPSG) are not available, the scale can help the clinician diagnose OSA, especially when it happens to be severe. The scale has questions that pertain to night snoring, pauses in breathing, gasping and choking sounds, night sweats, frequent awakenings, sleeping with the neck extended, daytime behavior, and so on. With regard to episodic phenomena, such as cataplexy, nocturnal seizures, and parasomnias,

Table 2.2 The pediatric sleep history

	SIFT		BEARS
Situation	When does the patient feel sleepy/tired?	**B**edtime problems	Do you have problems falling asleep at bedtime?
Impairment	To what extent does sleepiness interfere with daily life?	**E**xcessive daytime sleepiness	Do you feel sleepy a lot during the day? While driving?
Frequency	How often does the patient feel sleepy?		Do you wake up a lot at night?
Tools	Use tools such as the ESS to assess degree of sleepiness	**A**wakening at night	What time do you usually go to bed on school nights? At weekends? How much sleep do you usually get?
		Regularity and duration of sleep	Parent: Does your child usually snore at night?
		Sleep-disordered breathing	Patient: Has anyone ever told you that you snore loudly at night?

Reproduced with permission from Ref. [2].

provision of video clips of the spells by the parents is priceless in arriving at a diagnosis.

Survey Tools for Assessing Sleep-Wake Disorders

1. *Sleep Diary*

This is maintained by the parent, and in some cases, by the teenage patient. Ideally, the diary should be produced by the patient at the time of the initial sleep consultation. The diary records sleep-wake behaviors occurring over a 24-hour period for 2 to 3 successive weeks. Recording of bedtime (weeknights and weekends), sleep onset time, the number and length of night awakenings, morning wake-up times on school days and on weekends, frequency and length of daytime naps, how alert one feels during the day (on a 1–5 sliding scale), exercise, and use of caffeinated beverages and medications is documented.

2. *Epworth Sleepiness Scale*

ESS is a widely used, self-administered questionnaire for older teens and adults [12]. It has been validated in a variety of clinical scenarios and proven to be reliable [21–23]. Eight questions estimate the patient's chance of dozing off on a 0 to 3 scale during common activities such as while sitting and reading, watching television, sitting inactively in a public place (as a passenger in a car), lying down in the afternoon, sitting and talking to somebody, after lunch, and while driving after stopping for a few minutes in a traffic light. The maximum score is 24; values up to 10 are physiologic, and those above 12 correlate with pathologic daytime sleepiness. In the original description by Johns, the questionnaire was administered to 188 adults, including 30 healthy controls and 150 patients with sleep disorders consisting of primary snoring, OSA, narcolepsy, idiopathic hypersomnia, insomnia, and periodic limb movement disorder [12]. The ages of the subjects ranged from 18 to 78, with men outnumbering women in the snoring, OSA, and periodic leg movements disorder groups. The controls showed a mean ESS score of 5.9 ± 2.2, with no significant gender difference. All patients with narcolepsy and idiopathic hypersomnia had higher ESS scores (>10) than controls. Scores greater than 16 were felt to reflect severe sleepiness. One drawback of the ESS is that patients frequently underestimate the severity of their own sleepiness. Others have difficulty distinguishing sleepiness from fatigue.

As the conventional ESS contains questions pertaining to the use of alcohol and driving, a modified pediatric version of ESS created by Melendres et al from which mention of alcohol and driving by the subject has been removed can be used [24], with scores greater than 10 suggesting daytime sleepiness (Table 2.1).

3. *Karolinska Sleepiness Scale*

Developed in 1990 by Akerstedt et al [25], this scale has been frequently applied in occupational health field. It uses a 9-point scale that ranges from 1 being very alert to 9 being very sleepy and trying hard to stay awake. Patients are asked to rate their sleepiness in the 5 minutes immediately before taking the test. A score of 7 or more denotes pathologic sleepiness.

4. *Pittsburgh Sleep Quality Index*

This is a 19-item, self-rated questionnaire. Seven "component" scores are generated in subjective sleep quality, sleep latency, sleep duration, habitual sleep efficiency, sleep disturbances, use of sleeping medications, and daytime dysfunction. A global score of greater than 5 has a diagnostic sensitivity of 89.6% and specificity of 86.5% from the standpoint of distinguishing good sleepers from poor sleepers [26]. The test can be used for baseline and longitudinal follow-up of a cohort. The Pittsburgh Sleep Quality Index has good internal consistency and a Cronbach reliability coefficient of 0.83.

5. *Children's Sleep Habits Questionnaire*

This is a popular parent questionnaire that is designed for use in children aged 4 to 12 years. The questionnaire was validated in a sample of 469 children of 4 to 10 of years age [27]. There are 45 questions that pertain to 8 domains of sleep-wake function—bedtime resistance, sleep onset delay, sleep duration, sleep anxiety, night awakenings, parasomnias, breathing disturbance, and daytime sleepiness. Questions pertain to issues such as "child sleeps too little" or "the child suddenly falls asleep in the middle of active behavior." Responses are rated as rarely (occurrence none or once weekly; assigned 1 point), sometimes (occurring 2–4 nights per week; assigned 2 points), or usually (occurring 5–7 nights per week; assigned 3 points). The higher the score, the more disturbed the sleep; scores of 41 or greater correlate with presence of a sleep disorder. The internal consistency estimate for this questionnaire in a community sample of 4- to 10-year olds was 0.36 to 0.70, whereas the test-retest reliability over a 2-week period was 0.62 to 0.79 [27]. The shortcomings of the Children's Sleep Habits Questionnaire (CSHQ) are that it is a retrospective assessment by the parent. Although the total score provides a reliable cutoff for determining presence or absence of a sleep disorder, there has been no validation of the significance of scores in the various subscales. Nevertheless, the CSHQ is a simple and widely used survey tool in school-age children.

6. *Sleep Habits Survey*

The survey was validated by Wolfson et al in a sample of 302 high school students aged 13 to 19 years [28]. The survey asked about the sleeping and waking behaviors of the subjects in the preceding 2 weeks. During the subsequent week, they wore an actigraph on the nondominant wrist and kept a diary of sleep-wake function. Total sleep time and total awake time obtained by the survey were matched against those obtained by sleep diaries and actigraphy. The Pearson coefficient correlate for total sleep time, Sleep Habits Survey (SHS) versus actigraphy on school nights, was 0.53 and on weekends it was 0.31. Correlation coefficient of the sleep onset/bed onset time, SHS versus actigraphy on school nights, was 0.70, and on weekends it was 0.48. The correlation coefficient for wake time/sleep offset time, SHS versus actigraphy, was 0.77 on school days and 0.52 on weekends. All correlates were statistically significant at $P < .01$. The survey has 63 questions, many of which delve in depth into sleeping and waking behavior of teens.

7. *Cleveland Adolescent Sleepiness Questionnaire*

This questionnaire applies to adolescents aged 11 to 17 years [29]. Normative data were gathered from 411 adolescents who were predominantly Caucasian (74.4%) or African American (21.3%). Subjects were recruited from informational meetings at churches and schools. The average age of the subjects was 13.9 ± 1.6 years. The finalized questionnaire consists of 16 items that address daytime sleepiness in environments commonly encountered by teenagers. Each test item is assigned a score of 1 (never) to 5 (almost everyday). The mean sleepiness score for these healthy subjects was 35.2 (SD 11) and the median score was 34 (interquartile range 26–43). There was good internal consistency of the test items, with a Cronbach alpha score of 0.89. There were no significant differences of the scores from the standpoint of ethnic background of the subjects.

8. *The Pediatric Sleep Questionnaire*

This questionnaire was developed by Chervin et al after study of children and adolescents aged 2 to 18 years [30]. There were 54 patients with a sleep-related breathing disturbance (SRBD) (mean age, 9.3 ± 4.1 years) and 108 control subjects (mean age, 7.0 ± 3.8 years) from the general pediatric clinics. The questionnaire is completed by the parent or guardian. There are 22 items in the questionnaire that address snoring during sleep, periods of observed apnea, mouth breathing, bed wetting, waking up feeling unrefreshed, daytime sleepiness, headaches, overweight, inattentiveness, and so on. Responses to questions are in the yes/no/don't know format. The optimal cutoff score to diagnose SRBD would be 0.33, that is, 33% of the 22 questions answered positively. The sensitivity of the questionnaire for diagnosing SRBD is approximately 86% and specificity is 87%.

Sleep Laboratory Diagnostic Tests

Actigraphy

The actigraph is a wristwatch-shaped portable device for assessing sleep onset and offset times in the home environment, longitudinally over a 1- to 3-week period. It is conventionally strapped over the left wrist. Recording of signals is based on the premise that bodily movements are frequent during wakefulness and infrequent during sleep. The device measures linear acceleration from muscle activity and translates physical motion into a numeric representation that is sampled frequently, for example, every 0.1 second, and is aggregated at a constant interval or epoch, to be then displayed graphically [31]. To draw valid conclusions, data should be recorded for 1 to 3 weeks at a time and matched with simultaneously maintained logs of sleep-wake function. Visual inspection of the raw actigraphy data is necessary before generating a printout. On the basis of the presence or absence of muscle activity, one can determine whether an individual is awake or asleep at a given time. When combined with the sleep logs, indices such as total time in bed, total sleep time, sleep efficiency, sleep onset time, and awakening time can be reliably estimated [31]. There is good correlation with polysomnogram-based estimates of sleep and wakefulness; a trained actigraph scorer can distinguish sleep from wakefulness with 91% to 93% accuracy in adults (ages 20–30 years) and 91.4% to 96.5% accuracy in children and adolescents aged 10 to 16 years [31,32]. The level of agreement may diminish as sleep becomes more fragmented because of intrinsic sleep disorders. Wrist actigraphy is a useful adjunct in the assessment of insomnia, circadian rhythm sleep disorders, daytime sleepiness, and RLS/periodic limb movement disorder, as it provides longitudinal, qualitative and semiquantitative information about sleep-wake function in the home environment [32]. It also has utility in measuring the outcome in intervention trials of sleep disorders of children and adults. One limitation is not being able to distinguish wakefulness from sleep if the patient is awake, but lying immobile without movement, as this state may be mistaken by the instrument as sleep. Actigraphy is also not able to distinguish the various stages of sleep and also may be invalid during continuous involuntary activity such as tremor.

Overnight Oximetry

Overnight oximetry analysis is a screening tool for sleep-disordered breathing [33]. Oximetry data must be visually inspected and interpreted by clinicians knowledgeable in distinguishing movement artifact from the "saw-toothed" (cyclical) oscillations in the oxyhemoglobin saturation that are caused by apneas-hypopneas. Gries and Brooks, in a normative study of 350 healthy subjects [34], noted a mean overnight oxygen saturation (Sat_{50}) of 96.5%, with values decreasing slightly with age. The Sat_{50} values ranged from 96.8% in the 1- to 10-year age group to 95.1% in subjects older than 60 years. It was not influenced by age, gender, or ethnicity. The mean value of the lowest overnight oxygen saturation in healthy children is 92%. There is no difference in saturation values obtained from applying the sensors over the ear or the fingertip, but values recorded from over the toes may be lower. The sensitivity and specificity of oximetry in the diagnosis of OSA is dependent on its severity. Brouilette et al studied 349 patients who had been referred to a pediatric sleep center for possible OSA using both NPSG and overnight oximetry [33]. Oximetry was abnormal in approximately 25% of patients with OSA. When the oximetry study was abnormal, its positive predictive value of the test was 97%. Of note, an abnormal oximetry test in conjunction with history suggests that OSA can help establish the diagnosis, but a normal oximetry test does not exclude the possibility of mild or moderate OSA.

Nocturnal Polysomnography

The definitive test for an SRBD is NPSG (simultaneous evaluation of multiple physiologic parameters in sleep) that is conducted in a sleep laboratory. Consultation with a sleep specialist before the NPSG is recommended to optimally tailor the study to the clinical question, for example, using a 16-channel electroencephalogram (EEG) montage in a child with suspected parasomnias/nocturnal seizures rather than the 3-channel EEG recording used in standard polysomnography.

Polysomnography is indicated for the diagnosis of primary disorders of vigilance such as narcolepsy and idiopathic hypersomnia, for OSA, hypoventilation syndromes, central sleep apnea syndrome, and suspected Cheyne-Stokes breathing [35]. There are also a number of other disorders with SRBD in which polysomnography provides additional clinical perspective and assistance in management. These include asthma, cystic fibrosis, and myopathies such as myotonic dystrophy, spinal muscular atrophy, and poliomyelitis [35]. NPSG is also indicated for determining optimal continuous positive airway pressure (CPAP) settings in patients with confirmed OSA—generally when the baseline NPSG shows a respiratory disturbance index greater than 5 per hour. Follow-up polysomnography may be needed if there is a greater than 10% weight gain or weight loss and CPAP seems to be losing effectiveness [35]. Traditionally, a full-night diagnostic polysomnogram is performed for the evaluation of SRBD and followed, if necessary, by a full-night titration of CPAP or B-level positive airway pressure breathing. Because polysomnography is expensive and inconvenient, alternatives continue to be sought. One validated modification is split-night polysomnography, which combines an initial diagnostic segment with a latter-half CPAP titration during the same night—the first half serves as baseline or the diagnostic segment, whereas the second half is for titrating CPAP to an optimum level [36]. The initial diagnostic segment should include rapid eye movement (REM) sleep in the supine position. The CPAP titration segment should ideally be about 180 minutes in duration, with documentation of elimination/near elimination of sleep-disordered breathing by adjustments in positive airway pressure levels. The practice standards that have been developed pertain to adults [36] but are likely applicable to older children and adolescents as well (author's opinion).

In the investigation of disorders leading to daytime sleepiness such as narcolepsy, idiopathic hypersomnia, and periodic hypersomnia (Kleine-Levin Syndrome), the nocturnal polysomnogram is helpful in excluding disorders such as OSA that may also be accompanied by daytime sleepiness. Ideally, the patient should have been tapered off of REM-suppressing agents such as tricyclic agents or selective serotonin reuptake inhibitors for a minimum of 2 to 3 weeks before polysomnography. Patients with narcolepsy may exhibit a sleep-onset REM period (SOREMP), which is defined as REM sleep within 15 minutes of sleep onset. Others may show a short nocturnal REM latency of less than 70 minutes. During the symptomatic phase, patients with periodic hypersomnia may show decreased sleep efficiency, decreased slow-wave sleep, and a shortened initial REM latency. Patients with REM sleep behavior disorder may show persistence of tonic electromyographic activity (REM sleep without atonia) during REM sleep.

NPSG is also used for investigating nocturnal spells such as seizures, REM, and NREM parasomnias. The hypermotor clinical semiology of nocturnal frontal lobe can mimic parasomnias such as sleep terrors. An expanded, 16-channel EEG montage with synchronized digital video monitoring should be used when evaluating nocturnal spells [15]. During the record review process, the EEG tracing should be observed at a screen display of 10 seconds per frame to detect epileptiform transients such as spikes and sharp waves that may otherwise appear compressed and difficult to visualize at the traditional polysomnogram review speed of 30 seconds per frame.

During polysomnography, the EEG, eye movements, chin and leg electromyogram (EMG), electrocardiogram, oxygen saturation, nasal pressure/nasal airflow, and thoracic and abdominal respiratory effort are monitored simultaneously. Esophageal pressure monitoring, though a reliable tool in suspected upper airway resistance syndrome, is somewhat invasive and for the most part has been supplanted by nasal pressure transducers. End tidal CO_2 measurements are useful in children with suspected hypoventilation related to obesity, neuromuscular disorders, Down syndrome, and Prader-Willi syndrome. Hypoventilation is defined as end tidal CO_2 greater than 50 mm of mercury for more than 25% of the total sleep time [37].

Although standard polysomnographic measurements such as elevated apnea-hypopnea index and obstructive apnea index predict daytime sleepiness, the study of respiratory cycle–related electroencephalographic changes may be an additional measure of sleep fragmentation [38].

Multiple Sleep Latency Test

When used in conjunction with sleep history, clinical examination, and NPSG, the Multiple Sleep Latency Test (MSLT) is considered the "gold standard" for the assessment of daytime sleepiness in children and adults [39]. The strengths of the test lie in its intuitive design (sleepy individuals are likely to fall asleep more quickly than those who are not sleepy), its reliability, and the availability of normative data across various ages. The MSLT has also been validated in conditions such as sleep loss, sleep disruption, and hypnotic and alcohol use [40]. One major indication for the MSLT is suspected narcolepsy or idiopathic hypersomnia. For the MSLT to be valid, the procedure must have a polysomnogram performed the night before to exclude disorders such as OSA and periodic limb movement disorder, which can also be associated with sleepiness. The lower age limit till which one can apply the MSLT seems be around 6 years; physiologic daytime napping can occur up to 3 to 5 years. As far as possible, the total sleep time on the NPSG must approximate that observed at home. Wrist actigraphy obtained over the 1 to 2 weeks before the MSLT helps ensure that the patient has been receiving adequate sleep at night on a regular basis. All medications that impact sleep such as benzodiazepines, psychostimulants, antidepressants, and barbiturates must be stopped 2 weeks before the MSLT [39]. Drugs with very long half-lives such as fluoxetine may need to be discontinued for 3 to 4 weeks owing to their tendency for suppressing REM sleep for many days after discontinuance. Because sleep latency in children and adolescents is closely linked to the Tanner stage of sexual development, physical examination to evaluate the stage of sexual maturation is important. Tanner sleep stage–specific reference values for the mean sleep latency (MSL) are shown in Table 2.3 [41].

The MSLT is commenced 1.5 to 3 hours after the final morning awakening. At least 6 hours of sleep must have been recorded on the nocturnal polysomnogram if the MSLT is being conducted to rule out narcolepsy. The patient is dressed in street clothes. The test consists of the provision of 5 nap opportunities at 2-hourly intervals, for example, 09:00 hours, 11:00 hours, 13:00 hours, 15:00 hours, and 17:00 hours. A shorter, 4 naps MSLT can be employed if 2 or more SOREMPs have already occurred. Central and occipital EEG (C3-O1, C4-O2), eye movements (right outer canthus to left outer canthus), and chin EMG need to be recorded. One of the eye movement sensors is placed slightly above the outer canthus and the other slightly below the outer canthus. This arrangement facilitates capture of both horizontal and vertical eye movements. The time constant for the electrooculogram should be long enough to allow for the recording of slow rolling movements that typically herald the onset of NREM sleep. Baseline biocalibration signals are recorded before commencing each trial. At the designated hour, lights are turned off and the patient is advised to relax, close the eyes, and to try to fall asleep while the electrophysiologic parameters are being monitored. If no sleep occurs, the nap opportunity is terminated 20 minutes following "lights out," and the patient is designated as having a sleep latency of 20 minutes (the maximum). If the patient falls asleep, the test is continued for 15 minutes after sleep onset. Sleep is scored in 30-second epochs. The time interval between "lights out" and electroencephalographic sleep onset is designated

Table 2.3 Age-specific normal values for the Multiple Sleep Latency Test

Age/Tanner Stage of Sexual Development	Mean Sleep Latency (time in minutes)	SD (minutes)
Tanner stage I	18.8	1.8
Tanner stage II	18.3	2.1
Tanner stage III	16.5	2.8
Tanner stage IV	15.5	3.3
Tanner stage V	16.2	1.5
Older adolescents	15.8	3.5
Adults	13.3	4.3

Data for children and adolescents adapted from the first night of 3 successive nocturnal polysomnographic recordings. Adapted with permission from Ref. [41].

the sleep latency. MSL is derived from averaging the sleep latency of the 4 to 5 nap opportunities. Reference values for the MSL at various ages are listed in Table 2.3. If clinically indicated, a urine drug screen may be obtained in between the MSLT nap opportunities to exclude the possibility of drug-induced sleepiness.

Besides serving as an objective measure of sleep propensity, the MSLT also helps in determining whether the transition from wakefulness is into NREM or REM sleep. A SOREMP is defined as the occurrence of REM sleep within 15 minutes of sleep onset. About 80% of patients with narcolepsy show 2 or more SOREMPs during the MSLT. False positives may occur in patients with severe OSA who have suppression of nocturnal REM sleep with a consequent daytime REM sleep rebound. False negatives may occur in the early stages of evolution of narcolepsy in childhood when the patient may manifest daytime sleepiness but not the requisite 2 or more SOREMPs [40]. The diagnostic sensitivity of the MSLT for the diagnosis of narcolepsy has been estimated to be around 61%, whereas the diagnostic specificity when 2 or more SOREMPs are present is around 94%. If the presence of 2 or more SOREMPs was combined with an MSL of less than 5 minutes, the diagnostic specificity rises to 97%.

One drawback is that the MSL in preadolescent children may actually be more than 20 minutes, and the artificial truncation of the nap opportunity at 20 minutes may limit adequate assessment of the sleep propensity in this age group. Another limitation of the MSLT is its "floor" effect.For example, in pathologically sleepy subjects with MSL less than 5 minutes, it cannot help assess whether an individual with an MSL of 1 minute is more sleepy than an individual with MSL of 3 minutes. The normal values for the MSLT were derived from the study of healthy subjects, and thus, its application to subjects with sleep disorders also poses limitations. The MSLT can control for environmental variables such as light, ambient temperature, and noise, but it cannot control for internal psychological factors such as motivation and anxiety that might also impact sleep latency [40].

Maintenance of Wakefulness Test

This test is the mirror-image opposite of the MSLT [39,41]. It measures daytime alertness and the ability to stay awake during the daytime in a darkened, quiet environment. Electrodes are applied for monitoring the EEG, eye movements, and chin EMG in a manner identical to the MSLT. The patient is provided 4 opportunities to stay awake in a darkened quiet room at 2-hourly intervals, starting at 1.5 to 3 hours after the final morning awakening. The patient sits in street clothes and is advised to "sit still and remain awake for as long as possible." Sleep is scored in 30-second epochs. Each trial ends after 40 minutes if no sleep occurs, or after 3 epochs of unequivocal sleep. As in the MSLT, patients undergoing the Maintenance of Wakefulness Test (MWT) show their shortest MSL around 13:00 hours. The physiologic MSL on the MWT is 30.4 ± 11.2 minutes. The upper limit of the 95% confidence limit is 40 minutes. Using 20-minute MWT trials, Mitler et al [42] found that subjects with narcolepsy were able to stay awake only for an average of 6 minutes as compared to 19 minutes in normal control subjects. The MWT is useful in monitoring response to therapy in daytime sleepiness when the patient is being treated with psychostimulants (narcolepsy) or receiving CPAP for OSA and in instances where one needs to ensure adequate daytime alertness for occupational reasons (airline pilots, truck drivers, etc.). The drawback is that normative data are limited. It is unclear whether the MWT correlates reliably with alertness in the real-life, day-to-day setting.

Conclusions

Normal values for various sleep-related physiologic parameters change with age. Standards of practice have now been developed for a variety of sleep disorders [35,36,39] and for diagnostic studies such as pediatric polysomnography [37]. Certification of sleep specialists through the American Board of Medical Specialties and of sleep laboratories through the American Academy of Sleep Medicine has facilitated quality control at sleep centers. Optimal service to patients, however, demands that all clinicians who care for handicapped children integrate sleep-wake assessment into their overall patient management plans.

Acknowledgment

The sections on survey tools and diagnostic tests have been modified from Ref. [43].

References

1. Sheldon SH. Diagnostic methods in pediatric sleep medicine. *Sleep Med Clin*. 2007;2:343–351.
2. Kothare SV, Kaleyias J. The clinical and laboratory assessment of the sleepy child. *Semin Pediatr Neurol*. 2008;15:61–69.
3. Ivanenko A. Sleep and mood disorders in children and adolescents. In: Ivanenko A, ed. *Sleep and Psychiatric Disorders in Children and Adolescents*. New York, NY: Informa Healthcare; 2008: 279–291
4. Eliasson A, Eliasson A, King J, et al. Association of sleep and academic performance. *Sleep Breath*. 2002;6(1):45–48.
5. Snow A, Dayyat E, Montgomery-Downs HE, et al. Pediatric obstructive sleep apnea: a potential late consequence of respiratory syncytial virus bronchiolitis. *Pediatr Pulmonol*. 2009;44(12): 1186–1191.
6. Halbower AC, Ishman SL, McGinley BM. Childhood obstructive sleep-disordered breathing: a clinical update and discussion of technological innovations and challenges. *Chest*. 2007;132(6):2030–2034.
7. Jenni OG, Carskadon MA. Sleep behavior and sleep regulation from infancy through adolescence: normative aspects. *Sleep Med Clin*. 2007;2:321–329.
8. Blunden S, Hoban TF, Chervin RD. Sleepiness in children. *Sleep Med Clin*. 2006;1:105–118.
9. Kothare SV, Kaleyias J. Narcolepsy and other hypersomnias in children. *Curr Opin Pediatr*. 2008;20(6):666–675.
10. Nevsimalova S. Narcolepsy in childhood. *Sleep Med Rev*. 2009;13(2):169–180.
11. Drake C, Nickel C, Burdvall E, et al. The Pediatric Daytime Sleepiness Scale (PDSS): sleep habits and school outcomes in middle school children. *Sleep*. 2003;26(4):455–458.
12. Johns, MW. A new method for measuring daytime sleepiness: the Epworth sleepiness scale. *Sleep*. 1991;14:540–545.
13. Fiorino EK, Brooks LJ. Obesity and respiratory diseases in childhood. *Clin Chest Med*. 2009;30(3):601–608.
14. Kotagal S, Krahn LE, Slocumb N. A putative link between childhood narcolepsy and obesity. *Sleep Med*. 2004;5(2):147–150.
15. Tiinuper P, Provini F, Bisulli F, et al. Movement disorders in sleep: guidelines for differentiating epileptic from non-epileptic motor phenomena arising from sleep. *Sleep Med Rev*. 2007;11(4):255–267.
16. Owens JA, Dalzell V. Use of the "BEARS" sleep screening tool in a pediatric residents' continuity clinic: a pilot study. *Sleep Med*. 2005;6 (1):63–69.
17. Gosalakkal JA. Sleep disordered breathing in Chiari malformation type I. *Pediatr Neurol*. 2008;39(3):207–208.
18. Arens R, Muzumdar H. Sleep, sleep disordered breathing, and nocturnal hypoventilation in children with neuromuscular diseases. *Pediatr Respir Rev*. 2010;11(1):24–30.
19. Gonzalez C, Ferris G, Diaz J, et al. Kyphoscoliotic ventilatory insufficiency: effects of long term, intermittent positive pressure ventilation. *Chest*. 2003;124(3):857–862.
20. Goldstein NA, Pugazhendhi V, Rao SM, et al. Clinical assessment of pediatric obstructive sleep apnea. *Pediatrics*. 2004;114;33–43.
21. Johns, MW. Reliability and factor analysis of the Epworth Sleepiness Scale. *Sleep*.1992;15: 376–381.
22. Johns, MW. Daytime sleepiness, snoring, and obstructive sleep apnea. The Epworth Sleepiness Scale. *Chest*. 1993;103:30–36.
23. Johns, MW. Sleepiness in different situations measured by the Epworth Sleepiness Scale. *Sleep*. 1994;17:703–710.
24. Melendres CS, Lutz JM, Rubin ED, Marcus CL. Daytime sleepiness and hyperactivity in children with suspected sleep-disordered breathing. *Pediatrics*. 2004;114:768–775.
25. Akerstedt T, Gillberg M. Subjective and objective sleepiness in the active individual. *Int J Neurosci*. 1990;52:29–37.
26. Buysse DJ, Reynolds CF III, Monk TH, Berman SR, Kupfer DJ. The Pittsburgh Sleep Quality Index: A New Instrument for psychiatric practice and research. *J Psychiatric Res*. 1989;28(2):193–213.
27. Owens JA, Spirito A, McGuinn M. Children's Sleep Habits Questionnaire. *Sleep*. 2000;23(8):1–9.
28. Wolfson AR, Carskadon MA, Acebo C, et al. Evidence for the validity of a sleep habits survey for adolescents. *Sleep*. 2003;2:213–216.
29. Spilsbury JC, Drotar D, Rosen CL, et al. The Cleveland Adolescent Sleepiness Questionnaire: a new measure to assess excessive daytime sleepiness in adolescents. *J Clin Sleep Med*. 2007;3(6): 603–612.
30. Chervin RD, Hedger K, Dillon JE, et al. Pediatric sleep questionnaire (PSQ): validity and reliability of scales for sleep-disordered breathing, snoring, sleepiness and behavioral problems. *Sleep Med*. 2000;1:21–32.
31. Sadeh A, Sharkey KM, Carskadon MA. Activity based sleep-wake identification: an empirical test and methodological issues. *Sleep*. 1994;17: 201–207.
32. Ancoli-Israel S, Cole R, Alessi C, et al. The role of actigraphy in the study of sleep and circadian rhythms. *Sleep*. 2003; 26(3): 342–392.
33. Brouilette RT, Morielli A, Leimanis A, et al. Nocturnal pulse oximetry as an abbreviated testing modality for pediatric obstructive sleep apnea. *Pediatrics*. 2000;105;140–142.
34. Gries RE, Brooks LJ. Normal oxyhemoglobin saturation during sleep. How low does it go? *Chest*. 1996;110:1489–1492.

35. Kushida CA, Littner MR, Morgenthaler T, et al. Practice parameters for the indications for polysomnography and related procedures: an update for 2005. *Sleep*. 2005;28(4):499–521.
36. Kushida CA, Littner MR, Hirschkowitz M, Morgenthaler TA, et al. Practice parameters for the use of continuous and bi-level positive airway pressure devices to treat adult patients with sleep related breathing disturbances. *Sleep*. 2006;29(3):375–380.
37. Iber C, Ancoli-Israel S, Chesson A, et al for the American Academy of Sleep Medicine. *The AASM Manual for the Scoring of Sleep and Associated Events: Rules, Terminology, and Technical Specifications*. 1st ed. Westchester, IL: American Academy of Sleep Medicine; 2007.
38. Chervin RD, Weatherly RA, Ruzicka DL, et al. Subjective sleepiness and polysomnographic correlates in children scheduled for adenotonsillectomy vs. other surgical care. *Sleep*. 2006;29:495–503.
39. Littner MR, Kushida C, Wise M, et al. Practice parameters for clinical use of the multiple sleep latency test and the maintenance of wakefulness test. *Sleep*. 2005;28(1):113–121.
40. Kotagal S, Goulding P. The laboratory assessment of daytime sleepiness in childhood. *J Clin Neurophysiol.* 1996;13(3):208–218.
41. Carskadon MA. The second decade. In: Guilleminault C, ed. *Sleeping and Waking Disorders. Indications and Techniques*. Menlo Park, CA: Addison-Wesley; 1982:99–125.
42. Mitler MM, Gujavarty KS, Browman CP. Maintenance of wakefulness test: a polysomnographic technique for evaluation and treatment efficacy in patients with excessive somnolence. *EEG Clin Neurophysiol.* 1982;53(6): 658–661.
43. Mendez J, Kotagal S. Diagnostic tools for hypersomnias. In: Kushida CA, ed. *Handbook of Sleep Disorders*. New York, NY: Informa Healthcare; 2009:265–276.

CHAPTER 3

Sleep and ADHD: Daytime and Nighttime Phenotypes

Karen Spruyt and David Gozal

"There are no eternal facts, as there are no absolute truths . . . only interpretations"

Nietzsche (1867)

Introduction

The attention-deficit/hyperactivity disorder (ADHD) was described at least as long ago as Shakespeare's ". . . *It is the disease of not listening, and the malady of not marking* . . ."(*King Henry IV*, Act I, II). Over the past century, ADHD has been termed minimal brain damage; hyperkinetic syndrome; hyperkinetic reaction in childhood (*Diagnostic and Statistical Manual of Mental Disorders, Second Edition [DSM-II]*, APA 1968); attention-deficit disorder (ADD; *DSM-III*, APA 1980) with and without hyperactivity; and ADHD [1] with subtypes: ADHD predominantly inattentive (PIA), predominantly overactive (PHI), and combined type (C) (*DSM-IV*, APA 1994 [2]). The child with ADHD is therefore typically characterized by developmentally inappropriate symptoms of inattention, hyperactivity, and impulsivity and is diagnosed by an onset of symptoms before the age of 7 years and presence for at least 6 months of cross-situational impaired functioning (eg, school and home). Of note, potential changes are likely to be implemented in the forthcoming *DSM-V*, for instance, in the subtyping categories, age at onset [3], or in the diagnostic separation toward 2 variants.

ADHD is generally perceived as a neurodevelopmental condition potentially resulting from the interaction of multiple genetic and socioenvironmental factors exerting via multiple pathways symptoms marked and mediated by different phenotypes [4–6]. As such, comorbidity is not unlikely, and indeed 59% to 87% of children diagnosed with ADHD have at least 1 and 20% have 3 or more comorbid conditions or symptoms [7]. The latter include learning disabilities (15%–25%), language disorders (30%–35%), social adaptive dysfunction (eg, 10% autistic spectrum disorders), emotional lability (eg, 15%–20% mood disorder and 20%–25% anxiety disorder), motor coordination and balance deficits (60%) [8], obesity [9,10], sleep problems [11,12], and later in life, potential risks of oppositional deviant disorder (ODD; 40%), conduct disorder (CD; 20%), substance abuse (15%), and criminal behavior [13–19]. Interestingly, the potential link between ADHD and sleep was first published in 1971 [20]. Although the exact causes of ADHD are unknown, the growing literature on genetics [6,21,22], neuroimaging [23], and neuropsychology suggests features consistent with a neurodevelopmental disorder in which multiple socioenvironmental and biological factors interact to produce an abnormal brain condition that manifests as cognitive and neurobehavioral deficits throughout childhood, adolescence, and adulthood. To date, ADHD is seen as a complex, inherited neurological syndrome with a pooled estimate of 76% heritability in twin studies [6]. ADHD is currently viewed as a lifelong condition with onset during childhood, either diagnosed prospectively or retrospectively. Barkley [24] indicated that the disorder persists in 50% to 80% through adolescence and to adulthood in 30% to 50%, though its manifestations may change [3] through maturation, the latter exerting modifications in the clinical presentation. Noteworthy, the evidence of a genetic basis for ADHD posits the involvement of many genes, each contributing a small individual effect [6,21,22,25]. Additionally socioenvironmental factors might interact as well. For instance, the degree of acceptance of externalizing behavioral characteristics might differ among sociocultural groups or families and warrants cross-informant report or impressions, which might be further biased by a parent with ADHD (eg, more tolerant toward ADHD behavior). Noteworthy, an increased likelihood of ADHD-like behavior is observed in work-related tasks or behaviorally restricted settings as compared with unrestricted or free play situations [26], yet potentially biased by the observer. Although epidemiological studies indicate that ADHD is more commonly found among boys than girls, this also might be a biased ratio, because girls tend to exhibit higher level of inattentiveness, internalizing symptoms, or comorbid disorders such as anxiety, and because gender difference is mostly observed for those children presenting with aggression or hyperactivity without inattention [7]. The clinical phenotype is further complicated by the great within-subject variability, especially but not exclusively with respect to reaction time task behavior [27]. As such, the diagnostic rates may differ among countries, even if the prevalence appears to be rapidly increasing (eg, a 700% increase rate in the diagnosis of ADHD in UK children [28] or ~5 million affected school-aged children in the United States) [29,30]. Despite difficulties in operationalization, and subsequently assessment, ADHD affects about 4% to 12% of school-aged children. ADHD is thus the contemporary label for one of the most prevalent and intensively studied disorders in childhood, albeit potentially the most controversial.

Neuropathophysiology: "What" To Do—"How" To Do It—"When" To Do It

The brain is a highly flexible system of interacting centers whose activity and interrelationships shift dynamically with changing experience, of which the frontal lobe may be particularly vulnerable because of its late maturation. This brain region is constantly activated by both external and internal stimuli and is known to be involved in the representation and execution of actions, or the higher order cognitive processes. Basically, the frontal cortex exhibits massive connectivity with other brain regions and receives parietal, temporal, limbic, brainstem, basal ganglia, and cerebellum projections that can be dopaminergic, noradrenergic, and serotoninergic in their neuromodulatory inputs. Stated in a more simplified fashion, dopamine plays a role in reward-related functions and modulates movement and cognition, whereas noradrenaline modulates stress responses, central and peripheral arousal, and learning and memory and serotonin plays a role in sleep, mood, appetite, perception, and hormone secretion [31]. Pharmacogenomic research within psychiatric disorders focusing on genes that are involved with dopaminergic and serotoninergic transmission are therefore an area of intense scrutiny and research.

During the First World War, it was observed that the sequelae of von Economo's encephalitis included the hypokinetic symptoms of Parkinson disease, a neurodegenerative disorder of the fronto-striatal system in adults, but manifesting as hyperkinesias in children. Many years later, the role of the basal ganglia was assumed as the link between impulsivity, hyperactivity, and inattention. Joel and Weiner [32] proposed the existence of 5 semi-independent, parallel, frontal-subcortical circuits running through the basal ganglia; that is, they suggested the existence of 3 closed indirect pathways, each connecting the corresponding functional (motor, associative, and limbic) regions of the striatum, pallidum, subthalamic nucleus, and substantia nigra pars reticulata, as well as of 2 open indirect pathways, one connecting the associative striatum to the motor subregions of the basal ganglia and the other connecting the associative striatum to the limbic subregions of the basal ganglia, subserving several neurodevelopmental or psychiatric disorders. Without detailing these pathways, the motor circuit has been related to akinesia and bradykinesia (as seen in Parkinson disease); the oculomotor circuit moderates voluntary fixational control; the dorsolateral prefrontal cortical circuit has been associated with the "dysexecutive syndrome" characterized by problems in maintaining or shifting sets, generating organizational strategies, retrieving memory, fluidity of activity, whereas the lateral orbitofrontal cortical circuit relates to personality, empathy, disinhibition and irritability, or self-monitoring; and lastly the anterior cingulated circuit involves maintenance of drive and motivation or response intention (ie, the propensity to respond via behavioral readiness, anticipation, and response maintenance) [31,33–37]. All these separate yet integrated circuits could potentially nourish ADHD and its daytime and nighttime comorbidities. Evidence for a widely distributed frontal hypoactivity (eg, reduced intensity of activity or spatial extent of activity) is seen in ADHD children [38]. However, applying tasks known to produce consistent patterns of activity in other regions considered putative sources of dysfunction (eg, cerebellum, ventral striatum, parietal cortices) are advocated, and there may be more frontostriatal circuits than those described as mediating motor, cognitive, and emotional aspects. Likewise, a nighttime point of view, rather than just a daytime focus on manifestations and mechanisms could generate new insights into ADHD.

The ADHD Umbrella, Comorbidities, and Confounders

The executive-arousal and attention umbrella of ADHD has been commonly described as characterized by inappropriate or premature responses, recklessness, lack of patience, or inability to inhibit or delay responses, or *impulsivity*; whereas *hyperactivity* manifests as fidgetiness, restlessness, motility, or excessive locomotion; and *inattention* has been described as distractibility or failure to attend to details. Furthermore, there may be excessive attention to immediate gratification, while symptoms may be ameliorated in controlled, challenging, or novel situations. Symptoms related to impulse control may be the first to emerge, but dissipate with maturation, and thus ADHD may be a disorder of inhibitory control (and hence attention problems might be secondary). Commonalities to disinhibition such as poor self-control, aggressive or delinquent tendencies, and conduct problems as well as overreaction, low self-esteem, and distractibility might therefore lead to misdiagnosis. Such poor control also relates to motor overactivity and fidgetiness as seen in the child with ADHD. Attention on the other hand is considered a highly complex and multidimensional construct that is not secondary to the existence of other potential comorbid conditions (eg, anxiety, depression, CD, ODD). Accordingly, it is presumed that children with ADHD exhibit poor vigilance, sustained attention with characteristically errors of omission, or to a certain extent a range of behaviors commonly ascribed to posterior parietal activity. The potential overly attentionally disrupted child may show traits such as mental "fogginess," sluggishness, withdrawal, poor concentration, and reduced processing speed. Not unrelated to inattention is the association with problems involving working memory, especially spatial memory (please note that ADHD symptomatology has been related to potentially right hemisphere dysfunction). Subsequent impediment of acquisition of basic academic skills (eg, reading, spelling, math) results that by puberty about 80% of ADHD children are 2 or more grades behind their peers [39]. The list of behavioral impairments descriptive of the umbrella appears eternal, with more than a dozen ADHD models to explain this umbrella, each having roots in either bio-psycho-(and/or)-social paradigms.

More recently, efforts to subtype the existing subtypes is being attempted to deal with the heterogeneity of this ADHD umbrella [3,40] and potential circuits. Whereas the ADHD-C traits likely are social dysfunction, associated cognitive problems, and impairment in scholastic performance, the ADHD-PHI might be its precursor. Although not all ADHD-PHI children may develop the ADHD-C, some preschoolers may develop ODD, and others remain an ADHD-PHI with subthresholds of ADHD-C symptoms. The latter might also be seen with ADHD-PIA or the ADHD-C type that develops into the ADHD-PIA. ADHD-PIA traits are sluggish cognitive tempo such as easy confusion, daydreaming, or mental spaciness with hypoactivity, slow-moving, sluggish motor function [3,41]. These subtypes and their performance profiles have been suggested to be associated with separate and distinct underlying neurobiological mechanisms (eg, ADHD-C might be associated with dopamine transporter gene *DAT1*), but are likely to also reflect a gender-developmental inflexibility of the diagnostic criteria [42–44]. In fact, concurrent or successive comorbidities [45] are also incorporated, and as such, ADHD might be best understood as a concept of homuncular properties [46], whereby comorbidities related to these frontostriatal circuits are depression, obsessive compulsive disorder, Tourette syndrome, schizophrenia, and autism [5,31,47] but are also affected by genetic and sociocultural factors, such as parental ADHD, or parental psychopathology, and others. Hitherto, the more severe the ADHD symptomatology, and the earlier in life the signs surface, the more detrimental externalizing and/or internalizing problems later in life [48]. Indeed, although ADHD does not follow a uniform developmental course, it potentially crystallizes toward adulthood in general anxiety disorder (53%), alcohol dependence (34%), drug abuse (30%), and other psychiatric disorders [3].

Of particular interest to this discussion is the relationship between ADHD and sleep (Table 3.1). Thus far, the "waking" brain-behavior relationships of ADHD have been previewed; however, the same neurobiological as well as socioenvironmental factors are shared at nighttime. In other words, in the last 2 decades, the "sleeping" brain-behavior relationships of ADHD have become a substantial topic of research, partially because of its questionable role in the previous diagnostic criteria (*DSM-III*) but also because of the disorder itself and/or the other factors associated with ADHD, all of which will be discussed in greater detail below. Because sleep is regarded as the window on brain development, sleep research findings might propel forward our understanding on missing links toward the homogenization and integration of the ADHD umbrella.

In summary, the understanding of ADHD has evolved from one of universal minimal brain dysfunction toward ADD with and without hyperactivity (*DSM-III*), and thus, in this multidimensional disorder, the emphasis has shifted toward primarily attention instead of (the original signs of) hyperactivity and impulse control. This approach has resulted eventually in the attention-deficit/hyperactivity disorder label, in which ADHD subtypes have emerged, namely predominantly inattentive (PIA), predominantly hyperactive/impulsive (PHI), and combined (C) type (*DSM-IV* [2]) all of which have been studied in greater detail. Perhaps through biological and/or socioenvironmental factors, ADHD has long been associated with an increased risk of comorbid psychosocial disorders (rather the externalizing type). Although the presence of substantial heterogeneity within the ADHD literature might be ascribed to differences in assessed behaviors, diagnostic criteria, comorbidity and confounds characteristic to biomedical and/or sociocultural paradigms, and brain-behavior relationships may also emerge through the interaction of gender- and age-related differences across the lifespan, which might further complicate the clinical phenotype of ADHD. In recent years, growing attempts to identify the nighttime phenotype of ADHD have been made, with the anticipation that these studies on sleep might fill some of our blanks on our understanding of ADHD.

The Child With ADHD and Its Sleep Phenotypes

The guesstimated prevalence of sleep problems in ADHD children is about 5-fold that of healthy controls [19,49]. Conceptually, sleep problems in

Table 3.1 Subjective and objective reports of sleep problems in children with attention-deficit/hyperactivity disorder

Subjective	Objective
Bedtime resistance	Prolonged sleep onset latency (ACT)
Sleep onset difficulties	More stage shifts per hour of sleep (NPSG)
Nocturnal awakenings	Higher apnea-hypopnea index (NPSG)
Difficult morning awakenings	Lower sleep efficiency index (NPSG)
Sleep disordered breathing	Less total sleep time (ACT)
Daytime sleepiness	Shorter sleep latency (MSLT)

Abbreviations: ACT, actigraphy; NPSG, overnight polysomnography; MSLT, multiple sleep latency test.
From Ref. [126].

the ADHD child are likely multifactorial; that is, they might be because of the ADHD itself or the associated comorbidity or result from issues such as sleep quantity and quality of the child with ADHD, and as such, they might have a bio-psycho-social origin or even result from treatment of ADHD.

ADHD Per Se

Both parents of children with ADHD and children themselves commonly report sleep complaints [50,51]. Such complaints involve bedtime resistance, difficulty falling asleep, nocturnal awakenings, sleep-related anxiety, snoring, head banging, restlessness, or sleep-related involuntary movements, bad dreams, and the presence of leg jerks during sleep, the latter being particularly frequent in comparison with any other psychiatric disorder [52–56]. Sleep problems of children with ADHD were also associated with mental health of the caregivers, their work attendance, and overall family functioning [57]. Furthermore, children with ADHD may have a differential sensitivity to an altered sleep environment, and possibly they as well as their parents may have a characteristic way of perceiving sleep quality disturbances [58,59]. Indeed, polysomnographic (PSG) findings have been discrepant from self-reports and parent reports. Even among PSG studies, there is little consistency [57]. Some studies have found REM sleep abnormalities in children with ADHD; that is, either increased or decreased REM latency or REM sleep duration. Despite the inconsistencies on REM sleep findings in ADHD children, dysregulation of eye movements during waking hours and differences in eye movements during REM sleep have been reported in children with ADHD [60]. This might be an intriguing venue for further exploration considering the previously proposed frontostriatal comorbidities, such as autism or tics and may be of interest as well in the context of sustained attention and learning difficulties.

Despite the disparity in PSG sleep patterns among ADHD [61–63], a recent meta-analysis by Sadeh et al [11] nicely illustrates the moderating effect of age and gender, alongside the conceptual and methodological discrepancies. Eventually, these investigators conclude that the current evidence is primarily suggestive toward a periodic limb movement disorder (PLMS) in children with ADHD. Looking at the microstructure of sleep, children with ADHD showed a lower cyclic alternating pattern rate (CAP) and a lower number of CAP sequences, supporting the hypothesis of the existence of a hypoarousal state in these patients [64]. This is in contrast with the hyperactivity/impulsivity and attention deficits, such as found in the daytime brain-behavior relationship. Indeed, multiple sleep latency test (MSLT) studies, which assess sleepiness, have shown that children with ADHD are about 8 times more likely to fall asleep in comparison to controls [65]. Movements may thus assist in keeping the child awake (ie, fighting off sleepiness). Interestingly, sleep findings with respect to ADHD subtypes have not been thoroughly explored. For instance, impaired sleep efficiency and fragmented sleep could be more likely to occur in ADHD-C, greater daytime sleepiness could be present in the ADHD-PI, and therefore, the strategies required for treatment success may further delineate the nighttime ADHD umbrella [57]. In other words, the amalgamation of altered sleep in terms of increased nighttime motor activity, rapid eye movement differences, significant daytime somnolence, longer sleep latency, higher number of sleep cycles, and many other features reported in children with ADHD [57,66] leads to the obvious conclusion that more rigorous studies are clearly needed to identify the putatively distinct nighttime umbrella of ADHD. To date, the precarious and fragmented evidence would suggest that despite high rates of parental reports of sleep disturbances in medicated and unmedicated children with ADHD, objective sleep measurements do not seem to corroborate the extent of such disturbances as derived from parental reports [66].

The ADHD Comorbidities

In the following section, we will briefly review the sleep problems associated with the most prevalent ADHD comorbidities. Obviously, discussion of sleep issues as they relate to each of the neurodevelopmental or psychiatric disorders is beyond the scope of this book [67,68]. Ivanenko et al [53] reported a high frequency of sleep problems among children with psychiatric disorders. For example, 61.5% exhibited delayed sleep onset, 63% reported nocturnal awakenings, 67.8% complained of restless sleep, 57.5% of leg jerks, 66.7% had daytime sleepiness, 49.4% of fear of the dark, 62.6% of bedtime struggles, 55.7% of snoring during sleep, and 58.6% had frequent nightmares. Therefore, children with ADHD and comorbidities may have altered sleep architecture, different sleep-wake patterns, and sleep problems, which might further obscure the daytime and nighttime brain-behavior interactions, and thus alter the phenotypic presentation. Such interactions between disrupted sleep in the context of a comorbidity may interact in an additive, subtractive, or synergistic fashion with the underlying ADHD. In fact, among developmental neuropsychologists, viewpoints dealing with "masking" comorbid disorders have been proposed, illustrating the fact that the brain-behavior relationship is immensely developing throughout childhood, and is dealt with by heuristic concepts such as brain plasticity, "growing into (deficit)" and "fail to acquire (the skill)." Future studies should carefully elucidate the impact of comorbidities and the contribution of sleep to these interactions.

ODD and CD

A guesstimated 50% to 60% of children with ADHD meet criteria for ODD, even in the preschool period [8]. Suggested associations of ADHD/ODD and sleep behaviors are the presence of limit-setting sleep disorder, which is characterized by the inadequate enforcement of bedtimes by a caretaker, with resultant stalling or refusal to go to bed at an appropriate time, bedtime resistance, and delayed sleep onset [65]. The impact of gender is also present considering the recent findings that girls with ADHD may develop differently. Indeed, compared with girls who had ADHD only, those girls with ADHD + ODD at baseline had a significantly increased risk for ODD and major depression at follow-up [69]. Additionally, conduct problems have sociocultural or familial underpinnings [70] and are gaining importance in the study of sleep-disordered breathing (SDB). For example, Chervin et al [71] found associations with symptoms of SDB, RLS/PLMS and conduct problems, aggressive behavior, and bullying.

Mood

In major depression disorder, sleep complaints are commonly reported (~90%) [72], and include insomnia, delayed sleep onset, hypersomnia, awakenings, daytime sleepiness, and circadian reversal, even though objective sleep results are lacking [73]. The findings of longer sleep onset latency and shorter REM latency are more consistent in the context of adolescent sleep research and might be ascribed to neurodevelopmental stages. Conversely, misperception of sleep is possible and should not be discarded. The distinction between pediatric bipolar disorder (BPD) and ADHD is difficult because of their shared clinical features such as motor agitation, distractibility, impulsivity or irritability, and associated cognitive deficits. Studies focusing on pediatric BPD [68,74] are hampered by conceptual issues [75], though there is preliminary objective evidence of poorer sleep efficiency and more awakenings, less REM sleep, and longer periods of slow-wave sleep than matched controls [76], which substantial overlap among the reported subjective complaints.

Anxiety

Subjective studies indicate delayed sleep onset, bedtime resistance, disorders of maintaining sleep, involuntary movements, whereas objective studies suggest alterations in sleep architecture and higher density of periodic leg movements [65]. From a neurobiological standpoint, the increased vigilance and arousal associated with anxiety is plausible toward the increased frequency of nocturnal arousals in these children [53]. However, environmental determinants should also be assessed with respect to this comorbidity. Parent-reported sleep problems are as high as 95% in children with anxiety disorders [77]. Most studies focus on generalized anxiety disorders, though sleep-related problems, such as later bedtimes and less sleep, are common. But also here the comorbidities need to be disentangled, considering the proposed dysregulation of hypothalamic-pituitary-adrenal axis and the environmental and biological factors that can also play a role.

Learning

ADHD ratings have been significantly related to underachievement and have been a crucial reason for clinical referral. A more controversial topic remains intelligence, with the relationships between intelligence and cognitive vulnerabilities ascribed to ADHD varying in strength [78].

In this context, the issue of comorbidities needs to be carefully analyzed. For example, poor overnight sleep quality, that is, apneas, low desaturation rates, and awakenings in combination with limb activity and snoring, was found in children with ADHD and associated with low verbal IQ [79]. It has been suggested that reading disabilities may be attributed to failures in attentional focalization for incoming stimuli [80], and again frontoparietal pathways are suggested with respect to lesser preparation and reduced alertness to detect significant stimuli, as illustrated by event-related potential studies [81]. Conversely, sleep spindle activity and reading abilities in developmental dyslexia have been reported supporting the hypothesis of a role for NREM sleep and spindles in sleep-related neurocognitive processing [82]. Although Marcotte et al [83] did not find any differences in the parental report of sleep-related problems in children with ADHD when compared with those with learning disabilities, their reciprocal existence as a comorbidity might result in a unique phenotype. Sleep plays a significant and important role in memory consolidation, that is, learning. In terms of subtypes, Alloway et al [84] found that children with ADHD could be identified on the basis of oppositional and hyperactive behaviors, whereas those with working memory deficits were more inattentive. This dimensionality might be further explored in terms of objective sleep studies, for which no data are currently available.

Tourette Syndrome or Tic Disorder

Evidence of sleep problems in children with TS is quite limited, though overall quality of life was lower when ADHD symptoms were present [85,86]. The estimated rate of TD symptoms in ADHD is 10% to 30%. Kirov et al [62] focused on motor hyperactivity, which is typically identified in TD and ADHD. The core symptoms in TD are multiple motor and/or phonic tics, waxing and waning in form, frequency, intensity, and localization. Interrelation with sleep of both disorders has been hypothesized by the restlessness reported at night in ADHD and TD, although as mentioned, studies are scarcely available. Common mechanisms underpinning the hyperkinetic sleep pattern and differences in REM sleep regulation have been proposed, but the independent effect of ADHD or TD on sleep cannot be established.

Substance Abuse

Especially in adolescence, a dose-dependent relationship between sleep problems and use of substances of abuse, such as alcohol, cigarettes, and drugs, has been put forward [87]. The odds ratios varied from 1.5 to 3.8 for use of cigarettes, alcohol, and any illicit drug, with adolescents reporting having frequent sleep problems, even after adjusting for age, sex, race, and family income. When controlling for psychiatric problems, some reduction in the magnitude of the associations between sleep problems and substance abuse was noted, suggesting that part of the association is attributable to psychiatric problems. There is thus a latent multicollinearity between substance abuse, psychopathological problems, and sleep disorders. Increased sleep latency, awakenings, diminished sleep efficiency, irregular sleep schedules, perceived tiredness with potential use of stimulants during daytime (eg, ADHD medication, caffeine) and further inadequate sleep leading toward aggression, or shared emotional dysregulation have all been reported [87–90]. As part of a longitudinal study on the development of risk for alcohol and other substance-use disorders, sleep problems in early childhood were related to the onset of drug use in adolescence among 257 boys from a community-recruited sample of high-risk families, even after such associations were further analyzed for attention problems, anxiety/depression, and aggression in late childhood. If sleep problems were present, these children were indeed 2.3 times more likely to have used alcohol by age 12 to 14 years, 2.3 times more likely to have smoked, 2.6 times more likely to have used marijuana, and 2.2 times more likely to have tried illicit substance abuse [88]. Abuse of substances, school absences, and concurring eating disorders have been related to increased risks for abuse of stimulant medication as in ADHD [91].

To summarize the aforementioned issues, the subjectively reported problems illustrated for ADHD (see Table 3.1) commonly resurface among other comorbidities of ADHD. However, lack of solid objective evidence precludes delineation of specific nighttime phenotypes for each condition.

The Sleeping Child, Its ADHD Phenotypes

The prefrontal and frontal cortices are suggested to play a critical role in the regulation of arousal, sleep, affect, and attention [92,93]. Indeed, the neuromodulatory mechanisms of the sleep-wake cycle are closely associated with excitatory and inhibitory processes across the sleep-wake continuum [92,94,95]. In addition, the social environment will influence sleep. Thus, given that sleep problems are associated with cognitive and neurobehavioral problems, conceptualization of the sleep-ADHD link as opposed to the ADHD-sleep link may further elucidate clinical phenotypes. Unfortunately, the conceptual and methodological heterogeneity in ADHD not only adversely impacts ADHD-related research but also hampers the research on the links between sleep and ADHD. Nonetheless, we advocate elaborative neuropsychological testing of children with any sleep disorder, to identify complaints and symptoms that might further expose nighttime variants of the daytime brain-behavioral relationships such as ADHD, but also its subtypes and comorbidities.

Sleep Per Se

Nonoptimal sleep is unmistakably associated with decrements in neurobehavioral performance, and sleep complaints often comprise core features of psychiatric disorders. However, sleep problems are still too often perceived as part of the psychopathological symptomatology, and thus not as a primary disorder.

Bedtime issues, such as unstable bedtime [96,97] difficulties in settling down in the evening [57], have been universally reported and are frequent occurrences in otherwise healthy children. On the one hand, the child might be sent to bed when not yet sleepy, because of a delayed endogenous circadian rhythm potentially expressed as bedtime refusal and daytime somnolence, whereas on the other hand there might be a limit-setting problem, or inadequate enforcement of bedtimes by a caregiver, with resultant stalling or refusal to go to bed at the appropriate time. Furthermore, confounding factors such as medication and comorbid status, chaotic family schedules, and many others may further obscure the causal relationships. O'Brien [98] tabulated published associations of daytime effects in sleep problems, including poor sleep hygiene, sleep restriction, circadian rhythm problems, SDB, RLS/PLM, narcolepsy, and insomnia. Inattention was common to all these sleep conditions, whereas hyperactivity/impulsivity was related to disrupted sleep. Sleep disruption and insufficient sleep can lead to excessive daytime sleepiness, which not only could interfere with daytime performance but also likely affect mood, attention, self-regulation, and subsequently impede scholastic performance [57].

Although most of the findings with respect to sleep fragmentation are extrapolated from children with SDB, an emerging literature has recently originated from children with restless legs syndrome (RLS), with both potentially presenting with symptoms that strikingly resemble ADHD [99,100]. As such, symptoms of ADHD may be more strongly correlated with sleep-related breathing problems, nighttime involuntary movements, sleepiness secondary to bedtime resistance behaviors, or some combination of sleep-related factors. In other words, more meticulous studies investigating sleep quantity and quality are needed, ideally controlling for confounders, and also incorporating ADHD subtypes to address pertinent questions with respect to sleep duration, sleep initiating and maintaining problems, and parasomnias, that is, the sleep phenotype.

The Sleep Disorder

A retrospective study by Goraya et al [101] of PSG data of 3–16-year-olds with ADHD revealed that 24% had obstructive sleep apnea, 30% had PLMS and 24% had upper airway resistance syndrome, and 15% had obstructive sleep hypoventilation syndrome. Furthermore, those with SDB were more obese and had more architectural sleep abnormalities, which drastically and adversely impact the quality and quantity of their sleep. Because sleep disorders and symptoms are likely to coexist [102], the clinician and researcher need to be very attentive when facing ADHD symptomatology or even a specific phenotype.

Daytime Sleepiness

A common underestimation of frequency involves daytime sleepiness in children because it may present as irritability and hyperactivity rather than tiredness or lethargy. Consistent with the hypoarousal theory of ADHD, hyperactive children will be sleepier and as such excessive motor activity would de facto represent a strategy to stay awake and alert. MSLT studies are suggestive toward such reduced alertness [65]. However, we should also remember that in addition to intrinsic sleepiness, daytime sleepiness may also result from erratic sleep-wake patterns, as well as from SDB or periodic leg movement disorder of sleep (PLMD).

Sleep-Disordered Breathing

It has been estimated that 2% to 3% of children suffer from obstructive sleep apnea, characterized by repeated events of partial or complete upper airway obstruction during sleep and resulting in disruption of normal ventilation, hypoxemia, and sleep. However, about 12% to 20% report habitual snoring, which constitutes evidence for increased upper airway resistance. Chervin et al [103] suggested that snoring and other symptoms of SDB are not only strong risk factors for future emergence of behavior problems but also might exacerbate hyperactive behaviors. In fact, Beebe and Gozal [104] postulated a working model of the dysfunction of prefrontal regions of the brain cortex caused by sleep disruption and blood gas abnormalities that would prevent sleep-related restorative processes and further induce chemical and structural central nervous system cellular injury. The resultant phenotype from this model would be very ADHD-look-alike; that is, a child having cognitive and behavioral deficits such as sluggishness, hyperactivity, and inattentiveness [105–107]. Hyperactivity, inattention, as well as aggressive (ie, bullying, quarrelsome, cruel) [71] and emotional problems such as mood disturbances [108], scholastic underperformance [109], memory problems [107] have all been reported in the context of SDB and should alert us on their daytime behavioral phenotypes. Even though such neurobehavioral associations have been advanced, that is, symptoms of ADHD in children with SDB [110–114], patterns are less clear when examining the association between SDB severity and the magnitude of neurobehavioral problems. The contributions of intrinsic susceptibility characteristics and environmental issues will need to be incorporated to enable improved predictability of what child is at risk for neurobehavioral and cognitive pathology. In addition, treatment studies may further provide evidence of causality. Indeed surgical treatment of the adenotonsillar hypertrophy, or adenotonsillectomy, being the first-line treatment of SDB, improves neurobehavioral performance of these children. Lately, overweight and obesity are reported in children with SDB [115], and also in ADHD research [9,10], a venue that may place sleep in a more prominent place with respect to our understanding of diseases such as ADHD.

Restless Legs Syndrome and PLMS

RLS refers to the disagreeable leg sensations, usually before sleep onset, which cause an almost irresistible urge to move the legs, and PLMD refers to periodic episodes of repetitive and highly stereotypic limb movements that occur during sleep. Ped Rest study by Picchietti et al [116] revealed that RLS criteria were met by 1.9% of children aged 8 to 11 years and by 2% of adolescents aged 12 to 17 years. Because increased frequency of body movements during sleep has been reported in children with ADHD [117] and because RLS/PLMD and ADHD may share neural pathways [118,119] as well as share comorbidities (eg, parasomnias, ADHD, ODD, anxiety, and depression found in more than 20% of the cases with RLS/PLMD), the connection between daytime and nighttime brain-behavior umbrellas needs to be further emphasized. For example, night-to-night variability has been suggested in RLS/PLMD [120], which in turn appears to exert an influence on the associations with related symptoms of mood, fatigue, and inattention. Of interest, within-subject variability has also been reported in children with ADHD [27] in the realm of disinhibition and task performance. Thus, sleep disruption caused by the RLS/PLMD and the underlying dopaminergic pathway dysfunction ascribed to RLS/PLMD may reveal important insights into sleep and wake behaviors in ADHD.

Other sleep disorders that could affect ADHD phenotype include enuresis [121], delayed sleep phase syndrome [122], rhythmic movement disorders, and partial arousal parasomnias (eg, sleep terrors, confusional arousals, sleep walking) [123]. Unfortunately, such scarce studies have been limited by the size of the cohorts or have solely relied on subjective parental reports of sleep in the child. Based on aforementioned considerations, arousal deficits could contribute to both enuresis and inattentive ADHD, and therefore, nocturnal enuresis could be a potential clinical marker in the process of identifying ADHD-PIA [121].

A Short Note on Medications and Daytime and Nighttime Behaviors

Because ADHD is contextualized within various disciplines, for example, biomedical, psychological, and sociological, interventions using discipline-oriented tools have been developed. However, ADHD symptoms are primarily treated with medication, that is, methylphenidate and amphetamines. Stimulants have been associated with either no changes or with increased sleep complaints in children with ADHD [66], whereas treatment of underlying SDB, PLMD, and RLS have led to improved neurobehavioral functioning [99]. Additionally, management of sleep-wake patterns may improve the quality of life of children with ADHD. For example, promotion of sleep hygiene, as well as melatonin adjustments of the sleep-wake patterns in children with the light-dark cycle have yielded favorable results [57]. Melatonin seemed effective in abating chronic sleep onset insomnia but interestingly did not result in improvement of daytime sleepiness [124,125].

Taken together, psychotropic medications may impose either a negative effect, no effect, or a positive effect on ADHD, its comorbid diagnosis, or both, and thus potentially further complicate the ADHD-sleep links. Conversely, evaluation of children presenting with ADHD-look-alike symptoms should include child and parent reports of a sleep history; a thorough review of sleep schedules, behaviors, and habits surrounding sleep; assessment of sleep environment and the specific frequency, severity, and duration of sleep difficulties, alongside the current clinical standards for evaluation of ADHD. In addition, monitoring of sleep quality and quantity should accompany any intervention for ADHD.

Conclusions

The story of ADHD epitomizes the discrepant and many times nonoverlapping approaches by the various disciplines. Depending on the discipline paradigm, or alternatively the wake or sleep point of view, differing opinions will result on the mechanisms and thereby approaches needed for diagnosing and treating ADHD. We would advocate unity rather than divide. In such context, careful consideration of the age, gender, and subtype of ADHD alongside precise planning of sleep-ADHD studies might help unravel the wake and sleep phenotypes of ADHD in the future. Additionally, commonalities and dissimilarities throughout the day-night cycle of ADHD-like behaviors may cluster into new genotypes and phenotypes. As such, increased awareness of the sleep-ADHD associations will be essential. Strikingly, most of the past studies have relied on comparisons of frequencies rather than examine severity of day- and nighttime brain-behavior relationships. It is, however, possible that some components of ADHD symptoms may relate to severity rather than to frequency or relate to night rather than daytime events. As such, daytime inattention, hyperactivity

Practice Points

Potential issues of studies assessing links between ADHD and sleep

1. Professionally oriented bias
2. Definition and diagnosis of ADHD
3. ADHD-based diagnostic paradigm
4. Age and gender distribution
5. Treatment confounders
6. Comorbidity, that is, common underlying etiology which leads to 2 or more different disorders, or one disorder leads to another; 2 unrelated disorders co-occur
7. Respondent, that is, observer and recall bias and subjective assessment tool
8. Sleep (objective-subjective) assessment method
9. Sample generalizability, that is, clinical, community, referral
10. Consider each sleep behavior complaint and nigh-to-night variability
11. Monitor sleep when ADHD medication is given
12. Time of day and night, that is, assessment and medication

Abbreviation: ADHD, attention-deficit/hyperactivity disorder.

and impulsivity, and nighttime restless and motor activities during sleep may represent different portions of the same spectrum. We therefore advocate that day and nighttime researchers listen to each other and cooperate in delineation of an ADHD continuum in the wake-sleep cycle.

References

1. Barkley RA. *Attention Deficit-Hyperactivity Disorder: A Handbook for Diagnosis and Treatment*. New York, NY: Guildford Press; 1990.
2. American Psychiatric Association. *Diagnostic and Statistical Manual of Mental Disorders*. 4th ed. Washington, DC: American Psychiatric Association; 1994.
3. Stefanatos GA, Baron IS. Attention-deficit/hyperactivity disorder: a neuropsychological perspective towards DSM-V. *Neuropsychol Rev.* 2007;17:5–38.
4. Xu X, Mill J, Sun B, et al. Association study of promoter polymorphisms at the dopamine transporter gene in attention deficit hyperactivity disorder. 2009 *BMC Psychiatry* 9, art. no. 3.
5. Williams HJ, Owen MJ, O'Donovan MC. Schizophrenia genetics: new insights from new approaches. *Br Med Bull.* 2009;91(1):61–74.
6. Faraone SV, Perlis RH, Doyle AE, et al. Molecular genetics of attention-deficit/hyperactivity disorder. *Biol Psychiatry*. 2005;57:1313–1323.
7. Rowland AS, Lesesne CA, Abramowitz AJ. The epidemiology of attention-deficit/hyperactivity disorder (ADHD): a public health view. *Ment Retard Dev Disabil Res Rev.* 2002;8(3):162–170.
8. Kadesjo B, Gillberg C. The comorbidity of ADHD in the general population of Swedish school-age children. *J Child Psychol Psychiatry*. 2001;42(4):487–492.
9. Waring ME, Lapane KL. Overweight in children and adolescents in relation to attention-deficit/hyperactivity disorder: results from a national sample. *Pediatrics*. 2008;122(1):e1–e6.
10. Cortese S, Konofal E, Bernardina BD, Mouren MC, Lecendreux M. Does excessive daytime sleepiness contribute to explaining the association between obesity and ADHD symptoms? *Med Hypotheses*. 2008;70(1):12–16.
11. Sadeh A, Pergamin L, Bar-Haim Y. Sleep in children with attention-deficit hyperactivity disorder: a meta-analysis of polysomnographic studies. *Sleep Med Rev*. 2006;10(6):381–398.
12. Kirov R, Kinkelbur J, Banaschewski T, Rothenberger A. Sleep patterns in children with attention-deficit/hyperactivity disorder, tic disorder, and comorbidity. *J Child Psychol Psychiatry*. 2007;48(6):561–570.
13. Mayes SD, Calhoun S, Bixler EO, Vgontzas AN. Sleep problems in children with autism, ADHD, anxiety, depression, acquired brain injury, and typical development. *Sleep Med Clin*. 2009;4(1):19–25.
14. Jarrett MA, Ollendick TH. A conceptual review of the comorbidity of attention-deficit/hyperactivity disorder and anxiety: implications for future research and practice. *Clin Psychol Rev*. 2008;28(7):1266–1280.
15. Von Aster MG. The problem of the comorbidity in the calculation disorders. *ANAE—Approche Neuropsychologique des Apprentissages chez l'Enfant*. 2009;21(102):152–157.
16. Wells KC, Epstein JN, Hinshaw SP, et al. Parenting and family stress treatment outcomes in attention deficit hyperactivity disorder (ADHD): an empirical analysis in the MTA study. *J Abnorm Child Psychol*. 2000;28(6):543–553.
17. Pfiffner LJ, Calzada E, McBurnett K. Interventions to enhance social competence. *Child Adolesc Psychiatr Clin N Am*. 2000;9(3):689–709, x.
18. Zepf FD. Attention deficit-hyperactivity disorder and early-onset bipolar disorder: two facets of one entity? *Dialogues Clin Neurosci*. 2009;11(1):63–72.
19. Nutt DJ, Fone K, Asherson P, et al. Evidence-based guidelines for management of attention-deficit/hyperactivity disorder in adolescents in transition to adult services and in adults: recommendations from the British Association for Psychopharmacology. *J Psychopharmacol*. 2007;21(1):10–41.
20. Small A, Hibi S, Feinberg I. Effects of dextroamphetamine sulfate on EEG sleep patterns of hyperactive children. *Arch Gen Psychiatry*. 1971;25:369–380.
21. Gizer IR, Ficks C, Waldman ID. Candidate gene studies of ADHD: a meta-analytic review. *Hum Genet*. 2009;126(1):51–90.
22. Coghill D, Banaschewski T. The genetics of attention-deficit/hyperactivity disorder. *Expert Rev Neurother*. 2009;9(10):1547–1565.
23. Quintero J, Navas M, Fernandez A, Ortiz T. Advances in attention deficit hyperactivity disorder. What does neuroimaging provide us with? *Actas Esp Psiquiatr*. 2009;37(6):352–358.
24. Barkley RA. Behavioral inhibition, sustained attention, and executive functions: constructing a unifying theory of ADHD. *Psychol Bull*. 1997;121:65–94.
25. Asherson P, Kuntsi J, Taylor E. Unravelling the complexity of attention-deficit hyperactivity disorder: a behavioural genomic approach. *Br J Psychiatry*. 2005;187:103–105.
26. Biederman J. Attention-deficit/hyperactivity disorder: a selective overview. *Biol Psychiatry*. 2005;57(11):1215–1220.
27. Lijffijt M, Kenemans JL, Verbaten MN, van Engeland H. A meta-analytic review of stopping performance in attention-deficit/hyperactivity disorder: deficient inhibitory motor control? *J Abnorm Psychol*. 2005;114(2):216–222.
28. Lloyd G, Norris C. Including ADHD. *Disability & Society*. 1999;14(4):505.
29. Rafalovich A. Exploring clinician uncertainty in the diagnosis and treatment of ADHD. *Sociol Health Illn*. 2005;27(3):305–323.
30. Centers for Disease Control and Prevention. Mental Health in the United States: prevalence of diagnosis and medication treatment for

ADHD—United States. *Morb Mortal Wkly Rep.* 2005;54(4):842–847.
31. Bradshaw JL. *Developmental Disorders of the Frontostriatal System.* New York, NY: Psychology Press; 2006.
32. Joel D, Weiner I. The connections of the primate subthalamic nucleus: indirect pathways and the open-interconnected scheme of basal ganglia-thalamocortical circuitry. *Brain Res Rev.* 1997;23 (1–2):62–78.
33. Leh SE, Ptito A, Chakravarty MM, Strafella AP. Fronto-striatal connections in the human brain: a probabilistic diffusion tractography study. *Neurosci Lett.* 2007; 419(2):113–118.
34. Watts RL, Koller WC. *Movement Disorders: Neurologic Principles & Practice.* The McGraw-Hill Companies; 2004. ISBN 0-07-137496-5 chapter 2: Neurobehavioral Aspects of Movement Disorders, pp. 17 by MM Swanberg, D. Foti, and J. Cummings.
35. Zald DH, Kim SW. Anatomy and function of the orbital frontal cortex, I: anatomy, neurocircuitry; and obsessive-compulsive disorder. *J Neuropsychiatry Clin Neurosci.* 1996;8(2):125–138.
36. Awh E, Gehring WJ. The anterior cingulate cortex lends a hand in response selection. *Nat Neurosci.* 1999;2(10):853–854.
37. Turken AU, Swick D. Response selection in the human anterior cingulate cortex. *Nat Neurosci.* 1999;2(10):920–924.
38. Dickstein SG, Bannon K, Castellanos FX, Milham MP. The neural correlates of attention deficit hyperactivity disorder: an ALE meta-analysis. *J Child Psychol Psychiatry.* 2006;47(10):1051–1062.
39. Forness SR, Swanson JM, Cantwell DP, Youpa D, Hanna GL. Stimulant medication and reading performance: follow-up on sustained dose in ADHD boys with and without conduct disorders. *J Learn Disabil.* 1992;25(2):115–123.
40. Volk HE, Todorov AA, Hay DA, Todd RD. Simple identification of complex ADHD subtypes using current symptom counts. *J Am Acad Child Adolesc Psychiatry.* 2009;48(4):441–450.
41. Carlson CL, Booth JE, Shin M, Canu WH. Parent-, teacher-, and self-rated motivational styles in ADHD subtypes. *J Learn Disabil.* 2002;35(2): 104–113.
42. Stevenson J, Asherson P, Hay D, et al. Characterizing the ADHD phenotype for genetic studies. *Dev Sci.* 2005;8(2):115–121.
43. Lahey BB, Pelham WE, Loney J, Lee SS, Willcutt E. Instability of the DSM-IV subtypes of ADHD from preschool through elementary school. *Arch Gen Psychiatry.* 2005;62(8):896–902.
44. Berwid OG, Curko Kera EA, Marks DJ, Santra A, Bender HA, Halperin JM. Sustained attention and response inhibition in young children at risk for attention deficit/hyperactivity disorder. *J Child Psychol Psychiatry.* 2005;46(11):1219–1229.
45. Rommelse NNJ, Altink ME, Fliers EA, et al. Comorbid problems in ADHD: degree of association, shared endophenotypes, and formation of distinct subtypes. Implications for a future DSM. *J Abnorm Child Psychol.* 2009;37(6):793–804.
46. Band GPH, Scheres A. Is inhibition impaired in ADHD? *Br J Dev Psychol.* 2005;23(4):517–521.
47. Yerys BE, Wallace GL, Sokoloff JL, Shook DA, James JD, Kenworthy L. Attention deficit/ hyperactivity disorder symptoms moderate cognition and behavior in children with autism spectrum disorders. *Autism Res.* 2009;2(6): 322–333.
48. Connor DF, Edwards G, Fletcher KE, Baird J, Barkley RA, Steingard RJ. Correlates of comorbid psychopathology in children with ADHD. *J Am Acad Child Adolesc Psychiatry.* 2003;42(2): 193–200.
49. Corkum P, Tannock R, Moldofsky H. Sleep disturbances in children with attention-deficit/ hyperactivity disorder. *J Am Acad Child Adolesc Psychiatry.* 1998;37(6):637–646.
50. O'Brien LM, Gozal D. Sleep in children with attention deficit/hyperactivity disorder. *Minerva Pediatr.* 2004;56(6):585–601.
51. O'Brien LM, Holbrook CR, Mervis CB, et al. Sleep and neurobehavioral characteristics of 5- to 7-year-old children with parentally reported symptoms of attention-deficit/hyperactivity disorder. *Pediatrics.* 2003;111(3):554–563.
52. Corkum P, Tannock R, Moldofsky H, Hogg-Johnson S, Humphries T. Actigraphy and parental ratings of sleep in children with attention-deficit/hyperactivity disorder (ADHD). *Sleep.* 2001; 24(3):303–312.
53. Ivanenko A, Crabtree VM, O'Brien LM, Gozal D. Sleep complaints and psychiatric symptoms in children evaluated at a pediatric mental health clinic. *J Clin Sleep Med.* 2006;2(1):42–48.
54. Ming X, Walters AS. Autism spectrum disorders, attention deficit/hyperactivity disorder, and sleep disorders. *Curr Opin Pulm Med.* 2009;15(6): 578–584.
55. Mayes SD, Calhoun SL, Bixler EO, et al. ADHD subtypes and comorbid anxiety, depression, and oppositional-defiant disorder: differences in sleep problems. *J Pediatr Psychol.* 2009;34(3): 328–337.
56. Gaultney JF, Terrell DF, Gingras JL. Parent-reported periodic limb movement, sleep disordered breathing, bedtime resistance behaviors, and ADHD. *Behav Sleep Med.* 2005;3(1):32–43.
57. Gruber R. Sleep characteristics of children and adolescents with attention deficit-hyperactivity disorder. *Child Adolesc Psychiatr Clin N Am.* 2009;18(4):863–876.
58. Owens JA. The ADHD and sleep conundrum: a review. *J Dev Behav Pediatr.* 2005; 26(4): 312–322.
59. Wiggs L, Montgomery P, Stores G. Actigraphic and parent reports of sleep patterns and sleep disorders in children with subtypes of attention-deficit hyperactivity disorder. *Sleep.* 2005;28(11): 1437–1445.
60. Grissom EM, Brubaker B, Capdevila OS, Hawley WR, Gozal D. Eye movement during REM sleep in children with attention deficit hyperactivity disorder. *Dev Neuropsychol.* 2009;34(5):552–559.

61. Kirov R, Banaschewski T, Uebel H, Kinkelbur J, Rothenberger A. REM-sleep alterations in children with co-existence of tic disorders and attention-deficit/hyperactivity disorder: impact of hypermotor symptoms. 2007 *European Child and Adolescent Psychiatry* 16(8), pp. 536.
62. Kirov R, Kinkelbur J, Banaschewski T, Rothenberger A. Sleep patterns in children with attention-deficit/hyperactivity disorder, tic disorder, and comorbidity. 2007 *Journal of Child Psychology and Psychiatry and Allied Disciplines* 48(6), pp. 561-570.
63. Kirov R, Kinkelbur J, Heipke S, et al. Is there a specific polysomnographic sleep pattern in children with attention deficit/hyperactivity disorder? *J Sleep Res*. 2004;13(1):87–93.
64. Miano S, Donfrancesco R, Bruni O, et al. NREM sleep instability is reduced in children with attention-deficit/ hyperactivity disorder. *Sleep*. 2006;29(6):797–803.
65. Cortese S, Konofal E, Yateman N, Mouren MC, Lecendreux M. Sleep and alertness in children with attention-deficit/hyperactivity disorder: a systematic review of the literature. *Sleep*. 2006;29(4):504–511.
66. Cohen-Zion M, Ancoli-Israel S. Sleep in children with attention-deficit hyperactivity disorder (ADHD): a review of naturalistic and stimulant intervention studies. *Sleep Med Rev*. 2004;8(5):379–402.
67. Barnett R, Maruff P, Vance A. Neurocognitive function in attention-deficit-hyperactivity disorder with and without comorbid disruptive behaviour disorders. *Aust N Z J Psychiatry*. 2009;43(8): 722–730.
68. Biederman J, Petty CR, Byrne D, Wong P, Wozniak J, Faraone SV. Risk for switch from unipolar to bipolar disorder in youth with ADHD: a long term prospective controlled study. *J Affect Disord*. 2009; 119(1-3):16–21.
69. Biederman J, Petty CR, Monuteaux MC, et al. The longitudinal course of comorbid oppositional defiant disorder in girls with attention-deficit/ hyperactivity disorder: findings from a controlled 5-year prospective longitudinal follow-up study. *J Dev BehavPediatr.* 2008;29(6):501–507.
70. Anney RJL, Lasky-Su J, Ò'Dúshláine C, et al. Conduct disorder and ADHD: evaluation of conduct problems as a categorical and quantitative trait in the international multicentre ADHD genetics study. *Am J Med GenetB: Neuropsychiatr Genet*. 2008;147(8):1369–1378.
71. Chervin RD, Dillon JE, Archbold KH, Ruzicka DL. Conduct problems and symptoms of sleep disorders in children. *J Am Acad Child Adolesc Psychiatry*. 2003;42(2):201–208.
72. Ryan ND, Puig-Antich J, Ambrosini P, et al. The clinical picture of major depression in children and adolescents. *Arch Gen Psychiatry*. 1987;44(10):854–861.
73. Ivanenko A, Crabtree VM, Gozal D. Sleep and depression in children and adolescents. *Sleep Med Rev*. 2005;9(2):115–129.
74. Biederman J, Petty CR, Monuteaux MC, et al. wwThe child behavior checklist-pediatric bipolar disorder profile predicts a subsequent diagnosis of bipolar disorder and associated impairments in ADHD youth growing up: a longitudinal analysis. *J Clin Psychiatry*. 2009;70(5):732–740.
75. Baroni A, Lunsford JR, Luckenbaugh DA, Towbin KB, Leibenluft E. Practitioner review: the assessment of bipolar disorder in children and adolescents. *J Child Psychol Psychiatry*. 2009;50(3):203–215.
76. Mehl RC, O'Brien LM, Jones JH, Dreisbach JK, Mervis CB, Gozal D. Correlates of sleep and pediatric bipolar disorder. *Sleep*. 2006;29(2):193–197.
77. Alfano CA, Gamble AL. The Role of Sleep in Childhood Psychiatric Disorders. *Child Youth Care Forum*. 2009;38(6):327–340.
78. Antshel KM. Attention-deficit hyperactivity disorder in the context of a high intellectual quotient/ giftedness. *Dev Disabil Res Rev*. 2008;14(4): 293–299.
79. Andreou G, Karapetsas A, Agapitou P, Gourgoulianis K. Verbal intelligence and sleep disorders in children with ADHD. *Percept Mot Skills*. 2003;96(3, pt 2):1283–1288.
80. Silva-Pereyra J, Bernal J, Rodriguez-Camacho M, et al. Poor reading skills may involve a failure to focus attention. *Neuroreport*. 2010;21(1):34–38.
81. Spronk M, Jonkman LM, Kemner C. Response inhibition and attention processing in 5- to 7-year-old children with and without symptoms of ADHD: an ERP study. *Clin Neurophysiol*. 2008;119(12): 2738–2752.
82. Bruni O, Ferri R, Novelli L, et al. Sleep spindle activity is correlated with reading abilities in developmental dyslexia. *Sleep*. 2009;32(10):1333–1340.
83. Marcotte AC, Thacher PV, Butters M, Bortz J, Acebo C, Carskadon MA. Parental report of sleep problems in children with attentional and learning disorders. *J Dev Behav Pediatr*. 1998;19(3): 178–186.
84. Alloway TP, Gathercole SE, Holmes J, Place M, Elliott JG, Hilton K. The diagnostic utility of behavioral checklists in identifying children with ADHD and children with working memory deficits. *Child Psychiatry Hum Dev*. 2009;40(3): 353–366.
85. Bernard BA, Stebbins GT, Siegel S, et al. Determinants of quality of life in children with Gilles de la Tourette syndrome. *Mov Disord*. 2009;24(7):1070–1073.
86. Debes N, Hjalgrim H, Skov L. The presence of attention-deficit hyperactivity disorder (ADHD) and obsessive-compulsive disorder worsen psychosocial and educational problems in tourette syndrome. *J Child Neurol*. 2010;25(2):171–181.
87. Johnson EO, Breslau N. Sleep problems and substance use in adolescence. *Drug Alcohol Depend*. 2001;64(1):1–7.
88. Wong MM, Brower KJ, Fitzgerald HE, Zucker RA. Sleep problems in early childhood and early onset of alcohol and other drug use in adolescence. *Alcohol Clin Exp Res*. 2004;28(4):578–587.

89. Haynes PL, Bootzin RR, Smith L, Cousins J, Cameron M, Stevens S. Sleep and aggression in substance-abusing adolescents: results from an integrative behavioral sleep-treatment pilot program. *Sleep*. 2006;29(4):512–520.
90. Bootzin RR, Stevens SJ. Adolescents, substance abuse, and the treatment of insomnia and daytime sleepiness. *Clin Psychol Rev*. 2005;25(5):629–644.
91. Williams RJ, Goodale LA, Shay-Fiddler MA, Gloster SP, Chang SY. Methylphenidate and dextroamphetamine abuse in substance-abusing adolescents. *Am J Addict*. 2004;13(4):381–389.
92. Muzur A, Pace-Schott EF, Hobson JA. The prefrontal cortex in sleep. *Trends Cogn Sci*. 2002;6(11):475–481.
93. Dahl RE. Regulation of sleep and arousal: comments on part VII. *Ann N Y Acad Sci*. 2004;1021:292–293.
94. Dahl RE, Lewin DS. Pathways to adolescent health sleep regulation and behavior. *J Adolesc Health*. 2002;31(suppl 6):175–184.
95. Viggiano D, Vallone D, Sadile A. Dysfunctions in dopamine systems and ADHD: evidence from animals and modeling. *Neural Plast*. 2004;11 (1–2):97–114.
96. Gruber R, Sadeh A. Sleep and neurobehavioral functioning in boys with attention-deficit/hyperactivity disorder and no reported breathing problems. *Sleep*. 2004;27(2):267–273.
97. Gruber R, Sadeh A, Raviv A. Instability of sleep patterns in children with attention-deficit/hyperactivity disorder. *J Am Acad Child Adolesc Psychiatry*. 2000;39(4):495–501.
98. O'Brien LM. The neurocognitive effects of sleep disruption in children and adolescents. *Child Adolesc Psychiatr Clin N Am*. 2009;18(4): 813–823.
99. Picchietti DL, Underwood DJ, Farris WA, et al. Further studies on periodic limb movement disorder and restless legs syndrome in children with attention-deficit hyperactivity disorder. *Mov Disord*. 1999;14(6):1000–1007.
100. Cortese S, Konofal E, Lecendreux M, et al. Restless legs syndrome and attention-deficit/hyperactivity disorder: a review of the literature. *Sleep*. 2005;28(8):1007–1013.
101. Goraya JS, Cruz M, Valencia I, et al. Sleep study abnormalities in children with attention deficit hyperactivity disorder. *Pediatr Neurol*. 2009;40(1):42–46.
102. Spruyt K, O'Brien LM, Cluydts R, Verleye GB, Ferri R. Odds, prevalence and predictors of sleep problems in school-age normal children. *J Sleep Res*. 2005;14(2):163–176.
103. Chervin RD, Ruzicka DL, Archbold KH, Dillon JE. Snoring predicts hyperactivity four years later. *Sleep*. 2005;28(7):885–890.
104. Beebe DW, Gozal D. Obstructive sleep apnea and the prefrontal cortex: towards a comprehensive model linking nocturnal upper airway obstruction to daytime cognitive and behavioral deficits. *J Sleep Res*. 2002;11(1):1–16.
105. Honaker SM, Gozal D, Bennett J, Capdevila OS, Spruyt K. Sleep-disordered breathing and verbal skills in school-aged community children. *Dev Neuropsychol*. 2009;34(5):588–600.
106. Spruyt K, Capdevila OS, Kheirandish-Gozal L, Gozal D. Inefficient or insufficient encoding as potential primary deficit in neurodevelopmental performance among children with OSA. *Dev Neuropsychol*. 2009;34(5):601–614.
107. Kheirandish-Gozal L, de Jong MR, Spruyt K, Chamuleau SA, Gozal D. Obstructive sleep apnoea is associated with impaired pictorial memory task acquisition and retention in children. 2010 *European Respiratory Journal* 36(1), pp. 164-169
108. Crabtree VM, Varni JW, Gozal D. Health-related quality of life and depressive symptoms in children with suspected sleep-disordered breathing. *Sleep*. 2004;27(6):1131–1138.
109. Gozal D. Sleep-disordered breathing and school performance in children. *Pediatrics*. 1998;102(3, pt 1):616–620.
110. Chervin RD, Archbold KH, Dillon JE, et al. Associations between symptoms of inattention, hyperactivity, restless legs, and periodic leg movements. *Sleep*. 2002;25(2):213–218.
111. Chervin RD, Archbold KH, Dillon JE, et al. Inattention, hyperactivity, and symptoms of sleep-disordered breathing. *Pediatrics*. 2002; 109(3):449–456.
112. O'Brien LM, Mervis CB, Holbrook CR, et al. Neurobehavioral correlates of sleep-disordered breathing in children. *J Sleep Res*. 2004;13(2): 165–172.
113. Gozal D, O'Brien L, Row BW. Consequences of snoring and sleep disordered breathing in children. *Pediatr Pulmonol Suppl*. 2004;26:166–168.
114. Ali NJ, Pitson DJ, Stradling JR. Snoring, sleep disturbance, and behaviour in 4-5 year olds. *Arch Dis Child*. 1993;68(3):360–366.
115. Spruyt K, Gozal D. Mr. Pickwick and his child went on a field trip and returned almost empty handed . . . What we do not know and imperatively need to learn about obesity and breathing during sleep in children! *Sleep Med Rev*. 2008;12(5):335–338.
116. Picchietti D, Allen RP, Walters AS, Davidson JE, Myers A, Ferini-Strambi L. Restless legs syndrome: prevalence and impact in children and adolescents—the Peds REST study. *Pediatrics*. 2007;120(2):253–266.
117. Golan N, Shahar E, Ravid S, Pillar G. Sleep disorders and daytime sleepiness in children with attention-deficit/hyperactive disorder. *Sleep*. 2004;27(2):261–266.
118. Picchietti DL, Stevens HE. Early manifestations of restless legs syndrome in childhood and adolescence. *Sleep Med*. 2008;9(7):770–781.
119. Picchietti DL, Rajendran RR, Wilson MP, Picchietti MA. Pediatric restless legs syndrome and periodic limb movement disorder: parent-child pairs. *Sleep Med*. 2009;10(8):925–931.

120. Picchietti MA, Picchietti DL, England SJ, et al. Children show individual night-to-night variability of periodic limb movements in sleep. *Sleep*. 2009;32(4):530–535.
121. Elia J, Takeda T, Deberardinis R, et al. Nocturnal enuresis: a suggestive endophenotype marker for a subgroup of inattentive attention-deficit/hyperactivity disorder. *J Pediatr*. 2009;155(2); 239–244.
122. Gruber R, Grizenko N, Joober R. Delayed sleep phase syndrome, ADHD, and bright light therapy. *J Clin Psychiatry*. 2007;68(2):337–338.
123. Walters AS, Silvestri R, Zucconi M, Chandrashekariah R, Konofal E. Review of the possible relationship and hypothetical links between attention deficit hyperactivity disorder (ADHD) and the simple sleep related movement disorders, parasomnias, hypersomnias, and circadian rhythm disorders. *J Clin Sleep Med*. 2008; 4(6):591–600.
124. Van der Heijden KB, Smits MG, Van Someren EJW, Gunning WB. Idiopathic chronic sleep onset insomnia in attention-deficit/hyperactivity disorder: a circadian rhythm sleep disorder. *Chronobiol Int*. 2005;22(3):559–570.
125. Weiss MD, Wasdell MB, Bomben MM, Rea KJ, Freeman RD. Sleep hygiene and melatonin treatment for children and adolescents with ADHD and initial insomnia. *J Am Acad Child Adolesc Psychiatry*. 2006;45(5):512–19.
126. Cortese S, Faraone SV, Konofal E, Lecendreux M. Sleep in children with attention-deficit/hyperactivity disorder: meta-analysis of subjective and objective studies. *J Am Acad Child Adolesc Psychiatry*. 2009; 48(9):894–908.

CHAPTER 4

Restless Legs Syndrome

Daniel L. Picchietti and Matthew A. Picchietti

Key Points

- Pediatric restless legs syndrome (RLS) is not rare, occurring to a moderate or severe degree in about 1 of 125 school-age children in the United States.
- There is a strong genetic component to pediatric RLS, as well as evidence for several environmental factors.
- Negative impact of RLS on sleep, cognitive function, and mood has been documented in both children and adults.
- Pediatric-specific diagnostic criteria, vocabulary to describe RLS, and differential diagnosis have been defined.
- Common comorbid conditions are attention-deficit/hyperactivity disorder (ADHD), anxiety, and depression.
- Lifestyle changes and iron supplementation are important treatment considerations.

Introduction

The first detailed report of pediatric restless legs syndrome (RLS) did not appear in the medical literature until 1994 [1]. Since then, a substantial literature in both children and adults has characterized epidemiology, pathophysiology, impact, diagnosis, severity assessment, and treatment. RLS is defined by a maladaptive urge to move the legs, usually accompanied by significant sleep disruption and periodic limb movements in sleep (PLMS), which together can impair cognition, mood, daily activities, and quality of life. The urge to move is typically worst at rest, relieved by movement, and more severe at night.

Epidemiology

Multiple population-based studies of RLS in adults have shown a 5% to 10% prevalence in the United States and Western Europe, with 2% to 3% of the population affected to a moderate or severe degree. Fewer studies in Asian populations and in India have suggested a somewhat lower prevalence in those populations [2]. A large pediatric population–based study of more than 10,000 families in the United States and United Kingdom found a prevalence of 2.0% in 8- to 17-year-olds, with about one-third of these positive cases reporting moderate-to-severe symptoms [3]. Detailed questions helped to eliminate false-positive responses caused by potential mimics of RLS. In addition, these findings correlate well with retrospective adult RLS studies, which report childhood onset of RLS in about 25% of cases [4,5]. These results suggest that more than one-quarter of a million children are affected moderately or severely in the United States. By comparison, the overall prevalence of nonfebrile seizure disorders is approximately 0.5% of children, and a similar 2% are affected by pediatric obstructive sleep apnea. More women than men are reported to have RLS, by a ratio of 2:1, but this was not the case in the population-based pediatric study, where boys and girls were equally as likely to meet RLS criteria. A history of pregnancy is considered a major factor in explaining the gender difference in adults [6], perhaps mediated by the long-term effect of pregnancy on iron stores.

Clinic-based studies have shown a 1.3% prevalence of RLS in 12 pediatric practices [7] and 5.9% in a large pediatric sleep disorders clinic [8]. Specific conditions associated with a higher than expected prevalence of pediatric RLS are ADHD [9] and chronic kidney disease [10], approximately 12% to 35% and 27% to 35%, respectively. During pregnancy, there is a 2- to 3-fold increased risk for RLS, peaking in the third trimester but with resolution of RLS symptoms in about 75% by 1 month postpartum [11].

Pathophysiology

Genetic factors, central nervous system dopamine dysfunction, and brain iron deficiency have all been implicated in the pathophysiology of RLS. Based on current evidence, it is likely that RLS clinical manifestations are mediated by both genetic and environment influences.

Genetics

Familial aggregation of RLS has been shown in multiple studies with a 40% to 92% familial prevalence when the onset of RLS symptoms is before the age of 40 years [12]. A positive parental RLS history of 77% was found in a large pediatric RLS population–based study, with both parents reporting RLS in 16% of 8- to 17-year-olds [3]. Family history studies suggest an autosomal-dominant pattern of inheritance, with variable penetrance. However, linkage and genomewide studies suggest that a few, fairly common gene variants contribute to an individual's "genetic load" for RLS [13,14]. *BTBD9* is one of the gene variants associated with RLS and is estimated to account for 50% of the population-attributable risk for RLS [15]. Interestingly, serum ferritin levels were progressively lower in those with each additional *BTBD9* allele. Also, *BTBD9* is strongly associated with PLMS greater than 5/h. This and other evidence suggests that "RLS with PLMS" is a significant endophenotype, as compared with "RLS without PLMS" [16,17].

Neuroanatomy

Supraspinal and spinal influences are likely involved in RLS, with key roles played by the hypothalamic dopaminergic A11 cell group and a spinal cord generator for periodic motor activity [18]. Unlike in narcolepsy, REM sleep behavior disorder, and Parkinson disease, no degeneration of neural structures has been found.

Neurotransmitter Dysfunction

Central dopamine and opioid transmitter dysfunction have been implicated, based mainly on the therapeutic response of RLS to dopaminergic medications and opioids [19,20]. In addition, dopamine antagonists can aggravate RLS symptoms, but brain imaging studies using positron emission tomography with dopamine receptor binding have been inconsistent. Opioid studies suggest possible altered central processing of pain in RLS [20].

Iron

Autopsy data, magnetic resonance imaging, brain sonography, and cerebrospinal fluid analysis all support a role for brain iron deficiency in the pathophysiology of RLS [14,19]. Extensive basic research has shown iron to be important in brain dopamine production, dopamine synaptic density, myelin synthesis, and brain energy production [21]. In addition, iron may influence norepinephrine and serotonin neurotransmitter systems [22]. Although iron deficiency is typically defined as iron-deficiency anemia, body iron stores are not saturated until well above the iron intake needed to correct anemia, with functional iron deficits in some tissues caused by relative iron deficiency [23,24]. This nonanemic but not fully saturated range correlates with serum ferritin levels of 12 to 70 mcg/L [25–27]. In adult RLS studies, serum ferritin below 50 mcg/L has been associated with more severe RLS, and blinded treatment trials with both intravenous and oral iron have shown benefit for RLS, when baseline serum ferritin levels were below 50 mcg/L. Similar pediatric RLS data are beginning to emerge [14,28]. Interestingly, more severe ADHD in children has also been associated with lower serum ferritin [29,30], and treatment with oral iron has shown benefit [31]. All these data suggest that "low normal" ferritin levels are not enough for optimal brain function.

Hypertension, Heart Disease, and Stroke

Recent evidence has indicated a positive association between RLS, hypertension, coronary artery disease, and cardiovascular disease (including stroke) [32]. A large population-based study comparing adults with RLS to those without RLS found odds ratios of 2.05 (95% confidence interval 1.38%–3.04%) for coronary artery disease and 2.07 (95% CI 1.43%–3.00%) for cardiovascular disease [33]. In addition, several studies, including some with children, document PLMS-related heart rate and blood pressure spikes, which are possible mediators in the physiology of this association [32,34,35].

Impact

Extensive data on the impact of RLS in adults and children are available from both population-based and clinical studies [3,36–39]. The 4 specific domains that are typically affected in moderate-to-severe RLS are sleep, daily activities, mood, and energy/vitality. It is not yet known to what extent the impact on sleep mediates impact on the other 3 domains. Subjective and objective data demonstrate that sleep onset, sleep maintenance, and sleep quality are disrupted. Commonly affected are tedious or monotonous daily activities, such as sitting in class, doing schoolwork or homework, and reading. Children describe feeling sad, angry, and annoyed because of RLS, whereas their parents typically report the children as irritable and easily frustrated. In addition, fatigue and tiredness are a common complaint. However, as with adults who have RLS, significant sleepiness is unusual, even though sleep quantity and quality are significantly compromised. In adults, quality-of-life measures have found RLS to result in a decreased quality of life comparable to that experienced in other medical conditions such as type 2 diabetes and clinical depression. As noted above, RLS in adults has also been found to be associated with increased risk for hypertension, coronary artery disease, and stroke, potentially because of the sympathetic nervous system surges seen with PLMS [32,33].

Clinical Course

The clinical course of early-onset RLS, defined as onset before age 45 years, has been described as slowly progressive in about two-thirds of cases [4,40–42]. This is consistent with a gradual increase in prevalence with age [36]. A stable course over time is described by most of the remaining third. However, remission has been described in some early-onset cases. Also, after delivery in pregnancy-related RLS and after renal transplantation in chronic renal failure, remission is typical. Most of the reports of RLS natural history are based on retrospective analysis of clinical cases. It remains to be seen if in mild cases where medical care is not sought, the course is different. Perhaps in mild presentations, symptom presence is more intermittent, elicited by prolonged immobility (eg, automobile travel, airline travel, theatre events) or other exacerbating factors as described in this chapter.

Available information on pediatric RLS also suggests a slowly progressive course in clinical cases. In addition, clinical sleep disturbance and periodic limb movement disorder (PLMD) may precede the development of typical RLS sensory symptoms by months or years [43]. In some cases, this is related to language development, which needs to be sufficient to describe the sensory component. Adequate language skills are usually developed by age 6 to 8 years. However, in other cases, children who are capable of describing the sensory symptoms report either no sensory symptoms or atypical symptoms, such as worse symptoms during the day. These data and a poor correlation between RLS severity and PLMS severity in adults [44] suggest that there is complex relationship between the sensory, motor, and sleep components of RLS.

Diagnostic Criteria

Pediatric RLS Diagnostic Criteria

Definite RLS

As part of a workshop at the National Institutes of Health (NIH), in Bethesda, MD, the International RLS Study Group (IRLSSG) developed a set of diagnostic criteria for pediatric RLS [45]. Two categories of "definite" RLS were developed that are intended for children 2 to 12 years of age (Table 4.1), in addition to research criteria for ages 0 to 18 years (see Research Criteria section). Adolescents, ages 13 to 18 years, are considered to have definite RLS if they meet the adult RLS criteria. For younger children, definite RLS, subtype 1, specifies that the child describes

Clinical Pearls

Definite RLS—subtype 1 or 2?
Subtype 1 is much more common in children because, if given the opportunity, most children with definite RLS will provide significant detail in their own words. This will meet the criteria for subtype 1 and not require the presence of supportive criteria.

RLS sensations in his/her own words. It is assumed in the adult criteria that the patient will describe his/her own sensory symptoms. However, because parents often report symptoms for children in a medical setting, the criterion was formulated to require the child's own description. For this subtype, it is also required that the child report sensations of urge to move *and* discomfort, whereas adults need to only describe the urge component. This was added, not because there was evidence that children were different in this respect, but because there was uncertainty about descriptors for "urge" that children might use and the committee preferred to err on the side of underdiagnosis rather than overdiagnosis. Nonetheless, research since then has determined that school-age children can describe the "urge to move" (see Diagnostic Interview section) and, on the average, can use 3 or more descriptors for the RLS sensations [38,46]. Definite RLS, subtype 2 is composed of the adult criteria and at least 2 of 3 supportive features. However, subsequent research has shown that most children with definite RLS will meet criteria for subtype 1. In addition, access to biological family history may not be available for some children, diminishing uniform application of the criteria.

With minor revisions of the diagnostic criteria for the *International Classification of Sleep Disorders*, 2nd edition, in 2005 [47], a diagnostic criterion to rule out "mimics" of RLS was added for children and adults (see Differential Diagnosis section), stating, "Symptoms must not be better explained by another neurological, medical, mental, or other sleep disorder, or by the use of a medication or drug." More recently, based on work at an IRLSSG meeting in Baltimore, MD, in 2008, a specifier for clinical significance has been proposed, requiring that, "The symptoms of RLS cause significant distress or impairment in social, occupational, or other important areas of functioning, typically due to impact on sleep,

Table 4.1 National institutes of Health/International RLS Study Group Workshop Criteria for the Diagnosis of Definite RLS in Children and Adolescents*

Definite RLS in children 2–12 yrs old		
All 4 adult essential criteria are met: 1. An **urge to move** the legs that: 2. begins or worsens when sitting or lying down; 3. is partially or totally relieved by movement; and 4. is worse in the evening or night than during the day or only occurs in the evening or night.		
AND		
Definite RLS—subtype 1 There is a description in the child's own words consistent with leg discomfort.	OR	Definite RLS—subtype 2 At least 2 supportive criteria are met: • clinical sleep disturbance • biological parent or sibling has definite RLS • the child has a sleep study documenting a periodic limb movement index ≥5/h of sleep
Definite RLS in adolescents 13–18 yrs old		
All 4 adult essential criteria are met		

Abbreviation: RLS, restless legs syndrome.
*See text for additional criteria/specifiers regarding differential diagnosis and clinically significant RLS.

mood, cognition, daily activities, or energy/vitality." This is suggested because of the recognition of mild cases of RLS, especially those found in population-based prevalence studies and familial risk studies. The areas of impact have been defined for both adults and children [3,38,48]. Academic functioning is an additional, specific area for impairment in children, with impact on behavior as another concern [38].

Supportive Criteria

Although not found in all cases of pediatric RLS, the following are commonly present and considered supportive of an RLS diagnosis: (1) clinical sleep disturbance; (2) a family history of RLS in a first-degree biological relative (a parent or sibling); and (3) PLMS occurring ⩾5/h [45]. These supportive criteria can particularly increase diagnostic certainty for a young child or when there are atypical features. Although polysomnography (PSG) is not indicated for typical RLS in adults, documentation of disturbed sleep and/or PLMS in children with suspected RLS provides objective evidence to compliment the historically obtained subjective evidence. PLMS ⩾5/h are found in about 80% of adults with RLS on a single-night sampling [5], and in 91% when 5 nights are sampled [49]. Similarly, about two-thirds of children have been found to have PLMS ⩾5/h on single-night sampling [14]. However, unlike in adults, PLMS ⩾5/h are rarely found in controls and are thus more specific for pediatric RLS. In addition, there is evidence that "RLS with PLMS" is an important RLS subtype, sharing clinical, genetic, and treatment response characteristics, in contrast to an "RLS-like syndrome" [14,17]. There is considerable night-to-night variability of PLMS in both children and adults [50,51]. As a result, several nights should be monitored in research studies when PLMS is to be used as a severity measure applied to individual cases. Leg accelerometers are available for use over multiple nights in adults, but have not yet been validated for children. PLMS may or may not reflect the same aspects of severity as assessed by the sensory component of RLS [44]. However, PLMS do provide a measure that is much less affected by placebo response [52].

Research Criteria

A set of pediatric RLS research criteria for ages 0 to 18 years were developed at the NIH workshop in 2002 because there appeared to be gaps in the understanding of pediatric RLS [45]. These include "probable RLS" for 2 groups: those children who report that RLS symptoms are worse during the day and children who are cognitively impaired. For each group, a positive family history of RLS is required. "Possible RLS" is applied to children with PLMD who have a positive family history of RLS. Reconsideration of these criteria is warranted based on new data. Children who sit in class for prolonged periods of time may complain of symptoms being worse during the day but may report the more classic "worse at night" pattern on nonschool days or when sedentary activities are later in the day. This "possible RLS" category probably represents an important variant of RLS in childhood [14,43] and is likely to remain a useful concept for genetic research (see Pathophysiology section).

Periodic Limb Movement Disorder

The 4 diagnostic criteria for PLMD are listed in Table 4.2 [47,53]. PSG must show PLMS with specific characteristics (a–d) (Table 4.2 and Figure 4.1), the PLMS index must exceed 5 per hour in pediatric cases, clinical sleep disturbance or daytime fatigue must be present, and PLMS must not be better accounted for. Other etiologies include apneas or hypopneas (PLMS at the termination of these events), medication-induced PLMS (especially with serotonergic antidepressants), and REM sleep behavior disorder. Importantly, PLMD should not be diagnosed if the child meets criteria for RLS, although "RLS with PLMS" is worth noting, because this may be a common RLS subtype/endophenotype. Nonetheless, PLMD is particularly useful as a diagnosis for children less than 6 years of age or for cognitively impaired children, who do not have sufficient language skills to describe RLS sensations. Furthermore, evidence indicates that PLMD is often related to RLS in childhood, given the high prevalence of RLS in families of children with PLMD and the documentation of children with PLMD who later developed the sensory symptoms of RLS [37,43].

Table 4.2 Criteria for the diagnosis of PLMD

1. Polysomnography shows repetitive, stereotyped limb movements that are:
   a. 0.5 to 10 s in duration;
   b. minimum amplitude of 8 mV above resting electromyogram (EMG);
   c. in a sequence of 4 or more movements; and
   d. separated by an interval of more than 5 s (from limb-movement onset to limb-movement onset) and less than 90 s (typically there is an interval of 20–40 s).
2. The PLMS index exceeds 5/h in pediatric cases.
3. There is clinical sleep disturbance or a complaint of daytime fatigue.
4. The PLMS are not better explained by another current sleep disorder, medical disorder, mental disorder, medication use, or substance-use disorder (eg, exclude from PLMS counts the movements at the termination of apneas).

Abbreviations: PLMD, periodic limb movement disorder; EMG, electromyogram; PLMS, periodic limb movements in sleep; RLS, restless legs syndrome.
Note: An individual can have a diagnosis of RLS (with PLMS), but not RLS and PLMD; a diagnosis of RLS supersedes a PLMD diagnosis.

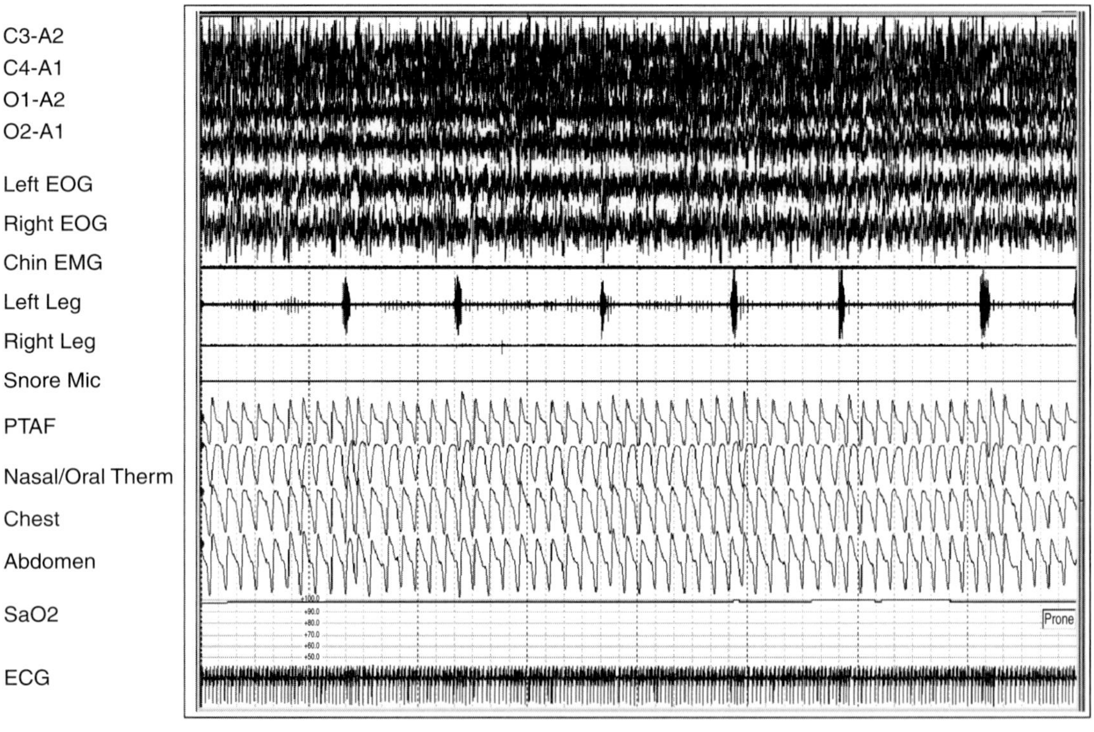

Figure 4.1 This 4-min sleep study segment demonstrates periodic limb movements in sleep involving the left leg of a 10-yr-old boy with restless legs syndrome.

Differential Diagnosis of RLS

The identification of conditions that cause leg discomfort and might appear to be RLS but are not (mimics) is a very important part of the diagnostic process [54,55]. Inclusion of questions about mimics is now part of several structured diagnostic interviews in adults and has been found to significantly improve specificity [56–58]. Common and less common pediatric RLS mimics are listed in Table 4.3. Careful assessment for the essential characteristics of RLS can rule out some mimics. For example, "better with movement" is characteristic of RLS but not common with sore muscles, sprains, cramps, arthritis, or most other

Table 4.3 Differential diagnosis of pediatric restless legs syndrome

Common mimics
- Positional discomfort
- Sore leg muscles
- Ligament sprain/tendon strain
- Positional ischemia (numbness)
- Dermatitis
- Bruises
- "Growing pains"

Less common mimics
- Leg cramps
- Arthritis
- Other orthopedic disorders
- Peripheral neuropathy
- Radiculopathy
- Myelopathy
- Myopathy
- Fibromyalgia
- Sickle cell disease

orthopedic problems. Some of the mimics will have skin changes, for example, dermatitis and bruises. Others, such as peripheral neuropathy, myelopathy, and myopathy, will have findings on neurological examination. In many, focus on the "urge to move" feature of RLS and the descriptors of RLS other than pain (bugs, ants, weird feelings, wiggly feelings) will help differentiate mimics because many of the mimics have pain as the main characteristic, without "urge to move" or these other descriptors.

"Growing pains" are a common diagnosis in children, estimated to affect about 37% of 4- to 6-year-olds [59,60]. Although many of the characteristics of growing pains are similar to pediatric RLS, growing pains do not have an "urge to move" component or many other characteristics of RLS, such as other uncomfortable feelings, sleep disturbance, PLMS, and a family history of RLS. Thus, if these RLS features are assessed, a more specific diagnosis of RLS can be reached. It is now clear that some cases of growing pains represent a misdiagnosis and are actually RLS [3,61,62].

Of course, it is possible for an individual child to have both RLS and a mimic, particularly a common one. Two of the most common mimics can be differentiated by additional characteristics. Positional discomfort may be related to a specific body position such as crossed legs and is relieved by simple repositioning. One simple movement does not relieve RLS. Sore muscles are typically tender to touch, worse with movement, and related to overexertion, whereas RLS is not. Of note is when both RLS and a mimic are present, it is important to focus back on the RLS feelings when assessing other characteristics and impact. Restating the child's most specific descriptor for RLS is helpful, for example, "Does the feeling like bugs in your legs make it hard to fall asleep?"

Diagnostic Interview

Establishing rapport directly with the child greatly enhances the chance of accurately assessing the sensory component of pediatric RLS. As with migraine headache, the child's own description of symptoms is critical for an accurate diagnosis. It is important to not ask leading questions or let the parent answer questions about leg sensations for the child. By age 6 to 8 years most children will have sufficiently developed language and cognitive skills for accurate clinical assessment of RLS.

The interview may start out with a nonspecific prompt, such as, "How did you sleep last night?" or a more specific prompts, such as, "Do your legs bother you at night?" or "Do your legs bother you at school?" If the child responds with insufficient detail, then the prompt, "Tell me more" is suggested. The use of age-appropriate vocabulary is important, because most young children do not understand the words "urge" or "unpleasant" (see Clinical Pearl, The vocabulary of pediatric RLS). If RLS-like feelings are reported, the next step is to assess for criteria 2, 3, and 4 (prominent sitting/lying, relieved with

Clinical Pearls

The vocabulary of pediatric RLS—how do children describe it?

- *Urge to move*: want to move, have to move, got to kick
- *Uncomfortable/unpleasant sensations*: bad feeling, bugs/ants, pain/hurts, tingling, shaky, wiggly feeling, can't get comfortable

movement, and worse evening/night). In addition, it is important to differentiate RLS from potential mimics of RLS (Table 4.3). If a child reports a mimic, then redirection back to the RLS sensations is important when assessing criteria 2 to 4 and severity. Finally, having the child make a drawing of the RLS feelings can provide additional information, as well as provide a visual description for the medical record to compliment the verbal report.

Severity Assessment

The severity of RLS symptoms should be assessed to help determine clinical significance and the need for treatment. Assessment of severity includes determining the frequency and intensity of symptoms, as well as the impact on functioning at school and home. As described above, the typical domains of impact are sleep, daily activities, mood, and energy/vitality. Questioning the parent/caregiver in addition to the child can provide complimentary information. For example, the child may be better able to relate frequency and intensity of sensory symptoms, while the parent or caregiver may be better able to assess irritability and behavioral consequences. PSG (to assess sleep pattern and PLMS), actigraphy (to assess sleep pattern), and leg accelerometry (to assess PLMS) can provide objective data about severity. For research, a pediatric-specific severity scale has been developed [38]. If ADHD, depression, and/or anxiety are comorbid conditions, severity assessment for these conditions can be done by clinical interview and/or appropriate pediatric severity scales.

Comorbidity

Comorbidity is defined as the coexistence of 2 or more disease processes in the same individual (eg, asthma and diabetes or ADHD and learning disability). It emphasizes the concept of "and" not "or." Thus, it is a distinctly different concept than differential diagnosis. Comorbidity does not necessarily indicate significant interaction between the conditions but helps alert the clinician to that possibility. Conditions that are considered to have potentially important comorbidity with pediatric RLS are ADHD, depression, anxiety, and chronic renal failure [14].

Of these, ADHD has been best characterized. About one-quarter of children and adults with RLS meet criteria for ADHD, whereas 12% to 35% with ADHD meet criteria for RLS [14,63]. Both of these prevalence rates are notably higher that general population rates. However, the relationship is likely complex. Because leg sensations (urge or discomfort) are not components of ADHD diagnostic criteria, ADHD should not be misdiagnosed as RLS. Conversely, RLS could influence ADHD diagnosis, because restlessness of RLS can lead to hyperactivity and RLS-related sleep disturbance can increase inattentiveness during the day. In addition, both could independently or jointly have impact on daily activities such as schoolwork. However, another consideration is that there may be a common underlying pathophysiology for both, related to dopamine and/or iron [14]. Nonetheless, it may be very difficult to determine causality of symptoms or impact in an individual case. Consequently, it is likely to be more fruitful to assess each condition by standard diagnostic and severity measures, and then focus on how the conditions might interact. Interestingly, children with both ADHD and RLS did not describe qualitative differences in RLS concepts, symptoms, or impact, when compared with children with only RLS [38]. However, this study did not assess for quantitative differences.

In adults, depression and anxiety disorders are commonly comorbid with RLS, with one population-based study showing odds ratios of 4.7 for major depressive disorder and 12.9 for panic disorder [64]. Interestingly, chronic insomnia is a strong risk factor for subsequent development of mood and anxiety disorders in adults and children [65–67]. In a pediatric RLS case series where children were followed longitudinally, 8 of 18 children with RLS developed anxiety and/or depression after the historical onset of clinical sleep disturbance [43].

As in adults, RLS is common in pediatric chronic kidney disease (CKD) [10,68,69]. Poor mental health, depression, decreased quality of life, and increased mortality are associated with RLS in adult CKD studies [70], suggesting that better recognition of RLS in this pediatric population is also important.

Treatment

Lifestyle Changes

Lifestyle habits significantly impact symptom severity in some cases and are an essential component of assessment and treatment. In mild cases, behavioral interventions alone may be a sufficient form of treatment. Exacerbating factors listed in Table 4.4 should be avoided. A regular sleep schedule of sufficient quantity for age is important. The recommended duration of sleep each night is 11 hours for 5-year-olds, 10 hours for 10-year-olds, and 9 hours for adolescents. The bedroom should be quiet and comfortable, without electronic distractions at bedtime such as a TV or computer. Physical exercise increases deep sleep and may improve both RLS symptoms and benefit mental health disorders such as depression [71–73]. Caffeine and tobacco can exacerbate symptoms and should be avoided. Medications suspected to aggravate RLS include serotonergic antidepressants, neuroleptics, and sedating antihistamines. In more severe cases of RLS, behavioral interventions are typically not sufficient to treat symptoms but are an important adjunct to other interventions.

Iron Supplementation

A promising treatment for RLS is the use of iron supplementation to attain "mid-normal" serum ferritin levels as described above in the Pathophysiology section. For adults, treatment is indicated for a serum ferritin of less than 50 mcg/L [74,75] and this is a reasonable approach for children [14]. Studies have shown improvement in pediatric PLMS and ADHD with increases in serum ferritin from 40.8 to 74.1 and 29.1 to 55.7 mcg/L, respectively [31,76,77]. Important to consider clinically is that serum ferritin is an acute-phase reactant and is not accurate to assess iron stores within 4 weeks of a febrile illness [78,79]. For children 6 years or older with documented serum ferritin levels of less than 50 mcg/L, we typically recommend ferrous sulfate at a dose of 50 to 65 mg of elemental iron, once or twice a day, with a follow-up assessment of serum ferritin in 2 to 3 months. Careful initial screening and monitoring of serum ferritin is recommended to prevent administration of therapeutic iron doses to children who may be at risk for hemochromatosis [80]. In many children, we have found it difficult to attain and maintain serum ferritin levels in the 50- to 100-mcg/L range because of depletion of iron stores due to growth, and in adolescent girls because of the additional factor of menses. To avoid accidental overdosage, the secure storage of iron is important.

Table 4.4 Potential exacerbating factors for restless legs syndrome

- Immobility
- Boring or monotonous situations
- Insufficient sleep for age
- Irregular sleep schedule
- Low body iron stores
- Pain
- Caffeine
- Nicotine
- Alcohol
- Medications

Clinical Pearls

Evaluation of iron status—serum ferritin.

- For RLS the optimal range is a ferritin value >50 mcg/L, well above 12 mcg/L, the typical value below which anemia develops.
- Serum ferritin is an acute-phase reactant. False elevation of ferritin is common within 4 weeks of an acute febrile illness and in the setting chronic inflammation (eg, rheumatoid arthritis).
- Do not assess ferritin within 4 weeks of an acute illness.
- For a child with chronic inflammation, less sensitive measures of iron status, such as percent iron saturation, may be helpful.

Medication

In moderate-to-severe cases of pediatric RLS, where there is significant impact on function, consideration of medication should involve a detail discussion of risks versus benefits with the family. For pediatric sleep disorders, there are no Food and Drug Administration (FDA)–approved medications, a situation that is common for many other pediatric disorders. However, there is medical literature that does support the careful use of medication for pediatric RLS [81–84]. We emphasize nonpharmacologic treatment in addition to medication and suggest treatment in the setting of long-term specialty care.

Clonidine, a medication developed for treatment of hypertension, has had extensive use in children for sleep-onset problems [85–87]. The typical dose is 0.2 to 0.4 mg before bedtime. Hypotension is uncommon in children, as opposed to the elderly, but nightmares or night terrors can be seen occasionally as an adverse effect at higher doses. Clonazepam has a long history of use as an anticonvulsant in children and can help with sleep maintenance at a low dose of 0.25 to 0.5 mg at bedtime. Gabapentin has been shown to be beneficial for RLS in adults [88] and has been used in children as an anticonvulsant. A low dose of 100 to 500 mg at bedtime is typically effective in children. Both clonazepam and gabapentin can cause irritability or hyperactivity in some children, which resolves promptly on discontinuation.

Dopaminergics

Medications that increase dopamine levels are considered the treatments of choice for adults with moderate-to-severe RLS [89]. Ropinirole and pramipexole are currently FDA approved in the United States. Placebo-controlled studies have also shown carbidopa/levodopa to be effective. There have been several published studies reporting benefit with these medications in children [14]. Potential adverse effects include augmentation and the development of impulse control problems. Augmentation is the worsening of RLS symptoms after starting dopaminergic medication for RLS, particularly with dosage increases, and should be monitored for. It is more common in the setting of low serum ferritin levels [90,91]. Impulse control problems have been reported in adults and include problem gambling and compulsive shopping [92,93].

Comorbid ADHD

Stimulant medication has been found to not adversely effect RLS, PLMS, or sleep if the alerting effect has worn off by bedtime [14]. Conversely, improved sleep can diminish ADHD symptoms [94].

Comorbid Depression or Anxiety

Serotonergic medications can worsen RLS or PLMS, so these should be avoided or used cautiously [14]. Dopaminergic or noradrenergic antidepressants are preferred, such as bupropion, if antidepressant medication is needed.

Monitoring and Reassessment

Careful monitoring for medication-related adverse effects is recommended, with periodic reassessment of treatment once iron stores have been optimized. Families should be cautious about the secure storage and proper administration of all medications.

Family Involvement of Treatment Section: Positive family support and understanding are crucial for children with RLS. Because of the common challenges with limit setting and sleep routines, parents/guardians should work to develop advanced parenting skills. Advocacy for the child in medical and school settings is often needed because pediatric RLS and its impact are frequently misunderstood. At school, accommodations may be beneficial such as preferential seating in the back of the classroom, so that the child may move around or occasionally stand up without disturbing others; avoidance of losing recess or physical education as a behavioral consequence; and additional time for exams, to stand up and walk, if needed. Importantly, adolescents should be involved in decisions about their own treatment plan. Finally, it is common for biological parents themselves to be affected by RLS, with depression and anxiety as potential comorbid conditions. If their symptoms are severe enough to need treatment, the child

Clinical Pearls

RLS is highly familial.

Assessment for a family history of RLS can provide support for the diagnosis in a child, as well as provide an opportunity to improve family dynamics if a parent or sibling is significantly affected and might benefit from treatment.

may benefit considerably by a parent's successful treatment.

Directions for Future Research

Simplification and refinement of the pediatric RLS diagnostic criteria are expected based on recent literature. Field testing and validation will enhance the utility of any changes, particularly in special pediatric populations where there are more complicated mimics and/or comorbid conditions, such as rheumatoid arthritis and chronic renal failure. Further genetic research is needed, with consideration of environmental factors such as iron, which may modify clinical expression. Additional study of the comorbidity of RLS and ADHD could provide insights into the pathophysiology of each. Periodic limb movements as an objective measure of RLS warrants further investigation. To economically assess PLMS on multiple nights, the validation of leg accelerometry for children would be valuable. Importantly, pediatric clinical trials of promising treatments are needed.

References

1. Walters AS, Picchietti DL, Ehrenberg BL, Wagner ML. Restless legs syndrome in childhood and adolescence. *Pediatr Neurol.* 1994;11(3):241–245.
2. Cho SJ, Hong JP, Hahm BJ, Jeon HJ, Chang SM, Cho MJ, Lee HB. Restless legs syndrome in a community sample of Korean adults: prevalence, impact on quality of life, and association with DSM-IV psychiatric disorders. *Sleep.* 2009;32(8):1069–1076.
3. Picchietti D, Allen RP, Walters AS, Davidson JE, Myers A, Ferini-Strambi L. Restless legs syndrome: prevalence and impact in children and adolescents—the Peds REST study. *Pediatrics.* 2007;120(2):253–266.
4. Walters AS, Hickey K, Maltzman J, et al. A questionnaire study of 138 patients with restless legs syndrome: the 'Night-Walkers' survey. *Neurology.* 1996;46(1):92–95.
5. Montplaisir J, Boucher S, Poirier G, Lavigne G, Lapierre O, Lespérance P. Clinical, polysomnographic, and genetic characteristics of restless legs syndrome: a study of 133 patients diagnosed with new standard criteria. *Mov Disord.* 1997;12(1):61–65.
6. Berger K, Luedemann J, Trenkwalder C, John U, Kessler C. Sex and the risk of restless legs syndrome in the general population. *Arch Intern Med.* 2004;164(2):196–202.
7. Kinkelbur J, Hellwig J, Hellwig M. Frequency of RLS symptoms in childhood. *Somnologie.* 2003;(7)(suppl 1):34.
8. Kotagal S, Silber MH. Childhood-onset restless legs syndrome. *Ann Neurol.* 2004;56(6):803–807.
9. Silvestri R, Gagliano A, Arico I, et al. Sleep disorders in children with Attention-Deficit/Hyperactivity Disorder (ADHD) recorded overnight by video-polysomnography. *Sleep Med.* 2009;10(10):1132–1138.
10. Sinha R, Davis ID, Matsuda-Abedini M. Sleep disturbances in children and adolescents with non-dialysis-dependent chronic kidney disease. *Arch Pediatr Adolesc Med.* 2009;163(9):850–855.
11. Manconi M, Govoni V, De Vito A, et al. Pregnancy as a risk factor for restless legs syndrome. *Sleep Med.* 2004;5(3):305–308.
12. Winkelmann J, Polo O, Provini F, et al. Genetics of restless legs syndrome (RLS): state-of-the-art and future directions. *Mov Disord.* 2007;22:S449–S458.
13. Winkelmann J, Schormair B, Lichtner P, et al. Genome-wide association study of restless legs syndrome identifies common variants in three genomic regions. *Nat Genet.* 2007;39(8):1000–1006.
14. Picchietti MA, Picchietti DL. Advances in pediatric restless legs syndrome: iron, genetics, diagnosis and treatment. *Sleep Med.* 2010; 11:643–651.
15. Stefansson H, Rye DB, Hicks A, et al. A genetic risk factor for periodic limb movements in sleep. *N Engl J Med.* 2007;357(7):639–647.
16. Winkelman JW. Periodic limb movements in sleep—endophenotype for restless legs syndrome? *N Engl J Med.* 2007;357(7):703–705.
17. Bassetti CL, Kretzschmar U, Werth E, Baumann CR. Restless legs and restless legs-like syndrome. *Sleep Med.* 2006;7(6):534.
18. Clemens S, Rye D, Hochman S. Restless legs syndrome: revisiting the dopamine hypothesis from the spinal cord perspective. *Neurology.* 2006;67(1):125–130.
19. Allen R. Dopamine and iron in the pathophysiology of restless legs syndrome (RLS). *Sleep Med.* 2004;5(4):385–391.
20. Walters AS, Ondo WG, Zhu W, Le W. Does the endogenous opiate system play a role in the Restless Legs Syndrome? A pilot post-mortem study. *J Neurol Sci.* 2009;279(1–2):62–65.
21. Beard JL, Connor JR. Iron status and neural functioning. *Annu Rev Nutr.* 2003;23:41–58.
22. Burhans MS, Dailey C, Beard Z, et al. Iron deficiency: differential effects on monoamine transporters. *Nutr Neurosci.* 2005;8(1):31–38.
23. Cook JD. Defining optimal body iron. *Proc Nutr Soc.* 1999;58(2):489–495.
24. Suominen P, Punnonen K, Rajamäki A, Irjala K. Serum transferrin receptor and transferrin receptor-ferritin index identify healthy subjects with subclinical iron deficits. *Blood.* 1998;92(8):2934–2939.
25. Guyatt GH, Oxman AD, Ali M, Willan A, McIlroy W, Patterson C. Laboratory diagno-sis of iron-deficiency anemia: an overview. *J Gen Intern Med.* 1992; 7(2):145–153.
26. Coenen JL, van Dieijen-Visser MP, van Pelt J, et al. Measurements of serum ferritin used to predict concentrations of iron in bone marrow in

anemia of chronic disease. *Clin Chem*. 1991;37(4):560–563.
27. Lichtman MA, Williams WJ. *Williams Hematology*. New York, NY: McGraw-Hill, Medical Pub. Division; 2006.
28. Picchietti D. Is iron deficiency an underlying cause of pediatric restless legs syndrome and of attention-deficit/hyperactivity disorder? *Sleep Med*. 2007;8:693–694.
29. Cortese S, Konofal E, Bernardina BD, Mouren MC, Lecendreux M. Sleep disturbances and serum ferritin levels in children with attention-deficit/hyperactivity disorder. *Eur Child Adolesc Psychiatry*. 2009;18(7):393–399.
30. Oner O, Alkar OY, Oner P. Relation of ferritin levels with symptom ratings and cognitive performance in children with attention deficit-hyperactivity disorder. *Pediatr Int*. 2008;50(1):40–44.
31. Konofal E, Lecendreux M, Deron J, et al. Effects of iron supplementation on attention deficit hyperactivity disorder in children. *Pediatr Neurol*. 2008;38(1):20–26.
32. Walters AS, Rye DB. Review of the relationship of restless legs syndrome and periodic limb movements in sleep to hypertension, heart disease, and stroke. *Sleep*. 2009;32(5):589–597.
33. Winkelman JW, Shahar E, Sharief I, Gottlieb DJ. Association of restless legs syndrome and cardiovascular disease in the Sleep Heart Health Study. *Neurology*. 2008;70(1):35–42.
34. Walter LM, Foster AM, Patterson RR, et al. Cardiovascular variability during periodic leg movements in sleep in children. *Sleep*. 2009;32(8):1093–1099.
35. Wing YK, Zhang J, Ho CKW, Au C-T, Li AM. Periodic limb movement during sleep is associated with nocturnal hypertension in children. *Sleep*. 2010; In press.
36. Allen RP, Walters AS, Montplaisir J, et al. Restless legs syndrome prevalence and impact: REST general population study. *Arch Intern Med*. 2005;165(11):1286–1292.
37. Picchietti DL, Rajendran RR, Wilson MP, Picchietti MA. Pediatric restless legs syndrome and periodic limb movement disorder: parent-child pairs. *Sleep Med*. 2009;10:925–931.
38. Arbuckle R, Abetz L, Durmer JS, et al. Development of the pediatric restless legs syndrome severity scale (P-RLS-SS): a patient-reported outcome measure of pediatric RLS symptoms and impact. *Sleep Med*. 2010; 11:897-906.
39. Winkelman JW, Redline S, Baldwin CM, Resnick HE, Newman AB, Gottlieb DJ. Polysomnographic and health-related quality of life correlates of restless legs syndrome in the sleep heart health study. *Sleep*. 2009;32(6):772–778.
40. Winkelmann J, Wetter TC, Collado-Seidel V, et al. Clinical characteristics and frequency of the hereditary restless legs syndrome in a population of 300 patients. *Sleep*. 2000;23(5):597–602.
41. Trenkwalder C, Seidel VC, Gasser T, Oertel WH. Clinical symptoms and possible anticipation in a large kindred of familial restless legs syndrome. *Mov Disord*. 1996;11(4):389–394.
42. Bassetti CL, Mauerhofer D, Gugger M, Mathis J, Hess CW. Restless legs syndrome: a clinical study of 55 patients. *Eur Neurol*. 2001;45(2):67–74.
43. Picchietti D, Stevens HE. Early manifestations of restless legs syndrome in childhood and adolescence. *Sleep Med*. 2008;9:770–781.
44. Hornyak M, Hundemer HP, Quail D, Riemann D, Voderholzer U, Trenkwalder C. Relationship of periodic leg movements and severity of restless legs syndrome: a study in unmedicated and medicated patients. *Clin Neurophysiol*. 2007;118(7):1532–1537.
45. Allen RP, Picchietti D, Hening WA, Trenkwalder C, Walters AS, Montplaisir J. Restless legs syndrome: diagnostic criteria, special considerations, and epidemiology: a report from the restless legs syndrome diagnosis and epidemiology workshop at the National Institutes of Health. *Sleep Med*. 2003;4(2):101–119.
46. Picchietti DL, Arbuckle R, Abetz L, et al. Pediatric restless legs syndrome: analysis of symptom descriptions and drawings. 2010; submitted.
47. American Academy of Sleep Medicine. *International Classification of Sleep Disorders: Diagnostic and Coding Manual*. 2nd ed. Westchester, IL: American Academy of Sleep Medicine; 2005.
48. Hening W, Walters AS, Allen RP, Montplaisir J, Myers A, Ferini-Strambi L. Impact, diagnosis and treatment of restless legs syndrome (RLS) in a primary care population: the REST (RLS epidemiology, symptoms, and treatment) primary care study. *Sleep Med*. 2004;5(3):237–246.
49. Trotti LM, Bliwise DL, Greer SA, et al. Correlates of PLMS variability over multiple nights and impact upon RLS diagnosis. *Sleep Med*. 2009;10(6):668–671.
50. Picchietti MA, Picchietti DL, England SJ, et al. Children show individual night-to-night variability of periodic limb movements in sleep. *Sleep*. 2009;32(4):530–535.
51. Hornyak M, Kopasz M, Feige B, Riemann D, Voderholzer U. Variability of periodic leg movements in various sleep disorders: implications for clinical and pathophysiologic studies. *Sleep*. 2005;28(3):331–335.
52. Fulda S, Wetter TC. Where dopamine meets opioids: a meta-analysis of the placebo effect in restless legs syndrome treatment studies. *Brain*. 2008;131(pt 4):902–917.
53. Iber C, Ancoli-Israel S, Chesson A, Quan SF, eds. *The AASM Manual for the Scoring of Sleep and Associated Events: Rules, Terminology and Technical Specifications*. 1st ed. Westchester, IL: American Academy of Sleep Medicine; 2007.
54. Hening WA, Allen RP, Washburn M, Lesage SR, Earley CJ. The four diagnostic criteria for Restless Legs Syndrome are unable to exclude confounding conditions ("mimics"). *Sleep Med*. 2009;10(9):976–981.
55. Möller C, Wetter TC, Köster J, Stiasny-Kolster K. Differential diagnosis of unpleasant sensations in

the legs: prevalence of restless legs syndrome in a primary care population. *Sleep Med.* 2010; 11(2):161–166.
56. Hening WA, Allen RP, Washburn M, Lesage S, Earley CJ. Validation of the Hopkins telephone diagnostic interview for restless legs syndrome. *Sleep Med.* 2008;9(3):283–289.
57. Allen RP, Burchell BJ, MacDonald B, Hening WA, Earley CJ. Validation of the self-completed Cambridge-Hopkins questionnaire (CH-RLSq) for ascertainment of restless legs syndrome (RLS) in a population survey. *Sleep Med.* 2009;10(10):1097–1100.
58. Popat RA, Van Den Eeden SK, Tanner CM, et al. Reliability and validity of two self-administered questionnaires for screening restless legs syndrome in population-based studies. *Sleep Med.* 2010;11: 154–160.
59. Evans AM. Growing pains: contemporary knowledge and recommended practice. *J Foot Ankle Res.* 2008;1(1):4.
60. Evans AM, Scutter SD. Prevalence of "growing pains" in young children. *J Pediatr.* 2004;145(2):255–258.
61. Walters AS. Is there a subpopulation of children with growing pains who really have Restless Legs Syndrome? A review of the literature. *Sleep Med.* 2002;3(2):93–98.
62. Rajaram SS, Walters AS, England SJ, Mehta D, Nizam F. Some children with growing pains may actually have restless legs syndrome. *Sleep.* 2004;27(4):767–773.
63. Zak R, Fisher B, Couvadelli BV, Moss NM, Walters AS. Preliminary study of the prevalence of restless legs syndrome in adults with attention deficit hyperactivity disorder. *Percept Mot Skills.* 2009;108(3):759–763.
64. Lee HB, Hening WA, Allen RP, et al. Restless legs syndrome is associatedwith DSM-IV major depressive disorder and panic disorder in the community. *J Neuropsychiatry Clin Neurosci.* 2008; 20(1):101–105.
65. Taylor DJ, Lichstein KL, Durrence HH, Reidel BW, Bush AJ. Epidemiology of insomnia, depression, and anxiety. *Sleep.* 2005;28(11):1457–1464.
66. Ong SH, Wickramaratne P, Tang M, Weissman MM. Early childhood sleep and eating problems as predictors of adolescent and adult mood and anxiety disorders. *J Affect Disord.* 2006;96(1–2):1–8.
67. Gregory AM, Caspi A, Eley TC, Moffitt TE, Oconnor TG, Poulton R. Prospective longitudinal associations between persistent sleep problems in childhood and anxiety and depression disorders in adulthood. *J Abnorm Child Psychol.* 2005;33(2):157–163.
68. Applebee GA, Guillot AP, Schuman CC, Teddy S, Attarian HP. Restless legs syndrome in pediatric patients with chronic kidney disease. *Pediatr Nephrol.* 2009;24(3):545–548.
69. Davis ID, Baron J, O'Riordan MA, Rosen CL. Sleep disturbances in pediatric dialysis patients. *Pediatr Nephrol.* 2005;20(1):69–75.
70. Szentkiralyi A, Molnar MZ, Czira ME, et al. Association between restless legs syndrome and depression in patients with chronic kidney disease. *J Psychosom Res.* 2009;67(2):173–180.
71. Aukerman MM, Aukerman D, Bayard M, Tudiver F, Thorp L, Bailey B. Exercise and restless legs syndrome: a randomized controlled trial. *J Am Board Fam Med.* 2006;19(5):487–493.
72. Deslandes A, Moraes H, Ferreira C, et al. Exercise and mental health: many reasons to move. *Neuropsychobiology.* 2009;59(4):191–198.
73. Dworak M, Wiater A, Alfer D, Stephan E, Hollmann W, Struder HK. Increased slow wave sleep and reduced stage 2 sleep in children depending on exercise intensity. *Sleep Med.* 2008;9(3):266–272.
74. Silber MH, Ehrenberg BL, Allen RP, et al. An algorithm for the management of restless legs syndrome. *Mayo Clin Proc.* 2004;79(7):916–922.
75. Wang J, O'Reilly B, Venkataraman R, Mysliwiec V, Mysliwiec A. Efficacy of oral iron in patients with restless legs syndrome and a low-normal ferritin: a randomized, double-blind, placebo-controlled study. *Sleep Med.* 2009;10(9):973–975.
76. Simakajornboon N, Gozal D, Vlasic V, Mack C, Sharon D, McGinley BM. Periodic limb movements in sleep and iron status in children. *Sleep.* 2003;26(6):735–738.
77. Simakajornboon N, Kheirandish-Gozal L, Gozal D, Sharon D, Murry L, Abraham M. A long-term follow-up study of periodic limb movement disorders in children after iron therapy (abstract). *Sleep.* 2006;29:A76–A77.
78. Hulthén L, Lindstedt G, Lundberg PA, Hallberg L. Effect of a mild infection on serum ferritin concentration—clinical and epidemiological implications. *Eur J Clin Nutr.* 1998;52(5):376–379.
79. Eskeland B, Baerheim A, Ulvik R, Hunskaar S. Influence of mild infections on iron status parameters in women of reproductive age. *Scand J Prim Health Care.* 2002;20(1):50–56.
80. Barton JC, Wooten VD, Acton RT. Hemochromatosis and iron therapy of Restless Legs Syndrome. *Sleep Med.* 2001;2(3):249–251.
81. Pelayo R, Chen W, Monzon S, Guilleminault C. Pediatric sleep pharmacology: you want to give my kid sleeping pills? *Pediatr Clin North Am.* 2004;51(1):117–134.
82. Pelayo R, Dubik M. Pediatric sleep pharmacology. *Semin Pediatr Neurol.* 2008;15(2):79–90.
83. Simakajornboon N, Kheirandish-Gozal L, Gozal D. Diagnosis and management of restless legs syndrome in children. *Sleep Med Rev.* 2009;13(2):149–156.
84. Picchietti MA, Picchietti DL. Restless legs syndrome and periodic limb movement disorder in children and adolescents. *Semin Pediatr Neurol.* 2008;15(2):91–99.
85. Newcorn JH, Schulz K, Harrison M, DeBellis MD, Udarbe JK, Halperin JM. Alpha 2 adrenergic agonists. Neurochemistry, efficacy, and clinical guidelines for use in children. *Pediatr Clin North Am.* 1998;45(5):1099–1022, viii.
86. Owens JA, Rosen CL, Mindell JA. Medication use in the treatment of pediatric insomnia: results

of a survey of community-based pediatricians. *Pediatrics*. 2003;111(5, pt 1):e628–e635.
87. Prince JB, Wilens TE, Biederman J, Spencer TJ, Wozniak JR. Clonidine for sleep disturbances associated with attention-deficit hyperactivity disorder: a systematic chart review of 62 cases. *J Am Acad Child Adolesc Psychiatry*. 1996;35(5):599–605.
88. Garcia-Borreguero D, Larrosa O, de la Llave Y, Verger K, Masramon X, Hernandez G. Treatment of restless legs syndrome with gabapentin: a double-blind, cross-over study. *Neurology*. 2002;59(10):1573–1579.
89. Trenkwalder C, Hogl B, Winkelmann J. Recent advances in the diagnosis, genetics and treatment of restless legs syndrome. *J Neurol*. 2009;256(4):539–553.
90. Frauscher B, Gschliesser V, Brandauer E, et al. The severity range of restless legs syndrome (RLS) and augmentation in a prospective patient cohort: association with ferritin levels. *Sleep Med*. 2009;10(6):611–615.
91. Trenkwalder C, Högl B, Benes H, Kohnen R. Augmentation in restless legs syndrome is associated with low ferritin. *Sleep Med*. 2008;9(5):572–574.
92. Cornelius JR, Tippmann-Peikert M, Slocumb NL, Frerichs CF, Silber MH. Impulse control disorders with the use of dopaminergic agents in restless legs syndrome: a case-control study. *Sleep*. 2010;33(1):81–87.
93. Tippmann-Peikert M, Park JG, Boeve BF, Shepard JW, Silber MH. Pathologic gambling in patients with restless legs syndrome treated with dopaminergic agonists. *Neurology*. 2007;68(4):301–303.
94. Walters AS, Mandelbaum DE, Lewin DS, Kugler S, England SJ, Miller M. Dopaminergic therapy in children with restless legs/periodic limb movements in sleep and ADHD. Dopaminergic Therapy Study Group. *Pediatr Neurol*. 2000;22(3):182–186.

CHAPTER 5

Sleep and Epilepsy

Joseph Kaleyias and Sanjeev V. Kothare

Introduction

The complicated and reciprocal relationship between sleep and epilepsy is a topic that has been intriguing to physicians and researchers for many years [1]. Epilepsy and sleep disorders are considered by many to be common bedfellows. The question as to whether sleep affects epilepsy or epilepsy modifies sleep has been extensively evaluated [2].

Sleep disorders frequently coexist in patients with epilepsy [3]. According to a questionnaire-based survey, the prevalence of subjectively reported sleep disturbance among adults with epilepsy (39%) was found to be significantly higher than that among controls (18%) [4]. The prevalence of sleep disorders in children with epilepsy is underrecognized. Children with epilepsy experience alterations in total sleep, sleep architecture, sleep latency, and spontaneous arousals with a higher incidence of sleep fragmentation and daytime drowsiness [5–8].

The etiology of sleep disruption in children with epilepsy is multifactorial and includes factors such as the epilepsy per se, seizure frequency, as well as the effect of antiepileptic medications. A variety of treatable sleep disorders such as sleep-disordered breathing (SDB) including obstructive sleep apnea (OSA), and periodic limb movements of sleep (PLMS) can be present in patients with epilepsy, leading to sleep fragmentation with resultant excessive daytime sleepiness (EDS), which in turn could lead to poor seizure control. Thus, sleep deprivation has seizure-provoking effects, whereas frequent seizures may in turn lead to sleep fragmentation. Furthermore, evidence suggests that the presence of seizures can disturb sleep, even when they occur during wakefulness, and interestingly enough, epilepsy per se can disrupt sleep [9]. Antiepileptic drugs (AEDs) can alter sleep, both beneficially and detrimentally, and these effects appear independent of their anticonvulsant actions. AEDs may lead to weight changes in children as well [10]. The resultant sleep fragmentation along with the obesity in itself may lead to EDS.

Not only quantity but also good quality sleep is important for optimal functioning in all people but is particularly essential in patients with epilepsy who may find themselves in a cycle of worsening seizures, further sleep disruption, and intractable epilepsy [3]. Treatment of sleep disorders in this population of children with epilepsy is likely to improve the quality of life and daily functioning along with improved seizure control [11].

Effect of Sleep on Epilepsy

The occurrence of seizures during sleep has been noted since the time of Hippocrates and Aristotle [12]. In 1885, Gower found that 21% of patients had seizures solely during sleep, 42% only during the awake state, and 37% had seizures during both the awake and asleep states [13]. The amount of baseline rhythmicity occurring in the brain differs considerably

Key Points

- The relationship of sleep and epilepsy in any one patient is complex: Independent sleep disorders frequently coexist with epilepsy, and seizures themselves can cause sleep disturbances. The clinician should approach these patients in a logical manner to determine the underlying etiologies that are contributing to the sleep complaints.
- Sleep fragmentation with resultant excessive daytime sleepiness is very common in the epilepsy population.
- Study of patients with epilepsy by the use of video-electroencephalogram polysomnography may be indicated.
- The commonest treatable comorbidity associated with epilepsy is obstructive sleep apnea.
- Awareness of these sleep comorbidities along with effective screening measures to appropriately detect and treat them will lead to overall improved seizure control, sleep quality, daytime functioning, and quality of life.
- Antiepileptic drugs can be contributors as well as be effective treatment measures for sleep fragmentation.
- Sleep-related epilepsy syndromes are an important subset of epilepsy. Occurrence of seizures in relation to the sleep-wake has important diagnostic implications in several syndromes.
- Although parasomnias are generally benign, frequent or unusual episodes may sometimes be confused with epilepsy, particularly nocturnal frontal lobe epilepsy. Clinical history and videotapes of suspected parasomnias provided by the family can provide valuable diagnostic clues. Onset of events within 30 minutes of sleep onset is suggestive of seizures, whereas onset at 2 hours after sleep onset is more suggestive of non-rapid eye movement parasomnias.

between the states of sleep and wakefulness. It is therefore not surprising that various seizure types begin preferentially in specific sleep states [9,14].

Sleep-Related Epilepsy

Although most seizure subtypes have the potential to occur during sleep or wakefulness, sleep has a well-documented and strong association with specific epilepsy syndromes. The term sleep-related epilepsy (SRE) has been coined to categorize those epileptic syndromes with more than 70% occurrence during sleep [15]. The most important among these SRE syndromes are the following.

1. **Partial seizures** tend to occur in both sleep and wakefulness, although the semiology varies according to the site of onset. Several studies have evaluated the influence of sleep on the incidence of partial seizures and have concluded that FLS began during sleep more often than temporal lobe seizures but TLS were more likely to secondarily generalize when they began during sleep (Table 5.1) [16–22]. Epileptic seizures appear to conform to circadian rhythms. This varies according to the cortical region involved, with frontal lobe seizures peaking in the very early morning and mesial temporal lobe seizures having a bimodal distribution with a primary peak in the late afternoon and a secondary peak in the early morning [19].

Frontal lobe epilepsy (FLE) is more likely to occur during sleep than temporal lobe seizures [18,19]. The seizures may show bizarre semiology with posturing, ambulation, violent outbursts, and complex behavior [23,24]. They are often misdiagnosed as OSA or a parasomnia because of the accompanying prominent choking or motor activity [14,25]. Only a third show clear epileptiform abnormalities on routine electroencephalogram (EEG) [26]. A form of FLE with seizures occurring almost exclusively during sleep has been described, and the term nocturnal frontal lobe epilepsy (NFLE) has been adopted [27]. NFLE may exist in sporadic, familial, idiopathic, cryptogenic, or symptomatic forms [23,27,28].

Autosomal-dominant nocturnal frontal lobe epilepsy (ADNFLE) is the first idiopathic epilepsy for which a genetic basis has been identified [29]. Approximately 25% of patients have family history of seizures [23]. Few families have 2 or more family members with the same seizure type consistent with ADNFLE [23]. Linkage studies have indentified genes for ADNFLE that encodes nicotinic

Table 5.1 Trials evaluating the occurrence of partial seizures by wake-sleep cycle and by day/night timing

Trial	Sample	Results
Crespel et al [16], 1998	$N = 30$ adults 15: FLE; 15: TLE VEM	61% of FLE occur during sleep; sleep organization was normal. 89% of TLE occur during wakefulness; sleep organization was characterized by a low efficiency index. The difference in seizure distribution persisted under all conditions investigated.
Bazil and Walczak, [17], 1997	$N = 188$ adults (1116 seizures) VEM	35% of complex partial seizures starting during sleep underwent secondary generalization compared with 18% in wakefulness ($P < .0001$). FLE were more likely to occur during sleep (37%) than were temporal lobe seizures (26%; $P = .0068$). FLE secondarily generalized at equal rates during sleep (22%) and wakefulness (20%). TLE generalized much more frequently during sleep (45%) than in wakefulness (19%; $P < .0001$).
Herman et al [18], 2001	$N = 133$ adults (613 seizures) VEM	43% of all partial seizures began during sleep. Sleep seizures began during stages 1 (23%) and 2 (68%) but were rare in slow-wave sleep; no seizures occurred during REM sleep. TLE were more likely to secondarily generalize during sleep (31%) than during wakefulness (15%), but FLE were less likely to secondarily generalize during sleep (10% vs 26%; $P < .005$).
Durazzo et al [19], 2008	$N = 131$ adults (669 seizures) Intracranial VEM	FLE: unimodal distribution (peaking 4:00 AM-7:00 AM). Mesial TLE were distributed bimodally, with the primary peak during 16:00–19:00 h and secondary peak during 7:00–10:00 h. Neocortical TLE peaked slightly before the primary peak observed in the mesial TLE ($P =$ NS). OLE peaked between16:00 and 19:00 h; PLE peaked between 4:00 and 7:00 h.
Hofstra et al [20] 2009	$N = 176$ patients (76 children, 100 adults) VEM	Significantly more seizures from 11:00 to 17:00 h, and significantly fewer from 23:00 to 05:00 h. The daytime peak incidences were observed in overall seizures, complex partial seizures (in children and adults), seizures of extratemporal origin (in children), and seizures of temporal origin (in adults). Incidences significantly lower during 23:00–05:00 h in seizures overall, complex partial seizures (in children and adults), and in tonic seizures (in children). In addition, significantly fewer seizures of temporal (in children and adults) and extratemporal origin (in children) were observed in this period.
Hofstra et al [21], 2009	$N = 33$ adults 450 seizures Intracranial VEM	TLE seizures occurred between 11:00 and 17:00 h; FLE between 23:00 and 05:00 h, and PLE between 17:00 and 23:00 h. In the awake state, larger proportions of clinical seizures were seen from 05:00 to 11:00 h and from 17:00 to 23:00 h. During sleep, larger proportions occurred from 11:00 to 17:00 h and from 23:00 to 05:00 h.
Pavlova et al [22], 2004	$N = 26$ adults 90 seizures 15: TLE; 11: XTLE VEM	In TLE, 50% of seizures occurred between the hours of 15:00 and 19:00. In XTLE, there was a peak between 19:00 and 23:00 h. The effect of time on seizures was least pronounced in the XTLE patients who had more than one epileptogenic region. The proportion of seizures occurring from sleep was significantly less in TLE (19%) than in XTLE patients (41%).

Abbreviations: FLE, frontal lobe epilepsy; TLE, temporal lobe epilepsy; OLE, occipital lobe epilepsy; PLE, parietal lobe epilepsy; XTLE, extratemporal lobe epilepsy; VEM, video-electroencephaloram monitoring; REM, rapid eye movement; NS, not significant.

acetylcholine receptor subunits (CHRNA4/CHRNB2) [30]. At least one-third of patients do not have identified genetic mutations (genetic heterogeneity) [31]. There is no difference between sporadic nocturnal FLE and ADNFLE in the clinical and neurophysiological findings. Paroxysmal arousals, episodic nocturnal wanderings (ENW), and nocturnal paroxysmal dystonia (NPD) are 3 characteristic manifestations of nocturnal FLE [23,32] (Table 5.2).

ENWs can mimic sleepwalking and confusional arousals, but has accompanying motor patterns and an abnormal EEG not seen with parasomnias [33]. NPD, which was initially thought to be a parasomnia with dystonic posturing out of sleep, is now believed to be a variant of frontal lobe epilepsy from a deep focus, with minimal to no EEG changes during the event, and normal EEGs in between attacks [34,35]. Episodes of NPD begin as a paroxysmal arousal, but are subsequently associated with more complex movements including bipedal automatisms, rhythmic twisting movements of the trunk and pelvis, vocalization, and tonic or dystonic posturing lasting less than a few minutes [32]. NPD are accordingly classified as hyperkinetic motor subtype or asymmetric bilateral tonic seizure subtype [36]. Clinical characteristics of NPD are summarized in Table 5.3 [23,37,38]. Recently, we have started recognizing the co-occurrence of NFLE with parasomnias. Onethird of patients with NFLE have a history of parasomnia (mostly arousal disorders), whereas the prevalence of arousal disorders in the general population is 1% to 6% [23]. Almost 50% of patients with NFLE have family history of parasomnia including arousal disorder, rapid eye movement (REM) behavior disorder (RBD), primary enuresis, and rhythmic movements disorders [23].

Hyperkinetic seizures associated with affective symptoms are considered a typical manifestation of NFLE [39]. Patients with nocturnal temporal lobe epilepsy (NTLE) with mainly sleep-related seizures have been described; however, they commonly lack hyperkinetic activity and their daily seizure frequency out of sleep is low. Mai et al [40] examined 25 patients with sleep-related hyperkinetic epileptic seizures, with a frontal lobe onset in 18 cases and a temporal lobe onset in 7. Patients with sleep-related hyperkinetic seizures with temporal lobe origin had anamnestic and clinical features strikingly similar to those with a frontal onset, with agitated movements, high seizure frequency, and no history of febrile convulsions. The authors confirmed that this kind of epileptic manifestation is thus not peculiar to frontal lobe epilepsy only. The comparison between NFLE and NTLE is shown in Table 5.4 [40].

Sleep-related seizures similar to those observed in people with NLFE may have an extrafrontal origin and the etiologic substrate may play a role in facilitating the occurrence of seizures during sleep [41–43]. In both frontal

Table 5.2 Nocturnal frontal lobe epilepsy: seizure types

	Paroxysmal Arousals (PA)	Nocturnal Paroxysmal Dystonia (NPD)	Episodic Nocturnal Wandering (ENW)
Onset	Abrupt, recurring arousals from non-rapid eye movement sleep	Begins as PA; then complex movements	Starts as PA, then NPD
Description	Vocalizations with stereotyped movements. Patients raise head, sit up in bed, look around, scream, occasionally with dystonic posturing	Kicking, bicycling, trunk rocking, tonic or clonic asymmetric, dystonic or ballistic movements with flailing of limbs	Patients jump out of bed, ambulate, appear agitated
Consequences	Sleep disruption and daytime sleepiness	Sleep disruption and daytime sleepiness	May lead to injuries
Duration	<20 s	<2 min	<3 min
% of recorded seizures	75%	23%	2%

From Refs. [23,32].

Table 5.3 Clinical features of nocturnal paroxysmal dystonia

Feature	
Mean age at onset (range)	14 years (1–64 yrs)
Male: female ratio	7:3 (high male prevalence)
Seizure type	Usually more than one type; occur in clusters
Clinical presentation	Patients may awaken with choking sensation, shortness of breath
Mean seizure frequency (range)	20 per month (range 1–20 per night)
Diurnal and secondarily generalized seizures	1/3 of patients
Unawareness of seizures	>70%; complaints brought by families
Consequences	Daytime sleepiness, sleep fragmentation, poor sleep quality reported by many; improves with antiepileptic drug therapy
Neurologic examination	Normal in 92%
Neuroradiologic examination	Normal in 86%

From Refs. [37,38].

Table 5.4 Comparison between nocturnal frontal and nocturnal temporal lobe epilepsy

	Nocturnal frontal lobe epilepsy ($N = 18$)	Nocturnal temporal lobe epilepsy ($N = 7$)
Male:female	10:8	2:5
Mean age of onset (yrs) (range)	6.3 (1−24)	5.6 (1−17)
Neurologic examination	2 with low IQ	Normal
Family history of epilepsy	7 (38.8%)	2 (28.5%)
Median frequency of seizures per month	35	42
EEG background activity normal	14 (77.8%)	1 (14.3%)
EEG focal spikes/sharp waves	7 (38.8%)	7 (100%)
EEG ictal		
Negative	5 (27.8%)	1 (14.3%)
Frontal uni- or bilateral fast activity	5 (27.8%)	0
Frontotemporal fast activity	8 (44.4%)	3 (42.9%)

Abbreviation: EEG, electroencephalogram.
From Ref. [40].

and extrafrontal cases of surgically treated drug-resistant SRE, Taylor's type focal cortical dysplasia (TFCD), a disorder of cortical malformation [44], has been shown to be the most frequent finding at the histopathologic examination [28,41]. Nobili et al [45] have statistically confirmed a strong association between SRE and TFCD in a population of drug-resistant epileptic patients. In particular, despite a significantly higher proportion of TFCD in the frontal lobe (67.6% in the frontal lobe vs 33.3 and 37.5 in the temporal and posterior quadrant, respectively) 1 of every 2 patients with a TFCD, independent of its location, had an SRE, confirming the effect of TFCD as an independent risk factor for SRE. The diagnosis of TFCD increases 14-fold the risk of SRE. The investigators concluded that when evaluating a drug-resistant patient with SRE, the presence of TFCD as the etiologic factor, even if occult on MRI, must be taken into account, in addition to considering that surgical treatment of TFCD-associated SRE provides excellent results [28,41].

2. **Juvenile myoclonic epilepsy** (JME) is a prototype of idiopathic generalized epilepsy and is characterized by a strong genetic predisposition [46], commonly presenting with early

morning myoclonic jerks during adolescence. Generalized tonic-clonic seizures can occur independently or precede the myoclonus. These tend to occur in early morning hours shortly after awakening, with a second peak of occurrence in some patients in the early evening. Myoclonic seizures can be subtle and overlooked for many years as simple clumsiness [14]. These patients also have daytime absence seizures with staring spells, which can mimic daytime sleep attacks. Patients may be exceedingly sensitive to sleep deprivation and alcohol consumption. Badawy et al [47], very recently using transcranial magnetic stimulation to investigate the effect of diurnal variability on cortical excitability in patients with epilepsy, showed that cortical excitability increases early in the morning in patients with idiopathic generalized epilepsy, particularly in JME, but not in subjects with focal epilepsy or controls without epilepsy. This finding may explain the increased seizure susceptibility in these patients in the early morning. Labate et al [48] found early morning awake EEGs to be more useful in detecting generalized epileptiform activity in comparison with an afternoon session.

3. **Benign epilepsy with centrotemporal spikes (BECT; benign rolandic epilepsy)** is the most common partial epilepsy syndrome in the pediatric age group, with an onset between age 3 and 13 years and remission in adolescence [49]. The typical presentation is a partial seizure with paresthesia and tonic or clonic activity of the lower face, associated with drooling and dysarthria. The seizures are mostly nocturnal, with 55% to 59% of patients having seizures exclusively during sleep [2]. EEG shows characteristic central and temporal spikes bilaterally but independently, potentiated during non-rapid eye movement (NREM) sleep. The discharge rate is increased during drowsiness and light sleep as compared with the waking record, with no change in spike morphology. Despite the increased frequency of seizures and IEDs during sleep, the sleep architecture is not affected, and no sleep disruption is seen in these children. The response to medications is excellent, and the prognosis is universally benign from an epilepsy perspective. However, these children often have deficits in visuo-spatial short-term memory, attention and cognitive flexibility, picture naming, visuo-perceptual skills, and visuo-motor coordination. These deficits may be related to nocturnal spiking, but interestingly have not been associated in other epilepsy syndromes with daytime spiking and lack of nocturnal sleep potentiation of these spikes. Attempts at reducing the nocturnal spike index has resulted in improved cognition, albeit at the cost of significant side effects [50].
4. **Landau-Kleffner syndrome (LKS)** is an acquired disorder with epileptic aphasia in which children, usually 3 to 8 years of age, who have developed age-appropriate speech, experience language regression with verbal auditory agnosia, abnormal epileptiform activity, behavioral disturbances, and sometimes overt seizures [51]. **Electrical status epilepticus in slow-wave sleep (ESES)** is primarily an EEG diagnosis and secondarily a clinical one, the principal criterion being the occurrence of spike wave (SW) complexes "continuously" during NREM sleep but not during the awake state or in REM sleep [52]. The term continuous is applied only to EEG abnormalities with a spike index usually >85% during SWS persistent on 3 or more recordings over a period of 1 month. There are several similarities between ESES and LKS. Both conditions demonstrate a normal EEG background during wakefulness, with generalized SW discharges or sometimes focal epileptiform activity. However, in ESES, discharges during sleep are generalized, whereas in LKS, SW activity is more temporally located. In ESES, epileptiform activity becomes virtually continuous during NREM sleep, such that it may be impossible to distinguish sleep stages [14,25].
5. **Infantile spasms** is an example of a catastrophic epilepsy syndrome characterized by a triad of epileptic spasms of the body, variable extent of intellectual disability, and hypsarrhythmic EEG, with onset between ages 3 and 18 months. Interestingly, these spasms tend to cluster on awakening in the morning [1].
6. **Infantile variant of benign epilepsy of childhood with occipital paroxysms (BECOP; Panayiotopoulos syndrome)** is an interesting benign epilepsy syndrome seen in children

of ages 2 to 6 years, characterized by prolonged periods of eye deviation and autonomic instability (temperature, heart rate, respiration, blood pressure), hemi-convulsive and generalized tonic-clonic seizures in sleep, with vomiting on waking up. Interictal EEGs show occipital spikes, whereas ictal EEGs show electrographic seizures emanating from the occipital region in sleep during these events [53].

The Effect of Different Sleep Stages on Seizures and IEDs

Seizures in sleep tend to occur during NREM sleep [2]. They are most frequently observed in stage 2 NREM sleep, followed by stage 1 and then stage 3 and 4 NREM sleep in that order [12]. Minecan et al [54] examined seizure rates in various stages of sleep in epilepsy patients undergoing overnight video-EEG polysomnography. A total of 55 patients having 117 seizures were included in that study. Ninety-five percent of seizures occurred in NREM sleep (61% stage 2, 20% stage 1, 14% stage 3 and 4) and only 5% in REM sleep. The authors concluded that both IEDs and seizures are facilitated by NREM sleep. Whereas deeper stages of NREM sleep activate IEDs, lighter stages of NREM sleep promote seizures at least for a single seizure occurring per night in adults.

IEDs are generally activated by NREM stages 3 and 4 in adults with focal epilepsy, and relatively suppressed by REM sleep [55]. Using the change of log delta power as a measure of deepening sleep, Malow et al [56] found that IEDs occurred more frequently as sleep deepened (N3 sleep). In contrast, focal IEDs that occur during REM sleep are more accurate for seizure localization as compared with other sleep states [57]. Interestingly in children, several Italian studies using cyclical alternating patterns (CAP) and spectral analysis on the EEG have shown that IEDS in BECT and BECOP are more prevalent in stage 1 and 2 sleep, coinciding with sigma (12–16 Hz) activity, and occurrence of spindles, rather than with slow waves of sleep (0.5–4 Hz). These studies postulate that the neural mechanism underlying spindles also facilitate IEDs and that this is a maturational effect, and an age-dependent phenomenon. The immature brain combined with the hypersynchronizing functions of NREM sleep may lead to a regional hyperexcitability of the cortex, thus facilitating thalamo-cortical volleys to transform from spindles into spikes [58–61].

Seizure and spike rate in different stages of sleep in adults are shown in Figure 5.1 [54].

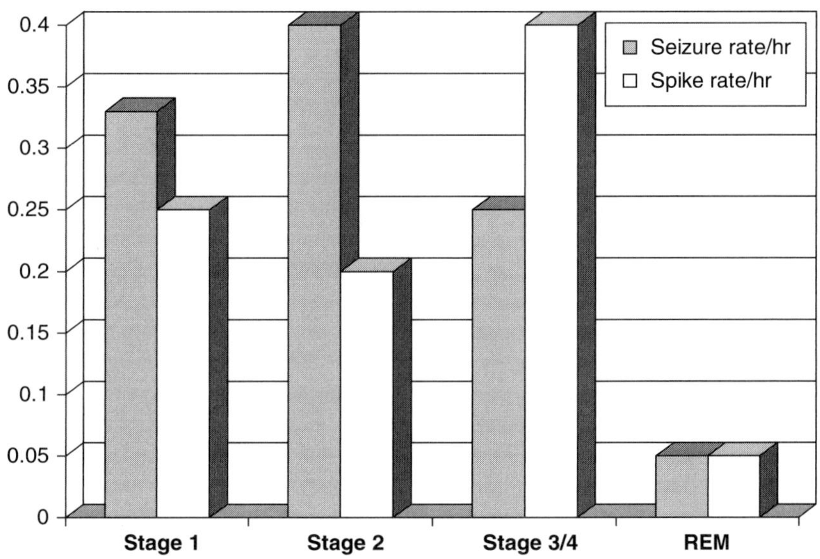

Figure 5.1 Seizure and spike rate/hour in different stages of sleep.

The Effect of Sleep Deprivation on Epilepsy and IEDs

Gibbs and Gibbs [62] have shown that sleep deprivation and recording of sleep increase the yield of detecting IEDs during an EEG. However, there is a continued debate whether sleep deprivation increases IEDs independent of increased likelihood of recording sleep. In a retrospective report comparing routine sleep EEG and subsequent sleep-deprived EEG with sleep, a 52% activation rate of IEDs was seen in the latter group independent of sleep duration or depth [63]. Thus, sleep deprivation became established as an activating method to elicit epileptiform activity while performing EEGs [64]. Studies comparing sleep-deprived EEGs with drug-induced sleep EEGs have reported conflicting findings [12].

Even though sleep is well known to facilitate seizures and epileptiform activity, it can also be protective against the occurrence of seizures in some cases [64].

How Sleep Affects Epilepsy

The neurophysiologic process involved in the deepening of NREM sleep may also facilitate both seizures and IEDs, although the exact level of sleep depth that is maximally facilitatory probably differs by age, epilepsy syndromes, and specific seizure subtypes and IEDs [54]. NREM sleep represents a state of synchronization between the brainstem reticular activating system, thalamus, and cortex (pyramidal neurons). The process of deepening NREM sleep is associated with reduction of the effect of acetylcholine, with progressive hyperpolarization of thalamo-cortical neurons [65]. Varying levels of hyperpolarization may facilitate IEDs and seizures. In contrast, REM sleep and wakefulness, 2 brain-activated behavioral stages, are opposed to the resting EEG-synchronized sleep [65]. REM sleep is characterized by inhibition of thalamocortical synchronizing mechanisms [66], a desynchronized EEG pattern, inhibition of spread of epileptiform discharges, and skeletal muscle paralysis.

Arousals from sleep result in transitions to lighter sleep, followed by a return to deeper levels of sleep. On the descent back to the deeper levels of sleep, seizures are more likely to occur. This model is consistent with work showing that patients with epilepsy have impaired sleep continuity, with more fragmentation of sleep, even in the absence of seizures [67]. Thus, seizures tend to occur more in sleep during CAP, a pattern commonly seen with sleep fragmentation [68].

Therefore, patients with epilepsy may be more susceptible to the neurophysiologic changes associated with sleep stage transitions. This model may also explain why pathophysiologic processes that fragment sleep such as OSA have been associated with worsening seizure frequency, and why treatment of these disorders may potentially improve seizure control [58,69,70]. In one series, those with medically refractory epilepsy and OSA were more likely to have seizures during sleep than those without OSA, supporting the premise that sleep fragmentation caused by OSA facilitates seizures [14]. The literature also supports that AEDs may exert their beneficial actions on seizures not only via direct effects on neuronal excitability but also via stabilization of sleep and reduction of sleep transitions [49].

The exact mechanism of how sleep and sleep deprivation activate seizures is unclear and may be related to γ-aminobutyric acid modulation and/or the offset of adenosine (AD) with sleep onset [71]. AD has long been thought to play a role in sleep, because caffeine, the major stimulant used around the world, was found to act as an antagonist at AD receptors. AD antagonists increase waking and decrease sleep EEG slow-wave activity in humans and rodents [72]. Conversely, AD and its analogs increase sleep and enhance slow-wave activity in a way suggesting that AD could serve as an endogenous sleep-promoting substance [71]. It is postulated that AD levels rise in the brain after prolonged wakefulness, thus signaling the brain of reduced brain energy levels that develop during wakefulness, and that sleep is induced as an energy-restorative state. The inhibitory neuromodulator and endogenous anticonvulsant AD is largely regulated by astrocytes and its key metabolite enzyme AD kinase (ADK) [73]. AD acts as an antiepileptogenic agent, whereas ADK acts as a pro-epileptogenic agent. Thus, at the transition of wakefulness to sleep, there is a dramatic drop in AD levels, along with high ADK levels, with lowered seizure threshold. Several studies support the ADK hypothesis of epileptogenesis; astorgliosis in the hippocampus associated with epilepsy with upregulation of ADK activity. This may have therapeutic implications in effective treatment of epilepsy via AD agonists or ADK antagonists [74].

Melatonin has been shown to enhance hippocampal excitability [75] and thus acting as proconvulsant at high doses, but may also have antiepileptic properties in lower doses [76,77]. There is conflicting evidence regarding the baseline levels of melatonin in people with epilepsy. Elevated melatonin levels have been reported in untreated patients with active epilepsy [78]. Yalýn et al [79] assessed serum melatonin levels and melatonin circadian rhythm in patients with diurnal and nocturnal complex partial epilepsy and showed that the nadir of melatonin levels was at 10:00 AM coinciding with the morning peak in TLE seizures recently reported by Durazzo et al [19], whereas the nocturnal peak of melatonin levels at 3:00 AM to 4:00 AM coincides with the peak of FLE.

Baseline levels of melatonin in patients with epilepsy increase after a seizure [80]. Bazil et al [80] measured salivary melatonin, at baseline and following seizures, in patients with intractable temporal lobe epilepsy and controls. Melatonin was reduced in patients with epilepsy at baseline compared with controls, and increased 3-fold following seizures.

Exposure to light affects subsequent expression of melatonin. Although sunlight suppresses melatonin expression during the daytime, it also allows adequate expression of melatonin in the evenings and the nighttime. Baxendale [81] examined 1715 seizures recorded over a 1-year period and showed that the epileptic seizures, particularly partial seizures from the temporal lobe, were less likely to occur on bright sunny days than dull days and winter season, and this correlation remained stable when seasonal patterns were controlled for. The author noticed "... it is possible that the reduction in partial seizures we observed on sunny days were due to the protective effects of adequate nocturnal melatonin expression following exposure to bright sunlight during the day, or the disruptive effects of a dull day on nocturnal melatonin expression."

There have been conflicting reports on seizure control when prescribing melatonin for people with epilepsy [82–84]. The effects of ramelteon, a selective melatonin receptor agonist, were evaluated in 2 animal models of epilepsy, and the results of this study showed that it possesses anticonvulsant properties in a chronic epilepsy model [85].

In a recent study, decreased levels of hypocretin-1 in the cerebrospinal fluid of patients with repetitive GTC seizures or status epilepticus have been demonstrated [85]. The results of this study suggest that the hypocretin-1 system deficiency may contribute to the typical somnolence after generalized tonic-clonic seizures. The exact mechanism of this observation is unclear and needs additional studies for confirmation of this finding.

Effect of Epilepsy on Sleep

Epilepsy per se and/or seizures themselves promote sleep disruption and affect significantly the quality, quantity, and the architecture of sleep [86]. Patients with epilepsy generally have sleep abnormalities such as increased number and duration of awakenings during sleep, reduced sleep efficiency, reduced or abnormal K-complexes and sleep spindles, reduced and fragmented REM sleep, and increased stage shifts [87].

Seizures may acutely disrupt the sleep-wake state, with the clinical consequence of nocturnal insomnia and EDS [14,17]. Sleep is disrupted in patients with epilepsy on seizure-free nights as well, when compared with non-epileptic controls. A possible explanation for this phenomenon could be that IEDs may cause sleep disruption, preventing normal progression though sleep stages [11].

Patients with seizures not only have a reduction in total sleep time but also REM sleep, when compared with patients without seizures [86]. Reduced REM sleep is seen with seizures occurring during the day as well at night, more so when seizures happen at night during sleep. Increased REM sleep on the other hand is seen with good seizure control [64].

Alterations in total sleep time, sleep latency, and spontaneous arousals have also been reported in children with epilepsy [11]. Sleep abnormalities are more common in children with generalized seizures than in those with simple or complex partial seizures. Like in adults, REM sleep may be decreased by 50% in children with generalized tonic-clonic seizures [11].

The authors of an interesting study noticed several possible reasons for decreased REM sleep in patients with epilepsy. The first was that sleep was more disrupted, with more frequent awakenings and less time spent asleep, including in REM sleep. A second explanation was that seizures affect the circadian pattern responsible for REM sleep, thus delaying its onset. Seizures may also have a direct REM suppressant effect without disruption of circadian rhythms. Finally AEDs may alter REM sleep [88].

Prevalence of Sleep Complaints in Patients With Epilepsy

Patients with epilepsy in general appear to have a greater prevalence of sleep disturbance than normal controls [86]. Stores et al [89] using parental questionnaires assessed sleep disturbances in 79 school children with epilepsy and 73 healthy control children. They found that children with epilepsy showed much higher rates of sleep disorders, particularly poor quality sleep and anxieties about sleep, in comparison with the normal controls. They also found a significant association between seizure frequency and anxieties about sleeping. Cortesi et al [90] evaluated the presence of sleep problems and their association with behavioral and adjustment problems in children with idiopathic epilepsy and found that children with epilepsy had significantly more sleep problems than did both siblings and healthy controls. Within the epileptic group, children with current seizures complained more of sleep problems than did seizure-free children.

Potential Causes of Sleep Disruption in Patients With Epilepsy

There are many causes of sleep disruption in epilepsy patients, including inadequate sleep hygiene, coexisting sleep disorders, and circadian rhythm disturbances. Seizures themselves can disrupt sleep, even when they occur during wakefulness [88] (for details please read section Effect of Epilepsy on Sleep). AEDs can also alter sleep in positive and negative ways, and these effects are independent of the anticonvulsant actions. The end result of sleep disruption is EDS, worsening seizures, and poor quality of life (Figure 5.2).

Polysomnographic Findings in Patients With Epilepsy

A variety of treatable sleep disorders have been shown to coexist during sleep studies (polysomnography [PSG]) in patients with epilepsy.

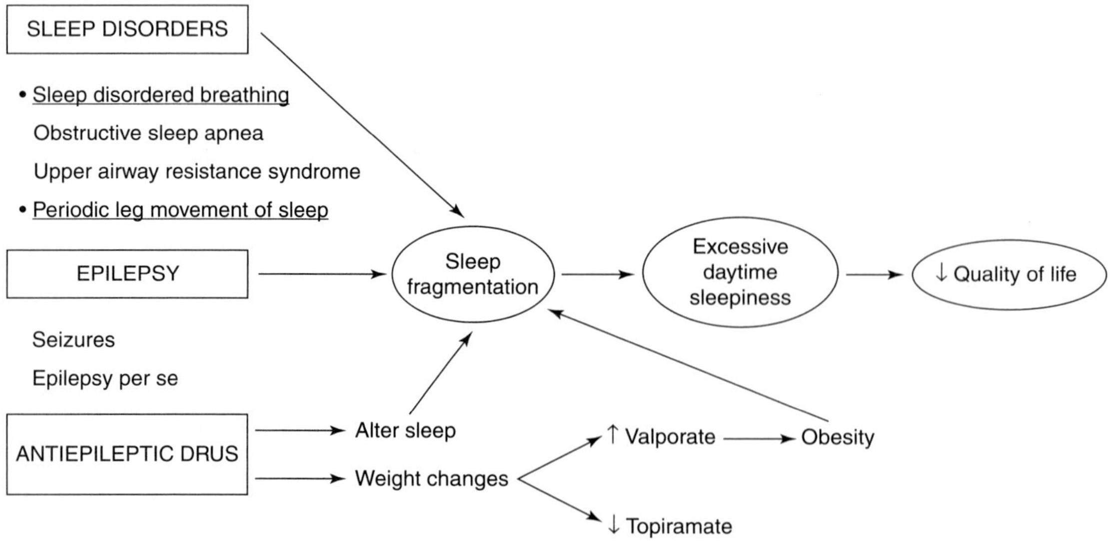

Figure 5.2 Sleep disruption in patients with epilepsy.

Table 5.5 Polysomnographic findings in children with epilepsy

Study	Sample	Results/conclusions
Maganti et al [91], 2005	11 children (5–18 yr old) with primary generalized epilepsy and 8 age- and sex-matched controls	Children with epilepsy had longer stage 1 sleep % and latency to REM sleep compared with controls. *Sleep architecture was abnormal in children with primary generalized epilepsy.*
Nunes et al [87], 2003	17 children with partial refractory epilepsy (subdivided into 2 subgroups based on the presence or absence of ictal episodes during the recording night)	↓ of total time in bed and total sleep time in both subgroups. ↑ number of stage shifts per hour in the control group; ↓ % of stage 2 shifts and ↑ % of stage 3–4 shifts in patients with epilepsy and seizures during the night; ↓ % of REM sleep and first REM latency is increased in both epileptic subgroups, compared with normal controls (P = NS). *Children with partial refractory epilepsies have only mild sleep structure abnormalities.*
Becker et al [92], 2004	N = 30 children with epilepsy and sleep-disordered symptoms	80% of children with epilepsy exhibited sleep disruption because of clinically significant OSA, disturbance of sleep architecture, or sleep fragmentation. *The daytime behavior problems encountered in children with epilepsy may be attributed to specific disruptions in sleep regulation.*
Nagarajan et al [93], 2003	N = 7 children with epilepsy on VNS	↓ effort and tidal volume occurred concordant with VNS activation. *Respiratory pattern changes in sleep occur in most children with refractory epilepsy on VNS.*
Kothare et al [94], 2008	N = 51 children (40 with epilepsy and 11 with OSA without epilepsy)	Primary snoring 42%, OSA 20%, obstructive hypoventilation 12.5%, UARS 8%, PLMS 10%. Children with poor seizure control had ↓ sleep efficiency arousal index, and ↑ REM. Patients with epilepsy with OSA had ↑ BMI, ↑sleep latency, and ↑arousal index. *A significant proportion of children with epilepsy manifest sleep-disordered breathing, including OSA syndrome.*
Bruni et al [95], 2010	N = 10 children with BERS, drug free at the time of the study and 10 age-matched normal controls	Sleep architecture in BERS showed only few significant differences vs controls (reduction of total sleep time, sleep efficiency, and REM %). CAP analysis revealed several significant differences: reduced total CAP rate, mainly in sleep stage 2, and reduced EEG slow oscillations and arousals during stages N1 and N2. *Sleep architecture is not importantly affected in BERS but CAP analysis reveals a decrease of NREM instability, mainly in sleep stage 2.*

Abbreviation: AHI, apnea hypopnea index; BERS, benign epilepsy with rolandic spikes; CAP, cyclical alternating pattern; PLMS, periodic leg movement syndrome; OSA, obstructive sleep apnea; REM, rapid eye movement; NREM, non-rapid eye movement; UARS, upper airway resistance syndrome; VNS, vagal nerve stimulator; EEG, electroencephalogram; BMI, body mass index; ↑, increase; ↓, decrease.

Available literature describing PSG abnormalities in children with epilepsy is scarce but has been summarized in Table 5.3 [87,91–95] (Table 5.5).

Recently, we have evaluated PSG abnormalities in a cohort of 40 children with epilepsy who underwent a sleep study for various sleep complaints [94]. Forty percent of the patients showed SDB, 42% primary snoring, 10% PLMS, and only 8% had a normal sleep study. Furthermore, children with poor control of epilepsy were more obese, had lower sleep efficiency, and higher arousal index in comparison with children with good seizure control or children free of seizures. We also compared the subgroup of children with epilepsy who were diagnosed with OSA with a subgroup of children with OSAs without epilepsy. Children with epilepsy with OSAs had longer sleep latency and higher arousal index in comparison with the nonepilepsy OSAs group. Even though the children with epilepsy had lower Apnea-Hypopnea Index than children with uncomplicated OSAs, they desaturated more significantly with lower nadir oxygen desaturation. Whether the epilepsy syndrome, effects of AEDs, obesity, or upper airway anatomy contributed to this observation was unclear. We have also discussed our experience in scoring sleep stages during sleep studies in patients with frequent IEDs. All attempts must be made at best to differentiate NREM from REM sleep and not try very hard to further attempt differentiation of N1–3 stages of NREM sleep. Data on sleep fragmentation caused because of partial vs generalized seizures in children are varied [87,91–95]. In our study, sleep fragmentation on PSGs was independent of seizure subtypes.

In a recent study, 970 healthy children from the general population and with no previous history of seizures or any other medical conditions underwent overnight PSG studies [96]. In 14 children (prevalence 1.45%), evidence of epileptiform activity was seen in the absence of any additional abnormality in the PSG. Epileptiform patterns found were either spike or spike and wave and were more prominent during NREM sleep, with 11 patients presenting with spike and wave patterns in the centro-temporal regions consistent with benign rolandic spikes, and 3 with generalized spike wave discharges. The authors concluded that the epileptiform activity in otherwise healthy children from the community is not uncommon and needs confirmation with formal EEGs. They also emphasize the need for PSG montages that includes temporal leads and >2 standard EEG leads to facilitate the detection of epileptiform activity in children.

Breathing Disorders in Patients With Epilepsy

Obstructive Sleep Apnea

OSA is particularly important, as it is frequently overlooked in patients with epilepsy, but appropriate treatment of OSA can result in reduced frequency or resolution of seizures. In some patients, OSA can also be the primary reason of intractability of epilepsy [69,97]. The postulated mechanisms explaining worsening of seizures with coexisting OSA could include the following.

Sleep loss: OSA is well known to cause sleep deprivation and sleep fragmentation. The effect of this sleep disruption deprives the patient from attaining restorative sleep, as well as increases the time spent in stages of sleep vulnerable to seizure induction, thus overall reducing the threshold for seizures.

Oxygen desaturation: The effect of hypoxia on lowering the seizure threshold seems to be most prominent in the developing brain [98]. Hypoxia induces a hyperexcitable state in the immature hippocampus [99]. Animal studies have shown that hypoxia produces a profound effect on glutamate synapses and leads to the cascade of events that ends in cell death and reorganization that promotes epileptogenesis [100].

Many reports show that treatment of OSA by tonsillectomy and adenoidectomy or use of nasal continuous positive airway pressure (CPAP) has resulted in better control of the seizures secondary to improved sleep fragmentation [101]. In contrast, CPAP use has been responsible for precipitating parasomnias secondary to a slow-wave sleep rebound with use of CPAP. A recent paper also showed that use of CPAP in an otherwise normal child resulted in activating a new-onset of frontal lobe seizures, and the authors postulate mechanisms to explain the same [102].

On the other hand, the increased prevalence of OSA in patients with epilepsy may be from several etiologies:

Factors inherent to the epilepsy syndrome: Epilepsy may affect the regulation of respiration during sleep [103]. Foldvary-Schaefer et al [104] described a case in which clinically significant OSA disappeared after left frontal lobe resection that produced a near–seizure-free state. The pathophysiology of OSA in patients with epilepsy may be related to the effect of frequent IEDs and/or seizures altering upper airway control. Abnormal upper airway anatomy in epilepsy with onset in early childhood may be another explanation.

Factors associated with the treatment of the epilepsy: AEDs may lead to obesity which is a commonly accepted risk factor for OSA [105]. VNS affects respiration during sleep and has been shown to worsen preexisting OSA [106] (for more details, please read the section Effect of Epilepsy Treatment on Sleep).

Central Sleep Apnea

CSA during epileptic seizure may be multifactorial [107]. The link between CSA and seizures is reciprocal and complex. CSA may trigger a seizure because of the hypoxia caused by the central apnea reducing the seizure threshold [88]. On the other hand, seizures may trigger a CSA (107) or CSA may be an event at the end of the seizure [108].

Ictal hypoxemia occurs often in patients with localization-related epilepsy, and the hypoxemia may be pronounced and prolonged even with seizures that do not progress to generalized convulsions [109]. Ictal desaturations are significantly more likely to be associated with temporal lobe seizures than with extratemporal seizures.

Tezer et al [107] recently documented the epileptic origin of ictal CSA in patients with right temporal and parasagittal epilepsy with EEG-video monitoring and placement of both noninvasive and invasive electrodes and concomitant PSG recording. The authors emphasize the importance of an epileptic origin of CSA in the differential diagnosis of breathing abnormalities.

Blum et al [110] examined the occurrence of hypoxemia in adults with partial seizures. During long-term video-EEG monitoring, patients underwent monitoring of oxygen saturation using a digital SpO2 (pulse oximeter) transducer. The results of this study showed that partial seizures may be associated with prominent oxygen desaturations. The comparable duration of each seizure and its subsequent desaturation suggest a close mechanistic (possibly causal) relationship. SpO2 monitoring thus provides an additional measure of seizure detection. These observations also raise the possibility of ictal ventilatory dysfunction playing a role in certain cases of sudden unexpected death in epilepsy population (SUDEP) in adults with partial seizures [111].

O'Regan and Brown [108] examined changes in cardiac and respiratory function that occurred during 101 seizures (40 partial, 21 generalized tonic-clonic, and 40 absences) in 37 children and found that partial seizures were frequently associated with significant respiratory abnormalities (tachypnea in 56%, apnea in 30%, frequent respiratory pauses in 70%, and severe hypoxemia in 40%). Catastrophic apnea with severe hypoxemia necessitating repeated cardiopulmonary resuscitation could be the presentation of a seizure with epileptic activity on the EEG preceding the apnoea. Sleep PSGs in patients with LGS show central apneas during generalized paroxysmal activity in sleep in LGS and has been suggested as a possible diagnostic criterion [112].

A recent study linked occurrence of central apneas with hypoxemia to spread of seizures to the contralateral side in patients with temporal lobe epilepsy, thus suggesting that spread of seizures from both temporal lobes to the respiratory centers in the brain stem may be necessary to induce sleep-related respiratory disturbances [109].

Several possible mechanisms could explain how the seizures can cause breathing abnormalities:

- The partial seizures may spread from the limbic structures and the temporal lobes to the brainstem respiratory center inducing a CSA.
- The generalized tonic seizures may cause diaphragmatic and glottis spasm thus inducing CSA.
- Hypoventilation and/or ventilatory instability may occur during the seizure with resultant CSA.
- Hyperventilation during seizures leading to CO2 washout with postarousal prolonged CSA [113].
- Cardiac autonomic instability with tachycardia may occur during seizures.
- Components of OSA may occur in addition to CSA during a seizure.
- Lying prone with resultant suffocation.
- Neurogenic pulmonary edema.

Overall, these possibilities may explain mechanisms for SUDEP.

The Effect of Epilepsy Treatment on Sleep

1. **Antiepileptic drugs:** The effects of AEDs on sleep have been studied independent of seizures showing both detrimental and beneficial effects. AEDs can induce sedation or

insomnia [86]. AEDs can also affect sleep architecture. Several studies have shown that some AEDs can produce sleep stability [114]. This naturally poses the question of whether the improvement in sleep patterns is a direct consequence of the use of the AED or the consequence of a suppression of epileptic manifestations. It is possible that sleep improvement plays a role in the therapeutic effects of these drugs. The beneficial effect may be expressed as the occurrence of more regular cycles of sleep. The restoration of sleep stability in successfully treated patients may be seen as a decrease in time spent awake during the sleep cycle after the use of an AED and may be a consequence of an increased arousal threshold [114–116]. In addition, some AEDs can be weight inducing, thus fragmenting sleep, along with predisposing the individual to OSA [10]. Benzodiazepines and barbiturates may cause increased upper airway musculature relaxation and alter responsiveness to changes in carbon dioxide and oxygen saturation [117]. The effects of AEDs on sleep are summarized in Table 5.6 [9,25,86,114–116].

2. **Vagus nerve stimulation** (VNS) therapy, a US Food and Drug Administration–approved adjunctive therapy for refractory epilepsy, affects respiration during sleep and has been shown to worsen preexisting OSA. Consistent sleep-related decreases in airflow and effort coinciding with VNS activation have been documented, with apneas and hypopneas found to be more frequent during VNS activation than during nonactivation. VNS may also interfere with effective CPAP titration [118]. A retrospective chart review was conducted on 26 children who had VNS implantation for refractory epilepsy by Khurana et al [119]. Four patients (15%) had OSA detected after placement of VNS. Therefore, performing PSGs before implantation of VNS should be considered to identify patients with preexisting OSA.
3. **Ketogenic diet** (KD) is a high-fat, low-carbohydrate diet used to treat patients with medically intractable epilepsy. Although the mechanisms underlying the clinical effects of the KD remain unclear, there are emerging links between circadian rhythms and the KD [120]. Hallböök et al [121] have recently evaluated sleep during KD treatment in children with therapy-resistant epilepsy to correlate possible alterations in sleep architecture with changes in clinical effects on seizure reduction, seizure

Table 5.6 Effects of antiepileptic drugs on sleep architecture and sleep complaints

Drug	Total sleep time	Sleep latency	Arousals	% Stage 1	% Stage 2	% Slow-wave sleep	% Rapid eye movement	Sleep efficiency	Sleep complaint
Carbamazepine	0	↓	↓	0	0	↑	↓/0	↑	Sleepiness
Ethosuximide	?	?	↑	↑	0	↓	↑	↓	Insomnia
Gabapentin	↑	?	↓	↓	0	↑	↑	↑	Sleepiness
Lamotrigine	0	0	0	0	0	?	↑	0	Insomnia
Levetiracetam	0	0	0	0	↑	↓	0	0	Sleepiness
Phenobarbital	0	↓	↓	↑	↑	0	↓	↓	Sleepiness
Phenytoin	0	↓	↓	↑	↑	↓	0	↓	Sleepiness
Tiagabin	?	?	?	?	?	?	?	?	Insomnia
Topiramate	?	?	?	?	?	?	?	?	Sleepiness
Valproate	0	0	↑	↓	0	↑	↓	0	Sleepiness
Vigabatrin	?	0	?	?	?	?	?	?	Sleepiness
Zonisamide	?	?	?	?	?	?	?	?	Insomnia

↑, increase; ↓ ,decrease; 0, no change; ?, unknown.
From Refs. [9,25,86,114–116].

severity, quality of life (QOL), and behavior. The results of this study showed that KD decreases sleep time but improves sleep quality in children with therapy-resistant epilepsy. The improvement in sleep quality, with increased REM sleep, seems to contribute to the improvement in QOL. The reduction of IEDs and seizures on KD could also contribute to improved sleep, with reduced EDS and improved quality of life.

Sleep Phenomena Mimicking Seizures

Several sleep phenomena may occur during nighttime, taking a wide variety of forms, and can mimic seizures. Sleep-related paroxysmal disorders in infancy and childhood represent a significant challenge for the clinician, with the distinction of nocturnal epilepsy from nonepileptic sleep disorders often being the primary concern [32]. Although in some patients, diagnosis is easy to achieve, at times a video-EEG recording of the episodes is required because of the similarity of the nonepileptic events to epileptic seizures [122].

With the *International Classification of Sleep Disorders*, 2nd edition, developed by the American Academy of Sleep Medicine in 2005, these disorders mimicking epilepsy can be broadly grouped into parasomnias, sleep-related breathing disorders, sleep-related movement disorders, and "others" [15]. In addition certain sleep phenomenon can occur in wakefulness in the daytime also, thus mimicking epilepsy.

These phenomena have been summarized in Table 5.7 [15,32]).

Parasomnias: More than 80% of preschool-age children experience parasomnias, which are a big source of confusion in differentiating them from nocturnal seizures [123,124]. The various parasomnias have been summarized in a chapter in this issue. Features differentiating them from seizures will be addressed here and have been summarized in Table 5.8 [32,125].

Parasomnias Predominately Associated With NREM Sleep

NREM arousal parasomnias are paroxysmal behaviors without conscious awareness, usually arising from stage 3 or 4 NREM sleep. Based on the occurrence of motor activity and the autonomic involvement, they are classically subdivided into 3 main forms: confusional arousals (little motor or autonomic involvement), somnambulism (mainly motor activity but little autonomic involvement), and sleep terrors (prominent autonomic involvement with variable motor activity) [15]. Although parasomnias are generally benign, frequent or unusual episodes may sometimes be confused with epilepsy, particularly NFLE [23,38,125,126].

Confusional arousals (sleep drunkenness), seen in young children, are characterized by sudden arousals usually from deeper NREM sleep stages, with disorientation and prolonged confusion on awakening, sometimes accompanied with complex behaviors, but without conscious awareness. They are very common, but under-recognized by non–sleep physicians, and are frequently misinterpreted as nocturnal seizures.

Somnambulism (sleep walking), seen in adolescents, consists of leaving the bed and performing complex activities such as walking, but with no memory of the event. It occurs during slow-wave sleep and is of various duration and complexity. Some patients can be agitated during the episode [32].

Sleep terrors, seen in toddlers, are the most dramatic of the arousal disorders, characterized by prominent autonomic and affective features. The individual will suddenly arouse from deep sleep, usually with a "blood-curdling" scream, and appear pale and terrified. Often agitated behavior is seen, and sometimes the individual will attempt to leave the room; extreme agitation may result in injuries from jumping out of windows or falling down stairs [32]. They can usually be distinguished from seizures by their exclusive occurrence in sleep combined with the expression of extreme fear on the face. Multiple episodes per night, abnormal rhythmic movements, posturing of extremities, eye deviation, shorter duration of event but prolonged confusion, drooling, and tongue biting are suspicious for seizures [14]. However, it must be reemphasized that occurrence only out of sleep, expression of fear on the face, and accompanying aggressive behavior can also be seen in FLE and has been further discussed under the sleep-related epilepsy section in this chapter. In a recent paper, Derry et al [125] evaluated systematically the semiological features

Table 5.7 Paroxysmal disorders of sleep mimicking epilepsy (ASDA, 2005)

Nighttime sleep episodes

Daytime sleep episodes

Narcolepsy with cataplexy
Episodic hypersomnia with narcolepsy

PARASOMNIAS	SLEEP-RELATED MOVEMENT DISORDERS	OTHER
Non-REM arousal disorders		
Confusional arousals	Periodic limb movements of sleep	Sleep starts Somniloquy Benign sleep myoclonus of infancy
Sleep walking	Sleep bruxism	Nocturnal psychogenic nonepileptic seizures (PNES) Nocturnal panic attacks
Sleep terrors	Nocturnal leg cramps	Sleep-related breathing disorders (obstructive sleep apnea) Gastroesophageal reflux
REM sleep disorders		
Nightmares REM behavior disorder Parasomnia overlap syndrome Sleep paralysis	Rhythmic movement disorders	Narcolepsy (hypnogogic/hypnopompic hallucinations, sleep paralysis) Sleepenuresis Newly recognized conditions Excessive fragmentary myoclonus Propriospinal myoclonus at sleep onset Rhythmic sleep movements while falling asleep Alternating leg muscle activation during sleep and arousals
Others		
Catathrenia (nocturnal groaning)		

Abbreviation: REM, rapid eye movement.
From Refs. [15,32].

of 120 events recorded on video-EEG monitoring (57 parasomnias, 63 NFLE seizures) from 44 subjects to identify features that can be used to reliably distinguish parasomnias from NFLE. Elemental clinical features strongly favoring parasomnias included: interactive behavior, failure to wake after event, and indistinct offset. Although sleep stage at onset was discriminatory (82% of seizures occurred during stage 1 or 2 sleep, with 100% of parasomnias occurring from stage 3 or 4 sleep), ictal EEG features were less useful. Video analysis of parasomnias identified 3 principal behavioral patterns: arousal behavior (92% of events), nonagitated motor behavior (72%), and distressed emotional behavior (51%). A diagnostic decision tree generated from these data correctly classified 94% of events. Although sleep stage at onset was discriminatory (82% of seizures occurred during stage 1 or 2 sleep, with 100% of parasomnias occurring from stage 3 or 4 sleep), ictal EEG features were less useful. During sleep, physiological stimuli (external or

Table 5.8 Comparison of clinical and video EEG/PSG features of parasomnias vs NFLE and important quantitative and qualitative features which can be used in the positive identification of parasomnias

	Parasomnias	**Nocturnal frontal lobe epilepsy (NFLE)**
Age at onset	Usually <10 yr	Variable; usually childhood or adolescence
Family history	60%–90%	≤40%
Attacks per night (mean)	1 or 2	>3
Episode frequency per month	<1 to 4	20–40
Clinical course (over years)	Trends to disappear by adolescence	Often stable with increasing age
Disease duration (mean)	~7 yr	~20 yr
Episode duration (mean)	Seconds to 30 min	Seconds to 3 min (often <2 min)
Semiology of movements *(for details see further down)*	Variable complexity; not highly stereotyped (on video)	Highly stereotyped on video monitoring; often vigorous movements
Trigger factors	Sleep deprivation, febrile illness, alcohol, stress	Often not identified
Associated conditions	Obstructive sleep apnea	Often not identified
Ictal EEG	Slow waves, no epileptiform features	Often normal or obscured by movements. Frankly epileptiform ictal rhythms in <10%
Time of episodes during sleep	First third of the night, but usually after 90 min of sleep	Any time, but may occur in first 30–60 min
Polysomnographic sleep stages when events occur	Non-rapid eye movement sleep stage 3 or 4	Usually non-rapid eye movement sleep stage 1, occasionally 3 or 4

Important quantitative and qualitative features which can be used in the positive identification of parasomnias

Features strongly favoring parasomnias	**Features moderately favoring parasomnias**	**Features which do not discriminate between parasomnias and NFLE**
Yawning Scratching and prominent nose rubbing Rolling over in bed Internal or external trigger (noise, cough, snore) Waxing and waning pattern Physical or verbal interaction Sobbing, sad emotional behavior Indistinct offset Failure to fully arouse after event with complex behavior Prolonged duration (>2 min) Discordance between severity and duration of *reported* event and *recorded* event	Tremor/trembling Myoclonic jerks Coughing Semipurposeful behaviors, fumbling, manipulation of nearby objects Variability/absence of stereotypy No events recorded on first night of monitoring Few events recorded in total (>3)	Brevity Sitting Standing or walking* Preceding "normal" arousal Brief arousals (up to 10 s) without definite semiological features of epilepsy Fearful emotional behavior *Standing and walking do not, in usual circumstances, discriminate between parasomnias and NFLE. However, in individuals who rouse to full wakefulness after their events, and in whom events have an indistinct offset, standing or walking suggests a diagnosis of parasomnias over NFLE

Abbreviation: EEG, electroencephalogram; PSG, polysomnography; NFLE, nocturnal frontal lobe epilepsy.
From Refs. [32,125].

internal) or subclinical seizure discharges can induce indistinguishable arousal behaviors. In parasomnias, these may evolve to a clinical parasomnia or terminate with return to sleep or full waking. In individuals with nocturnal epilepsy, clinically evident seizures with distinguishing characteristic behaviours and marked stereotypy may occur or the event may terminate with full

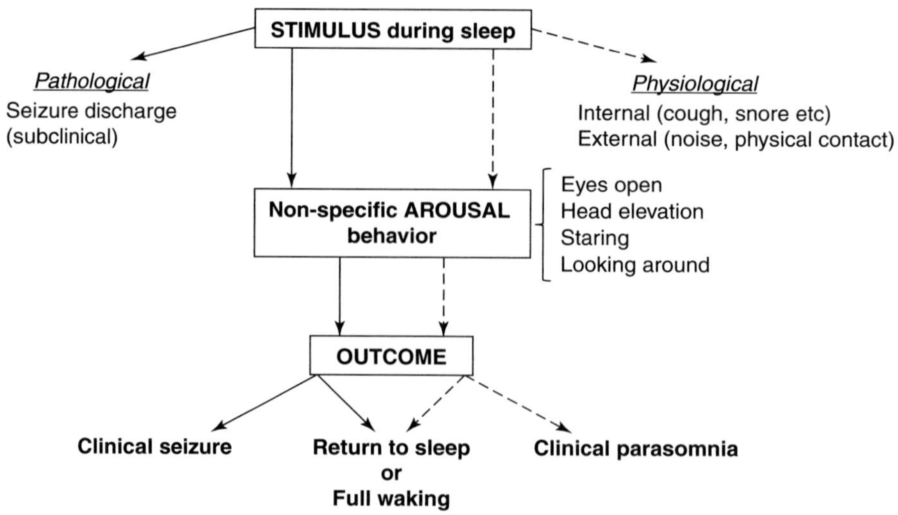

Figure 5.3 Stimulus during sleep can induce arousal behaviors. In parasomnia subjects (dashed arrows), these may evolve to a clinical parasomnia or terminate with return to sleep or full waking. In individuals with nocturnal epilepsy (heavy arrows), clinically evident seizures may occur, or the event may terminate with full waking or return to sleep [125].

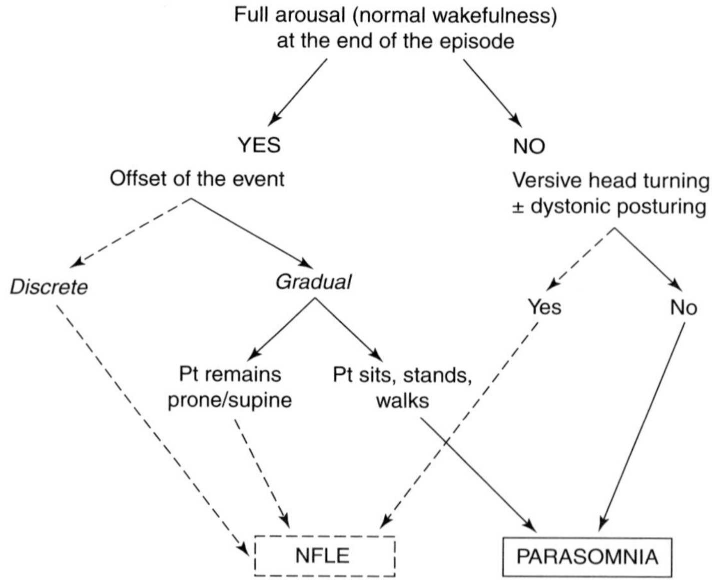

Figure 5.4 Diagnostic classification tree.

waking or return to sleep (Figure 5.3) [125]. The diagnostic classification tree, based on video features only, is shown in Figure 5.4. In the data set of this study, the algorithm correctly classified 113 of 120 (94%) events. The comparison of clinical and video-EEG/PSG features of parasomnias vs NFLE and important quantitative and qualitative features, which can be used in the positive identification of parasomnias, is shown in Table 5.8 [32,125].

Sleep deprivation, poor sleep hygiene, hypnotic use, or fragmented sleep (especially because of OSA) increases the frequency of these parasomnias [127]. Onset of events within 30 minutes of sleep onset is suggestive of seizures, whereas onset at 2 hours after sleep onset is more suggestive of NREM parasomnias.

Disorders Predominately Associated With REM Sleep

Nightmares, seen in toddlers and young children, consist of frightening dreams that often awaken the patient from sleep and can be accompanied by agitation. There is generally full alertness on awakening from a nightmare and intact recall of the dream experience. Unlike NREM phenomena such as sleep terrors, there is usually no thrashing or ambulation. As REM sleep is preponderant during the second half of the night, nightmares tend to occur in the early hours of the morning [124].

REM behavior disorder: The presence of REM sleep without atonia (RSWA), with prominent motor and behavioral manifestations associated with dreaming during REM sleep, is the key feature of a condition called REM sleep behavior disorder (RBD) [15], which may be idiopathic or associated with other neurological disease including narcolepsy and parkinsonian syndromes [128]. The bizarre movements, such as kicking, punching, vocalization, and running accompanying these, can mimic nocturnal seizures. Injury to extremities during these events is common, whereas injuries during seizures are uncommon. Video-PSG may help in differentiating seizures from RBD. In children, narcolepsy remains the leading cause of RBD [129], though an important but unrecognized precipitating factor is concomitant use of selective serotonin reuptake inhibitor (SSRI) antidepressants [130]. Other causes of RBD in children include cases of infiltrating tumors of the pons, postexcision of midline cerebellar astrocytomas, Tourette syndrome, autism, hereditary quivering chin syndrome, traumatic brain injury, juvenile Parkinson disease, posttraumatic stress disorder, xeroderma pigmentosa, West syndrome, and olivopontocerebellar atrophy. Recently in children, the entity of "subclinical RBD," with lack of REM atonia on PSG but without clinical features, has been recognized [131]. In addition, Ferri et al used quantitative and computerized methods of analysis of the EMG signals and found significant PSG evidence of motor dyscontrol among patients with narcolepsy/cataplexy compared with controls. They used REM sleep atonia index as a marker and found 38% of patients with narcolepsy/cataplexy to have RSWA related to short-lasting EMG activity [132].Overall, subclinical RBD may be more common in narcolepsy, but remains unrecognized [129].

Overlap parasomnias: These have the characteristics of both NREM and REM sleep parasomnias and may be considered in the differential diagnosis of nocturnal seizures.

Other parasomnias: Catathrenia (nocturnal groaning) is a newly recognized parasomnia with unclear effects on sleep and life quality, and which can mimic seizures [133]. It is characterized by repeated episodes of monotonous vocalization with prolonged expiration (episodes of bradypnea) occurring mostly in REM sleep. The hallmark of catathrenia is that inspiration is followed by protracted expiration during which a prolonged or fragmented sound is produced, and this recurs especially during REM sleep [134]. Video-PSG will help sort out this condition from nocturnal frontal lobe seizures, which is rare in REM sleep. However, this condition has yet to be described in the pediatric population.

Sleep-Related Movement Disorders

Periodic limb movements of sleep (PLMS) consist of repetitive cycles of rhythmic movement usually occurring in one or both legs but sometimes involving the arms, at 5 times per hour, 0.5 to 5 seconds in duration, in clusters of 4 or more leg movements, separated by 5 to 90 seconds [135]. Patients are usually unaware of the movements but may report frequent awakenings. They are rarely confused with seizures, but can cause daytime sleepiness. Actigraphy seems suitable in screening for PLMS over a few days time in an ambulatory setting [136].

Bruxism consists of teeth grinding and clenching movements of jaws during sleep. It is common in children and teenagers and may persist into adulthood. It is often seen in children with intellectual disabilities and with use of SSRIs. It may lead to sleep fragmentation with daytime hypersomnia and features similar to ADHD [137]. It has also been recently described as a manifestation of temporal lobe seizures [138].

Rhythmic Movement Disorders of Sleep

Jactatio capitis (headbanging) is characterized by rhythmic head banging, and head rolling, along with body rocking, occurring in wakefulness, during transition into sleep, or during sleep. They are seen in children with intellectual disability, pervasive developmental disorders, or even in normal children. They can mimic nocturnal seizures. Reassurance of the parents is vital; rare cases need pharmacological intervention with use of clonazepam [139]. When Rhythmic movement disorders persists into childhood and beyond, possibility of behavioral, psychiatric, and attentional issues as comorbid conditions should be evaluated for [140].

Other Paroxysmal Events

Sleep starts, also known as hypnic jerks, are an extremely common phenomenon and are essentially physiologic in nature. They consist of brief myoclonic jerks, usually affecting the whole body at the transition of wakefulness and sleep. They are often associated with sensory phenomena, most commonly a sensation of falling. Caffeine, stimulants, stress, and excessive exercise may increase their frequency in some individuals [15]. When they become frequent and are accompanied with awakenings, they are seen in children with migraines and those suffering from neurological impairments including cerebral palsy and epilepsy and can mimic epileptic spasms [122].

Somniloquy (sleep talking) usually occurs during light NREM sleep or during arousals from deeper sleep, but occasionally arises during REM sleep [32]. It usually consists of single words or short sentences, usually with minimal effective content and is sometimes associated with body movement [32]. Unlike seizures, speech during these episodes is random, whereas ictal speech tends to be stereotypical in a given individual. With somniloquy, there is usually a lack of abnormal body movements, drooling, tongue biting, or incontinence [125].

Benign sleep myoclonus of infancy is a common source of referral for video-EEG monitoring to rule out seizures. The myoclonus can be generalized or fragmented, whereas the infant and EEG monitoring is always normal.

Nocturnal psychogenic nonepileptic seizures (PNES) are not uncommon in childhood and adolescents. Video-EEG monitoring confirms that they arise out of wakefulness, even though they appear in sleep and are characterized by bizarre, nonrhythmic movements, with waxing-waning character and long durations. Common precipitating factors in children and teenagers include physical and sexual abuse [141].

Nocturnal panic attacks are characterized by brief awakening out of NREM sleep accompanied with choking sensation in the throat along with other respiratory symptoms and similar symptoms in the daytime consistent with panic attacks [142]. They are not uncommon in adolescent girls, and video-EEG monitoring is often necessary in differentiating them from orbitofrontal nocturnal seizures.

Sleep-related breathing disorder (obstructive sleep apnea) The symptoms such as choking, gasping, and abnormal postures in sleep accompanying OSA are sometimes confused with nocturnal frontal lobe seizures. In some patients, OSA can provoke seizures or be the primary reason for intractability of epilepsy [69,97]. Increasing evidence also suggests that OSA may trigger arousal parasomnias [143]. Interestingly, a recent paper found bursts of paroxysmal activity with embedded spikes on EEGs in children with OSA but not from children with habitual snoring, thus further complicating the issue of differentiating nocturnal events because of OSA from seizures. These bursts have been postulated to be responsible for the neurocognitive deficits observed in the daytime in children with OSA [144].

Narcolepsy is a chronic and potentially disabling REM sleep disorder resulting from the dysregulation of sleep-wake cycle [130] that affects 0.03% to 0.16% of the general population including children in various ethnic groups [145].

Sleep paralysis is characterized by brief episodes of inability to move, generally occurring on awakening, and relieved by touching or speaking to the child. Sleep paralysis can be accompanied by *hypnagogic* (during the transition from wakefulness to sleep) or *hypnopompic* (during the transition from sleep to wakefulness) *hallucinations,* which consist of vivid visual or auditory experiences, usually of a benign content [15]. However, both these symptoms can be unrecognized or misinterpreted by young children or their parents. They may seem to resemble nightmares in children and may be frightening and can also mimic nocturnal seizures. They can happen as an isolated phenomenon in variable frequency in normal children but can also occur in narcolepsy.

Gastroesophageal reflux (Sandifer syndrome) can present with nocturnal arousals and bizarre postures and paroxysmal movements, along with torticollis in the daytime [146,147]. It presents typically between the ages of 2 months and 5 years. The episodic nature of attacks often results in misdiagnosis of paroxysmal dystonia, or epilepsy [147].

Sleep enuresis can occur in NREM or REM and affects approximately 4% to 15% of school children [148]. As these episodes are typically unwitnessed, atypical characteristics of rhythmic body movements, tongue bite, or unexplained bruising warrant neurological evaluation and in some cases video-EEG monitoring to rule out unrecognized seizures [14].

Daytime Episodes

Cataplexy is the presence of REM intrusion in wakefulness in patients with narcolepsy, with sudden but brief flaccid drop attacks in the daytime. These can mimic atonic seizures. Recently Serra et al [149] have described features of cataplexy in children, emphasizing that isolated cataplexy without hypersomnia can present at the onset of narcolepsy in 10% of children. Atypical features are more common in childhood, with falls present in only 43% cases. Most have only partial cataplexy involving face, eyelids, slurred speech, tongue thrusting, and blank stares. The usual triggers of emotion are not present, and children are often unaware of these symptoms, thus making diagnosis difficult. The authors also describe "cataplectic facies" with semipermanent jaw and eyelid weakness. Video-PSG may be necessary to seperate these drop attacks of cataplexy from the tonic-atonic seizures of Lennox Gastaut syndrome or Doose syndrome (myoclonic astatic epilepsy syndrome).

Thus, from the above description, the *evaluation* of sleep phenomena mimicking seizures involves [44,45]

1. a detailed history
2. capture the events on home videos by encouraging family members
3. routine/sleep-deprived EEG
4. 24-hour ambulatory EEGs
5. video-EEG and video-PSGs

Summary and Conclusions

Epilepsy and sleep disorders are considered by many to be common bedfellows. Several sleep phenomena may occur during nighttime, taking a wide variety of forms, and which can mimic seizures. Although most seizure subtypes have the potential to occur during sleep or wakefulness, sleep has a well-documented and strong association with specific epilepsy syndromes. Seizures in sleep also tend to occur during lighter stages of NREM sleep. The neurophysiologic process involved in the deepening of NREM sleep may also facilitate both seizures and IEDs. Epilepsy per se and/or seizures themselves promote sleep disruption and affect significantly the quality, quantity, and the architecture of sleep. There are many causes of sleep disruption in patients with epilepsy, including inadequate sleep hygiene, coexisting sleep disorders, and circadian rhythm disturbances. Seizures themselves can disrupt sleep, even when they occur during wakefulness. AEDs can also alter sleep in positive and negative ways, and these effects are independent of the anticonvulsant actions. The result of sleep disruption is EDS, worsening seizures, and poor quality of life. Screening for sleep disorders in epilepsy population and appropriate intervention strategies will lead to overall improved quality of life and seizure control.

References

1. Malow B. Sleep and epilepsy. *Neurol Clin.* 1996; 14(4):765–789.
2. Mendez M, Radtke RA. Interactions between sleep and epilepsy. *J Clin Neurophysiol.* 2001;18(2): 106–127.
3. Bazil CW. Sleep and epilepsy. *Curr Opin Neurol.* 2000;13(2):171–175.
4. De Weerd A, de Haas S, Otte A, et al. Subjective sleep disturbance in patients with partial epilepsy: a questionnaire-based study on prevalence and impact on quality of life. *Epilepsia.* 2004;45(11):1397–1404.
5. Sterman MB, Shouse MN, Passouant P. Effects of epilepsy on sleep, overview. In: Sterman MB, Shouse MN, Passouant P, eds. *Sleep and Epilepsy.* New York, NY: Academic Press; 1982:325–327.

6. Hoeppner JB, Garron DC, Cartwright RD. Self-reported sleep disorder symptoms in epilepsy. *Epilepsia*. 1984;25(4): 434–437.
7. Declerck AC, Wauquier A, Sijben-Kiggen R. Normative study of sleep in different forms of epilepsy. In: Sterman MB, Shouse MN, Passouant P, eds. *Sleep and Epilepsy*. New York, NY: Academic Press; 1982:329–333.
8. Carney PR, Kohrman MH. Relation between epilepsy and sleep during infancy and childhood. In: Bazil CW, Malow BA, Sammaritano MR, eds. *Sleep and Epilepsy: The Clinical Spectrum*. Amsterdam: Elsevier Science; 2002:359–372.
9. Bazil CW. Epilepsy and sleep disturbance. *Epilepsy Behav*. 2003;(4)(suppl 2):S39–S45.
10. Kothare SV, Kaleyias J. The adverse effects of antiepileptic drugs in children. *Expert Opin Drug Saf*. 2007;6(3):251–265.
11. Becker DA, Fennell EB, Carney PR. Sleep disturbance in children with epilepsy. *Epilepsy Behav*. 2003;4(6):651–658.
12. Kotagal P, Yardi N. The relationship between sleep and epilepsy. *Semin Pediatr Neurol*. 2008;15(2): 42–49.
13. Passouant P. Historical aspects of sleep and epilepsy. *Epilepsy Res Suppl*. 1991;2:19–30.
14. Bazil CW. Nocturnal seizures. *Semin Neurol*. 2004;24(3):293–300.
15. American Academy of Sleep Medicine. International classification of sleep disorders. 2nd ed. In: *Diagnostic and Coding Manual*. Westchester, IL: American Academy of Sleep Medicine; 2005.
16. Crespel A, Baldy-Moulinier M, Coubes P. The relationship between sleep and epilepsy in frontal and temporal lobe epilepsies: practical and physiologic considerations. *Epilepsia*. 1998;39(2):150–157.
17. Bazil CW, Walczak TS. Effects of sleep and sleep stage on epileptic and nonepileptic seizures. *Epilepsia*. 1997;38(1):56–62.
18. Herman ST, Walczak TS, Bazil CW. Distribution of partial seizures during the sleep-wake cycle: differences by seizures onset site. *Neurology*. 2001;56(11):1453–1458.
19. Durazzo TS, Spencer SS, Duckrow RB, Novotny EJ, Spencer DD, Zaveri HP. Temporal distributions of seizure occurrence from various epileptogenic regions. *Neurology*. 2008;70(15):1265–1271.
20. Hofstra WA, Grootemarsink BE, Dieker R, van der Palen J, de Weerd AW. Temporal distribution of clinical seizures over the 24-h day: a retrospective observational study in a tertiary epilepsy clinic. *Epilepsia*. 2009;50(9):2019–2026.
21. Hofstra WA, Spetgens WP, Leijten FS, et al. Diurnal rhythms in seizures detected by intracranial electrocorticographic monitoring: an observational study. *Epilepsy Behav*. 2009;14(4):617–621.
22. Pavlova MK, Shea SA, Bromfield EB. Day/night patterns of focal seizures. *Epilepsy Behav*. 2004;5(1):44–49.
23. Provini F, Plazzi G, Tinuper P, Vandi S, Lugaresi E, Montagna P. Nocturnal frontal lobe epilepsy. A clinical and polygraphic overview of 100 consecutive cases. *Brain*. 1999;122(pt 6):1017–1031.
24. Ryvlin P, Rheims S, Risse G. Nocturnal frontal lobe epilepsy. *Epilepsia*. 2006;47(suppl 2):83–86.
25. Bazil CW. Sleep and Epilepsy. *Semin Neurol*. 2002;22(3):321–327.
26. Malow BA, Selwa LM, Ross D, Aldrich MS. Lateralizing value of Interictal spikes on overnight sleep-EEG studies in temporal lobe epilepsy. *Epilepsia*. 1999;40(11):1587–1192.
27. Scheffer IE, Bhatia KP, Lopes-Cendes I, et al. Autosomal dominant nocturnal frontal lobe epilepsy. A distinctive clinical disorder. *Brain*. 2005;118:61–73.
28. Nobili L, Francione S, Mai R, et al. Surgical treatment of drug-resistant nocturnal frontal lobe epilepsy. *Brain*. 2007;130:561–573.
29. Combi R, Dalpra L, Tenchini ML, Ferini-Strambi L. Autosomal dominant nocturnal frontal lobe epilepsy-a critical overview. *J Neurol*. 2004;251(8):923–934.
30. Scheffer IE, Bhatia KP, Lopes-Cendes I, et al. Autosomal dominant nocturnal frontal lobe epilepsy. A distinctive clinical disorder. *Brain*. 1995; 118(pt 1):61–73.
31. Phillips HA, Scheffer IE, Crossland KM, et al. Autosomal dominant nocturnal frontal-lobe epilepsy: genetic heterogeneity and evidence for a second locus at 15q24. *Am J Hum Genet*. 1998;63(4):1108–1116.
32. Derry CP, Duncan JS, Berkovic SF. Paroxysmal motor disorders of sleep: the clinical spectrum and differentiation from epilepsy. *Epilepsia*. 2006;47(11):1775–1791.
33. Plazzi G, Tinuper P, Montagna P, Provini F, Lugaresi E. Epileptic nocturnal wanderings. *Sleep*. 1995;18(9):749–756.
34. Provini F, Plazzi G, Lugaresi E. From nocturnal paroxysmal dystonia to nocturnal frontal lobe epilepsy. *Clin Neurophysiol*. 2000;111(suppl 2):S2–S8.
35. Lombroso CT. Nocturnal paroxysmal dystonia due to a subfrontal cortical dysplasia. *Epileptic Disord*. 2000;2(1):15–20.
36. Tinuper P, Provini F, Bisulli F, et al. Movement disorders in sleep: Guidelines for differentiating epileptic from non-epileptic motor phenomena arising from sleep. *Sleep Med Rev*. 2007;11(4):255–267.
37. Peled R, Lavie P. Paroxysmal awakenings from sleep associated with excessive daytime somnolence: a form of nocturnal epilepsy. *Neurology*. 1986;36(1):95–98.
38. Provini F, Plazzi G, Montagna P, Lugaresi E. The wide clinical spectrum of nocturnal frontal lobe epilepsy. *Sleep Med Rev*. 2000;4(4):375–386.
39. Salanova V, Morris HH, Van Ness P, Kotagal P, Wyllie E, Lüders H. Frontal lobe seizures: electroclinical syndromes. *Epilepsia*. 1995;36:16–24.
40. Mai R, Sartori I, Francione S, et al. Sleep-related hyperkinetic seizures: always a frontal onset? *Neurol Sci*. 2005;26(suppl 3):S220–S224.
41. Nobili L, Cossu M, Mai R, et al. Sleep-related hyperkinetic seizures of temporal lobe origin. *Neurology*. 2004;62:482–485.
42. Nobili L, Francione S, Cardinale F, Lo Russo G. Epileptic nocturnal wanderings with a temporal

lobe origin, a stereo-EEG study. *Sleep*, 2002;25: 669–671.
43. Dobesberger J, Ortler M, Unterberger I, et al. Successful surgical treatment of insular epilepsy with nocturnal hypermotor seizures. *Epilepsia*. 2008;49:159–162.
44. Taylor DC, Falconer MA, Bruton CJ, Corsellis JA. Focal dysplasia of the cerebral cortex in epilepsy. *J Neurol Neurosurg Psychiatry*. 1971;34: 369–387.
45. Nobili L, Cardinale F, Magliola U, et al. Taylor's focal cortical dysplasia increases the risk for sleep-related epilepsy. *Epilepsia*, 2009;50:2599–2604.
46. Pung T, Schmitz B. Circadian rhythm and personality profile in juvenile myoclonic epilepsy. *Epilepsia*. 2006;47(suppl 2):S111–S114.
47. Badawy RA, Macdonell RA, Jackson GD, Berkovic SF. Why do seizures in generalized epilepsy often occur in the morning? *Neurology*. 2009;73(3):218–222.
48. Labate A, Ambrosio R, Gambardella A, Sturniolo M, Pucci F, Quattrone A. Usefulness of a morning routine EEG recording in patients with juvenile myoclonicepilepsy. *Epilepsy Res*. 2007;77(11):17–21.
49. Wirrell EC. Benign epilepsy of childhood with centrotemporal spikes. *Epilepsia*. 1998;39(suppl 4): S32–S34.
50. Baglietto MG, Battaglia FM, Nobili L, et al. Neuropsychological disorders related to interictal epileptic discharges during sleep in benign epilepsy of childhood with centrotemporal or Rolandic spikes. *Dev Med Child Neurol*. 2001;43(6):407–412.
51. McVicar KA, Shinnar S. Landau-Kleffner syndrome, electrical status epilepticus in slow wave sleep, and language regression in children. *Ment Retard Dev Disabil Res Rev*. 2004;10(2):144–149.
52. Jayakar PB, Seshia SS. Electrical status epilepticus during slow-wave sleep: a review. *Clin Neurophysiol*. 1991;8(3):299–311.
53. Capovilla G, Striano P, Beccaria F. Changes in Panayiotopoulos syndrome over time. *Epilepsia*. 2009;50(suppl 5):S45–S48.
54. Minecan D, Natarajan A, Marzec M, Malow B. Relationship of epileptic seizures to sleep stage and sleep depth. *Sleep*. 2002;25(8):56–61.
55. Sammaritano M, Gigli GL, Gotman J. Interictal spikes during wakefulness and sleep and localization of foci in temporal lobe epilepsy. *Neurology*. 1991;41(2, pt 1):290–297.
56. Malow BA, Lin X, Kushwaha R, Alrich MS. Interictal spiking increases with sleep depth in temporal lobe epilepsy. *Epilepsia*. 1998;39(12):1309–1316.
57. Malow BA, Aldrich MS. Localizing value of rapid eye movement sleep in temporal lobe epilepsy. *Sleep Med*. 2000;1(1):57–60.
58. Ferrillo F, Beelke M, Nobili L. Sleep EEG synchronization mechanisms and activation of interictal epileptic spikes. *Clin Neurophysiol*. 2000;111 (suppl 2):S65–S73.
59. Terzano MG, Parrino I, Spiaggiari MC, Barusi R, Simeoni S. Discriminatory effect of cyclic-alternating pattern in focal lesional and benign rolandic interictal spikes during sleep. *Epilepsia*. 1991;32(5): 616–628.
60. Beelke M, Nobili L, Baglietto MG, et al. Relationship of sigma activity to sleep interictal epileptic discharges: a study in children affected by benign epilepsy with occipital paroxysms. *Epilepsy Res*. 2000;40(2–3):179–186.
61. Nobili L, Ferrillo F, Baglietto MG, et al. Relationship of sleep interictal epileptiform discharges to sigma activity(12–16 Hz) in benign epilepsy of childhood with rolandic spikes. *Clin Neurophysiol*. 1999;110(1): 39–46.
62. Gibbs E, Gibbs F. Diagnostic and localizing value of electroencephalographic studies in sleep. *Assoc Res Nerv Ment Dis*. 1947; 26,366–377.
63. Fountain NB, Kim JS, Lee SI. Sleep deprivation activates epileptiform discharges independent of the activating effects of sleep. *J Clin Neurophysiol*. 1998;15(1):69–75.
64. Touchon J, Badly-Mouliner M, Billiard M, Besset A. Cadilhac J. Sleep organization and epilepsy. *Epilepsy Res*. 1991;2(suppl):S73–S81.
65. Steriades M, Conteras D, Amzica F. Synchronized sleep oscillations and their paroxysmal developments. *Trends Neurosci*. 1994;17(5):199–208.
66. Shouse MN, Siegel JM, Wu MF, Szymusiak R, Morrison AR. Mechanisms of seizure suppression during rapid-eye movement sleep in cats. *Brain Res*. 1989;505(2):271–282.
67. Touchon J, Badly-Moulinier M, Billiard M, Besset A, Cadilhac J. Sleep organization and epilepsy. In: Degen R, Rodin EA, eds. *Epilepsy, Sleep and Sleep Deprivation*. New York, NY: Elsevier; 1991: 73–81.
68. Miano S, PiaVilla M, Blanco D, et al. Development of NREM sleep instability-continuity (cyclic alternating pattern) in healthy term infants aged 1 to 4 months. *Sleep*. 2009;32(1):83–90.
69. Devinsky O, Ehrenberg B, Barthlen GM, Abramson HS, Luciano D. Epilepsy and sleep apnea syndrome. *Neurology*. 1994;44(11):2060–2064.
70. Malow BA, Fromes GA, Aldrich MS. Usefulness of polysomnography in epilepsy patients. *Neurology*. 1997;48(5):1389–1394.
71. Jones BE. Glia, adenosine, and sleep. *Neuron*. 2009; 61(2):156–157.
72. Landolt HP. Sleep homeostasis: a role for adenosine in humans? *Biochem Pharmacol*. 2008; 75(11):2070–2079.
73. Boison D. The adenosine kinase hypothesis of epileptogenesis. *Prog Neurobiol*. 2008;84(3): 249–262.
74. Boison D, Stewart KA.Therapeutic epilepsy research: From pharmacological rationale to focal adenosine augmentation. *Biochem Pharmacol*. 2009;78(12):1428–1437.
75. Stewart LS, Leung LS. Hippocampal melatonin receptors modulate seizure threshold. *Epilepsia*. 2005;46(4):473–480.
76. Muñoz-Hoyos A, Sánchez-Forte M, Molina-Carballo A, et al. Melatonin's role as an anticonvulsant and neuronal protector: experimental and clinical evidence. *J Child Neurol*. 1998;13(10): 501–509.

77. Yildirim M, Marangoz C. Anticonvulsant effects of melatonin on penicillin-induced epileptiform activity in rats. *Brain Res.* 2006;1099(1):183–188.
78. Schapel GJ, Beran RG, Kennaway DL, McLoughney J, Matthews CD. Melatonin response in active epilepsy. *Epilepsia.* 1995;36:75–78.
79. Yalýn O, Arman F, Erdoğan F, Kula M. A comparison of the circadian rhythms and the levels of melatonin in patients with diurnal and nocturnal complex partial seizures. *Epilepsy Behav.* 2006;8(3):542–546.
80. Bazil CW, Short D, Crispin D, Zheng W. Patients with intractable epilepsy have low melatonin, which increases following seizures. *Neurology.* 2000;55(11):1746–1748.
81. Baxendale S. Seeing the light? Seizures and sunlight. *Epilepsy Res.* 2009;84(1):72–76.
82. Sheldon SH. Pro-convulsant effects of melatonin in neurologically disabled children. *Lancet.* 1998;351(9111):1254.
83. Jan JE, Hamilton D, Seward N, et al. Clinical trials of controlled-release melatonin in children with sleep-wake cycle disorders. *J Pineal Res.* 2000;29(1):34–39.
84. Peled N, Shorer Z, Peled E, Pillar G. Melatonin effect on seizures in children with severe neurologic deficit disorders. *Epilepsia.* 2001;42(9):1208–1212.
85. Rejdak K, Papuć E, Grieb P, Stelmasiak Z. Decreased cerebrospinal fluid hypocretin-1 (orexin A) in patients after repetitive generalized tonic-clonic seizures. *Epilepsia.* 2009;50(6):1641–1644.
86. Vaughn BV, D' Cruz OF. Sleep and epilepsy. *Semin Neurol.* 2004;24(3):301–313.
87. Nunes ML, Ferri R, Arzimanoglou A, Curzi L, Appel CC, Costa da Costa J. Sleep organization in children with partial refractory epilepsy. *J Child Neurol.* 2003;18(11):763–766.
88. Bazil CW, Castro LH, Walczak TS. Reduction of rapid eye movement sleep by diurnal and nocturnal seizures in temporal lobe epilepsy. *Arch Neurol.* 2000;57(3):363–368.
89. Stores G, Wiggs L, Campling G. Sleep disorders and their relationship to psychological disturbance in children with epilepsy. *Child Care Health Dev.* 1998;24(1):5–19.
90. Cortesi F, Giannotti F, Ottaviano S. Sleep problems and daytime behavior in childhood idiopathic epilepsy. *Epilepsia.* 1999;40(11):1557–1565.
91. Maganti R, Sheth RD, Hermann BP, Weber S, Gidal BE, Fine J. Sleep architecture in children with idiopathic generalized epilepsy. *Epilepsia.* 2005;46(1):104–109.
92. Becker DA, Fennell EB, Carney PR. Daytime behavior and sleep disturbance in childhood epilepsy. *Epilepsy Behav.* 2004;5(5):708–715.
93. Nagarajan L, Walsh P, Gregory P, Stick S, Maul J, Ghosh S. Respiratory pattern changes in sleep in children on vagal nerve stimulation for refractory epilepsy. *Can J Neurol Sci.* 2003;30(3):224–227.
94. Kaleyias J, Cruz M, Goraya JS, et al. Spectrum of polysomnographic findings in children with epilepsy. *Pediatr Neurol.* 2008;39(3):170–176.
95. Bruni O, Novelli L, Luchetti A, et al. Reduced NREM sleep instability in benign childhood epilepsy with centro-temporal spikes. *Clin Neurophysiol.* 2010;121(5):665–671.
96. Capdevila OS, Dayyat E, Kheirandish-Gozal L, Gozal D. Prevalence of epileptiform activity in healthy children during sleep. *Sleep Med.* 2008;9(5):303–309.
97. Malow BA, Levy K, Maturen K, Bowes R. Obstructive sleep apnea is common in medically refractory epilepsy patients. *Neurology.* 2000;55(7):1002–1007.
98. Jensen FE, Wang C, Stafstrom CE, Liu Z, Geary C, Stevens MC. Acute and chronic increases in excitability in rat hippocampal slices after perinatal hypoxia In vivo. *J Neurophysiol.* 1998;79(1):73–81.
99. Johnston MV. Excitotoxicity in neonatal hypoxia. *Ment Retard Dev Disabil Res Rev.* 2001;7(4):229–234.
100. Zgodziński W, Rubaj A, Kleinrok Z, Sieklucka-Dziuba M. Effect of adenosine A1 and A2 receptor stimulation on hypoxia-induced convulsions in adult mice. *Pol J Pharmacol.* 2001;53(1):83–92.
101. Oliveira AJ, Zamagni M, Dolso P, Bassetti MA, Gigli GL. Respiratory disorders during sleep in patients with epilepsy: effect of ventilatory therapy on EEG interictal epileptiform discharges. *Clin Neurophysiol.* 2000;111(suppl 2):S141–S145.
102. Miano S, Pelliccia A, Evangelisti M, Pagani J, Villa MP. Role of continuous positive airway pressure therapy on the pathogenesis of sleep-related frontal lobe epilepsy in a child with obstructive sleep apnea syndrome. *J Child Neurol.* 2008;23(1):124–128.
103. Larner AJ. Obstructive sleep apnoea syndrome presenting in a neurology outpatient clinic. *Int J Clin Pract.* 2003;57(2):150–152.
104. Foldvary-Schaefer N, Stephenson L, Bingaman W. Resolution of obstructive sleep apnea with epilepsy surgery? Expanding the relationship between sleep and epilepsy. *Epilepsia.* 2008;49(8):1457–1459.
105. Fiorino EK, Brooks LJ. Obesity and respiratory diseases in childhood. *Clin Chest Med.* 2009;30(3):601–608.
106. Marzec M, Edwards J, Sagher O, Fromes G, Malow BA. Effects of vagus nerve stimulation on sleep-related breathing in epilepsy patients. *Epilepsia.* 2003;44(7):930–935.
107. Tezer FI, Rémi J, Noachtar S. Ictal apnea of epileptic origin. *Neurology.* 2009;72(9):855–857.
108. O'Regan ME, Brown JK. Abnormalities in cardiac and respiratory function observed during seizures in childhood. *Dev Med Child Neurol.* 2005;47(1):4–9.
109. Seyal M, Bateman LM. Ictal apnea linked to contralateral spread of temporal lobe seizures: intracranial recordings in refractory temporal lobe epilepsy. *Epilepsia.* 2009;50:2557–2564.

110. Blum AS, Ives JR, Goldberger AL, et al. Oxygen desaturations triggered by partial seizures: implications for cardiopulmonary instability in epilepsy. *Epilepsia*. 2000;41(5):536–541.
111. Nashef L, Walker F, Allen P, Sander JW, Shorvon SD, Fish DR. Apnea and bradycardia during epileptic seizures: relation to sudden death in epilepsy. *J Neurol Neurosurg Psychiatry*. 1996;60(3):297–300.
112. Arzimanoglou A, French J, Blume WT, et al. Lennox-Gastaut syndrome: a consensus approach on diagnosis, assessment, management, and trial methodology. *Lancet Neurol*. 2009;8(1):82–93.
113. Abramo TJ, Wiebe RA, Scott S, Goto CS, McIntire DD. Noninvasive capnometry monitoring for respiratory status during pediatric seizures. *Crit Care Med*. 1997;25(7):1242–1246.
114. Sammaritano M, Sherwin A. Effect of anticonvulsants on sleep. *Neurology*. 2000;54(5)(suppl 1): S16–S24.
115. Legros B, Bazil CW. Effects of antiepileptic drugs on sleep architecture: a pilot study. *Sleep Med*. 2003;4(1):51–55.
116. De Haas S, Otte A, de Weerd A, van Erp G, Cohen A, van Gerven J. Exploratory polysomnographic evaluation of pregabalin on sleep disturbance in patients with epilepsy. *J Clin Sleep Med*. 2007;3(5):473–478.
117. Takhar J, Bishop J. Influence of chronic barbiturate administration on sleep apnea after hypersomnia presentation: case study. *J Psychiatry Neurosci*. 2000;25(4):321–324.
118. Ebben MR, Sethi NK, Conte M, Pollak CP, Labar D. Vagus nerve stimulation, sleep apnea, and CPAP titration. *J Clin Sleep Med*. 2008;4(5):471–473.
119. Khurana DS, Reumann M, Hobdell EF, et al. Vagus nerve stimulation in children with refractory epilepsy: unusual complications and relationship to sleep-disordered breathing. *Childs Nerv Syst*. 2007;23(11):1309–1312.
120. Allen CN. Circadian rhythms, diet, and neuronal excitability. *Epilepsia*. 2008;49(suppl 8): S124–S126.
121. Hallböök T, Lundgren J, Rosén I. Ketogenic diet improves sleep quality in children with therapy-resistant epilepsy. *Epilepsia*. 2007;48(1):59–65.
122. Fusco L, Specchio N. Non-epileptic paroxysmal manifestations during sleep in infancy and childhood. *Neurol Sci*. 2005;26(suppl 3):S 205–209.
123. Stores G. Aspects of parasomnias in childhood and adolescence. *Arch Dis Child*. 2009; 94(1):63–69.
124. Kotagal S. Parasomnias of childhood. *Curr Opin Pediatr*. 2008;20(6):659–665.
125. Derry CP, Harvey AS, Walker MC, Duncan JS, Berkovic SF. NREM arousal parasomnias and their distinction from nocturnal frontal lobe epilepsy: a video EEG analysis. *Sleep*. 2009;32(12): 1637–1644.
126. Montagna P. Nocturnal paroxysmal dystonia and nocturnal wandering. *Neurology*. 1992;42(7) (suppl 6):61–67.
127. Sheldon SH, Jacobsen J. REM-sleep motor disorder in children. *J Child Neurol. 1998;* 13(6):257–260.
128. Dauvilliers Y, Rompré S, Gagnon JF, Vendette M, Petit D, Montplaisir J. REM sleep characteristics in narcolepsy and REM sleep behavior disorder. *Sleep*. 2007;30(7):844–849.
129. Maski KP, Kothare SV. Searching for marker of REM sleep behavior disorder: submentalis muscle EMG amplitude analysis during sleep in patients with narcolepsy/cataplexy. *Sleep*. 2009;32(2):137.
130. Winkelman JW, James L. Serotonergic antidepressants are associated with REM sleep without atonia. *Sleep*. 2004;27(2):317–321.
131. Stores G. Rapid eye movement sleep behaviour disorder in children and adolescents. *Dev Med Child Neurol*. 2008;50(10):728–732.
132. Ferri R, Franceschini C, Zucconi M, et al. Searching for a marker of REM sleep behavior disorder: submentalis muscle EMG amplitude analysis during sleep in patients with narcolepsy/cataplexy. *Sleep*. 2008;31(10):1409–1417.
133. Ramar K, Olson EJ, Morgenthaler TI. Catarthrenia. *Sleep Med*. 2008;9(4):457–459.
134. Vetrugno R, Lugaresi E, Ferini-Strambi L, Montagna P. Catathrenia (nocturnal groaning): what is it? *Sleep*. 2008;31(3):308–309.
135. Pennestri MH, Whittom S, Adam B, Petit D, Carrier J, Montplaisir J. PLMS and PLMW in healthy subjects as a function of age: prevalence and interval distribution. *Sleep*. 2006;29(9): 1183–1187.
136. Kemlink D, Pretl M, Sonka K, Nevsimalova S. A comparison of polysomnographic and actigraphic evaluation of periodic limb movements in sleep. *Neurol Res*. 2008;30(3):234–238.
137. Herrera M, Valencia I, Grant M, Metroka D, Chialastri A, Kothare SV. Bruxism in children: effect on sleep architecture and daytime cognitive performance and behavior. *Sleep*. 2006;29(9): 1143–1148.
138. Meletti S, Cantalupo G, Volpi L, Rubboli G, Magaudda A, Tassinari CA. Rhythmic teeth grinding induced by temporal lobe seizures. *Neurology*. 2004;62(12):2306–2309.
139. Chisholm T, Morehouse RL. Adult headbanging: sleep studies and treatment. *Sleep*. 1996;19(4):343–346.
140. Stepanova I, Nevsimalova S, Hanusova J. Rhythmic movement disorder in sleep persisting into childhood and adulthood. *Sleep*. 2005;28(7):851–857.
141. Wyllie E, Glazer JP, Benbadis S, Kotagal P, Wolgamuth B. Psychiatric features of children and adolescents with pseudoseizures. *Arch Pediatr Adolesc Med*. 1999;153(3):244–248.
142. Craske MG, Tsao JC. Assessment and treatment of nocturnal panic attacks. *Sleep Med Rev*. 2005;9(3):173–184.
143. Guilleminault C, Palombini L, Pelayo R, Chervin RD. Sleepwalking and sleep terrors in prepubertal children: what triggers them? *Pediatrics*. 2003;111(1):e17–e25.
144. Miano S, Paolino MC, Peraita-Adrados R, Montesano M, Barberi S, Villa MP. Prevalence of EEG paroxysmal activity in a population of

children with obstructive sleep apnea syndrome. *Sleep*. 2009;32(4):522–529.
145. Guilleminault C, Zvonikina V, Tantrakul V, Kim JH. Advances in narcolepsy syndrome and challenges in the pediatric population. *Sleep Med Clin*. 2007;2(3):397–404.
146. Kotagal P, Costa M, Wyllie E, Wolgamuth B. Paroxysmal nonepileptic events in children and adolescents. *Pediatrics*. 2002;110(4):e46.
147. Somjit S, Lee Y, Berkovic SF, Harvey AS. Sandifer syndrome misdiagnosed as refractory partial seizures in an adult. *Epileptic Disord*. 2004;6(1): 49–50.
148. Erdogan A, Akkurt H, Boettjer NK, Yurtseven E, Can G, Kiran S. Prevalence and behavioral correlates of enuresis in young children. *J Paediatr Child Health*. 2008;44(5):297–301.
149. Serra L, Montagna P, Mignot E, Lugaresi E, Plazzi G. Cataplexy features in childhood narcolepsy. *Mov Disord*. 2008;23(6):858–865.

CHAPTER 6

Sleep-Potentiated Spike-Wave Discharges and Electrical Status Epilepticus of Slow-Wave Sleep

Tobias Loddenkemper and Prakash Kotagal

Introduction

Relationships between sleep and epilepsy have been included in the very first written descriptions of epilepsy [1,2]. A prominent effect of sleep on the timing of seizures has been shown by several studies [3–5], especially in primary or secondarily generalized seizures. These studies indicate that sleep increases seizure frequency, duration, and rate of secondary generalization in patients with focal epilepsy [6]. Furthermore, sleep-related variation in cerebral excitability has been demonstrated, as evidenced by sleep stage–dependent activation and potentiation of interictal epileptiform discharges [7]. An increase of spike and wave discharges during sleep has been shown in animals [8,9] and in humans [7]. Understanding of the basic mechanisms influencing sleep and epilepsy may help with furthering our knowledge of underlying circadian patterns of epilepsy, epileptic encephalopathy, and interictal spiking [10] and may provide future insights for additional treatment options [11].

Mechanisms of Sleep-Potentiated Spiking

Suprachiasmatic nuclei (SCN) and "pace maker": At this point, little is known about the underlying mechanisms of circadian patterns of epileptic seizures and interictal spiking. Several authors suggested a relationship with the circadian "pacemaker" in the SCN in the anterior hypothalamus [12–14]. Interestingly, neurons in the SCN fire in a 24-hour cycle, and this cycle persists even when the neurons are disconnected from each other in cell cultures [15]. A cell-based transcription and translation feedback loop comprising a core set of genes has been suggested as explanation [16]. A complex of genes encode proteins essential to circadian rhythm function, and these form a feedback loop involving both transcription and translation [17]. Fiber tracts from the SCN connect to the hypothalamus, pineal body, thalamus, and limbic system and therefore to some of the most important relay stations for epileptic networks. These connections may explain some of the individual circadian modulation of excitability and susceptibility for different seizure types and spiking.

Role of the thalamus: Thalamo-cortical circuits that oscillate during sleep are also involved in the generation of pathological oscillations in certain types of epilepsy [18]. Inhibitory thalamic neurons in the reticular nucleus and excitatory thalamocortical connections in the dorsal thalamic nuclei interact with cortical slow oscillations and may play a central role in the mechanisms underlying generation of sleep spindles [19,20]. Circuitry function relies on reciprocal synaptic connectivity between excitatory thalamocortical relay neurons and inhibitory thalamic reticular neurons [21]. These circuits are also suspected in the generation of generalized seizures, and state-dependent activation of circuits may influence diurnal seizure susceptibility and cortical excitability [18]. Early developmental or genetic lesions of this thalamo-cortical circuitry may lead to hyperexcitability and increased spiking, in particular during sleep [22,23]. In 147 patients with sleep-potentiated spiking, patients with thalamic lesions had a significantly higher spike wave index [22]. Early developmental lesions were more frequently seen in patients with sleep-potentiated spiking [22]. Disruption of normal sleep structures may lead to memory problems and possibly learning difficulties [24]. Thalamic modulation may serve as a treatment option of sleep and neurocognitive function in pediatric patients in the future, that is, with use of drugs such as sodium oxybate [25] or thalamic stimulation [26].

The adenosine hypothesis: Adenosine antagonists increase waking and reduce slow-wave sleep [27]. After prolonged wakefulness, brain adenosine levels rise as an indicator of reduced brain energy levels and thereby facilitate sleep as a restorative state [28]. Astrocytes modulate the anticonvulsant adenosine by the pro-epileptogenic adenosine kinase [29]. Adenosine falls off at the transition of wakefulness to sleep [30]. This may explain why some seizures and interictal spikes manifest more frequently at this time [30]. One proposed mechanism may involve adenosine-mediated GABA modulation of neuronal excitability [31].

Melatonin, serotonin, and cortisol: The pineal body produces melatonin in a circadian pattern, with a nocturnal peak and low daytime levels [12]. Some authors have suggested that melatonin may act as a proconvulsant, especially at higher doses, possibly through inhibition of dopaminergic activity [32]. However, lower dose trials of melatonin treatment in epilepsy patients have also shown some anticonvulsant properties and may act as a spike suppressant [33,34]. Furthermore, serotonin may also regulate sleep wake patterns [35]. Interictal epileptiform discharges and epileptic seizures may also be induced by 5-hydroxytryptamine (5-HT) attenuation, whereas augmentation of serotonin function may have anticonvulsant effects [36]. Additionally, cortisol levels follow a circadian rhythm. Infants with epileptic spasms have decreased levels, and ACTH is an established treatment option for these seizures [37].

Early developmental brain lesions and epileptogenesis: Epileptogenesis in infancy and during the first years of life in the developing brain is different than in the mature brain [38]. Experimental evidence from several animal models reveals markedly decreased seizure thresholds in the immature brain [38,39]. Excitation predominates overinhibition of neuronal networks in infancy and early childhood [40]. Excitatory ion channels and transporters are expressed at levels that promote excitation in early childhood, whereas inhibition is relatively underrepresentated as compared with older children [38]. Furthermore, whereas GABA is inhibitory and hyperpolarizing in the mature brain, it is excitatory and hyperpolarizing in the immature brain [41]. Evidence from postmortem human tissue samples supports the notion that early developmental lesions may interfere with the switch from excitatory to inhibitory receptor subunits, including regulatory subunits NKCC1 and KCC2 [42]. Interestingly, NMDA, AMPAR, and GABA receptor subunit ratios in human tissue samples from patients with electrical status epilepticus in sleep (ESES) differed significantly from postmortem controls [43]: in patients with ESES, NR2B/NR2A ratio and GluR1/GluR1 ratios were elevated as compared with postmortem controls, whereas no change in GABAα2/GABAα1 ratio as compared with postmortem controls was seen in ESES. However, the α2/α1 ratio showed a significant increase in human tissue from status epilepticus and chronic epilepsy patients, potentially suggesting a decreased upregulation of GABA subunits in ESES patients as compared with patients with status epilepticus and chronic seizures [43].

Many types of epilepsy present with sleep-potentiated spiking. Most prominently, benign seizure susceptibility syndromes, such as benign focal epilepsy of childhood or benign focal epilepsy with occipital spikes, ESES, and variants present with sleep-potentiated spiking. Although the underlying pathophysiology of sleep-potentiated spiking is not clear, several of the above outlined mechanisms may contribute. We now present an overview over some pediatric epilepsy syndromes with sleep-potentiated spiking and electrical status epilepticus in sleep.

Continuous Spikes and Waves During Sleep

History: The first description of ESES dates back to 1971 [44]. The initial term ESES was criticized because of a lack of epileptic seizures in some patients as well as lack of clinical signs of the presumed status epilepticus. Therefore, the term "Continuous spikes and waves during sleep" (CSWS) was introduced [45] and included in the revised classification of epilepsies in 1989 [46]. CSWS is characterized by simultaneous presentation of almost continuous spike-wave activity on electroencephalogram (EEG) during slow-wave sleep and by neuropsychological deficits. Some authors use ESES and CSWS interchangeably, but more recently CSWS has been suggested for the actual syndrome and ESES has been suggested for the EEG finding [47].

Epidemiology and definitions: CSWS is rare and an incidence of 0.5% among children with epilepsy has been published [48]. There are no data on prevalence of CSWS. Although a minimally higher rate of males was reported in one review, this was deemed not significant [49]. Upon review of incidence and available literature, Tassinari et al stated that "the parameters used for the definition were not the same for all authors, with a consequent variability of incidence and prognosis" [49]. Therefore, Tassinari et al suggested several clinical diagnostic features [50]. These include neuropsychological impairment presenting as global developmental delay and regression, or delay and regression of specific cognitive function, such as language. Additionally, motor impairment presenting as ataxia, dyspraxia, dystonia, or unilateral deficit may be seen. Furthermore, the patient may present with epilepsy with focal or apparently generalized seizures, including tonic-clonic seizures, absences, partial-motor seizures, complex partial seizures, or epileptic falls. EEG criteria include electrographic status epilepticus occurring during at least 85% of slow sleep and persisting on 3 or more records for at least 1 month [50].

Clinical presentation: CSWS occurs only in children and the course is related to age. Seizures start usually between 2 months and 12 years, with a peak around 5 years, and the typical EEG pattern may be detected between 3 and 14 years, usually a few years after the first seizure. The EEG pattern may be seen for a duration of 8 to 12 years and show improvement toward normalization in late teenage years. Other clinical features, such as perinatal distress and an abnormal neurological exam, such as hemiparesis, can be seen in up to 50% of cases [51]

Clinical seizures usually present with focal motor or generalized tonic-clonic seizures and occur frequently at night [49,50]. Tonic seizures are usually excluded [49]. Most patients present with seizures, although even in the first description only 5 out of 6 patients presented with epileptic seizures [44].

Neuroimaging and EEG findings: Early developmental lesions, in particular periventricular leukomalacia, strokes, and malformation of cortical development may be related to CSWS [52,53]. Abnormal magnetic resonance images (MRIs) are seen in about half of all patients [53].

Typical EEG findings include generalized sleep-potentiated spiking during 85% of slow-wave sleep [54]. Some authors also include patients with lower spike wave indices and with localized sleep-potentiated spiking [53]. Spikes and sharp waves present typically at a 1.5- to 2.5-Hz frequency and are predominantly seen during slow-wave sleep, particularly during the first sleep cycle [49,55] (Figure 6.1A–D).

There is preservation of physiological rapid eye movement (REM) sleep patterns. REM sleep can be identified because of prominent decrease or even complete discontinuation of CSWS. However, slow-wave sleep and sleep stages I and II are frequently disrupted. Occasionally, there are no normal sleep structures such as spindles, Vertex waves, and K-complexes. The cyclic sleep organization may be preserved, but larger and detailed studies are not available at this point.

Neuropsychological manifestations: Children frequently present with developmental regression, loss of developmental milestones, and deficits in language function, socialization skills, memory, global intellect, and motor function [50]. Developmental delay and regression have at least in part been attributed to interference of nocturnal spiking with sleep-related processes such as plasticity, learning, and memory consolidation [51]. Although seizures and ESES remit with age, cognitive deficits remain. The duration of ESES is thought to correlate with the severity and persistence of neuropsychological deficits [56].

A

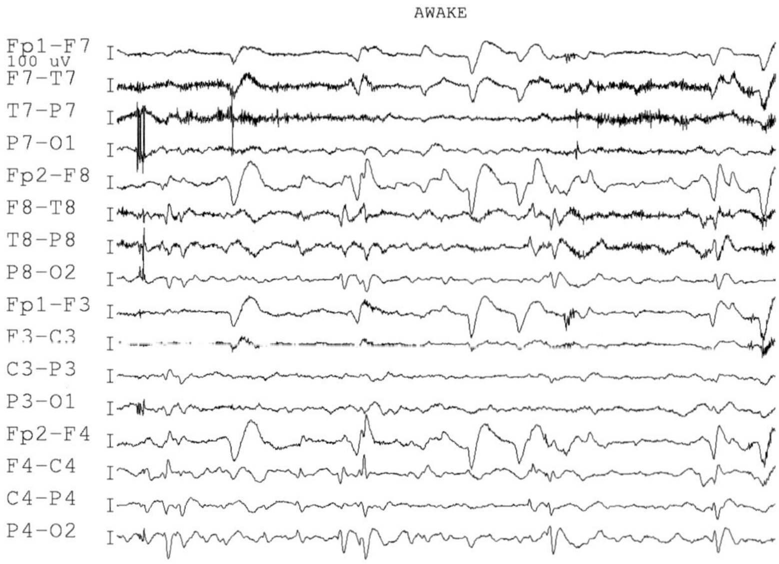

B

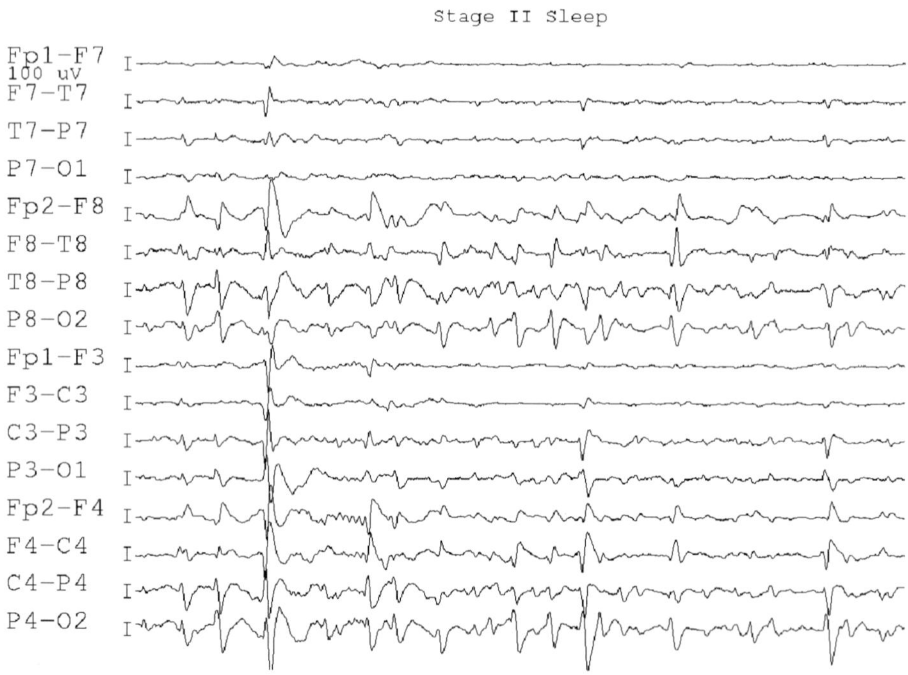

Figure 6.1 A, This awake electroencephalogram (EEG) demonstrates focal slowing and sharp waves in the right centro-temporal region. B, Stage II non-rapid eye movement sleep leads to potentiation of sharp waves. C, The field of the sharp waves becomes more widespread over both hemispheres during slow-wave sleep, more prominently over the left side. Sharp waves involve almost the entire EEG page (CSWS). D, This is an ictal EEG from the same patient. Clinically, seizures presented as axial myoclonic seizures while awake. On EEG, the seizure pattern appears lateralized right with a central maximum and only limited reflection over the left hemisphere. Reprinted with permission from Ref. [55].

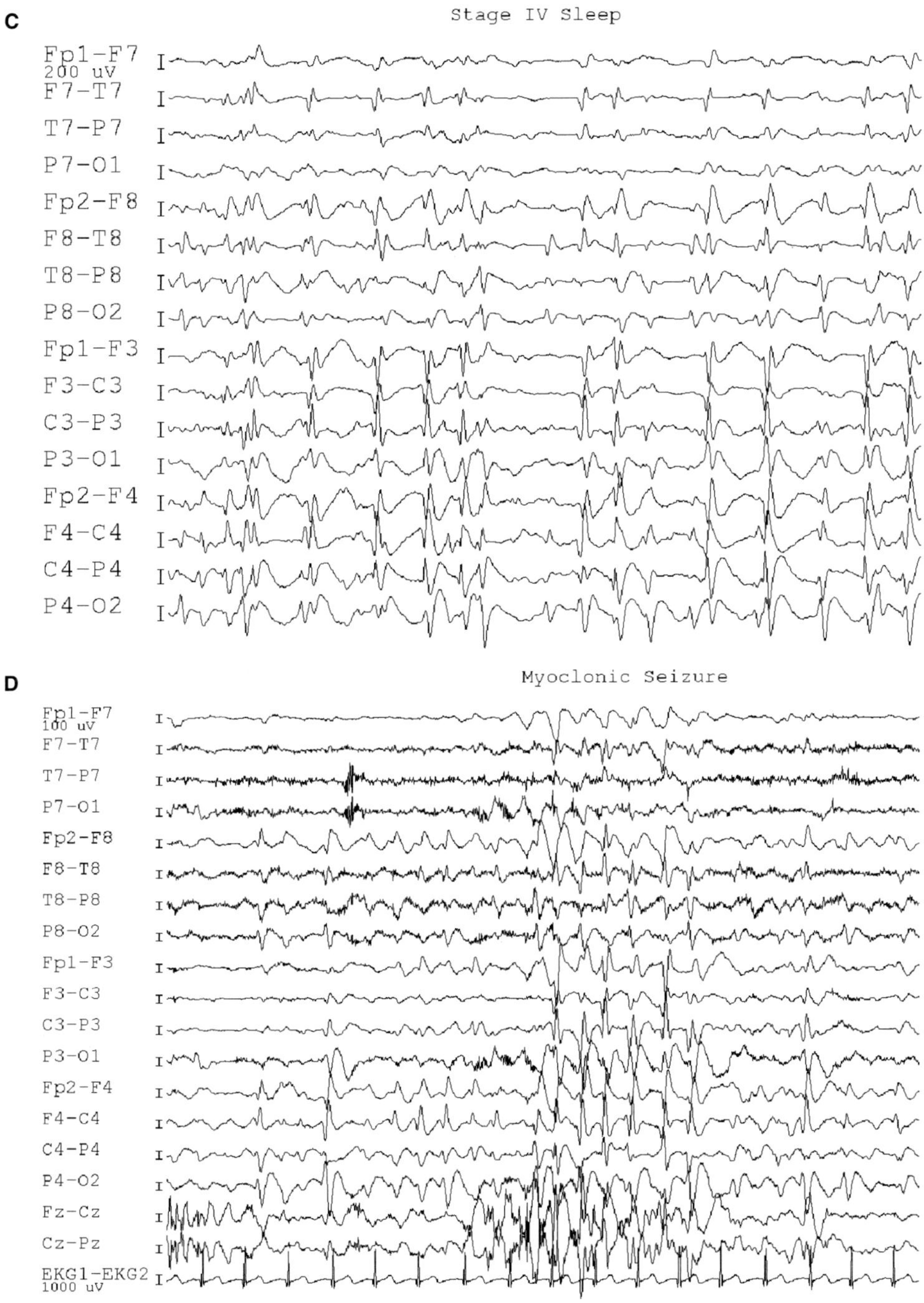

Figure 6.1 (*Continued*)

Treatment: There are no clear treatment guidelines and most recommendations are based on case reports or case series. Several authors have targeted the EEG pattern with antiepileptic medications on the basis of the assumption that neuropsychological regression and continuous status epilepticus during slow-wave sleep as well as frequent interictal epileptiform discharges are related [57–60]. Valproic acid, ethosuximide, and high-dose diazepam have been tried among others [57–60]. However, it remains unclear if frequent spiking is a cause of regression, is just a surface phenomenon of regression and developmental delay, or presents as an additional clinical presentation of a common underlying cause of epileptic activity and regression. Speech and occupational therapy are extremely important. In addition to anticonvulsants for seizures, encephalopathy has been treated with a 6- to 12-week trial of corticosteroids [61]. Furthermore, intravenous immunoglobulin application has been tried [62]. Medical treatment may provide some improvement in more than 50% of cases, but patients usually do not return to developmental baseline. It remains unclear whether treatment can influence the long-term outcome with language and cognitive delay [61,62].

Multiple subpial transection (MST) is a surgical treatment option [63], in particular when spiking is regional and when eloquent areas are involved. The technique consists of intracortical transverse fiber sectioning with sparing of the vertically directed pathways [64]. Because of the self-limiting process in many cases, surgical treatment has been controversial. Nonetheless, the devastating developmental outcome from CSWS and Landau-Kleffner spectrum has prompted the use of MST as a surgical option [63]. On the basis of the indications of a focal origin [48,65], resective epilepsy surgery has also recently been completed with good seizure outcome [52] (Figure 6.2A and B). Data on treatment outcome are limited and no detailed data on neuropsychological outcome are available to date.

Focal Epilepsy With Centrotemporal Spikes (BECTS)

Epidemiology: BECTS is the most frequent focal epilepsy syndrome among children [66–68]. It accounts for up to 23% of new-onset epilepsy in children [66–68]. In children under 16 years, a

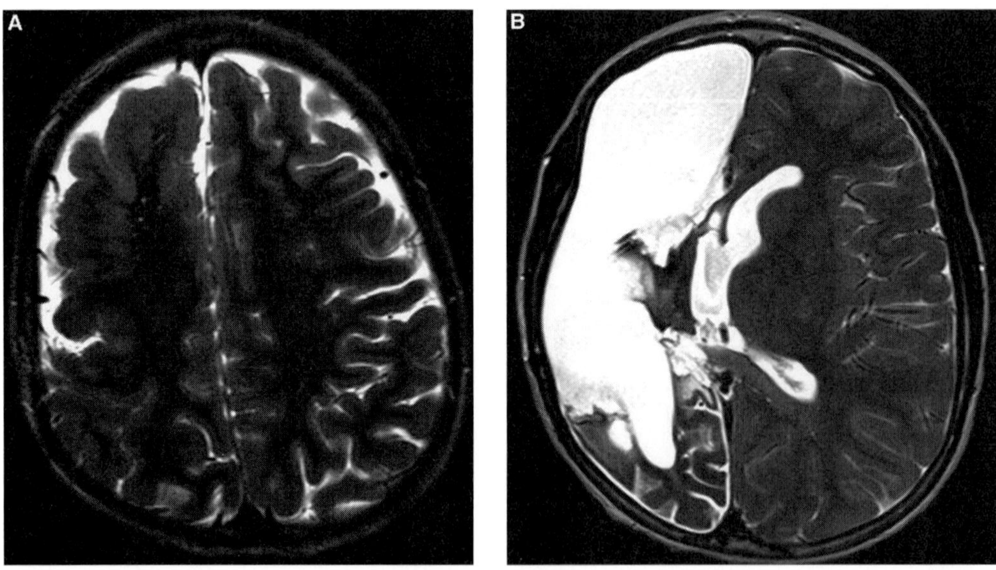

Figure 6.2 A, This axial T2-weighted brain magnetic resonance image (MRI) demonstrates an extensive malformation of cortical development of the anterior two-thirds of the right hemisphere. B, This is a postoperative T2-weighted axial MRI after right functional hemispherectomy. Reprinted with permission from Ref. [55].

BECTS incidence as high as 21 per 100 000 has been described [69]. Boys are slightly more frequently affected than girls [70,71]. Predisposition to febrile seizures (16%) and an increased frequency of seizures in infancy (1%–8%) [66] have been described.

Clinical presentation and seizure semiology: Seizures start at an average age of 8 years (range 1–13 years) [72]. There is almost complete remission by 16 years [73,74]. Seizures are most frequently seen out of sleep [70,75] and tend to occur at the transition between sleep and wakefulness [75]. Up to 17% develop status epilepticus [75].

Clinical seizures last seconds to minutes and present with a unilateral facial sensory aura, jaw and tongue stiffness, and at times a sensation of choking. Additionally, guttural noises, gargling, grunting, or even a "death rattle" [76] have been noted. Parents frequently highlight drooling. Speech arrest or inability to swallow has been ascribed to laryngeal and oropharyngeal involvment. Children frequently remain conscious during the initial phase of the seizure and are able to alert parents unless seizures become secondarily generalized [71]. In young children and during sleep-onset seizures, auras may not be noted [66].

Neuroimaging and EEG: Brain MRIs are usually not performed unless atypical features or focal neurological deficits are present [77]. Although a number of CNS abnormalities have been reported in patients with BECTS, these findings do not seem to influence the disease course [77].

EEG background activity is normal in most cases. Typical interictal EEG presentation consists of a high-voltage, diphasic spike followed by a prominent slow wave [78]. A dipole with a negative maximum at C3/T3 or C4/T4 and a positive frontal maximum is characteristic [79,80] (Figure 6.3A and D). It has been speculated that these spikes are generated by a single tangential source on the surface of the rolandic region [81]. Spikes may be central, central-temporal, mid-temporal, central-parietal, or parietal [78] and spikes may be uni- or bilateral [78] with equal distribution between the right and left hemispheres [82]. Additionally, an association with generalized spike and wave complexes has been described [83]. Spikes are often potentiated by non-REM sleep [78,84–86] and decrease during REM sleep [86]. Up to 30% of patients present with spike activation during sleep, that is, no spikes during wakefulness [84]. Only few ictal recordings have been reported to date [83]. Most studies report a regional centro-temporal seizure onset [83] and very rare cases of parietal ictal onset zones have been reported [87].

Neuropsychological manifestations: About half of all children with BECTS may exhibit neuropsychological abnormalities [88]. Auditory-verbal and visuospatial memory tasks, executive function, language, attention, learning, and behavior are predominantly affected [66,75,88–97]. Interestingly, the lateralization of interictal epileptiform discharges relates to the type of cognitive deficit [66].

Genetics and pathophysiology: A genomewide linkage scan suggested the Elongator Protein Complex 4 gene (ELP4) on chromosome 11p13 [98]. ELP4 has functions in transcription and tRNA modification. Decrease in elongator complex results in downregulation of genes implicated in neuronal cell motility and migration [98]. Additionally, genetic heterogeneity with linkage to a locus on chromosome 15q14 has been described [99]. Even before that, increased occurrence of BECTS has been described in family members of affected children [75,100,101]. Metrakos and Metrakos suggested variable penetrance on the basis of age [102]. A series on 8 twin pairs did not show co-twin concordance [103] and proposed possible environmental or epigenetic influences [104].

Management and prognosis: A diagnosis of BECTS does not necessarily require treatment with antiepileptic medications. Risks, benefits, and alternatives of treatment should be discussed with the family. Treatment may be warranted in children with early epilepsy onset, and in patients with atypical or more severe clinical seizure presentations, such as daytime seizures, prolonged and recurrent generalized tonic-clonic seizures, or status epilepticus [66,75]. If medication treatment is initiated, potential options include clobazam, clonazepam, sulthiame, levetiracetam, oxcarbazepine, carbamazepine, phenytoin, valproate, and phenobarbital and others [66]. Seizures may be controlled in up to 65% of patients [66,75]. Remission occurs in almost all patients by 18 years of age,

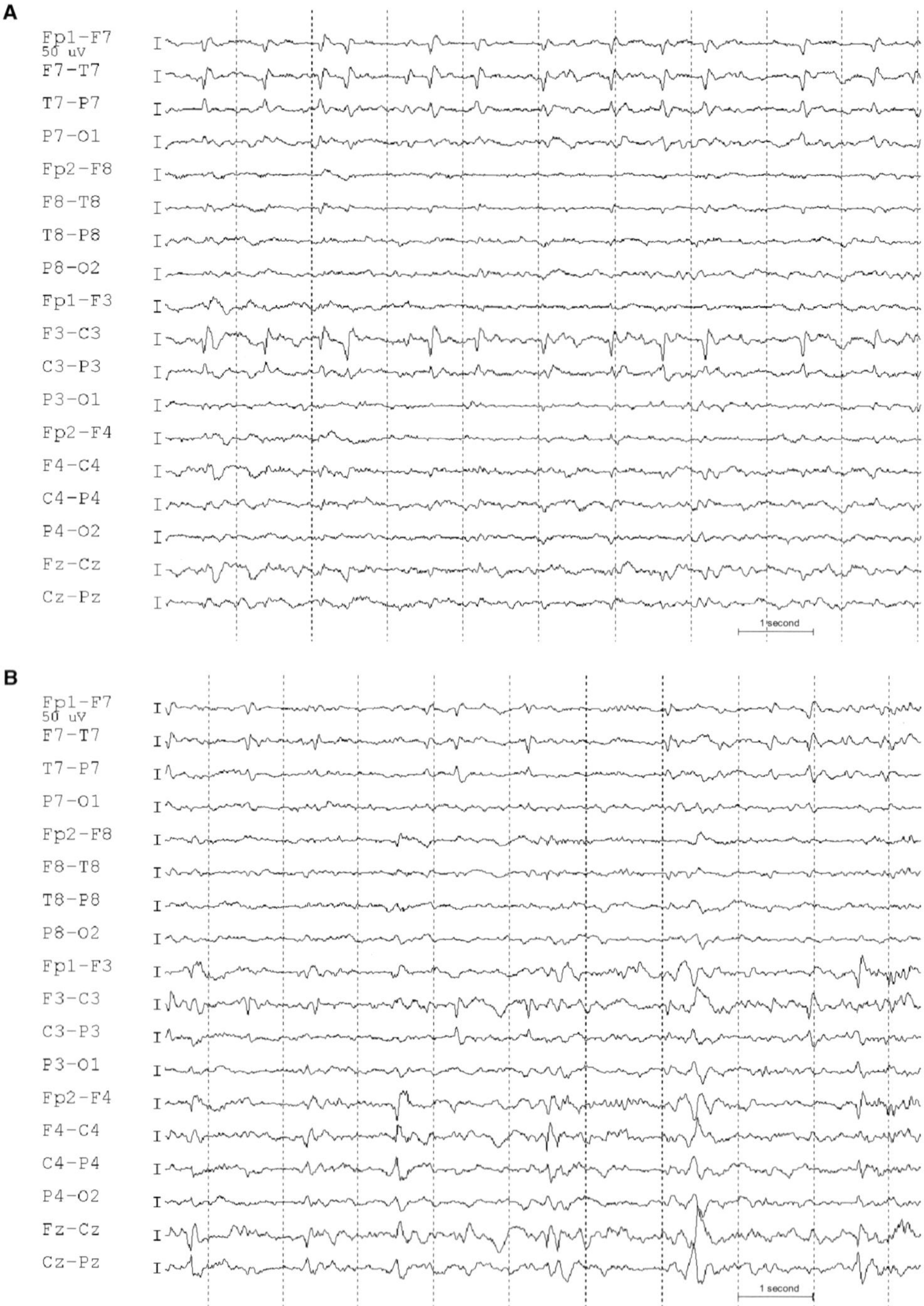

Figure 6.3 This electroencephalogram demonstrates A, frequent left centro-temporal benign focal epileptiform discharges and B, left and right independent centro-temporal epileptiform discharges. Reprinted with permission, from Ref. [82].

even if they are pharmacologically intractable [105]. Occasionally, BECTS exacerbation has been ascribed to some antiepileptic drugs (carbamazepine, phenytoin, valproate, and phenobarbital) [106,107].

Benign Focal Epilepsy With Occipital Spikes of Gastaut

Epidemiology: Benign focal epilepsy with occipital spikes of Gastaut is rare (0.15% of all focal epilepsies) [108]. Febrile seizures, migraine, and a history of BECTS have been reported in relationship to Gastaut syndrome [109].

Clinical presentation and seizure semiology: Mean seizure onset is at 8 years (range 3–16 years) [66,109,110]. Seizures occur on average 1 to 2 times per month [109] and usually last 1 to 2 minutes [110]. Up to 40% of patients may present with seizures up to 15 minutes [109,111,112]. Eighty percent of patients present with visual auras of simple visual patterns of circles or light flashes [109]. Additionally, more complex visual auras, ictal or postictal blindness occur [65,109,111,113]. Evolution into tonic eye deviation and head deviation, unilateral arm or leg motor seizures, bilateral eyelid clonic seizures, and generalized tonic-clonic seizures has been described in up to 60% [66,109]. Furthermore, headache, nausea, vomiting, and light sensitivity is seen in up to 50% of patients, and this can be observed in the ictal or postictal period [109,111]. Most seizures occur out of wakefulness, and concomitant seizures out of sleep are seen in about one-third of patients [109,110,114].

EEG findings: Typical interictal EEG findings consist of occipital sharp waves and these are frequently abolished by eye opening [109]. Generalized and centrotemporal sharp waves have also been noted [109]. Occipital spikes are sleep potentiated, and concomitant centro-temporal spikes are frequently activated and unmasked by sleep. Rare ictal EEGs were occipital [109].

Neuropsychological manifestations: To our knowledge, there is no information on neuropsychological manifestations.

Pathophysiology and genetics: Benign epilepsy of Gastaut has been described in families [115,116]. No gene locus has been identified to date.

Management and prognosis: Recommended medications include carbamazepine, oxcarbazepine, valproic acid, phenobarbital, and clobazam [66,113,117]. More than 90% of patients remit by the age of 19 years. Response rates to pharmacological therapies of up to 50% to 90% have been reported with treatment with higher rates in more recent studies [111–113].

Benign Focal Epilepsy With Occipital Spikes of Panayiotopoulos

Epidemiology and definition: Panayiotopoulos proposed a separation into an early-onset (Panayiotopoulos) and late-onset (Gastaut) benign focal epilepsy of childhood and suggested a more common subtype of benign focal occipital lobe epilepsy of childhood with onset under 8 years [118–120]. This epilepsy syndrome is seen in 6% of 1- to 15-year-old epilepsy patients with focal epilepsy [108,121]. Febrile seizures and migraine have been found in relationship with this syndrome [108,121–123].

Seizure semiology and clinical presentation: Age of onset peaks at 4 to 5 years (range 1–14 years) [110,114,122]. Up to 20% of seizures may be preceded by a visual aura [120,122,123]. Abdominal auras may occur in 15% of patients. Autonomic features are prominent and may present with pallor, emesis, retching, nausea, and even incontinence or syncope [66,108,114,120,121,123–125].

Motor features include tonic head and eye deviation and unilateral clonic seizures [66,108,114,123]. Consciousness is frequently preserved, unless evolution into a generalized tonic-clonic seizure is seen [120,121,123,124].

A few patients present with another "rolandic" seizure type presenting with typical features of drooling, unilateral sensory aura and motor features, and at times evolution into a generalized tonic-clonic seizure [110,123,124].

Two-third of seizures occur at night [121–123]. Seizures frequently last 5 minutes or longer. Status epilepticus may be the first presentation of this epilepsy in up to 20% of patients [123].

Neuroimaging and EEG findings: MRI is usually normal [123]. Interictal EEG findings include occipital (75%) and extraoccipital spikes (23%). Normal interictal EEGs are seen in up to 2% [123]. Most frequent locations of spikes in patients with extraoccipital interictal epileptiform discharges are temporal and frontal [123]. In up to 90% of patients, sleep potentiation or activation of spiking occurs [113,121,123]. Typical seizures start usually in the occipital regions [123].

Neuropsychological manifestations: A lower IQ during the peak phases of the disease has been described [126]. Additional neuropsychological deficits may involve tasks of global visual perception, visual-motor integration, and visual attention [127].

Pathophysiology and genetics: No genetic linkage has been described to date. A family history of seizures was found in up to 32% of patients, suggesting an underlying genetic predisposition [108,121–123,126]. Abnormalities during birth may also play a role.

Management and prognosis: Carbamazepine, valproic acid, phenobarbital, oxcarbazepine, and clobazam have been successfully tried [66]. Carbamazepine may lead to exacerbation in rare cases [128]. Seizure freedom rates of up to 90% are seen after pharmacological treatment [123]. Mean disease duration is 3 years, and almost all patients remit within 6 years after onset [111].

Landau-Kleffner and BFEC Variants

Landau-Kleffner Syndrome

William Landau and Frank Kleffner identified acquired language regression as the main feature of this syndrome [129] in 1957. At that time the authors suspected that interictal epileptiform discharges may have lead to a functional lesion of cortical areas important for language development [129]. Patry et al described an epilepsy syndrome defined by generalized and almost continuous electrical status epilepticus during slow-wave sleep of at least 85% [44]. Both syndromes share progressive cognitive dysfunction (and frequently ESES) as a common feature [130] and they were therefore included in the same spectrum of a single syndrome by the International League Against Epilepsy commission [131] (Table 6.1).

Overall, Landau-Kleffner syndrome (LKS) is rare. Typically, age of onset ranges from 2 to 14 years [132,133]. Specific clinical features include regression of developmental language milestones, in particular comprehension, after the first 2 years of life [132,133]. Other neuropsychological and behavioral abnormalities include hyperactivity and attention deficit, developmental motor deficits, and autism spectrum disorder and global developmental delay [94]. Up to 30% of patients do not have any epileptic seizures. Seizures frequently present with focal motor features and preserved consciousness [134], if they occur. Remission of seizures is seen around the third decade, but cognitive deficits are permanent [134]. EEG reveals sleep-potentiated centro-temporal spiking and slowing in this region. Neuroimaging is usually normal [133,134]. The prognosis and management is similar to CSWS, and antiepileptic medications such as valproate, ethosuximide, clobazam, oxcarbazepine, sulthiame, levetiracetam, topiramate, or lamotrigine have been reported in the LKS spectrum [135].

BFEC Variants

Several authors endorse atypical features of benign focal epilepsies of childhood in addition to the classic and better delineated benign focal epilepsy syndromes of childhood as outlined in this chapter. There are significant variations in definitions with a lot of overlap between different subcategories.

BECTS may present with atypical features, such as leg clonic seizures and versive seizures, status epilepticus, seizures only during daytime, and postictal Todd's palsy [88,136] or BFEC with myoclonic seizures. Additional overlap may exist with acquired epileptic opercular syndrome presenting with prolonged episodes of drooling and oromotor apraxia [137], continuous spike-waves during sleep syndrome [50,54], atypical benign partial epilepsy, pseudo-Lennox syndrome, and early-onset benign childhood seizure susceptibility syndrome with occipital or extra-occipital spikes [72].

Other atypical features may include changes in seizure semiology and seizure frequency, sleep potentiation and localization of interictal epileptiform discharges, and associated clinical symptoms and neurological or neuropsychological deficits. Additional subcategories that have been characterized by a variation in the benign focal epilepsies that differ on

Table 6.1 Comparison of LKS and CSWS

	LKS (Acquired epileptic aphasia)	CSWS
Epidemiology	0.2% among children with epilepsy	0.5% among children with epilepsy
Gender	Male-to-female ratio 1.7:1	Male preponderance
Clinical presentation		
Age of Onset	Usually 4–7 yrs; range 1–14 yrs	
Seizure semiology	Focal motor seizures, generalized tonic-clonic seizures, and atypical absences.	Frequently 2 or more seizure types: focal motor seizures; atypical absence seizures and atonic seizures (falls); occasional absence status; never tonic seizures
Seizure timing	Predominantly nocturnal seizures	
Seizure frequency	Up to numerous seizures per day; seizures are seen in 70%–90%	
Neuropsychological findings	Predominantly language regression	Language regression; reduced temporal-spatial orientation and memory function; apraxia; loss of IQ
Other clinical features	Behavioral problems may occur, including aggression, emotional liability, disinhibition, and hyperactivity.	
Duration	6–10 yrs	
Electrophysiology		
Interictal EEG	Focal and multifocal sharp waves and spikes; often temporal or parietal distribution; marked increase of discharges in sleep; at times more localized sleep potentiation	Focal or multifocal spikes and sharp waves; often frontal or frontocentral location; also generalized sharp waves; marked increase of discharges in sleep
ESES	10%–20% present with typical ESES, and additional 60%–70% with sleep potentiated spiking	ESES occupying <85% during sleep per definition (some authors use <50%)
Ictal EEG	More frequently localized EEG seizure patterns	Generalized and regional EEG seizure patterns
Imaging	Usually normal	Abnormal in 50%
Prognosis		
Epilepsy	Seizures usually disappear after age 16–18 yrs	
Neuropsychological deficits	Variable neuropsychological outcome; spectrum between permanent language loss and some language recovery; improved prognosis with later onset; relapsing and remitting course possible	Poor neuropsychological prognosis in about 50%

Comment: Some authors noted that LKS and CSWS have so many features in common that they are likely part of a spectrum.
Abbreviations: CSWS, continuous spikes and waves during sleep; EEG, electroencephalogram; ESES, electrical status epilepticus in sleep; LKS, Landau-Kleffner syndrome.

the basis of location of the discharge include, benign parietal lobe epilepsy and benign childhood focal seizures associated with frontal and midline spikes and others. Severe ends of this spectrum may be represented by LKS [129] and continuous spike and wave discharges during slow-wave sleep [44].

Outlook

Despite different clinical presentations, many pediatric epileptic encephalopathies can present with ESES or sleep-potentiated spiking [44,72, 129,138,139]. A complete list of all conditions is beyond the scope of this chapter. Depending on inclusion criteria and definitions, the associated group of clinical conditions is large and includes patients with epilepsy and/or cognitive delay or focal neurological deficits in a previously healthy child or in a child with a structural brain lesion.

It has been suggested that benign occipital epilepsies, benign focal epilepsy with centrotemporal spikes, LKS, and CSWS are an age-related continuum. Similarities include sleep potentiation, occurrence and resolution in childhood, and associated cognitive deficits. The clinical symptom complex (including febrile seizures) has therefore also been termed benign seizure susceptibility syndrome [111], although the term "benign" has recently been debated because of persistent cognitive deficits [140]. Interactions between brain development and maturation processes as well as genetic influences may play a role in the development of various childhood epileptic syndromes associated with language and cognitive deficits [141]. Recent discoveries including the possible involvement of the ELP4 and other genes with roles in cell motility, migration, and adhesion have provided first insights into the complex molecular bases of childhood focal epilepsies [98,142]. This gene and/or other genetic, epigenetic, or environmental factors may lead to delayed or incomplete maturation-related cortical hyperexcitability, possibly of cortico-thalamic circuitry in selected subtypes [18]. Maturation-related cortical hyperexcitability with sleep-potentiated spiking and/or ESES may be regulated by genetic influences as well as early developmental lesions involving subcortical neuronal migration [141].

The hypothesis of a spectrum is also supported by interesting interrelations with evolution from benign centro-temporal into benign occipital lobe epilepsy types [109], concomitant presentation of benign centro-temporal and occipital lobe epilepsy [143], and relationships between occipital lobe epilepsy, generalized absence epilepsy, BECTS, and ESES [66,83,109,144]. Efforts to determine additional pathophysiological and genetic causes of this unique group of developmental epileptic encephalopathies are underway.

Acknowledgments

The work presented was in part supported by the American Epilepsy Society and Milken Family Foundation Early Career Physician Scientist Award Program and by the Children's Hospital Boston and Harvard Medical School Faculty Development Fellowship Award Program (TL).

References

1. Wilson JV, Reynolds EH. Texts and documents. Translation and analysis of a cuneiform text forming part of a Babylonian treatise on epilepsy. *Med Hist.* 1990;34(2):185–198.
2. Temkin O. Epilepsy: the sacred disease. In: Temkin O, ed. *The Falling Sickness.* Baltimore and London: The Johns Hopkins University Press Ltd; 1994:3–27.
3. Janz D. The grand mal epilepsies and the sleeping-waking cycle. *Epilepsia.* 1962;3:69–109.
4. Touchon J, Baldy-Moulinier M, Billiard M, Besset A, Cadilhac J. Sleep organization and epilepsy. *Epilepsy Res Suppl.* 1991;2:73–81.
5. Hofstra WA, Grootemarsink BE, Dieker R, van der PJ, de Weerd AW. Temporal distribution of clinical seizures over the 24-h day: a retrospective observational study in a tertiary epilepsy clinic. *Epilepsia.* 2009;50(9):2019–2026.
6. Bazil CW, Walczak TS. Effects of sleep and sleep stage on epileptic and nonepileptic seizures. *Epilepsia.* 1997;38(1):56–62.
7. Malow BA, Lin X, Kushwaha R, Aldrich MS. Interictal spiking increases with sleep depth in temporal lobe epilepsy. *Epilepsia.* 1998;39(12):1309–1316.
8. Steriade M. Interneuronal epileptic discharges related to spike-and-wave cortical seizures in behaving monkeys. *Electroencephalogr Clin Neurophysiol.* 1974;37(3):247–263.
9. Guberman A, Gloor P. Cholinergic drug studies of generalized penicillin epilepsy in the cat. *Brain Res.* 1974;78(2):203–222.
10. Kotagal P. The relationship between sleep and epilepsy. *Semin Pediatr Neurol.* 2001;8(4):241–250.
11. Quigg M. Circadian rhythms: interactions with seizures and epilepsy. *Epilepsy Res.* 2000;42(1):43–55.
12. Hofstra WA, de Weerd AW. The circadian rhythm and its interaction with human epilepsy: a review of literature. *Sleep Med Rev.* 2009;13(6):413–420.
13. Hofstra WA, de Weerd AW. How to assess circadian rhythm in humans: a review of literature. *Epilepsy Behav.* 2008;13(3):438–444.
14. Saper CB, Scammell TE, Lu J. Hypothalamic regulation of sleep and circadian rhythms. *Nature.* 2005;437(7063):1257–1263.
15. Reppert SM, Weaver DR. Coordination of circadian timing in mammals. *Nature.* 2002;418(6901):935–941.
16. Bell-Pedersen D, Cassone VM, Earnest DJ, et al. Circadian rhythms from multiple oscillators: lessons from diverse organisms. *Nat Rev Genet.* 2005;6(7):544–556.

17. Lowrey PL, Takahashi JS. Mammalian circadian biology: elucidating genome-wide levels of temporal organization. *Annu Rev Genom Hum Genet.* 2004;5:407–441.
18. Beenhakker MP, Huguenard JR. Neurons that fire together also conspire together: is normal sleep circuitry hijacked to generate epilepsy? *Neuron.* 2009;62(5):612–632.
19. Steriade M, Nunez A, Amzica F. Intracellular analysis of relations between the slow <1 Hz neocortical oscillation and other sleep rhythms of the electroencephalogram. *J Neurosci.* 1993;13(8):3266–3283.
20. Steriade M, McCormick DA, Sejnowski TJ. Thalamocortical oscillations in the sleeping and aroused brain. *Science.* 1993;262(5134):679–685.
21. Huguenard JR, McCormick DA. Thalamic synchrony and dynamic regulation of global forebrain oscillations. *Trends Neurosci.* 2007;30(7):350–356.
22. Tas E, Takeoka M, Molino J, et al. Thalamic lesions increase the frequency of spiking during sleep. *Epilepsia.* 2009;11(50):479.
23. Guzzetta F, Battaglia D, Veredice C, et al. Early thalamic injury associated with epilepsy and continuous spike-wave during slow sleep. *Epilepsia.* 2005;46(6):889–900.
24. Stickgold R, Walker MP. Sleep-dependent memory consolidation and reconsolidation. *Sleep Med.* 2007;8(4):331–343.
25. Kothare SV, Adams R, Valencia I, Faerber EC, Grant ML. Improved sleep and neurocognitive functions in a child with thalamic lesions on sodium oxybate. *Neurology.* 2007;68(14):1157–1158.
26. Fisher R, Salanova V, Witt T, et al. Electrical stimulation of the anterior nucleus of thalamus for treatment of refractory epilepsy. *Epilepsia.* 2010;51(5):899–908.
27. Landolt HP. Sleep homeostasis: a role for adenosine in humans? *Biochem Pharmacol.* 2008;75(11):2070–2079.
28. Jones BE. Glia, adenosine, and sleep. *Neuron.* 2009;61(2):156–157.
29. Boison D. The adenosine kinase hypothesis of epileptogenesis. *Prog Neurobiol.* 2008;84(3):249–262.
30. Boison D, Stewart KA. Therapeutic epilepsy research: from pharmacological rationale to focal adenosine augmentation. *Biochem Pharmacol.* 2009;78(12):1428–1437.
31. Duy PM, Xia L, Bartlett D Jr, Leiter JC. An adenosine A(2A) agonist injected in the nucleus of the solitary tract prolongs the laryngeal chemoreflex by a GABAergic mechanism in decerebrate piglets. *Exp Physiol.* 2010;95(7):774–787.
32. Sandyk R, Tsagas N, Anninos PA. Melatonin as a proconvulsive hormone in humans. *Int J Neurosci.* 1992;63(1–2):125–135.
33. Peled N, Shorer Z, Peled E, Pillar G. Melatonin effect on seizures in children with severe neurologic deficit disorders. *Epilepsia.* 2001;42(9):1208–1210.
34. Gupta M, Aneja S, Kohli K. Add-on melatonin improves quality of life in epileptic children on valproate monotherapy: a randomized, double-blind, placebo-controlled trial. *Epilepsy Behav.* 2004;5(3):316–321.
35. Monti JM. The role of dorsal raphe nucleus serotonergic and non-serotonergic neurons, and of their receptors, in regulating waking and rapid eye movement (REM) sleep. *Sleep Med Rev.* 2010;14(5):319–327.
36. Gholipour T, Ghasemi M, Riazi K, Ghaffarpour M, Dehpour AR. Seizure susceptibility alteration through 5-HT(3) receptor: modulation by nitric oxide. *Seizure.* 2010;19(1):17–22.
37. Baram TZ, Mitchell WG, Brunson K, Haden E. Infantile spasms: hypothesis-driven therapy and pilot human infant experiments using corticotropin-releasing hormone receptor antagonists. *Dev Neurosci.* 1999;21(3–5):281–289.
38. Rakhade SN, Jensen FE. Epileptogenesis in the immature brain: emerging mechanisms. *Nat Rev Neurol.* 2009;5(7):380–391.
39. Silverstein FS, Jensen FE. Neonatal seizures. *Ann Neurol.* 2007;62(2):112–120.
40. Sanchez RM, Jensen FE. Maturational aspects of epilepsy mechanisms and consequences for the immature brain. *Epilepsia.* 2001;42(5):577–585.
41. LoTurco JJ, Owens DF, Heath MJ, Davis MB, Kriegstein AR. GABA and glutamate depolarize cortical progenitor cells and inhibit DNA synthesis. *Neuron.* 1995;15(6):1287–1298.
42. Robinson S, Mikolaenko I, Thompson I, Cohen ML, Goyal M. Loss of cation-chloride cotransporter expression in preterm infants with white matter lesions: implications for the pathogenesis of epilepsy. *J Neuropathol Exp Neurol.* 2010;69(6):565–572.
43. Loddenkemper T, Alexopoulos A, Joseph A, et al. Altered glutamate and GABA receptor expression in cortical tissue resected from pediatric patients with status epilepticus. *Epilepsia.* 2009;50(11):358–359.
44. Patry G, Lyagoubi S, Tassinari CA. Subclinical "electrical status epilepticus" induced by sleep in children. A clinical and electroencephalographic study of six cases. *Arch Neurol.* 1971;24(3):242–252.
45. Bureau M. Continuous spikes and waves during slow sleep (CSWS): definition of the syndrome. In: Beaumanoir A, Bureau M, Deonna T, Mira L, Tassinari CA, eds. *Continuous Spikes and Waves During Slow Sleep/Electrical Status Epilepticus During Slow Sleep. Acquired Epileptic Aphasia and Related Conditions.* Milan, Italy: Fondazione Pierfranco e Luisa Mariani; 1995:17–26.
46. Komatsu H, Wurtz RH. Modulation of pursuit eye movements by stimulation of cortical areas MT and MST. *J Neurophysiol.* 1989;62(1):31–47.
47. Galanopoulou AS, Bojko A, Lado F, Moshe SL. The spectrum of neuropsychiatric abnormalities associated with electrical status epilepticus in sleep. *Brain Dev.* 2000;22(5):279–295.

48. Morikawa T, Seino M, Osawa T, Yagi K. Clinical relevance of continuous spike-wave discharges duirng sleep. In: Manelis S, Bental E, Loeber JN, Dreifuss FE, eds. *Advances in Epileptology*. Vol 17. New York, NY: Raven Press; 1989:359–363.
49. Tassinari CA, Bureau M, Dravet C, Dalla Bernardina B, Roger J. Epilepsy with continuous spikes and waves during slow sleep—otherwise described as ESES (epilepsy with electrical status epilepticus during slow sleep). In: Roger J, Dravet C, Bureau M, Dreifuss FE, Wolf P, eds. *Epileptic Syndromes in Infancy, Childhood and Adolescence*. London, UK: John Libbey & Company; 1985:194–204.
50. Tassinari CA, Rubboli G, Volpi L, et al. Encephalopathy with electrical status epilepticus during slow sleep or ESES syndrome including the acquired aphasia. *Clin Neurophysiol.* 2000;111(suppl 2):S94–S102.
51. Tassinari CA, Cantalupo G, Rios-Pohl L. Encephalopathy with status epilepticus during slow sleep: "the Penelope syndrome." *Epilepsia.* 2009;50(suppl 7):4–8.
52. Loddenkemper T, Cosmo G, Kotagal P, et al. Epilepsy surgery in children with electrical status epilepticus in sleep. *Neurosurgery*. 2009; 64(2):328–337.
53. Hirtum-Das M, Licht EA, Koh S, Wu JY, Shields WD, Sankar R. Children with ESES: variability in the syndrome. *Epilepsy Res.* 2006;70(suppl 1):S248–S258.
54. Tassinari CA, Bureau M, Dravet C, Dalla Bernardina B, Roger J. Epilepsy with continuous spikes and waves during slow sleep. In: Roger J, Dravet C, Bureau M, Dreifuss F, Wolf P, eds. *Epileptic Syndromes in Infancy, Childhood and Adolescence*. London, UK: John Libbey Eurotext Ltd.; 1985:194–204.
55. Loddenkemper T, Kotagal P. The boy who seized every time he slept. In Foldvary-Schaefer N, Krishna J, Budur K: A case a week—Sleep Disorders from the Cleveland Clinic. Oxford University Press 2011:349–356.
56. De Negri M. Electrical status epilepticus during sleep (ESES). Different clinical syndromes: towards a unifying view? *Brain Dev.* 1997;19(7):447–451.
57. Inutsuka M, Kobayashi K, Oka M, Hattori J, Ohtsuka Y. Treatment of epilepsy with electrical status epilepticus during slow sleep and its related disorders. *Brain Dev.* 2006;28(5):281–286.
58. Ohtsuka Y, Amano R, Mizukawa M, Oka E, Ohtahara S. Treatment of intractable childhood epilepsy with high-dose valproate. *Epilepsia.* 1992;33(1):158–164.
59. Ribacoba R, Salas-Puig J, Solar DM, Otero B, Herranz JL. [The efficacy of the valproic acid-ethosuximide combination in the continuous slow point wave syndrome during sleep]. *Neurologia.* 1997;12(8):335–338.
60. De Negri M, Baglietto MG, Battaglia FM, Gaggero R, Pessagno A, Recanati L. Treatment of electrical status epilepticus by short diazepam (DZP) cycles after DZP rectal bolus test. *Brain Dev.* 1995;175):330–333.
61. Buzatu M, Bulteau C, Altuzarra C, Dulac O, Van Bogaert P. Corticosteroids as treatment of epileptic syndromes with continuous spike-waves during slow-wave sleep. *Epilepsia.* 2009;50(suppl 7): 68–72.
62. Arts WF, Aarsen FK, Scheltens-de Boer M, Catsman-Berrevoets CE. Landau-Kleffner syndrome and CSWS syndrome: treatment with intravenous immunoglobulins. *Epilepsia.* 2009;50(suppl 7):55–58.
63. Morrell F, Whisler WW, Smith MC, et al. Landau-Kleffner syndrome. Treatment with subpial intracortical transection. *Brain.* 1995;118 (pt 6):1529–1546.
64. Devinsky O, Perrine K, Vazquez B, Luciano DJ, Dogali M. Multiple subpial transections in the language cortex. *Brain.* 1994;117 (pt 2):255–265.
65. Hirsch E, Pierre M, Metz-Lutz MN, Motta J, Finck S, Marescaux C. The eponym "Landau-Kleffner syndrome" should not be restricted to childhood-acquired aphasia with epilepsy. In: Beaumanoir A, Bureau M, Deonna T, Mira L, Tassinari C, eds. *Continuous Spikes and Waves During Slow Sleep*. London, UK: John Libbey; 1995:57–62.
66. Chahine LM, Mikati MA. Benign pediatric localization-related epilepsies. *Epileptic Disord.* 2006;8(4):243–258.
67. Eriksson KJ, Koivikko MJ. Prevalence, classification, and severity of epilepsy and epileptic syndromes in children. *Epilepsia.* 1997;38(12): 1275–1282.
68. Cavazzuti GB. Epidemiology of different types of epilepsy in school age children of Modena, Italy. *Epilepsia.* 1980;21(1):57–62.
69. Heijbel J, Blom S, Bergfors PG. Benign epilepsy of children with centrotemporal EEG foci. A study of incidence rate in outpatient care. *Epilepsia.* 1975;16(5):657–664.
70. Beaussart M. Benign epilepsy of children with Rolandic (centro-temporal) paroxysmal foci. A clinical entity. Study of 221 cases. *Epilepsia.* 1972;13(6):795–811.
71. Ma CK, Chan KY. Benign childhood epilepsy with centrotemporal spikes: a study of 50 Chinese children. *Brain Dev.* 2003;25(6):390–395.
72. Gobbi G, Boni A, Filippini M. The spectrum of idiopathic Rolandic epilepsy syndromes and idiopathic occipital epilepsies: from the benign to the disabling. *Epilepsia.* 2006;47(suppl 2):62–66.
73. Bouma PA, Bovenkerk AC, Westendorp RG, Brouwer OF. The course of benign partial epilepsy of childhood with centrotemporal spikes: a meta-analysis. *Neurology.* 1997;48(2):430–437.
74. Kriz M, Gazdik M. [Epilepsy with centrotemporal (Rolandic) spikes. A peculiar seizure disorder of childhood]. *Neurol Neurochir Pol.* 1978;12(4):413–419.
75. Wirrell EC. Benign epilepsy of childhood with centrotemporal spikes. *Epilepsia.* 1998;39(suppl 4): S32–S41.
76. Panayiotopoulos CP, Michael M, Sanders S, Valeta T, Koutroumanidis M. Benign childhood focal

epilepsies: assessment of established and newly recognized syndromes. *Brain*. 2008;131(pt 9): 2264–2286.
77. Sarkis R, Wyllie E, Burgess RC, Loddenkemper T. Neuroimaging findings in children with benign focal epileptiform discharges. *Epilepsy Res*. 2010;90(1–2):91–98.
78. Holmes GL. Rolandic epilepsy: clinical and electroencephalographic features. *Epilepsy Res Suppl*. 1992;6:29–43.
79. Graf M, Lischka A, Gremel K. [Benign Rolandic epilepsy in children. Topographic EEG analysis]. *Wien Klin Wochenschr*. 1990;102(7):206–210.
80. Pan A, Luders HO. Epileptiform discharges in benign focal epilepsy of childhood. *Epileptic Disord*. 2000;2(suppl 1):S29–S36.
81. Gregory DL, Wong PK. Topographical analysis of the centrotemporal discharges in benign rolandic epilepsy of childhood. *Epilepsia*. 1984;25(6): 705–711.
82. Loddenkemper T, Burgess RC, Syed T, Pestana EM. Lateralization of interictal EEG findings. *J Clin Neurophysiol*. 2007;24(5):379–385.
83. Sarkis RA, Loddenkemper T, Burgess RC, Wyllie E. Childhood absence epilepsy in patients with benign focal epileptiform discharges. *Pediatr Neurol*. 2009;41(6): 428–434.
84. Blom S, Heijbel J. Benign epilepsy of children with centro-temporal EEG foci. Discharge rate during sleep. *Epilepsia*. 1975;16(1):133–140.
85. Dalla BB, Pajno-Ferrara F, Beghini G. Proceedings: rolandic spike activation during sleep in children with and without epilepsy. *Electroencephalogr Clin Neurophysiol*. 1975;39(5):537.
86. Rose D, Duron B. [Prognostic value of EEG abnormalities observed during sleep in epilepsy with rolandic spikes (RSE)]. *Rev Electroencephalogr Neurophysiol Clin*. 1984;14(3):217–226.
87. Saint-Martin AD, Carcangiu R, Arzimanoglou A, et al. Semiology of typical and atypical Rolandic epilepsy: a video-EEG analysis. *Epileptic Disord*. 2001;3(4):173–182.
88. Vinayan KP, Biji V, Thomas SV. Educational problems with underlying neuropsychological impairment are common in children with Benign Epilepsy of Childhood with Centrotemporal Spikes (BECTS). *Seizure*. 2005;14(3):207–212.
89. Pinton F, Ducot B, Motte J, et al. Cognitive functions in children with benign childhood epilepsy with centrotemporal spikes (BECTS). *Epileptic Disord*. 2006;8(1):11–23.
90. Saint-Martin AD, Seegmuller C, Carcangiu R, et al. [Cognitive consequences of Rolandic Epilepsy]. *Epileptic Disord*. 2001;3(spec No 2):SI59–SI65.
91. Sart ZH, Demirbilek V, Korkmaz B, Slade PD, Dervent A, Townes BD. The consequences of idiopathic partial epilepsies in relation to neuropsychological functioning: a closer look at the associated mathematical disability. *Epileptic Disord*. 2006;8(1):24–31.
92. Croona C, Kihlgren M, Lundberg S, Eeg-Olofsson O, Eeg-Olofsson KE. Neuropsychological findings in children with benign childhood epilepsy with centrotemporal spikes. *Dev Med Child Neurol*. 1999;41(12):813–818.
93. Ong HT, Wyllie E. Benign childhood epilepsy with centrotemporal spikes: is it always benign? *Neurology*. 2000;54(5):1182–1185.
94. Deonna T. Rolandic epilepsy: neuropsychology of the active epilepsy phase. *Epileptic Disord*. 2000;2(suppl 1):S59–S61.
95. Metz-Lutz MN, Filippini M. Neuropsychological findings in Rolandic epilepsy and Landau-Kleffner syndrome. *Epilepsia*. 2006;47(suppl 2):71–75.
96. Fejerman N. Atypical rolandic epilepsy. *Epilepsia*. 2009;50(suppl 7):9–12.
97. Volkl-Kernstock S, Bauch-Prater S, Ponocny-Seliger E, Feucht M. Speech and school performance in children with benign partial epilepsy with centro-temporal spikes (BCECTS). *Seizure*. 2009;18(5):320–326.
98. Strug LJ, Clarke T, Chiang T, et al. Centrotemporal sharp wave EEG trait in rolandic epilepsy maps to Elongator Protein Complex 4 (ELP4). *Eur J Hum Genet*. 2009;17(9):1171–1181.
99. Neubauer BA, Fiedler B, Himmelein B, et al. Centrotemporal spikes in families with rolandic epilepsy: linkage to chromosome 15q14. *Neurology*. 1998;51(6):1608–1612.
100. Doose H, Brigger-Heuer B, Neubauer B. Children with focal sharp waves: clinical and genetic aspects. *Epilepsia*. 1997;38(7):788–796.
101. Heijbel J, Blom S, Rasmuson M. Benign epilepsy of childhood with centrotemporal EEG foci: a genetic study. *Epilepsia*. 1975;16(2):285–293.
102. Metrakos K, Metrakos JD. Genetics of convulsive disorders. II. Genetic and electroencephalographic studies in centrencephalic epilepsy. *Neurology*. 1961;11:474–483.
103. Vadlamudi L, Harvey AS, Connellan MM, et al. Is benign rolandic epilepsy genetically determined? *Ann Neurol*. 2004;56(1):129–132.
104. Rudolf G, Valenti MP, Hirsch E, Szepetowski P. From rolandic epilepsy to continuous spike-and-waves during sleep and Landau-Kleffner syndromes: insights into possible genetic factors. *Epilepsia*. 2009;50(suppl 7):25–28.
105. Wirrell EC, Hamiwka LD. Do children with benign rolandic epilepsy have a higher prevalence of migraine than those with other partial epilepsies or nonepilepsy controls? *Epilepsia*. 2006;47(10):1674–1681.
106. Corda D, Gelisse P, Genton P, Dravet C, Baldy-Moulinier M. Incidence of drug-induced aggravation in benign epilepsy with centrotemporal spikes. *Epilepsia*. 2001;42(6):754–759.
107. Massa R, Saint-Martin A, Carcangiu R, et al. EEG criteria predictive of complicated evolution in idiopathic rolandic epilepsy. *Neurology*. 2001;57(6):1071–1079.
108. Oguni H, Hayashi K, Imai K, Hirano Y, Mutoh A, Osawa M. Study on the early-onset variant of benign childhood epilepsy with occipital paroxysms otherwise described as early-onset benign occipital seizure susceptibility syndrome. *Epilepsia*. 1999;40(7):1020–1030.

109. Caraballo RH, Cersosimo RO, Fejerman N. Childhood occipital epilepsy of Gastaut: a study of 33 patients. *Epilepsia*. 2008;49(2):288–297.
110. Covanis A. Panayiotopoulos syndrome: a benign childhood autonomic epilepsy frequently imitating encephalitis, syncope, migraine, sleep disorder, or gastroenteritis. *Pediatrics*. 2006;118(4):e1237–e1243.
111. Panayiotopoulos CP. Early-onset benign childhood occipital seizure susceptibility syndrome: a syndrome to recognize. *Epilepsia*. 1999;40(5):621–630.
112. Tsai ML, Lo HY, Chaou WT. Clinical and electroencephalographic findings in early and late onset benign childhood epilepsy with occipital paroxysms. *Brain Dev*. 2001;23(6):401–405.
113. Gastaut H. A new type of epilepsy: benign partial epilepsy of childhood with occipital spike-waves. *Clin Electroencephalogr*. 1982;13(1):13–22.
114. Kivity S, Ephraim T, Weitz R, Tamir A. Childhood epilepsy with occipital paroxysms: clinical variants in 134 patients. *Epilepsia*. 2000;41(12):1522–1533.
115. Kellerman K. Benign epilepsy of childhood with occipital paroxysms: familial occurence with three affected children. *Epilepsia*. 1993;34(suppl 2):65.
116. Nagendra K, Rossiter M. Benign occipital epilepsy of childhood: a family study. *J R Soc Med*. 1990;83:804–805.
117. Verrotti A, Domizio S, Guerra M, Sabatino G, Morgese G, Chiarelli F. Childhood epilepsy with occipital paroxysms and benign nocturnal childhood occipital epilepsy. *J Child Neurol*. 2000;15(4):218–221.
118. Panayiotopoulos CP. Vomiting as an ictal manifestation of epileptic seizures and syndromes. *J Neurol Neurosurg Psychiatry*. 1988;51(11):1448–1451.
119. Panayiotopoulos CP. Benign childhood epilepsy with occipital paroxysms: a 15-year prospective study. *Ann Neurol*. 1989;26(1):51–56.
120. Panayiotopoulos CP. Panayiotopoulos syndrome. *Lancet*. 2001;358(9275):68–69.
121. Lada C, Skiadas K, Theodorou V, Loli N, Covanis A. A study of 43 patients with panayiotopoulos syndrome, a common and benign childhood seizure susceptibility. *Epilepsia*. 2003;44(1):81–88.
122. Caraballo R, Cersosimo R, Medina C, Fejerman N. Panayiotopoulos-type benign childhood occipital epilepsy: a prospective study. *Neurology*. 2000;55(8):1096–1100.
123. Caraballo R, Cersosimo R, Fejerman N. Panayiotopoulos syndrome: a prospective study of 192 patients. *Epilepsia*. 2007;48(6):1054–1061.
124. Koutroumanidis M. Panayiotopoulos syndrome. *BMJ*. 2002;324(7348):1228–1229.
125. Ferrie CD, Grunewald RA. Panayiotopoulos syndrome: a common and benign childhood epilepsy. *Lancet*. 2001;357(9259):821–823.
126. Oguni H, Hayashi K, Funatsuka M, Osawa M. Study on early-onset benign occipital seizure susceptibility syndrome. *Pediatr Neurol*. 2001;25(4):312–318.
127. Germano E, Gagliano A, Magazu A, et al. Benign childhood epilepsy with occipital paroxysms: neuropsychological findings. *Epilepsy Res*. 2005;64(3):137–150.
128. Kikumoto K, Yoshinaga H, Oka M, et al. EEG and seizure exacerbation induced by carbamazepine in Panayiotopoulos syndrome. *Epileptic Disord*. 2006;8(1):53–56.
129. Landau W, Kleffner F. Syndrome of acquired aphasia with convulsive disorder in children. *Neurology*. 1957;7:523–530.
130. Van Bogaert P, Paquier PF. Landau-Kleffner syndrome: 50 years after. *Epilepsia*. 2009;50(suppl 7):1–2.
131. Engel J Jr. Report of the ILAE classification core group. *Epilepsia*. 2006;47(9):1558–1568.
132. Bishop DV. Age of onset and outcome in "acquired aphasia with convulsive disorder" (Landau-Kleffner syndrome). *Dev Med Child Neurol*. 1985;27(6):705–712.
133. Steinlein OK. Epilepsy-aphasia syndromes. *Expert Rev Neurother*. 2009;9(6):825–833.
134. Beaumanoir A. The Landau Kleffner syndrome. In: Beaumanoir A, Bureau M, Deonna T, et al., eds. *Epileptic Syndromes in Infancy, Childhood, and Adolescence*. London, UK: John Libbey; 1992:231–244.
135. Garcia-Penas JJ. [Antiepileptic drugs in the treatment of autistic regression syndromes]. *Rev Neurol*. 2005;40(suppl 1):S173–S176.
136. Wirrell EC, Camfield PR, Gordon KE, Dooley JM, Camfield CS. Benign rolandic epilepsy: atypical features are very common. *J Child Neurol*. 1995;10(6):455–458.
137. Roulet E, Deonna T, Despland PA. Prolonged intermittent drooling and oromotor dyspraxia in benign childhood epilepsy with centrotemporal spikes. *Epilepsia*. 1989;30(5):564–568.
138. Aicardi J, Chevrie JJ. Atypical benign partial epilepsy of childhood. *Dev Med Child Neurol*. 1982;24(3):281–292.
139. Nass R, Petrucha D. Acquired aphasia with convulsive disorder: a pervasive developmental disorder variant. *J Child Neurol*. 1990;5(4):327–328.
140. Berg AT, Berkovic SF, Brodie MJ, et al. Revised terminology and concepts for organization of seizures and epilepsies: report of the ILAE Commission on Classification and Terminology, 2005-2009. *Epilepsia*. 2010;51(4):676–685.
141. Rudolf G, Valenti MP, Hirsch E, Szepetowski P. From rolandic epilepsy to continuous spike-and-waves during sleep and Landau-Kleffner syndromes: insights into possible genetic factors. *Epilepsia*. 2009;50(suppl 7):25–28.
142. Roll P, Rudolf G, Pereira S, et al. SRPX2 mutations in disorders of language cortex and cognition. *Hum Mol Genet*. 2006;15(7):1195–1207.
143. Caraballo RH, Sologuestua A, Granana N, et al. Idiopathic occipital and absence epilepsies appearing in the same children. *Pediatr Neurol*. 2004;30(1):24–28.
144. De Tiege X, Goldman S, Verheulpen D, Aeby A, Poznanski N, Van Bogaert P. Coexistence of idiopathic rolandic epilepsy and CSWS in 2 families. *Epilepsia*. 2006;47(10):1723–1727.

CHAPTER 7

Childhood Parasomnias

Radhika Dhamija and Suresh Kotagal

Introduction

Parasomnias are paroxysmal events that occur predominantly at the sleep-wake interface or during sleep [1]. The American Academy of Sleep Medicine defines parasomnias as "undesirable physical events or experiences that occur during entry into sleep, within sleep or during arousals from sleep" [2,3]. They may be confused with other episodic nocturnal phenomena such as seizures and nocturnal panic attacks (NPAs) because of a similarity in semiology. Although generally not harmful to the child, the events can be distressing for the parents or caretaker to watch. Preschool children have the highest prevalence. The events are less common during the latter half of the first decade and the second decade [1,2]. Sleep-related bruxism and rhythmic movement disorder (RMD) were previously considered parasomnias, but have now been classified as movement disorders under the *International Classification of Sleep Disorders-2* (*ICSD-2*) [3]. They are retained in this discussion, however, as they still represent undesirable events that intrude on sleep.

Epidemiology

Petit et al conducted a prospective study of childhood parasomnias in Quebec, Canada, in which the subjects were followed up from 2.5 to 6 years [4]. The prevalence of individual parasomnias over the study period was as follows: somnambulism 14.5%, sleep terrors 39.8%, somniloquy 84.4%, enuresis 25.0%, bruxism 45.6%, and rhythmic movements 9.2% [5]. In a study of 1413 school children aged 6.2 to 10.9 years, Klackenberg found the prevalence of frequent sleepwalking to be 7% [5].

The events are generally less common before 2 years of age, manifest most commonly in preschool children, and then resolve by the end of the first decade of life. They are equally common in boys and girls [4–6].

Pathophysiology

Parasomnias appear to develop because of a combination of genetic predisposition and activation of subcortical central pattern generators (CPGs) [2]. CPGs can be defined as neural networks that have intrinsic rhythmicity and can lead to patterns of stereotyped motor behavior. They are composed of networks of interneurons that project onto the motor neurons of the ventral brainstem and spinal cord [7]. Central pattern generators can be activated by sleep-disordered breathing, sleep deprivation, gastroesophageal reflux, periodic limb movement activity, stress, fever, and epilepsy. The stage is set for activation of CPGs by an underlying instability of sleep that may be caused by triggers such as genetic predisposition, obstructive sleep apnea, and periodic limb movements in sleep. The activation of arousals from sleep by epileptiform discharges that are recordable on the intracerebral electroencephalogram (EEG) is further indication of parasomnias being caused by instability of the arousal mechanism(s) [8]. With maturation of intracortical pathways and descending inhibitory projections from the cortex to subcortical structures, there is progressive inhibition of central pattern generators, hence likely the gradual resolution of parasomnias with age [2]. Glutamate and serotonin are involved in the regulation of the function of CPGs [9]. This may explain why glutamate antagonists such as benzodiazepines are generally effective in the treatment of a number of parasomnias.

Classification of Parasomnias

Parasomnias can be classified as those occurring at the transition from wakefulness to sleep, events occurring during non-rapid eye movement (NREM) and those occurring in rapid eye movement (REM) of sleep (Table 7.1) [3].

Parasomnias Occurring at the Transition From Wakefulness to Sleep

Sleep Starts

Children may experience sudden and brief jerks of the extremities at the time of initial sleep onset, often accompanied by a subjective sensation of falling [10]. They do not consistently awaken the child and may only be noted by the caretaker. These events are also termed benign hypnic myoclonus or hypnic starts. They result from loss of inhibition exercised by the cerebral cortex on subcortical structures during wakefulness. These phenomena may be more intense following physical activity or excessive caffeine intake [3,6]. Infrequently, in children with developmental problems, there may be 2 to 3 successive jerks that can be confused with myoclonic seizures. A video-EEG that captures the events can help clarify the nonepileptic nature of the events, as it remains normal [3].

Table 7.1 Classification of parasomnias*

Sleep-Wake Transition Parasomnias
Sleep starts
Isolated sleep paralysis
Rhythmic movement disorder
Sleep talking
NREM Parasomnias
Confusional arousals
Sleepwalking
Night terrors
REM Parasomnias
Nightmares
Rapid eye movement sleep behavior disorder
Other Parasomnias
Sleep bruxism
Sleep enuresis
Status dissociates
Overlap parasomnia

*Adapted from the *ICSD* manual with permission from Ref. [3].

Isolated Sleep Paralysis

This disorder is associated with a transient inability to move on awakening, or at the time of falling asleep. Isolated sleep paralysis (ISP) is not accompanied by an underlying sleep disorder, and thus is distinct from the sleep paralysis that accompanies 30% to 50% of patients with narcolepsy [11]. In a survey of 8075 subjects aged more than 15 years, Ohayon et al found a prevalence rate for ISP of 6.2% [11]. The condition is probably more common in youth—using a questionnaire survey of college students from Kuwait, Sudan, and the United States, Awadalla et al found prevalence rates of sleep paralysis in the 3 groups of subjects to be 28.8%, 29.9%, and 24.5%, respectively [12]. The events usually last 5 to 10 minutes and can be frightening to patients, as inability to move is accompanied by fully preserved consciousness. Physiologically, sleep paralysis represents intrusion of atonia of REM sleep onto wakefulness (sleep state dissociation) [11]. Panic disorder may coexist with ISP [13]. Sleep deprivation is a common trigger. ISP should be distinguished from periodic paralysis, which is a disorder that generally occurs during wakefulness. Owing to the benign nature, treatment of ISP is generally not needed. On an empiric basis, one of the authors (SK) has successfully used the REM sleep–suppressing property of imipramine to prevent recurrent episodes of sleep paralysis.

Rhythmic Movement Disorder

Three phenomena are generally grouped under the term "rhythmic movement disorder"—head banging, body rocking, and head rolling. These events are considered to be developmentally physiologic in preschool-age children [14]. In a prospective study, Klackenberg found that 66% of infants of 9 months age showed RMD symptoms as compared with only 8% of 4-year-olds [15]. The events have a 4:1 male to female predominance [6]. The events stop with an extraneous distraction and once the child has fallen asleep. The child generally has no recollection of the events on awakening. To be considered pathological, the *ICSD-2* requires that the sleep-related rhythmic movements interfere "markedly with normal sleep, cause significant impairment in daytime function, or result in self-inflicted bodily injury that requires medical treatment or would result in injury if preventive measures were not used" [16]. Mechanistically, RMD represents activation of sets of central pattern generators at subcortical levels [2]. It should be distinguished from rhythmic movements that accompany neurodevelopmental disorders such as autism and severe mental retardation that are accompanied by rhythmic movements during wakefulness. Walters et al have suggested a potential link between RMD and attention deficit hyperactivity disorder. They posit that immaturity of premotor and striatal circuits may be involved in both disorders. [17]. No specific treatment is needed for most subjects with RMD. Clonazepam has been used empirically in problematic cases.

Parasomnias Occurring During NREM Sleep

Arousals occurring during NREM sleep can evolve into confusional arousals, sleepwalking, or night terrors. These 3 NREM parasomnias are because of partial arousal from N3 stage of sleep. They are most likely to occur in the first third of the night, as N3 is most prevalent at this time. The age of occurrence is generally between 2 and 12 years, with resolution by adolescence. Confusional arousals are the most common of the 3 arousal parasomnias and are encountered in children at the younger end of this age group.

Sleepwalking (Somnambulism)

Children with sleepwalking appear to arise out of stage 3 NREM sleep (slow-wave sleep) and act as if they are awake but respond only partially to the surroundings or stimuli. Sleepwalking can result in falls and injuries while attempting to "escape," or simply from walking into dangerous situations. Walking out of a door onto the street has been reported. There is generally no autonomic dysfunction in the form of sweating, flushing of the face, or piloerection. Other parasomnias such as sleep terrors can coexist [6]. The duration of the event is generally 5 to 20 minutes. The EEG shows generalized, rhythmic activity in the 2- to 7-Hz range. The patient is unaware of the event on awakening in the morning.

Night Terrors (Pavor Nocturnus)

Children with night terrors arise out of deep sleep seemingly terrified, often screaming with fright and eyes open wide. They have accompanying autonomic activation in the form of piloerection, flushing of the face, sweating, and tachycardia [6]. The events may be triggered by sleep deprivation, febrile illness, sleep-disordered breathing, periodic limb movements, or anxiety [2]. The duration is 5 to 20 minutes. Sleep terrors have a strong genetic predisposition. They can be sometimes difficult to differentiate from NPAs [2]. Cyclic alternating patterns are oscillatory patterns on the EEG that occur with a periodicity of 20 to 40 seconds and are a representation of the dynamic organization of sleep [18]. They are increased in patients with unstable sleep, and notably in patients manifesting sleep terrors [19].

Confusional Arousals

This NREM parasomnia is common in toddlers and become less frequent after the age of 5 to 7 years. The events develop out of slow-wave (N3) sleep and, thus, are most prevalent during the first third of night sleep. The child typically sits up in bed and moans or cries for a few minutes. Much to the exasperation of the parent, the child's agitation may increase further with attempts at soothing and comforting! Utterances such as "no" or "go away" are common. The parents may mistakenly feel that the child is experiencing pain or discomfort. The episodes are 5 to 15 minutes long, but can last up to a half hour. On most occasions, the child has no recollection of the event on awakening the following morning. The daytime behavior is generally unaffected, though the child may manifest behavioral problems if sleep has been fragmented because of underlying obstructive sleep apnea or periodic limb movements [20,21].

Management of NREM Arousal Parasomnias

Infrequently occurring (<1–2 times per month) confusional arousals, sleep terrors, and sleepwalking may not need to be treated. They are benign and self-limiting, and parents may be counseled that they will resolve gradually over the next few months. Toddlers should receive adequate napping time during the day because sleep deprivation can be a trigger. In the case of sleepwalking, environmental safety measures such installing dead bolts and motion sensors in the house should be discussed with the parents.

A low threshold should be maintained for adding a 16-channel EEG montage to the polysomnogram to exclude sleep-related seizures, which are the key consideration in the differential diagnosis. If sleep-disordered breathing, periodic limb movement disorder, or gastroesophageal reflux are identified as potential triggers for the NREM arousal parasomnias, treatment efforts should be directed at these underlying disorders. In a group of 51 children with sleep terrors or sleepwalking, Guilleminault et al found that treatment of underlying inciting factors such as sleep-disordered breathing or restless legs syndrome led to resolution of the underlying parasomnia in 45 of 51 (88%) subjects [22]. If no specific underlying triggers are found and the arousal parasomnia remains problematic, a low dose of benzodiazepine at bedtime is recommended, for example, clonazepam 0.125 to 0.5 mg [2].

Nocturnal Frontal Lobe Epilepsy, NPAs, and NREM Arousal Sleep Parasomnias: A Comparison

Nocturnal frontal lobe epilepsy (NFLE) is a partial epilepsy in which seizures characterized by hypermotor behavior or dystonic posturing appear during sleep. The events can be mistaken for psychogenic nonepileptic seizures or NREM arousal parasomnias [23]. Bicycling automatisms, pelvic thrusting, genital manipulation, thrashing around, and vocalizations may be seen. Case reports of ictal aggressive behavior with complex motor and vocal features and gelastic seizures in NFLE have been described [24–28]. Secondary generalization may occur after any of the above initial ictal manifestations.

NFLE has autosomal dominant transmission in some families. It is associated with mutations in the CHRNA2/CHRNA4/CHRNB2 genes that regulate the expression of neuronal nicotinic acetylcholine receptors [29–31]. Other etiologies include cortical dysplasia, trauma, and vascular malformations. Some cases remain cryptogenic and hence a challenge to treat as the epileptic focus is not amenable to surgical resection.

The seizure can originate from over the orbitofrontal region or the mesial frontal/temporal region. Epileptiform discharges may therefore not be consistently reflected on to the conventional scalp EEG recordings, which pose a diagnostic dilemma. An initial standard outpatient EEG may detect interictal epileptiform abnormalities in generally a third to one half of the patients. The diagnostic yield from the standpoint of capturing the events can be increased by prolonged inpatient monitoring in a specialized epilepsy unit [24–28]. Distinguishing nocturnal frontal lobe seizures from NREM parasomnias such as sleep terrors or confusional arousals may be difficult and sometimes impossible on clinical grounds alone. Further, a reliable clinical description of NFLE is often difficult to obtain as the events are brief, lasting 10 to 30 seconds. Further, NFLE and NREM parasomnias may coexist in the same patient [32]. Video-EEG or video-polysomnography, together with careful history-taking and high-resolution magnetic resonance neuroimaging (for symptomatic cases with structural lesions) is recommended for distinguishing NFLE from NREM parasomnias [26,33].

The features that distinguish NFLE from NREM arousal parasomnias are shown in (Table 7.2) and discussed in detail by Tinuper et al [33]. They include the occurrence of the former predominantly during stages 1 and 2 of NREM sleep with the EEG showing sharp waves, as compared with N3 and accompanied by rhythmic delta for arousal parasomnias. In a study of 30 patients with autosomal dominant frontal lobe epilepsy, 27 of 30 subjects had seizure onset after K-complexes [34]. The events of NFLE are typically shorter in duration (<1 minute) and can be multiple in the same night. They can occur at any time during the night, unlike the NREM arousal parasomnias that tend to cluster into the first third of the night. Seizures also show a clearly demarcated time of onset and offset—this is somewhat less apparent in arousal parasomnias.

Table 7.2 Comparison between nocturnal frontal lobe epilepsy and non-rapid eye movement parasomnias

Clinical features	Nocturnal frontal lobe epilepsy	NREM parasomnias
Age of onset	In the first 2 decades of life but may occur later as well.	2–12 years, with resolution by late adolescence
Peak time of occurrence	Any time during the night (stage 1 or 2 of NREM sleep)	Generally first third of the night
Ictal electroencephalogram	Normal or sleep-related frontal epileptiform discharges	Rhythmic delta activity over a generalized distribution
Semiology	Abrupt onset and offset, hypermotor	More gradual onset over seconds, may exhibit sleepwalking, night terrors and confusional arousals, and indistinct offset; increased autonomic activity in sleep terrors
Duration and frequency	Short, generally <5 min; may have multiple events on one night	Longer, 10–30 minutes; multiple events less common on one night

Derry et al studied 120 patient events to describe the semiological features of NREM arousal parasomnias in detail and identify features that could be used to reliably distinguish them from NFLE [23]. Elemental clinical features strongly favoring parasomnias included: interactive behavior, failure to awaken after event, and indistinct offset. While sleep stage at onset was discriminatory (82% of seizures occurred during stage 1 or 2 sleep, with 100% of parasomnias occurring from stage 3 sleep), ictal EEG features were less useful. Video analysis of arousal parasomnias identified 3 principal behavioral patterns: arousals (92% of events), nonagitated motor behavior (72%), and distressed emotional behavior (51%).

NPAs have been reported in 28% to 71% of adult panic disorder patients [35–37]. The diagnostic criteria for NPA are listed in (Table 7.3) [38]. NPAs are NREM events, usually occurring during transition from N2 to N3 sleep, without associated electroencephalographic abnormalities. Panic events are common in anxiety disorder, which often has its onset during adolescence. Patients may show disrupted sleep and suffer from insomnia. This disorder has not been systematically studied in children. As the name implies, there are attacks that awaken patients from sleep. As in the daytime panic attacks, NPA may be associated with sweating, tachycardia, shortness of breath, and a feeling of impending doom that lasts from minutes to hours. The events can be frightening for the child, who might subsequently develop a conditioned fear of going to sleep. Most events occur between 1 and 3 hours after sleep onset and rarely more than once per night. Patients are able to vividly recall their experiences.

Table 7.3 Diagnostic criteria for nocturnal panic attacks

An abrupt onset of intense fear or discomfort, in which 4 or more of the following symptoms develop out of sleep:

1. Sensation of shortness of breath or smothering
2. Feeling of severe choking
3. Fear of losing control
4. Fear of dying
5. Tachycardia
6. Sweating
7. Chest pain and discomfort
8. Stomach discomfort such as nausea
9. Dizziness, lightheadedness, or unsteadiness
10. Depersonalization or derealization
11. Hot flashes or cold chills
12. Trembling or shaking
13. Numbness or tingling

When not precipitated by a stressful circumstance and feelings of depersonalization, panic attacks can be mistaken for nocturnal seizures. Features that help distinguish nocturnal seizures from panic attacks include short duration of the former, with abrupt onset and stereotyped nature. Cognitive behavioral therapy (CBT) has been shown to ameliorate NPAs [39].

A number of randomized clinical trials comparing CBT with medications have established the clinical efficacy of the former in patients with panic disorder [39–41]. A meta-analysis of 11 trials that compared CBT with antidepressants for panic disorder demonstrated similar outcomes (decrease in symptoms by 50%) in the acute phase, though patients receiving CBT fared better in follow-up over 6 months [40].

Parasomnias of REM Sleep

Nightmares

Nightmares are dream anxiety attacks with strong emotional responses that include fear or horror. The dream may contain situations of danger, discomfort, or psychological or physical distress. The prevalence of nightmares is estimated at 10% to 50% in children between 3 and 5 years, with an equal sex ratio [6]. Nightmares tend to occur in the latter half of the night, when REM sleep is most prevalent. Children usually awaken immediately from a nightmare with full recall of the dream. They may find it hard to go back to sleep partly because of fear. Nightmares can have physical triggers such as sleeping in an uncomfortable position or new surroundings, becoming febrile, or develop on a psychological basis from anxiety, and may follow an emotionally traumatic experience [2]. Older children may benefit from CBT. On an empiric basis, one can also treat nightmares using REM sleep–suppressing agents such as imipramine. Nightmares generally seem to diminish in frequency and intensity over the course of years [6].

REM Sleep Behavior Disorder

This parasomnia is often associated with physical acting out of the dream in the form of violent punching, kicking, or running that can lead to injury to the patient or a bed partner. Yelling behavior is also common. REM sleep behavior disorder (RBD) is generally seen in adults with neurodegenerative conditions, especially synucleinopathies, but is underrecognized in children. Sheldon and Jacobsen have, however, described the clinical and polygraphic features of 5 children who met criteria for RBD [42]. Nevsimalova et al have reported the clinical and polysomnographic features of 2 girls, aged 7 and 9, who had combined RBD and narcolepsy-cataplexy [43]. The dreams often have a threatening quality to them, such as being attacked or pursued by a stranger. The polysomnogram shows persistence of muscle tone during REM sleep (REM sleep without atonia). The locus coeruleus contains cells that have receptors for hypocretin-1. These cells also serve a "REM-off" function as they actively inhibit muscle tone and movement during this stage of sleep [44]. It is possible that reduced activity of these REM-off cells in narcolepsy or other degenerative brainstem disorders leads to physical enactment of dreams. RBD may also develop as a consequence of treatment with selective serotonin reuptake inhibitors and tricyclic agents [45,46] and Tourette syndrome [47]. The long-term outcome of childhood RBD is unknown [2]. Treatment with clonazepam in low doses such as 0.125 to 0.25 mg at bedtime is generally effective in suppressing the events [42].

Other Parasomnias

Nocturnal Bruxism (Teeth Grinding)

This disorder is typically accompanied by repetitive clenching of the jaw during NREM sleep. The AASM diagnostic criteria for sleep bruxism include a complaint by the patient or family member of tooth grinding or tooth clenching in sleep, abnormal wear of the teeth, sounds associated with the bruxism, increased masseter electromyographic activity during sleep, and absence of simultaneous epileptiform activity on the EEG [48]. Bruxism can develop as early as infancy, soon after the eruption of incisors. Disorders such as obstructive sleep apnea and anxiety may coexist and exacerbate bruxism [2,6]. Complications include abnormal wear to the teeth, damage and inflammation of the gums and resorption of the alveolar bone, hypertrophy of the muscles of mastication, and temporomandibular joint disorders. From the pathophysiologic standpoint, the disorder is likely a consequence of activation of central pattern generators in the motor nucleus of the trigeminal nerve that is located in the pons [2]. There is no single accepted strategy for treating bruxism. Adenotonsillectomy has been reported to reduce the incidence of bruxism from 25% to 7% [49]. Provision of a mouth guard to minimize damage to the teeth has also been recommended [6]. Biofeedback has been used to manage coexisting anxiety [50].

Sleep Enuresis

Sleep enuresis is characterized by recurrent involuntary micturition during sleep. It is physiologic during infancy and early childhood, with resolution by the age of 5 years. Obstructive sleep apnea has been associated with enuresis, and often its correction leads to resolution of enuresis as well. Increased plasma levels of brain atrial natriuretic peptide that have been reported in some patients with OSA [51] may underlie the enuresis. Enuretic episodes can occur in all stages of sleep. Cystometrography during sleep reveals elevated intravesical pressure and detrusor contractions during bladder filling [6]. Enuresis gradually decreases with age. No treatment is needed for bed-wetting before the age of 5 or 6 years, subsequent to which conditioning devices with alarms have shown success. In refractory cases, medications such as imipramine and desmopressin can be tried, though the combination of conditioning device and medication seems to be the most effective [52].

Status Dissociatus

Structural brainstem lesions involving the pontomesencephalic tegmentum such as cavernomas have been associated with sleep talking, vigorous movements accompanied by vivid dreams, enuresis, and daytime sleepiness [53]. Nocturnal polysomnography shows ambiguous sleep with mixture of the polygraphic features of REM and NREM sleep, which might reflect regression to an immature form of sleep, such as the transitional sleep of the newborn. During REM sleep, a 36-year-old patient described by Provini et al [54] demonstrated persistence of tonic electromyographic tone (REM sleep without atonia) and violent motor behaviors that were consistent with RBD. It is possible that similar disturbances occur in rapidly progressive childhood neurodegenerative disorders also (author's opinion).

Overlap Parasomnia

This disorder is less recognized and perhaps overlooked in pediatric somnology. It was originally described by Schenck et al in a series of 33 young adults [55]. It manifested as combined sleepwalking (injurious), sleep terrors, and RBD. The mean age of onset in their series was 15 ± 16 years, which emphasizes the onset during childhood or adolescence. The subgroup of 22 idiopathic overlap parasomnia patients had a significantly earlier age of onset (9 ± 7 years) as compared with 11 patients in the symptomatic subgroup (27 ± 23 years), who had disorders such as Mobius syndrome, narcolepsy, multiple sclerosis, brain tumor, and head trauma. All subjects were responsive to treatment with clonazepam, alprazolam, and/or carbamazepine. Overlap parasomnia has also been described in the Harlequin syndrome [56] and Parkinson disease [57].

Conclusions and Possible Directions for Further Inquiry

Childhood parasomnias can range from those occurring at the sleep-wake transition to those associated with NREM and REM sleep. It is important to differentiate between parasomnias and other nocturnal events such as seizures and panic disorders as treatment and prognosis is different for all these conditions. A scheme for differentiating events such as arousal parasomnias and other nocturnal spells is shown in Figure 7.1.

The discovery of a link between the *BTBD9* homeobox gene complex and the rhythmic phenomenon of periodic limb movements has been a significant milestone in sleep medicine [58,59]. It may spur interest in population-based, whole-genome analyses for genetic markers relevant to other rhythmic or automatic nocturnal phenomena such as bruxism and sleepwalking [2]. As we move from phenomenology to physiology, the central role played by central pattern generators in pathogenesis of many parasomnias will likely receive more attention. Study of markers of unstable sleep

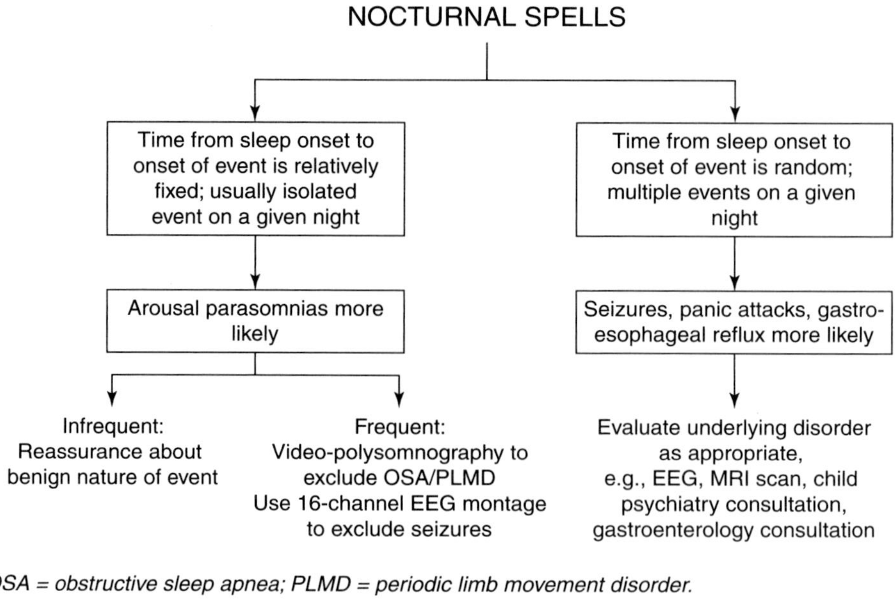

Figure 7.1 An algorithm for the evaluation of nocturnal spells. Adapted with permission from Ref. [38].

such as cyclic alternating patterns may garner more interest among sleep clinicians [58,60].

References

1. Mahowald MW, Schenck CH. Status dissociatus—a perspective on states of being. *Sleep*. 1991; 14(1):69–79.
2. Kotagal S. Parasomnias of childhood. *Curr Opin Pediatr.* 2008;(6):659–665.
3. American Academy of Sleep Medicine (2005). *International Classification of Sleep Disorders, 2nd ed.: Diagnostic and Coding Manual.* Westchester, IL:American Academy of Sleep Medicine.
4. Petit D, Touchette E, Tremblay RE, Boivin M, Montplaisir J. Dyssomnias and parasomnias in early childhood. *Pediatrics*. 2007;119:e1016–e1025.
5. Klackenberg G. Incidence of parasomnias in children in a general population. In: C. Guilleminault C, ed. *Sleep and Its Disorders in Children*. New York, NY: Raven Press; 1987:99–113.
6. Sheldon SH. Parasomnias in childhood. *Pediatr Clin North Am*. 2004;51:69–88.
7. Grillner S, Wallen P, Saitoh K, Kozlov A, Robertson B. Neural bases of goal directed locomotion in vertebrates–an overview. *Brain Res Rev.* 2008;57:2–12.
8. Nobili L, Sartori I, Terzaghi M, et al. Relationship of epileptic discharges to arousal instability and periodic leg movements in a case of nocturnal frontal lobe epilepsy: a stereo-EEG study. *Sleep*. 2006;29(5):701–704.
9. Hagglund M, Borgius L, Dougherty KJ, Kiehn O. Activation of groups of excitatory neurons in the mammalian spinal cord or hind brain evokes locomotion. *Nat Neurosci*. 2010;132):246–252.
10. Ramelli GP, Sozzo AB, Vella S, Bianchetti MG. Benign neonatal sleep myoclonus: an under-recognized, non-epileptic condition. *Acta Pediatr*. 2005;94(7):962–963.
11. Ohayon MM, Zulley J, Guilleminault C, Smirne S. Prevalence and pathologic associations of sleep paralysis in the general population. *Neurology*. 1999;52(6):1194–2000.
12. Awadalla A, Al-Favez G, Harville M, et al. Comparative prevalence of isolated sleep paralysis in kuwaiti, sudanese, and american college students. *Psychol Rep*. 2004;95(1):317–322.
13. Otto M, Simon NM, Powers M, Hinton D, Zalta AK, Pollack MH. Rates of isolated sleep paralysis in outpatients with anxiety disorders. *J Anxiety Disord*. 2006;20(5):687–693.
14. Khan A, Auger R, Kushida CA, Ramar K. Rhythmic movement disorder. *Sleep Med*. 2008;9(3):329–330.
15. Klackenberg G. A prospective longitudinal study of children. Data on psychic health and development up to 8 years of age. *Acta Paediatr Scand Suppl*. 1971;224:1–239.
16. American Academy of Sleep Medicine. *International Classification of Sleep Disorders, Pocket Version, Diagnostic and Coding Manual*. Westchester, IL: American Academy of Sleep Medicine; 2005: 138–139.

17. Walters AS, Silvestri R, Zucconi M, Chandrashekariah R, Konofal E. Review of the possible relationship and hypothetical links between attention deficit hyperactivity disorder (ADHD) and the simple sleep related movement disorders, parasomnias, hypersomnias, and circadian rhythm disorders. *J Clin Sleep Med.* 2008;4(6):591–600.
18. Terzano MG, Parino L. Origin and significance of cyclic alternating patterns (CAP). *Sleep Med Rev.* 2000;4:101–123.
19. Bruni O, Ferri R, Novelli L, Finotti E, Miano S, Guilleminault C. NREM sleep instability in children with sleep terrors: the role of slow wave interruptions. *Clin Neurophysiol.* 2008;119(5):985–992.
20. Mehlenbeck R, Spirito A, Owens J, Boergers J. The clinical presentation of childhood partial arousals parasomnias. *Sleep Med.* 2000;1(4):307–312.
21. Rosen GM, Mahowald MW. Disorders of arousal in children. In: Sheldon SH, Ferber R, Kryger MH, eds. *Principles and Practice of Pediatric Sleep Medicine*. Philadelphia, PA: Elsevier Saunders; 2005:293–304.
22. Guilleminault C, Palombini L, Pelayo R, Chervin RD. Sleep walking and sleep terrors in prepubertal children: what triggers them? *Pediatrics.* 2003;111:e17–e25.
23. Derry CP, Harvey AS, Walker MC, Duncan JS, Berkovic SF. NREM arousal parasomnias and their distinction from nocturnal frontal lobe epilepsy: a video EEG analysis. *Sleep.* 2009;32(12):1637–1644.
24. Williamson PD, Spencer DD, Spencer SS, Novelly RA, Mattson RH. Complex partial seizures of frontal lobe origin. *Ann Neurol.* 1985;18(4):497–504.
25. Shih JJ, Leslie-Mazwi T, Falcao G, Van Gerpen J. Directed aggressive behavior in frontal lobe epilepsy: a video-EEG and ictal SPECT case study. *Neurology.* 2009;73(21):1804–1806.
26. Manford M, Fish DR, Shorvon SD. An analysis of clinical seizure patterns and their localizing value in frontal and temporal lobe epilepsies. *Brain.* 1996;119(1):17–40.
27. Jobst BC, Siegel AM, Thadani VM, Roberts DW, Rhodes HC, Williamson PD. Intractable seizures of frontal lobe origin: clinical characteristics, localizing signs, and results of surgery. *Epilepsia.* 2000;41(9):1139–1152.
28. Cercy SP, Kuluva JE. Gelastic epilepsy and dysprosodia in a case of late-onset right frontal seizures. *Epilepsy Behav.* 2009;16(2):360–365.
29. Steinlein OK, Mulley JC, Propping P, et al. A missense mutation in the neuronal nicotinic acetylcholine receptor α-4 subunit is associated with autosomal dominant nocturnal frontal lobe epilepsy. *Nat Genet.* 1995;11(2):201–203.
30. Aridon P, Marini C, Di Resta C, et al. Increased sensitivity of the neuronal nicotinic receptor α-2 subunit causes familial epilepsy with nocturnal wandering and ictal fear. *Am J Hum Genet.* 2006;79(2):342–350.
31. Diaz-Otero F, Quesada M, Morales-Corraliza J, Martínez-Parra C, Gómez-Garre P, Serratosa JM. Autosomal dominant nocturnal frontal lobe epilepsy with a mutation in the CHRNB2 gene. *Epilepsia.* 2008;49(3):516–520.
32. Cornaggia CM, Beghi M, Giovannini S, Boni A, Gobbi G. Partial seizures with affective semiology versus pavor nocturnus. *Epileptic Disord.* 2010;12(1):65–68.
33. Tinuper PF, Provini FF, Bisulli F, et al. Movement disorders in sleep: guidelines for differentiating epileptic from non-epileptic motor phenomena arising from sleep. *Sleep Med Rev.* 2007;11:255–267.
34. El Helou J, Navarro V, Depienne C, et al. K-complex-induced seizures in autosomal dominant nocturnal frontal lobe epilepsy. *Clin Neurophysiol.* 2008;119(10):2201–2204.
35. Singareddy R, Uhde TW. Nocturnal sleep panic and depression: relationship to subjective sleep in panic disorder. *J Affect Disord.* 2009;112(1–3):262–266.
36. Sarísoy G, Böke O, Arík AC, Sahin AR. Panic disorder with nocturnal panic attacks: symptoms and comorbidities. *Eur Psychiatry.* 2008;23(3):195–200.
37. Albert U, Maina G, Bergesio C, Bogetto F. Nocturnal panic and recent life events. *Depress Anxiety.* 2005;22(2):52–58.
38. Craske MG, Tsao JC. Assessment and treatment of nocturnal panic attacks. *Sleep Med Rev.* 2005;9(3):173–184.
39. Overbeek T, Schruers K. Cognitive behavioural therapy reduces nocturnal panic in people with panic disorder. *Evid Based Ment Health.* 2006;9(1):13.
40. Mitte K. A meta-analysis of the efficacy of psycho-and pharmacotherapy in panic disorder with and without agoraphobia. *J Affect Disord.* 2005;88:27–45.
41. Barlow DH. Cognitive-behavioral therapy for panic disorder: current status. *J Clin Psychiatry.* 1997;58(suppl 2):32–36.
42. Sheldon SH, Jacobsen J. REM-sleep motor disorder in children. *J Child Neurol.* 1998;13:257–260.
43. Nevsimalova S, Prihodiva I, Kemlink D, Lin L, Migno E. REM behavior disorder (RBD) can be one of the first symptoms of childhood narcolepsy. *Sleep Med.* 2007;8:784–786.
44. Bourgin PS, Huitron-Resendiz S, Spier AD, et al. Hypocretin-1 modulates rapid eye movement sleep through activation of locus coeruleus neurons. *J Neurosci.* 2000;20:7760–7765.
45. Winkelmann JW, James L. Serotonergic antidepressants are associated with REM sleep without atonia. *Sleep.* 2004;27(2):317–321.
46. Stamenkovic M, Pezawas L, de Zwaan M, Aschauer HN, Kasper S. Mirtazapine in recurrent brief depression. *Int Clin Pharmacol.* 1998;13(1):39–40.
47. Trajanovic NN, Voloh I, Shapiro CM, Sandor P. Rem sleep behavior disorder in a child with tourette syndrome. *Can J Neurol Sci.* 2004;31(4):572–575.

48. American Academy of Sleep Medicine. Bruxism. In: *International Classification of Sleep Disorders, Pocket Version, Diagnostic and Coding Manual.* Westchester, IL: American Academy of Sleep Medicine; 2005:120–122.
49. Eftekharian A, Raad A, Gholami-Ghasri N. Bruxism and adenotonsillectomy. *Int J Pediatr Otorhinolaryngol.* 2008;72:509–511.
50. Funch DP, Gale EN. Factors associated with nocturnal bruxism and its treatment. *J Behav Med.* 1980;3:385–397.
51. Svatikova A, Shamsuzzman AS, Wolk R, Phillips BG, Olson LJ, Somers VK. Plasma brain atrial natriuretic peptide in obstructive sleep apnea. *Am J Cardiol.* 2004;94(4):529–532.
52. Kamperis K, Hagstroem S, Rittig S, Djurhuus JC. Combination of the enuresis alarm and desmopressin: second line treatment for nocturnal enuresis. *J Urol.* 2008;179(3):1128–1131.
53. Mason TBA, Pack AI. Pediatric parasomnias. In: Marcus CL, Carroll JL, Donnely DF, Loughlin GM, eds. *Sleep in Children.* New York, NY: Informa Health Care; 2008:223–241.
54. Provini F, Vetrugno R, Pastorelli F, et al. Status dissociatus after surgery for tegmental pontomesencephalic cavernoma: a state dependent disorder of motor control during sleep. *Mov Disord.* 2004;19(6):719–724.
55. Schenck CH, Boyd JL, Mahowald MW. A parasomnia overlap disorder involving sleepwalking, sleep terrors and REM sleep behavior disorder in 33 polysomnographically confirmed cases. *Sleep.* 1997;20:972–981.
56. Lombardi C, Vetrugo R, Provini F, et al. Harlequin syndrome: an association with overlap parasomnia. *J Neurol Neurosurg Psychiatry.* 2004;75:341–345.
57. Poryazova R, Waldvogel D, Bassetti CL. Sleep walking in patients with parkinson disease. *Arch Neurol.* 2007;64(10):1524–1527.
58. Stefansson H, Rye DB, Hicks A, Petursson H, et al. A genetic risk factor for periodic limb movements in sleep. *N Engl J Med.* 2007;357(7):639–647.
59. Winkelmann J, Schormair B, Lichtner P, et al. Genome-wide association study of restless legs syndrome identifies common variants in three genomic regions. *Nat Genet.* 2007;39(8): 1000–1006.
60. Tassinari CA, Cantalupo G, Hogl B, et al. Neuroethological approach to frontolimbic epileptic seizures and parasomnias: the same central pattern generators for the same behaviors. *Rev Neurol.* 2009;165(10):762–768.

CHAPTER 8

Smith-Magenis Syndrome

Gabor P. Szuhay and Andrea L. Gropman

Introduction

Children with the Smith-Magenis syndrome (SMS) display a unique combination of dysmorphic facial features, neurological, developmental, and behavioral profile of which sleep-related abnormalities, more specifically an inverted diurnal pattern of melatonin secretion, is most pathognomonic. Because children with SMS have other risk factors and disease processes that may independently cause sleep disruption, and not all children with sleep disturbances have altered melatonin secretion, it is likely that the sleep disturbance in this syndrome is multifactorial.

The SMS is a multiple congenital anomaly and mental retardation syndrome first recognized in 1982 by Smith and colleagues, in 2 severely impaired patients. Further cases had been ascertained and a full spectrum delineated [1], many of which are associated with a milder phenotype. SMS is due to either a deletion of genes on chromosome 17p11.2 (Figure 8.1) or a mutation in the RAI1 gene, a gene that is in the deletion region. The estimated prevalence of SMS deletion cases was reported to be 1 in 25,000 [2]. However, new cases have been identified in the last decade as a result of improved molecular cytogenetic techniques such as microarray technology, rather than increased awareness of the phenotype. It is therefore, not unreasonable to recommend repeating cytogenetic analysis in the face of a previously "normal" karyotype; if this was done more than 5 years ago as in deletion cases, the 2 to 3 MB deletion may be overlooked. Two genetic mechanisms cause SMS: an interstitial deletion involving chromosome 17p11.2 (including the retinoic acid–induced 1 [RAI1] gene) or a mutation in the RAI1 gene [3–5]. Patients with the full deletion tend to have a more severe phenotype. Therefore, in addition to recognition of cytogenetic deletion and use of FISH probes

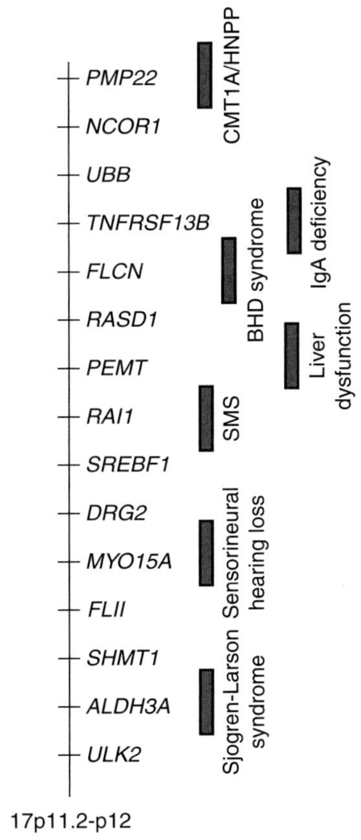

Figure 8.1 Ideogram of chromosome 17p11.2 showing the region containing the deleted genes involved in SMS.

specific for this deletion, RAI1 mutation testing can be used in the child with classic phenotype and "negative karyotype" [6]. On this basis, it is suggested that the incidence may be closer to 1 in 15 000 births [7].

SMS Phenotype

The phenotype of SMS becomes more pronounced and recognizable with advancing age, often leading to a delay in diagnosis in the early years when the child may come to clinical attention for hypotonia or developmental delay (DD). This is true both in terms of the dysmorphic and medical features, but especially with regard to the sleep and behavioral features [8] (Table 8.1 and 8.2). Infants with SMS present with a rather nonspecific clinical phenotype consisting of central hypotonia, a weak, hoarse cry, and decreased vocalizations including decreased babbling. Temperament is often described as easy and complacent [8–10]. Gross and fine motor skill development is delayed in the first year of life. Sensory integration problems are frequently noted, becoming more obvious in the toddler years. Because social skills are often age appropriate in infancy, the diagnosis is not entertained, and this leads to further investigation for an alternative cause as the motor delays are felt to be "transient" and felt to improve.

Table 8.1 Across the lifespan characteristic neurodevelopmental and behavioral features in infants and toddlers with SMS

Infant with SMS

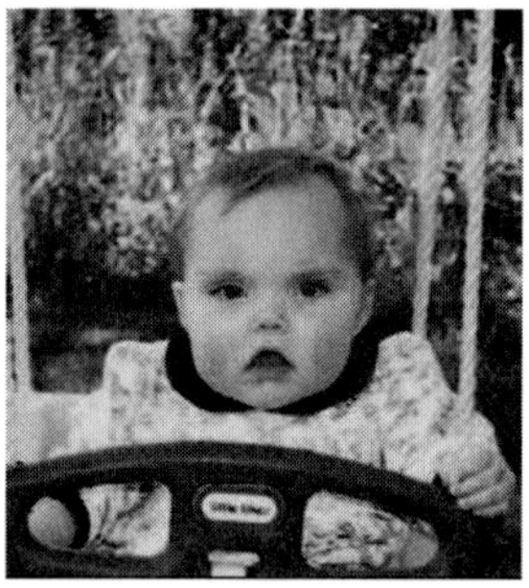

Dysmorphisms—diagnostic pearls

Down-turned mouth
Brachycephaly
Down-slanting palpebral fissures
Flat midface
Failure to thrive
Lethargic
Parent perception of "good sleeper"
"Quiet good babies"
Complacent
Diminished vocalizations and crying

Neurodevelopmental examination features/objective findings

Generalized hypotonia
Delayed gross/fine motor skills
Age appropriate social skills
Decreased total sleep for age

Toddler with SMS

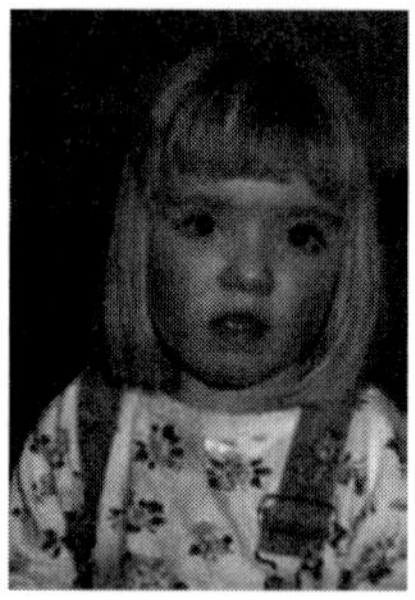

Dysmorphisms—diagnostic pearls

Down-turned mouth
Brachycephaly
Down-slanting palpebral fissures
Flat midface
Pes planus (flat) or pes cavus
Engaging personality
Frequent night awakenings and daytime naps
Sleep disturbance: short sleep cycle; early risers (5:30–6:30 AM)
Decreased pain sensitivity

Neurodevelopmental examination features/objective findings

Developmental delays
Gross/fine motor delays
Marked speech delay (expressive and receptive)
Delayed potty training
Sensory Integration issues
Stereotypic behaviors: self-hugging, lick and flip behaviors, head banging, skin picking

Table 8.2 Characteristic neurodevelopmental/behavioral features in children and adults with SMS

School age child with SMS	Adolescent/adult with SMS
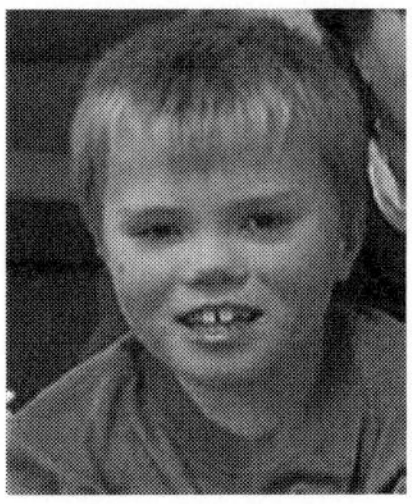	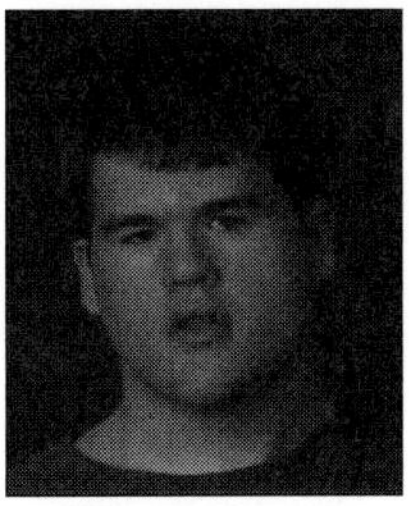
Dysmorphisms—diagnostic pearls	**Dysmorphisms—diagnostic pearls**
Coarsening of facial features	Coarsening of facial features
Relative prognathism	Relative prognathism
Chronic sleep disturbance	Chronic sleep disturbance
Behavior	Reports of exercise intolerance
Attention-seeking behaviors	**Behavior**
Frequent outbursts and tantrums	Major behavioral outbursts or rage behaviors, property destruction
Sudden mood shifts	Attention seeking behavior
Impulsivity/aggression	Aggressive/explosive outbursts
Stereotypic behaviors	Impulsive, disobedient
Self-injurious behaviors: hitting self, nail biting or pulling, object insertion into body orifices	Self-injurious behaviors (hitting self/nail yanking, object insertion)
Pes planus or pes cavus	Mood shifts (rapid) without major provocation attention deficits
Bedwetting	Argumentative
Neurodevelopmental findings	Self hug, upper body spasmodic squeeze
Cognitive delays, sensory integration issues	Mouthing of objects, bruxism. Lick and flip of pages in a book,
Excellent long term memory	Body rocking, spinning and twirling of objects
Very communicative	**Neurodevelopmental findings**
	Very communicative, excellent long term memory
	Cognitive delays
	Poor adaptive function
	Very communicative

Children with SMS have autistic features (because of language and communication delays) and may be classified as such without consideration of SMS as a potential underlying diagnosis, especially in cases where there is no familiarity with the clinical manifestations of SMS. Alternative genetic diagnoses may include Prader-Willi syndrome (obesity and hypotonia in some children with SMS), Down syndrome (up slanting palpebral fissures, hypotonia, and flat occiput), Velocardiofacial syndrome (language delays), Fragile X (stereotypies, language delays, and autism), or Angelman syndrome (toe walking, lack of early language) [8]. It is therefore important to maintain a high level of clinical suspicion for the diagnosis of SMS in a child presenting with dysmorphic facies, hypotonia, speech delays, autistic features, maladaptive behaviors, and especially with impaired nocturnal and daytime sleep patterns.

The most intriguing aspect of SMS, one that serves to distinguish it from the other genetic conditions and a subject of our ongoing research, is the circadian sleep disturbance that distinguishes this mental retardation disorder from many others and presents opportunities and challenges for treatment.

Sleep in SMS

Sleep disturbances in vulnerable pediatric subpopulations have been understudied, and SMS is an example of a neurogenetic syndrome with potentially multiple risk factors for sleep disturbance. In SMS, abnormal sleep patterns are described already in infancy. Smith et al reported on the sleep patterns of 39 individuals ranging from 1 to 32 years of age with mean age of 10.5 years based on parent surveys [11]. On average, bedtime ranged from 6:30 to 10:20 PM and wake up times from 2:00 to 7:00 AM. Total sleep time ranged from 3.5 to 10.5 hours, average of 7.8 hours. Night awakenings were 2.3/night, ranging from 0 to 18/night. Time to fall back to sleep was 31 minutes, ranging from 0 to 180 minutes. Naps ranged from 1 to 6/d, n average 1.4/d. Broken down by age, older individuals woke up more frequently at night, woke up earlier, took more but shorter naps, and slept less in total per day. However, there was no correlation between daytime sleepiness on the Sleep History Questionnaire and difficulty initiating or maintaining sleep and morning symptoms of an insufficient night sleep. Sleep times are plotted against that of healthy controls and other patient groups including those with unspecified mental retardation and Fragile X (Figure 8.2).

The infants with SMS are characterized as docile, even lethargic, some needing to be awakened to feed. They have decreased total sleep time in 24 hours and increased daytime napping. In contrast, school age children with SMS are described as temperamental (94%), aggressive (57%), attention seeking (100%), hyperactive (94%), and disobedient (97%). They manifest characteristic self-mutilating behaviors, which escalate and in adolescence they can become destructive (86%). Sleeping problems escalate beginning at 18 to 24 months of age and worsen again at school age and at puberty. If children were not brought to clinical attention because of developmental concerns, then they typically present due to parental concerns about their sleep [8].

In toddlers, sleep disturbances intensify, and 24-hour sleep is decreased. The sleep cycles remain shortened, with fragmented sleep from frequent and prolonged awakenings and early morning rising between 5 and 6 AM with more awakenings in the second half of the night in children under 10 years of age [8].

Infants and toddlers appear socially appropriate, thus it is not until early school age that children with SMS may come to medical attention as they become more attention seeking, moody, and aggressive displaying self-mutilating behaviors; however, they remain communicative within their limitations, and no autistic regression is noted. Previously mentioned chronic sleep disturbances also predominate in this age group, and primary enuresis becomes apparent. In adolescence, sleep-onset insomnia and maintenance is more evident with relatively increased awakenings and arousals in the first half compared to the second half of the night. Bruxism also becomes more prevalent which may suggest underlying anxiety. Their behavior continues to be aggressive even destructive, and self-mutilation does not cease [8].

Studying Sleep in Children With SMS

Three methods have been used to quantify the sleep of patients with SMS: clinical polysomnography (PSG), actigraphy, and subjective questionnaires or diaries. Each has its relative advantages and disadvantages, and the findings drawn from the use of each method should be considered in view of their strengths and weaknesses.

The study of sleep maintenance relies on parental report and objective assessments compared to normative values for age and sleep environment. Overnight PSG is the gold standard for sleep stage measurement, arousal assessment, respiratory disturbance and its role in sleep disruption, and seizure detection. Parental reports are important when instrumentation is not tolerated, sleep disruption varies from night-to-night with prolonged hypokinetic wakefulness, and in preschool age and younger children where wakefulness may not be accompanied by leg movements. Videosomnography (ie, video-recording analysis without instrumentation on the child) provides complimentary data and may be preferable if multiple night recordings at home and when the child's sleep is disturbed by being observed.

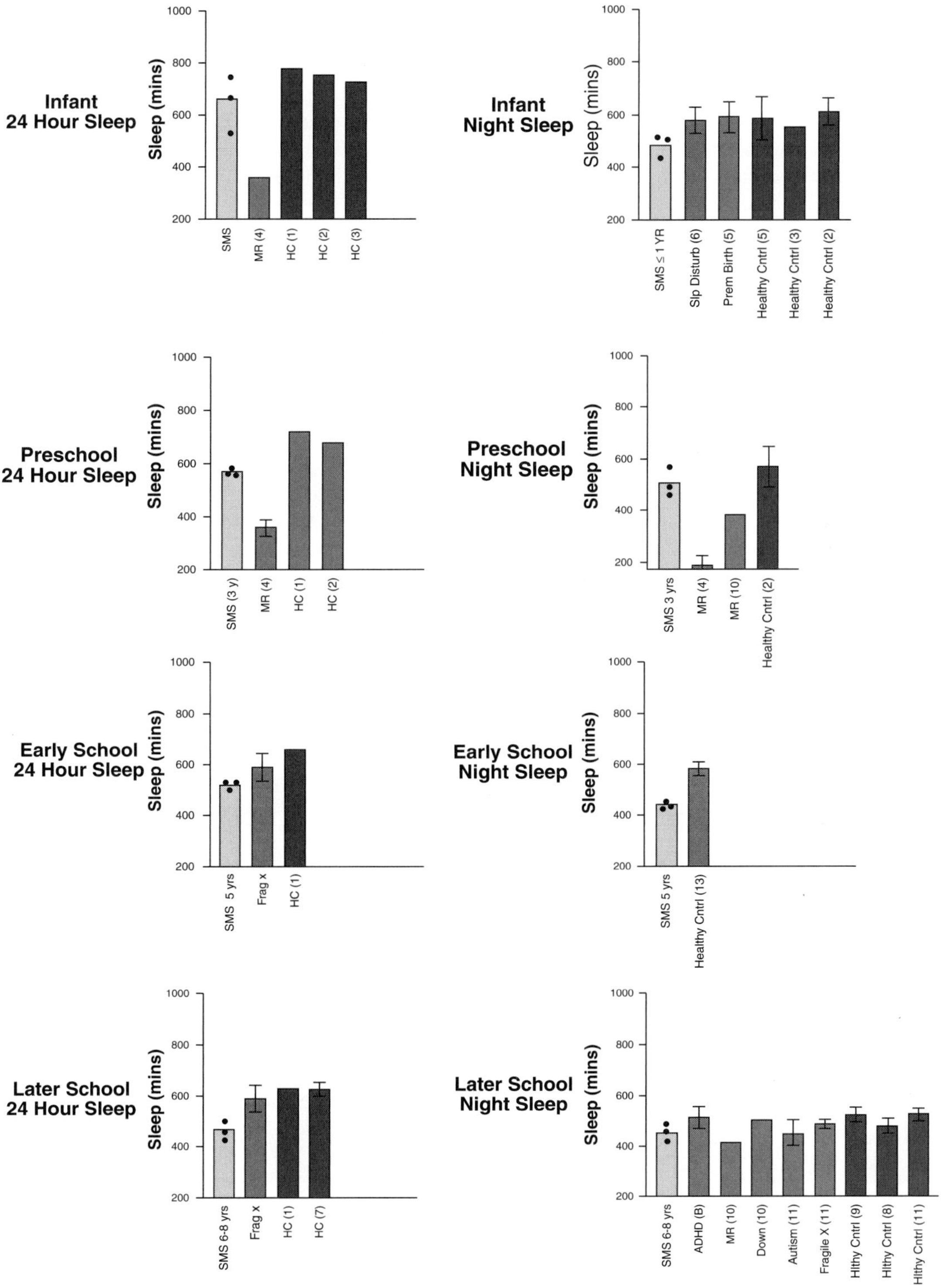

Figure 8.2 Comparison of 24-hour sleep in infants and children with SMS as compared to normal controls and other classes of mental retardation.

Actigraphy is an attractive method for sleep maintenance analysis especially in the developmentally delayed group because it is relatively better tolerated than PSG. However, actigraphy is not an accurate measure of electroencephalogram (EEG) or autonomic arousals, more subtle awakenings, and cannot differentiate nonrespiratory from respiratory arousals in a child with even mild sleep disordered breathing (ie, primary snoring) or central sleep apnea.

Actigraphy may underestimate awakenings in the younger age groups, where awakenings frequently manifest by sitting up with little movement of the lower leg and will not detect quiet wakefulness in any age group [12,13]. In periodic limb movement disorder, it will not accurately estimate sleep disruption because of leg movements, where subtle awakening or arousal often accompanies subtle movements. In an individual with very active rapid eye movement (REM) sleep, awakenings may also be overestimated. Movements of a fidgety co-sleeper may confound actigraphy as well. Comorbid DD, psychiatric disorders such as anxiety disorder, or ADHD as well as AUT are independently associated with increased sleep disruption from spontaneous awakenings.

Importantly, however, actigraphy is reliable to characterize sleep-wake cycles in all age groups and shows a unique persistence of daily sleep problems over time in SMS compared to children with DD, AUT, or ADHD (Figure 8.3). It is difficult to compare data between SMS individuals and these children, especially given that aspects of sleep worsen in older SMS patients, such as total sleep time in 24 hours.

Children with ADHD demonstrate significant night-to-night variability. This is appreciated mainly in older children [14]. When parent reports and actigraphy data were compared between preschool children from 2 to 5.5 years with DD, AUT typically developing children (TYP), children with AUT spent significantly less time sleeping in 24 hours than the other 2 groups, but at least 2.8 hours more than average SMS group. TYP awoke 3.7 times a night but could fall back asleep

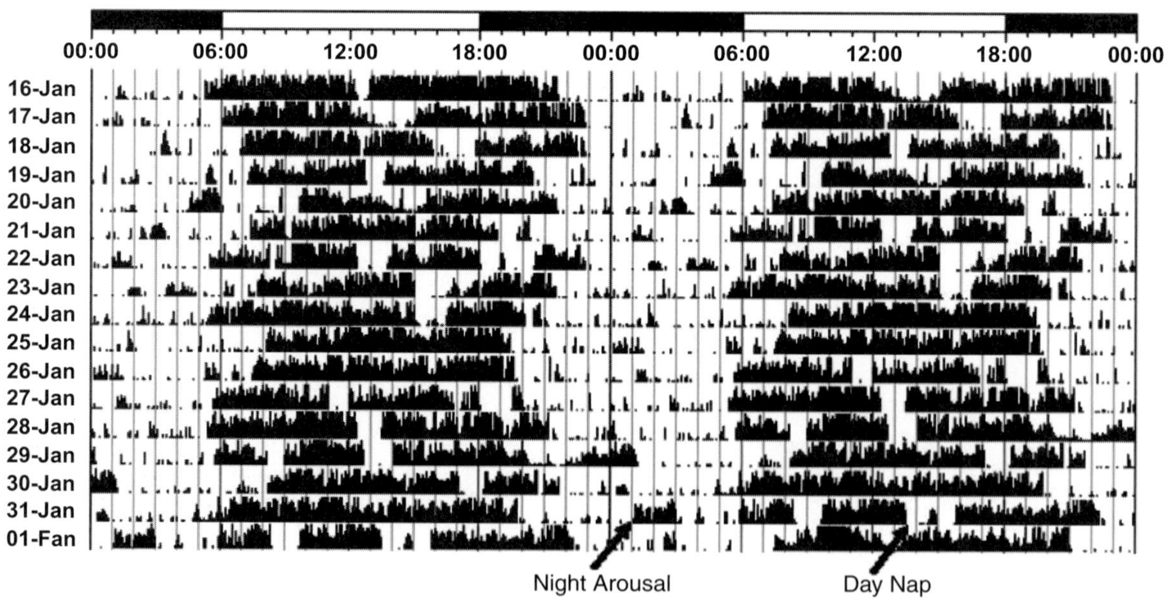

Figure 8.3 Seventeen days of continuous wrist activity are depicted from a boy 5 years of age with confirmed SMS. The clock time (48 hours) is indicated at the top of the panel; consecutive days are plotted beneath each other. Consecutive days are plotted adjacent to each other on the same horizontal line to view the nighttime transition from 1 day to the next. Vertical black bars indicate minute-to-minute activity counts. Rest is indicated by the absence of the vertical bars. Note that most rest occurs during the night, and most activities occur during the day. However, this pattern is often interrupted by episodes of night waking and daytime naps.

faster than the other 2 groups. Wake-time after sleep onset (WASO) was 18 minutes in AUT, 29 in DD, and 18 minutes in TYP, much less than in SMS. The number of naps were less than observed in SMS, 0.65 in AUT and DD, similar to TYP, but lower than in SMS, and the duration of naps were much shorter: 47 to 58 minutes [15].

In TYP, sleep onset or sleep maintenance problems can vary over time and generally improve into the school age period and thereafter. Some studies report about a fifth of problems recurring up to 3 years of age [16], whereas others note that 84% continue from 3 to 6 years of age [17]. This appears to be the case for most sleep insomnias in children with AUT and DD. Their problems may be intermittent, although not typically varying day by day. When a week of additional sleep was analyzed by actigraphy in 3 and 6 months following initial assessment, sleep problems lessened with the exception of awakenings in the DD group only. However, parents of autistic children continue to report sleep difficulties despite evidence to the contrary on actigraphs [18]. In older autistic children (5–16 years of age), sleepless children determined by parents' report on structures questionnaires, had similar actigraphy, with actigraph on the nondominant wrist, to the children with no sleeplessness, but as a whole parents reported that sleep maintenance improved from earlier years and sleep-onset insomnia remained a significant problem [13]. This is in sharp contrast to children with SMS, whose sleep problems are persistent from day to day and worsen over longer periods by parent reports and actigraphy [15,18].

PSG evaluations are difficult in children with SMS because they do not easily tolerate the monitoring equipment, thus "milder" forms of sleep disordered breathing such as upper airway resistance syndrome [19] may be missed. A systematic study of PSG in SMS is ongoing. From the available descriptions, Potocki et al [20] report PSG findings from age 32 months to 31 years, with an average of 9 years and 4 months. Total sleep time less than 7 hours was seen in 43%, REM sleep decrease in 39%, and increase in 25%. Few patients had absent REM sleep. More than 10 spontaneous awakenings were documented in 57% of PSGs. Respiratory parameters were not commented on in this report. As with the frequency of abnormal EEGs, there were differences in the frequencies of sleep disturbances between children with typical versus atypical size deletions. Total sleep time less than 7 hours, REM sleep percentage changes, spontaneous awakenings, sleepiness on multiple sleep latency test (MSLT), and reported modified ESS scores were higher among those with atypical deletions. Respiratory parameters are not frequently reported in SMS. Leoni et al report a 2-year-old with an atypical deletion and hypoventilation in REM and associated frequent REM arousals, and thus significant sleep disruption [21]. Hypoventilation in REM sleep is thought to be an early sign of sleep disordered breathing especially in children with neuromuscular diseases [22]. A 20-year-old woman had apnea hypopnea index (AHI) of 3.2/h on PSG [23]. Actigraphy in infants with SMS shows decreased total daily sleep; in children with SMS, a decrease of 1 to 2 h/d of total sleep was shown compared to controls and persist until 8 years studies and likely thereafter (personal observation). The modified Epworth Sleepiness Scale for children showed scores above 10 in 65%, at least mildly abnormal sleepiness [8].

Melatonin, Sleep, SMS, and AUT

Inverted melatonin secretion pattern in 2 independent cohorts of children has been identified [20,24] (Figure 8.4). Normal growth hormone and cortisol secretion and recently normal 24-hour temperatures [23] of children with SMS suggest dissociation and phase shift of melatonin rhythm from the biological clock rhythm.

Melatonin and Sleep

Melatonin is the most reliable marker of the endogenous physiologic clock rhythm and is highly resistant to stress, sleep disruption, or activity. It was first discovered by Aaron Lerner in 1958 from bovine pineal tissue. It is present in plants, bacteria, higher order animals, and humans and has important physiological roles. Melatonin is released mainly from the pineal gland into the CSF and systemic circulation, but it is also produced in other tissues such as the

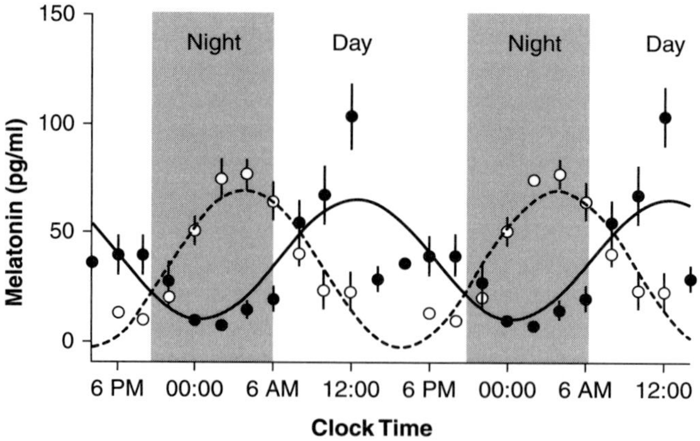

Figure 8.4 Inverted melatonin secretion pattern.

photoreceptor cells in the retina where it circulates locally. It is synthesized from l-tryptophan, and serotonin n-acetyltransferase (AANAT) is the rate-limiting enzyme. In mammals, the pineal AANAT activity is largely controlled by the circadian clock in the suprachiasmatic nucleus (SCN). The endogenous or free running sleep-wake cycle is longer on average than the 24-hour day (24.3 hours). Light is the most powerful negative controller of melatonin synthesis, and it entrains the sleep-wake cycle daily to the 24-hour day. The retinohypothalamic tract originating from type III melanopsin containing photoreceptors in the ganglionic layer of the retina projects to the SCN and retrains the endogenous circadian oscillator to the seasonal light/dark or day/night rhythm every day. Neighboring rod and cone cells also can influence the melanopsin containing photoreceptors, but in their absence, phase abnormality does not necessarily occur. Lockley et al [25] examined the relationship of light and nonlight vision, bilateral versus unilaterally enucleated patients from several different diseases (anophthalmia, micro-ophthalmia, retinal trauma, inflammatory, infectious or tumor induced damage, retinitis pigmentosa, Leber's hereditary optic neuropathy, or other neuropathies), and the presence of sleep phase abnormalities with measuring sulfatoxymelatonin (aMT6s) levels. They found that there was more shift delay among bilaterally enucleated patients and nonlight seeing patients, but was often normal in nonlight seeing patients with 1 eye. Therefore, 1 of 2 intact retinohypothalamic tracts is most important in entraining phase secretion and may remain intact even in some of the severe rod and cone diseases with nonlight sight [25]. The light signal is inhibitory on the signal relayed through the paraventricular nuclei of the hypothalamus, to the upper thoracic intermediolateral columns, to the upper cervical sympathetic ganglia, to the postganglionic adrenergic fibers, by the nervi conarii, into the pineal gland where noradrenaline would be released in the absence of light through activation of beta1 and alpha1 adrenergic receptors resulting in AANAT activity thus producing melatonin. In mammals, the increase in melatonin production at night is by norepinephrine's effect on phosphorylation of creb binding protein (CREB) and activation of AANAT gene translation. Norepinephrine release ceases at the end of the night and by light exposure, and enzymatic expression of arylalkylamine N-acetyltransferase (AANAT) diminishes. Norepinephrine also regulates hydroxyindole-O-methyl transferase (HIOMT) enzyme translation. This enzyme is more stable and plays a role in increasing the amount of melatonin with seasonal variations when the nights are longer. Several other pineal transmitters regulate melatonin secretion such as neurotransmitters, neuropeptides, and others [26].

There are 2 melatonin receptors currently identified in humans. MT1 is the most abundant, and both are most concentrated and abundant in the anterior pituitary and pars tuberalis. MT1 receptors are also found in the hypothalamus,

SCN, cerebral cortex, thalamus, hippocampus, cerebellum, cornea, and retina. MT2 receptors, apart from the anterior pituitary, are also found in the retina, hippocampus, and cerebellum. These are also located in the adrenal gland, the circulatory system, and other major organs as well as in lymphocytes. These tissues are in turn entrained to the daily, seasonal, or other cycles through cell-specific induction of their clock genes, which subsequently alter their physiologic function and activity. The clock gene products modulate their own production and activity largely by self-degradation and inactivation of protein production by forming cell-specific hetero or homodimers [27].

Circulating melatonin is broken down and deactivated in the liver through the P450 cytochrome, mainly the CYP1A2 isoform. 6-Hydroxymelatonin is conjugated with sulfate to sulfatoxymelatonin (aMT6s) and to a lesser extent with glucuronic acid and excreted in urine. This process is rapid, thus the half life of exogenous melatonin is 10 to 60 minutes. aMT6s in urine reflects plasma melatonin levels and is used to approximate plasma melatonin rhythm in humans [27]. There are several ways of measuring melatonin and establishing a melatonin phase estimate. The dim light (less than 10–30 lux) melatonin onset (DLMO) is established by 2SD rise above baseline, absolute rise above 3 ng/ml salivary or 10 ng/ml plasma melatonin values or the visual scoring of beginning of the rise of the fitted cosine curve to the melatonin levels. The termination of melatonin synthesis, melatonin synthesis offset (Synoff), is estimated to be at the top of the curve, and dimlight melatonin offset (DLMOff) is a measure of return to baseline levels similar to DLMO. Light exposure during testing, previous light exposure, and posture all influence melatonin levels. Urinary aMT6s is collected at certain intervals, usually between 2 and 8 hours, and the phase rhythm is calculated from establishing the peak and fitting other values into a cosine curve. Frequent sampling may be needed to fine-tune the phase curve, and this may be inconvenient. Overnight samples, however, are good estimators of nighttime melatonin secretion, but can be cumbersome and requires sleep disruption as well. Blood sampling is favorable if frequent overnight sampling is required. Plasma levels are usually 3 times salivary levels and should be used if low baseline melatonin synthesis is suspected with a lower sensitivity assay [28]. Saliva sampling requires a minimum amount of saliva (0.4 ml), so urinary sampling is favored until 2 months of age after which sufficient amount of saliva can be collected. Four-hour samples of urine and saliva collected at 4 hour intervals should be used in a day period [28,29].

The circadian rhythm of endogenous melatonin secretion shows highest plasma levels toward the middle of the night and a return to baseline levels toward the morning. A longer day shortens and shorter day lengthens the melatonin peak values. There is little variability between peak and low values in the individual, but these values differ significantly between individuals [27]. This rhythm is not present in newborns and young infants until approximately 3 months of age. In newborns, melatonin levels do not differ with respect to time of delivery and do not correlate with sleep-wake times, day/night, or activity/rest periods. However, feeding schedule dictates sleep-wake cycles, regardless of whether the newborn is breastfed. Toward the end of the first month, significant day/night variability was found in aMT6s that continued to be present until 24 months of age. At around 3 months of age, the relationship between urinary aMT6s, salivary aMT, and sleep-wake cycle is established in full-term infants but is delayed in premature infants. The rising median peak salivary aMT values between midnight and 8 AM (with the highest values at around 4 AM, median of approximately 20 pg/ml) account for most of the difference between day and night values in this range of ages. During the day, median salivary melatonin values between noon and 8 PM were close to zero, but several children had values at approximately 10 to 15 pg/ml. There is also a small elevation in average production toward the middle of the afternoon from 4 to 24 months, when a second smaller peak has been documented in older children and adults [30]. Melatonin production peaks between 1 and 3 years of age, then drops progressively by 80% to the adult values. The average adult plasma peak melatonin values are between 60 to 70 pg/ml. The decline with age is significant after 70 years and is thought to be secondary to SCN denervation or degeneration and not dysfunction of the pineal gland [28].

Melatonin has many critical physiologic functions. It is primarily involved in the cueing of sleep-wake functions of all cells of the body to the length of the day and to seasonal changes. Timing of puberty is influenced by melatonin levels and can be nonpermanently delayed by exogenous administration in rats by inhibiting GnRH induced luteinizing hormone. Prolactin secretion is also influenced by melatonin. Reducing core body temperature vasodilation, and thus increasing blood flow to the distal limbs in relation to the sleep-wake cycle, glucose homeostasis, retinal function, and even cardiovascular and immune functions are under melatonin's influence. More recently, its effect is becoming more evident in synaptic plasticity [26,31].

Melatonin is thought to be responsible for the non—24-hour free running circadian rhythm observed in blind individuals that can be entrained with exogenous melatonin and behavioral interventions. This type of sleep-wake cycle disorder is characterized by increased napping and reduced alertness during the day. Bilateral sympathectomy at the level of the second thoracic ganglion decreases plasma melatonin levels. Melatonin levels are altered in many conditions such as liver disease, renal failure, and in many psychiatric disorders such as seasonal depression, mania, and depression as well as premenstrual irritability, but not altered consistently in delayed sleep phase syndrome [30].

Endogenous melatonin production can be altered by several medications. Blocking sympathetic innervation of the pineal gland by B1-adrenergic blockers can decrease production of melatonin. Nonsteroidal anti-inflammatory drugs (NSAIDs) and aspirin can reduce nighttime melatonin levels, whereas selective serotonin reuptake inhibitors (SSRIs), fluvoxamine, and desipramine can increase plasma melatonin levels by inhibiting CYP1A2 catabolism by the latter. Exogenous melatonin (0.3–10 mg) can raise plasma levels hundred fold. Increased seizures have been reported with melatonin, usually with the administration of more than 9 mg/d. Melatonin receptor agonists are available [27].

In SMS, phase shifted melatonin secretion was discovered by Potocki et al and also evaluated by DeLeersnyder [20,32]. The time of onset of melatonin secretion is at 6 AM ± 2 hours and the peak is at noon ± 1 hour. A longer duration of melatonin synthesis to 15.5 ± 3.5 hours compared to 8 ± 1 hour in controls and the offset is at 8 PM ± 1 hour. Irregular plasma melatonin levels were recorded throughout the day, and a second peak was found to be delayed between 6 and 8 PM; however, this peak was not observed with salivary melatonin measurements in a later sample by Chik et al [33]. There is thus a 9.6 ± 0.9 hour shift phase of melatonin. So expectedly, some SMS children sleep at appropriate times when crossing time zones.

Although peak melatonin production can vary hundred fold between normal individuals, the utility of the previously reported peak in midday melatonin in SMS patients, using salivary melatonin, was examined as a biomarker for diagnosing SMS [33]. As expected, salivary melatonin was low in the youngest 2 children under 15 months, but was elevated on follow-up after they both were older than 17 months. Lower dose adrenergic blockers (with nighttime melatonin use), anticonvulsants, or antipsychotic had no effect on daytime values.

Although the authors did not comment on whether children with atypical deletions were more likely to have higher midday salivary melatonin levels, 90% of the 28 patients with del.17p11.2 from 90 samples, whereas 1 of the 2 patients with RAI1 point mutations from 20 samples had levels above 15.5 pg/ml. All 69% of SMS patients ranging from 4.5 months to 20 years had over 25 pg/ml of salivary melatonin on first measurement concentrations at midday just above the highest value in controls, with an increase to 76% if samples at multiple time points were collected or if patients taking melatonin within 24 hours were excluded [33].

Importantly, Ardura reported lower daytime salivary melatonin levels in normal children than the 2 youngest children at retesting at 17 and 23 months [33], so the utility of daytime salivary melatonin may also be useful between 1 and 2 years, despite peak in production normally observed at this age. However, in the overall sample, elevated midday salivary melatonin lacks specificity and sensitivity in distinguishing SMS children from normal children [33].

There was apparent uncoupling of melatonin rhythm from other hormonal rhythms; growth hormone, cortisol, and prolactin levels were not affected [24]. Body temperature followed a normal rhythm [34] and was not affected by fluctuating daytime salivary melatonin levels [33].

Abnormal behaviors also follow the plasma melatonin rhythm with temper tantrums in older infants at high melatonin levels at the beginning of the day, presumably from endogenous pressure to sleep versus social and environmental pressures to stay awake.

Current research is focusing on comparison of SMS children's daytime melatonin level to that in children with other causes of mental retardation and difficult behaviors. To date, there has been no study comparing SMS children's daytime melatonin level to equally temperamental children. Currently, a study comparing children with SMS to those with Cornelia deLang is underway.

A curious feature of SMS is that as plasma melatonin rises, SMS children nap midday, are awake until the second peak of melatonin as mentioned above, and may experience a sleep attack. Sleep attacks can be severe enough that the child falls asleep with food in his mouth. Children have difficulty falling asleep at night and stay awake for large portions of the night with wakefulness in early morning when endogenous melatonin levels are low.

Treatment of Sleep Disorders in SMS

Treatment with B1-adrenergic blockers and nighttime melatonin is effective in most children for the treatment of sleep and behavioral problems [35]. Our current research with supraphysiologic light therapy is underway. The treatment of melatonin phase shift with beta-blockers consists of blocking unwanted melatonin peak toward the later afternoon and facilitating a peak toward the second half of the night. The protocol developed by DeLeersnyder advocates screening children for cardiac and respiratory contraindications for B1-adrenergic blocking agents. Doses of 10 mg/kg of acebutolol are given in the morning by mouth was shown to significantly reduce plasma melatonin levels from 68 to 8 pg/ml, remaining low until 6 AM the next day and rising again until the morning dose was repeated. Daytime naps ceased and daytime behaviors markedly improved with a few temper tantrums per week. With the administration of controlled release melatonin in the evening, plasma levels rose from 12.7 ± 10.6 to 2189 ± 1800 pg/ml 2 hours after. As a result, sleep onset was delayed by 30 minutes, offset by 60 minutes, and total increase of sleep was 60 minutes per night and patients slept through the night. PSG showed more organized sleep architecture and increase in slow-wave and REM sleep percentage and stability. There was no desensitization over 4 years and no side effects were noted [36].

Melatonin and AUT

The intellectually normal autistic population represents the more genetically isolated autistic proband, and as sleep abnormality is notably a salient feature of AUT, it is best studied in this population [37]; however, most studies target mentally retarded or a mix of higher and lower functioning autistic children. Low nocturnal peak, delayed nocturnal phase, and increased daytime melatonin levels have been documented in children with developmental disorders, but studies are relatively small and their subjects are heterogeneous. In smaller studies, daytime urinary melatonin levels were higher and levels were normal at night in autistic children [38]. Others reported an abnormal or blunted nighttime melatonin levels. Nir et al [39] studied plasma melatonin levels in 10 males, from 16 to 30 years of age, with AUT and some with seizures, all off medications [including neuroleptics and antiepileptic drugs (AEDs)] and compared them to controls. They found that nocturnal melatonin levels were lower and daytime levels were higher in autistic children, but there was no phase shift. Ritvo et al also found higher daytime melatonin levels [38]. TSH levels were generally the same but overall tended to be higher. There were no differences in cortisol or prolactin levels [39]; however, earlier literature documents abnormalities in cortisol rhythm [40]. In Angelman syndrome, low peak nighttime melatonin levels were noted, 4/13 children had a phase delay in nocturnal melatonin [41]. Kulman et al [42] studied 14 (ages 5–10 years) autistic children's melatonin rhythm using 24-hour plasma levels and showed that none of them had a normal rhythm. An inverted melatonin rhythm was seen in 29% and no discernable rhythm in 71%. These autistic children's plasma melatonin was also lower than controls, but when inverted, nadir was at midnight and noon and peak was at around 8 PM, very similar to age-matched SMS children published by DeLeersnyder [35]. Behavioral/sleep disturbances were greater in the group with the inverted rhythm, but no specific observations were made [42]. A recent larger scale study by Tordjman et al [43] of 50 autistic children measured nocturnal urinary melatonin in the same season. Most differences from controls were observed in the prepubertal ages, among boys, because of higher values in normal prepubertal children compared to others, but this difference was considerable even when compared with postpubertal values. This decrease of over 50% of nocturnal melatonin was confirmed in plasma in similar proportion (65%) of autistic children [44] and correlated with acetylmelatonin methyltransferase (ASMT) enzymatic activity in AUT only. Additionally, parents (mothers especially) of autistic children also had reduced values arguing for genetic bases, explained in some by ASMT gene variation. There was no difference in IQ or communication between autistic children with normal and low melatonin levels [44]. Furthermore, Nir et al [39] report higher levels at night and daytime with more language delay. The lower nocturnal melatonin levels in autistic children may not correlate with sleep issues but with daytime deficiencies in communication and play [43]. In summary, studies agree on lower nocturnal melatonin levels and some show higher daytime levels in AUT with and without below average intellectual functioning. Some suggest that lower nocturnal melatonin levels are also present in some autistic children's parents. One study in AUT documented inverted melatonin rhythm, and another study in children with Angelman syndrome showed similar findings. Interestingly, abnormal electroretinograms were documented in 48% to 60% in 2 independent smaller groups of autistic children and in some of their first degree relatives (fathers) [44,45]. The effect of this on nocturnal melatonin is not known. While melatonin abnormalities in AUT may not correlate with sleep disturbances on parents' questionnaires or actigraphy, they seem to be more prominent in younger children and they may correlate with and/or have developmental/behavioral consequences on communication, play, and the ability to learn.

Exogenous melatonin has both hypnotic and chronobiologic effects. In healthy individuals, at physiologic doses (under 3 mg), melatonin elicits a dose-dependent sleep promotion with decreased sleep latency, increased sleep efficiency, increased REM sleep latency, increased REM sleep, increased stage 2 sleep, and decreased slow-wave sleep, but individual differences exist. At supraphysiologic doses (above 3 mg), the effect is not dose-dependent, and daytime dosages may interfere with alertness and reaction time. In individuals with delayed sleep phase and prolonged sleep onset (over 20 minutes), its effects will be more pronounced [46]. Plasma melatonin is documented to be lower in sleep in Angelman syndrome, Rett syndrome, and tuberous sclerosis. Therefore, it has been used to treat sleep insomnias frequently in the intellectually disabled children. A recent meta-analysis by Braam et al [46] indicated in 9 separate double-blind, placebo-controlled trials of 183 individuals with intellectual disabilities, mainly children, showed benefit from melatonin therapy. Actigraphy was used in 2 studies, one with Rett syndrome and another with undiagnosed developmentally delayed children [47,48] and may show more clinical benefit than objective changes on actigraph. In children with Angelman syndrome, after 1 to 2 days of 0.3 mg of melatonin 0.5 hours before bedtime, children's sleep improved both clinically and on actigraphy [41]. On average in this collection of studies by Braam et al, decreased sleep latency by 34 minutes, increased night sleep by 50 minutes, and significantly decreased nighttime awakenings were recorded with short period of follow-up (10–28/d). This is very similar to the benefit recorded in SMS. In the neurodevelopmentally delayed population, there is evidence that the positive response of melatonin can be independent or dependent of dose or timing which argues that both the hypnotic and chronobiologic effects may play a role in certain populations [46]. Studies by Wasdell et al [48] using 3 year and 9 month follow-up reported durable response of sleep phase delay and sleep maintenance insomnia to melatonin in intellectually disabled children. Seizures in sleep in SMS are thought to be more common than previously documented, and the effect of melatonin on seizures in this population has not been explored. Decreased sleep onset judged by sleep logs (without objective measurement) was reported in a double-blind, placebo-controlled trial in children with mental retardation with or without epilepsy. Only 30% of the patients were receiving less than 3 mg, 26% 9 to 12 mg, and dual effect on seizure frequency was noted, although it is unknown if higher melatonin dose was associated with seizure exacerbation [49]. Melatonin also has anticonvulsant effects [50,51] but doses above 9 mg may have proconvulsant effects (Kotagal, personal communication).

Genes Implicated in the Circadian Clock in SMS

Among the clock genes, PER1 and COP9 may be implicated in circadian rhythm abnormalities in SMS. PER1 gene is on chromosome 17p, outside of the gene deletion in SMS. Subunit 3 of the COP9 signal transduction complex maps to the region deleted in SMS [52]. However, since the original reports, 2 SMS individuals of the 28 studied showed a normal melatonin pattern. Both these individuals harbor an unusually large deletion encompassing the usual hemizygous 3.5 Mb interstitial deletion of chromosome 17p11.2. This region encompasses the COPS3 gene encoding subunit 3 of the COP9 signal transducing complex related to the 26S proteasome regulatory complex. This in turn controls N-acetyltransferase, the rate-limiting step in melatonin synthesis. Potocki et al [52], in the original report, described a 5-year-old girl whose mutation was later identified as a 5-Mb deletion of paternal origin [52,53]. Boudreau et al reported a 20-year-old woman who had a 6-Mb deletion from TNFRSF protein B to the centromere of chromosome 17 [23]. Importantly, both individuals had similar sleep habits, PSG, and actigraphy findings than the rest of the cohort. However, out of 2 individuals with RAI1 point mutations had documented inverted melatonin and complained of the sleep disturbance, only the 11 year old showed polysomnographic evidence of sleep cycle abnormalities [54]. Furthermore, several healthy individuals show no detectable plasma melatonin and have normal sleep-wake cycles [55]. Another possible explanation is a dysfunction in the retinohypothalamic tracts input to the SCN, signal transduction to the pineal gland, and regulation of the AANAT. With the demonstrated hypoperfusion on PET scans, smaller size of the lenticular nuclei, and insular cortices bilaterally in SMS, the melatonin dopamine interactions may be implicated [56]. Therefore, it is likely that the observed sleep disruption, excessive daytime somnolence, and behavioral abnormalities are not solely related to the inverted melatonin levels but may be at least exacerbated by sleep insufficiency.

The literature on the important effects of sleep disruption on daytime functioning is becoming more convincing. The literature on sleep-disordered breathing perhaps best approximates the daytime neurocognitive and behavioral effects of nighttime sleep disruption in children. Children with SMS are at risk for other processes that can disrupt the normal sleep-wake cycle. Although no report suggests sleep apnea or periodic limb movement disorder (PLMD) as features of SMS, the scoring criteria for these disorders changed since the publication of the original reports, so it is possible that they are in fact more prevalent as children with SMS have several risk factors for sleep disordered breathing (SDB): obesity (38%), maxillary hypoplasia (94%), cleft lip/palate (10%) [57], hypotonia (66%), laryngeal abnormalities, atopy (45%) breathing problems (27%), congenital heart defects (31%), reflux, oropharyngeal dysfunction, excessive drooling, and frequent ear infections (87%) [2,22,58]. Mouth breathing is common which may signal a degree of nasal obstruction and/or low oropharyngeal/mandible tone, which may put them at risk for high upper airway resistance in sleep and thus sleep-related respiratory obstruction. Pharyngeal hypotonia may cause intermittent upper airway obstruction in sleep in infancy, even without audible snoring. There is evidence of disordered breathing in sleep from increased snoring (69%), labored breathing in sleep (28%), apneas (24%), bedwetting (82%), bruxism (44%), jumping in sleep (18%), and failure to thrive (61%) [11].

It is thought that the robust improvements in behavior and learning after treatment of OSA with modest improvements in currently used measures of sleep disruption imply that these criteria underdetect arousals in children in SDB, and in fact it is sleep disruption that explains most of these disturbances [59,60]. The effect of even mild sleep disordered breathing, that is primary snoring, will cause decreased total sleep time [61] (disrupted sleep with frequent awakenings in infants) [62]. The neurobehavioral description of otherwise healthy snoring infants with sleep disordered breathing is said to be "moody and negative" on the Early Infancy Temperament Questionnaire [63] that is unlike the temperament of SMS, but clinical experience suggests that especially developmentally delayed infants can also appear docile. In addition to temperament changes, sleep disordered breathing can also affect development. Mental Developmental Index scores of snoring infants negatively correlated with snoring related arousals, that is not necessarily with snoring associated desaturations or airway obstructions [64].

Children with SMS have decreased working memory and concentration and are very poor learners. Their behaviors that may significantly contribute to their learning problems are similar to the common behavioral symptoms associated with sleep disordered breathing such as hyperactivity, rebelliousness, and aggression in otherwise normal children [60].

Poor learning has been documented in children with SDB; it may not be an accurate indicator of cognitive disturbance as behavioral issues are frequently confounding. Moreover, even in the otherwise healthy population, the severity of OSA explains less than half of neurocognitive affects in otherwise healthy children, which infers genetic susceptibility [65]. Short-term memory processes may be more vulnerable to SDB effects in younger children, which argues for a developmentally vulnerable period [60]. Nevertheless, 18% of normal 6-year-olds who were in the lower 10th percentile in academics have evidence of gas exchange abnormalities [66]. In children 6 to 11 years of age, respiratory disturbance indexes that are associated with even modest hypoxia (2% and 3% desaturations, with apneas or hypopneas of 0.5–2/h, ie, mild sleep apnea) were observed more frequently in children with snoring, excessive daytime somnolence, and learning disability [67].

In healthy children between 6 to 12 years of age with adenotonsillar hypertrophy (ATH), AHI/AI and snoring predicted vocabulary score, similarities, verbal, and general memory [68]. In 10- to 13-year-olds with ATH, memory and learning disability was found, with more severe language dysfunction [69]. Low performing 13- to 14-year-olds were more likely to snore between 2 to 6 years of age [70]. Habitual snoring independent of intermittent hypoxia was associated with poor academic performance, hyperactivity, inattentiveness, daytime sleepiness, conduct problems, emotionality, and peer problems [71]. Some studies report improved working memory after adenotonsillectomy [72,73], but academic performance may take longer to improve [70]. Since medical sleep history even with careful assessment for anatomical risk factors for SDB or PLMD by physical exam is inaccurate for SDB diagnosis, a systematic reevaluation of children with SMS by overnight PSG may be needed. We are currently conducting such studies.

Unrecognized Epilepsy and Sleep Disturbance

In addition to these factors, seizures may also contribute to the sleep disruption as well as to daytime cognitive and behavioral dysfunction. Epileptiform EEGs and seizures may be even more prevalent if prolonged video-EEG monitoring is used. Abnormal EEG was found in 52% of children with SMS and possibly even underreported when assessed by an 8-channel EEG montage during routine overnight polysomnograms; therefore, cortical excitability has become one of the major features of the syndrome. The most common feature was generalized epileptiform discharge in 45% of all children and 73% of those with epileptiform discharges; some children had both generalized and focal features and 43% had a purely focal pattern. All types of epileptiform discharges occurred predominantly in sleep. A third of the overall group of children studied by Goldman et al [74] had clinical seizures. In this series, 29% of the cases with epileptiform EEGs had clinical seizures, and the majority of the children with clearly epileptiform discharges who were not treated had staring spells. Interestingly, those with atypical size deletions had more epileptiform discharges and seizures: 75% of those with large deletions and 83% with smaller deletions had abnormal EEGs versus 49% of children with the common size deletion. Four of the 6 individuals with smaller deletions shared the proximal breakpoints, but the distal breakpoints were variable and obscured the genotype-epilepsy correlation [74].

The interaction between sleep and epilepsy is well known. Epileptic children frequently experience seizures in drowsiness before sleep, shortly after awakening, and in some epilepsy syndromes predominantly in sleep [75]. Epileptiform discharges in sleep are not common in healthy children and were seen in 1.45% of healthy children during routine PSG, most of which were centrotemporal spikes occurring in slow-wave sleep. The children with incidentally found abnormal discharges in sleep had behavioral and/or learning issues [76]. Others had similar finding of more frequent similar interictal discharges in a group of children with ADHD on routine PSG [77].

Prolonged sleep deprivation (48 hours) can elicit seizures in healthy adults without history of epilepsy [78]. Such studies in children are not available, but few hours of sleep deprivation the night before can assure sleep during and may also activate epileptiform discharges on the EEG [79]. Sleep deprivation is one of the most frequent causes of breakthrough seizures in children [80] may be a more commonly reported trigger by patients with generalized epilepsy [81]. Conversely, interictal epileptiform discharges may also disrupt sleep [82]. This may explain that even in the absence of sleep disorders, epileptics not taking antiepileptic medications (after treatment with AED and a sufficient seizure free period) had significantly more excessive daytime sleepiness on objective measures [83]. Similar findings were reported in children with cerebral palsy and epilepsy [84]. It is unknown whether epileptiform abnormalities in SMS are linked to the sleep disruption. Interestingly, in autistic children between 5 to 16 years of age, epilepsy (remote or active) was more common in sleepless autistic children, by parents' account, compared to normal sleeping autistic children, and it seemed to be better distinguishing these 2 groups than indicators of sleep disruption by actigraphy [13]. In support of this observation, Nir et al [39] recorded most blunted nocturnal melatonin and also daytime melatonin among patients with AUT and seizures compared to AUT without seizures and controls. Tordjman et al found no difference in urinary excretion of melatonin with or without lifetime history of epilepsy, but active epilepsy was not differentiated [43]. It is unknown how closely epileptiform abnormalities in SMS (or AUT) are linked to melatonin levels, sleep disruption, and abnormal behaviors, whereas several antiepileptic medications (valproic acid, carbamazapine) improved behaviors, no specific antiepileptic trials have been done.

Possible link of peripheral neuropathy and sleep disturbance: Furthermore, peripheral neuropathy is documented in 75% of the cases, but its significance is unknown as pes cavus/planus and hyporeflexia have been documented in its absence [2]. The presumed lower pain tolerance may be a function of sensory deficits, or part of the autistic-like phenotype, its presence, nature, and significance are uncertain. In addition, it is unknown whether this neuropathy is painful and may result in self-mutilation. Peripheral neuropathy has been documented to cause secondary restless legs syndrome (RLS) and may mimic the sleep disruption from RLS or periodic limb movement disorder; additionally, certain pain syndromes, including peripheral neuropathy, can have a circadian pattern with worse symptoms in the evening [85]. These 2 sleep conditions and pain [86] may independently disrupt sleep. Thus far, there have been no careful lab studies examining iron stores, a marker in children for RLS/PLMD susceptibility [85], or studies of periodic limb movements in SMS.

Conclusions and Future Directions

The study of sleep disorders in neurologically vulnerable populations is in its infancy. Children with SMS offer a unique opportunity for the study of melatonin rhythm and severe sleep disturbances in a neurogenetic syndrome. The pathophysiology of SMS is not known; however, the inverted melatonin rhythm is nearly universal, and this pattern has been only seldom documented in individuals with other neurodevelopmental disorders. This inverted melatonin rhythm is most likely linked to their chaotic sleep pattern, which may in large part account for some aspects of their behavioral phenotype.

In SMS between the typical and the atypical deletions, there may be significant clinical differences in the expression of the melatonin rhythm, sleep patterns, and seizures. The treatment protocol involving B1 antagonist and nighttime melatonin has promising results and is used extensively in Europe. Whether this treatment is effective because of melatonin alteration alone or through additional nonspecific hypnotic and/or antiepileptic effects of exogenous melatonin is unclear. In addition, other aspects of the SMS phenotype may also independently alter sleep and thus daytime functioning such as behavioral abnormalities, milder forms of sleep disordered breathing, seizures, and the epileptogenic brain. Sleep movement disorders or other possible effects of peripheral neuropathy have not been studied. In the future, specific therapies for the typical and atypical genotypes may be necessary and may allow new insights into the pathophysiology of SMS. A comparative study of sleep in Cornelia DeLange syndrome, a neurogenetic syndrome with similarly temperamental behavioral profile, is in progress. An ongoing study involving supraphysiologic light therapy will determine whether it can effectively normalize the melatonin rhythm and whether a normalized melatonin rhythm without exogenous melatonin will be sufficient to correct the sleep disturbances. In conclusion, sleep disturbances in SMS are likely multifactorial. Several studies are ongoing and will shed more light onto the nature of the severe sleep disturbance in this unique neurogenetic syndrome.

References

1. Smith AC, McGavran L, Robinson J, et al. Interstitial deletion of (17)(p11.2p11.2) in nine patients. *Am J Med Genet.* 1986;24:393–414.
2. Greenberg F, Lewis RA, Potocki L, et al. Multidisciplinary clinical study of Smith-Magenis syndrome (deletion 17p11.2). *Am J Med Genet.* 1996;62:247–254.
3. Greenberg F, Guzzetta V, Montes de Oca-Luna R, et al. Molecular analysis of the Smith-Magenis syndrome: a possible contiguous-gene syndrome associated with del(17)(p11.2). *Am J Hum Genet.* 1991;49:1207–1218.
4. Seranski P, Hoff C, Radelof U, et al. Rai1 is a novel polyglutamine encoding gene that is deleted in Smith-Magenis syndrome patients. *Gene.* 2001; 270:69–76.
5. Slager RE, Newton TL, Vlangos CN, Finucane B, Elsea SH. Mutations in rai1 associated with Smith-Magenis syndrome. *Nat Genet.* 2003;33: 466–468.
6. Yamamoto T, Ueda H, Kawataki M, et al. A large interstitial deletion of 17p13.1p11.2 involving the Smith-Magenis chromosome region in a girl with multiple congenital anomalies. *Am J Med Genet A.* 2006; 140:88–91.
7. Elsea SH, Girirajan S. Smith-Magenis syndrome. *Eur J Hum Genet.* 2008; 16:412–421.
8. Gropman AL, Duncan WC, Smith AC. Neurologic and developmental features of the Smith-Magenis syndrome (del 17p11.2). *Pediatr Neurol.* 2006; 34:337–350.
9. Martin SC, Wolters PL, Smith AC. Adaptive and maladaptive behavior in children with Smith-Magenis syndrome. *J Autism Dev Disord.* 2006; 36:541–552.
10. Wolters PL, Gropman AL, Martin SC, et al. Neurodevelopment of children under 3 years of age with Smith-Magenis syndrome. *Pediatr Neurol.* 2009;41:250–258.
11. Smith AC, Dykens E, Greenberg F. Sleep disturbance in Smith-Magenis syndrome (del 17 p11.2). *Am J Med Genet.* 1998;81:186–191.
12. Sitnick SL, Goodlin-Jones BL, Anders TF. The use of actigraphy to study sleep disorders in preschoolers: some concerns about detection of nighttime awakenings. *Sleep.* 2008;31(3):395–401.
13. Wiggs L, Stores G. Sleep patterns and sleep disorders in children with autistic spectrum disorders: insights using parent report and actigraphy. *Dev Med Child Neurol.* 2004;46(6):372–380.
14. Gruber R, Sadeh A, Raviv A. Instability of sleep patterns in children with attention-deficit/hyperactivity disorder. *J Am Acad Child Adolesc Psychiatry.* 2000;39:495–501.
15. Goodlin-Jones BL, Tang K, Liu J, Anders TF. Sleep patterns in preschool-age children with autism, developmental delay, and typical development. *J Am Acad Child Adolesc Psychiatry.* 2008;47(8):930–938.
16. Lam P, Hiscock H, Wake M. Outcomes of infant sleep problems: a longitudinal study of sleep, behavior, and maternal well-being. *Pediatrics.* 2003;111(3):e203–e207.
17. Kataria S, Swanson MS, Trevathan GE. Persistence of sleep disturbances in preschool children. *J Pediatr.* 1987;110(4):642–646.
18. Goodlin-Jones B, Schwichtenberg AJ, Iosif AM, Tang K, Liu J, Anders TF. Six-month persistence of sleep problems in young children with autism, developmental delay, and typical development. *J Am Acad Child Adolesc Psychiatry.* 2009;48(8):847–854.
19. Guilleminault C, Poyares D. Arousal and upper airway resistance (UAR). *Sleep Med.* 2002; 3(suppl 2):S15–S20.
20. Potocki L, Glaze D, Tan DX, et al. Circadian rhythm abnormalities of melatonin in Smith-Magenis syndrome. *J Med Genet.* 2000;37:428–433.

21. Leoni C, Cesarini L, Dittoni S, et al. Hypoventilation in rem sleep in a case of 17p11.2 deletion (Smith-Magenis syndrome). *Am J Med Genet A.* 2010; 152A(3):708–712.
22. Dhand UK, Dhand R. Sleep disorders in neuromuscular diseases. *Curr Opin Pulm Med.* 2006; 12(6):402–408.
23. Boudreau EA, Johnson KP, Jackman AR, et al. Review of disrupted sleep patterns in Smith-Magenis syndrome and normal melatonin secretion in a patient with an atypical interstitial 17p11.2 deletion. *Am J Med Genet A.* 2009;149A: 1382–1391.
24. De Leersnyder H, De Blois MC, Claustrat B, et al. Inversion of the circadian rhythm of melatonin in the Smith-Magenis syndrome. *J Pediatr.* 2001; 139:111–116.
25. Lockley SW, Skene DJ, Arendt J, Tabandeh H, Bird AC, Defrance R. Relationship between melatonin rhythms and visual loss in the blind. *J Clin Endocrinol Metab.* 1997;82(11):3763–3770.
26. Simonneaux V, Ribelayga C. Generation of the melatonin endocrine message in mammals: a review of the complex regulation of melatonin synthesis by norepinephrine, peptides, and other pineal transmitters. *Pharmacol Rev.* 2003;55(2): 325–395.
27. Zawilska JB, Skene DJ, Arendt J. Physiology and pharmacology of melatonin in relation to biological rhythms. *Pharmacol Rep.* 2009;61(3): 383–410.
28. Benloucif S, Burgess HJ, Klerman EB, et al. Measuring melatonin in humans. *J Clin Sleep Med.* 2008;4(1):66–69.
29. Ardura J, Gutierrez R, Andres J, Agapito T. Emergence and evolution of the circadian rhythm of melatonin in children. *Horm Res.* 2003;59: 66–72.
30. Kryger Meir H, Thomas Roth, Dement William C. *Principles and Practice of Sleep Medicine.* 2009; 4th ed. Philadelphia, PA: Elsevier Saunders.
31. Chaudhury D, Wang LM, Colwell CS. Circadian regulation of hippocampal long-term potentiation. *J Biol Rhythms.* 2005;20(3):225–236.
32. De Leersnyder H, de Blois MC, Bresson JL, Sidi D, Claustrat B, Munnich A. Inversion of the circadian melatonin rhythm in Smith-Magenis syndrome. *Rev Neurol (Paris).* 2003;159: 6S21–6S26.
33. Chik CL, Rollag MD, Duncan WC, Smith AC. Diagnostic utility of daytime salivary melatonin levels in Smith-Magenis syndrome. *Am J Med Genet A.* 2000;152A:96–101.
34. Duncan WE, Morse RS, Krasnewish D, Smith ACM. *Body Temperature and Sleep Disturbance in Smith-Magenis Syndrome.* Genetics, Toronto, ON, Canada: American Society of Human Genetics; 2004:A814.
35. De Leersnyder H, de Blois MC, Vekemans M, et al. Beta(1)-adrenergic antagonists improve sleep and behavioural disturbances in a circadian disorder, Smith-Magenis syndrome. *J Med Genet.* 2001;38: 586–590.
36. De Leersnyder H. Inverted rhythm of melatonin secretion in Smith-Magenis syndrome: from symptoms to treatment. *Trends Endocrinol Metab.* 2006;17(7):291–298.
37. Nicolson R, Szatmari P. Genetic and neurodevelopmental influences in autistic disorder. *Can J Psychiatry.* 2003;48(8):526–537.
38. Ritvo ER, Ritvo R, Yuwiler A, Brothers A, Freeman BJ, Plotkin S. Elevated dayime melatonin concentrations in autism: a pilot study. *Eur Child Adolesc Psychiatr.* 1993;2:75–78.
39. Nir I, Meir D, Zilber N, Knobler H, Hadjez J, Lerner Y. Brief report: circadian melatonin, thyroid-stimulating hormone, prolactin, and cortisol levels in serum of young adults with autism. *J Autism Dev Disord.* 1995;25(6):641–654.
40. Tordjman S, Anderson GM, Pichard N, Charbuy H, Touitou Y. Nocturnal excretion of 6-sulphatoxymelatonin in children and adolescents with autistic disorder. *Biol Psychiatry.* 2005;57(2):134–138.
41. Zhdanova IV, Lynch HJ, Wurtman RJ. Melatonin: a sleep-promoting hormone. *Sleep.* 1997; 20(10):899–907.
42. Kulman G, Lissoni P, Rovelli F, Roselli MG, Brivio F, Sequeri P. Evidence of pineal endocrine hypofunction in autistic children. *Neuro Endocrinol Lett.* 2000;21(1):31–34.
43. Tordjman S, Anderson GM, Pichard N, Charbuy H, Touitou Y. Nocturnal excretion of 6-sulphatoxymelatonin in children and adolescents with autistic disorder. *Biol Psychiatry.* 2005;57(2):134–138.
44. Ritvo ER, Creel D, Realmuto G, et al. Electroretinograms in autism: a pilot study of b-wave amplitudes. *Am J Psychiatry.* 1988; 145(2):229–232.
45. Realmuto G, Purple R, Knobloch W, Ritvo E. Electroretinograms (ERGs) in four autistic probands and six first-degree relatives. *Can J Psychiatry.* 1989;34(5):435–439.
46. Braam W, Smits MG, Didden R, Korzilius H, Van Geijlswijk IM, Curfs LM. Exogenous melatonin for sleep problems in individuals with intellectual disability: a meta-analysis. *Dev Med Child Neurol.* 2009;51(5): 340–349.
47. McArthur AJ, Budden SS. Sleep dysfunction in rett syndrome: a trial of exogenous melatonin treatment. *Dev Med Child Neurol.* 1998;40(3): 186–192.
48. Wasdell MB, Jan JE, Bomben MM, et al. A randomized, placebo-controlled trial of controlled release melatonin treatment of delayed sleep phase syndrome and impaired sleep maintenance in children with neurodevelopmental disabilities. *J Pineal Res.* 2008;44(1):57–64.
49. Coppola G, Iervolino G, Mastrosimone M, La Torre G, Ruiu F, Pascotto A. Melatonin in wake-sleep disorders in children, adolescents and young adults with mental retardation with or

without epilepsy: a double-blind, cross-over, placebo-controlled trial. *Brain Dev.* 2004; 26(6):373–376.
50. Gupta M, Aneja S, Kohli K. Add-on melatonin improves sleep behavior in children with epilepsy: randomized, double-blind, placebo-controlled trial. *J Child Neurol.* 2005;20(2):112–115.
51. Elkhayat HA, Hassanein SM, Tomoum HY, Abd-Elhamid IA, Asaad T, Elwakkad AS. Melatonin and sleep-related problems in children with intractable epilepsy. *Pediatr Neurol. 2010*;42(4): 249–254.
52. Potocki L, Chen KS, Lupski JR. Subunit 3 of the COP9 signal transduction complex is conserved from plants to humans and maps within the Smith-Magenis syndrome critical region in 17p11.2. *Genomics.* 1999;57:180–182.
53. Stankiewicz P, Shaw CJ, Dapper JD, et al. Genome architecture catalyzes nonrecurrent chromosomal rearrangements. *Am J Hum Genet.* 2003;72: 1101–1116.
54. Dang DX, Glaze D, Reiter RJ, Tan DX, Lupski JR, Potocki L. *Circadian Rhythm Abnormalities of Melatonin in Smith-Magenis Syndrome Patients With RAI1 Point Mutation.* San Diego, CA: The American Society of Human Genetics; 2007. 10/26/07
55. Arendt J, Deacon S, English J, Hampton S, Morgan L. Melatonin and adjustment to phase shift. *J Sleep Res.* 1995;4:74–79.
56. Boddaert N, De Leersnyder H, Bourgeois M, Munnich A, Brunelle F, Zilbovicius M. Anatomical and functional brain imaging evidence of lenticulo-insular anomalies in Smith Magenis syndrome. *Neuroimage.* 2004;21:1021–1025.
57. Andrieux J, Villenet C, Quief S, et al. Genotype phenotype correlation of 30 patients with Smith-Magenis syndrome (SMS) using comparative genome hybridisation array: cleft palate in SMS is associated with larger deletions. *J Med Genet.* 2007; 44:537–540.
58. Szuhay G, Rotenberg J. Sleep apnea in pediatric neurological conditions. *Curr Neurol Neurosci Rep.* 2009;9(2):145–152.
59. Lopes MC, Marcus CL. The significance of ASDA arousals in children. *Sleep Med.* 2007;9:3–8.
60. Beebe DW. Neurobehavioral morbidity associated with disordered breathing during sleep in children: a comprehensive review. *Sleep.* 2006;29: 1115–1134.
61. Kahn A, Groswasser J, Sottiaux M, Rebuffat E, Franco P. Mechanisms of obstructive sleep apneas in infants. *Biol Neonate.* 1994;65:235–239.
62. Montgomery-Downs HE, Gozal D. Sleep habits and risk factors for sleep-disordered breathing in infants and young toddlers in louisville, kentucky. *Sleep Med.* 2006;7: 211–219.
63. Kelmanson IA. Snoring, noisy breathing in sleep and daytime behaviour in 2–4-month-old infants. *Eur J Pediatr.* 2000;159:734–739.
64. Montgomery-Downs HE, Crabtree VM, Gozal D. Cognition, sleep and respiration in at-risk children treated for obstructive sleep apnoea. *Eur Respir J.* 2005;25:336–342.
65. Gozal D, Kheirandish-Gozal L. Neurocognitive and behavioral morbidity in children with sleep disorders. *Curr Opin Pulm Med.* 2007;13: 505–509.
66. Gozal D. Sleep-disordered breathing and school performance in children. *Pediatrics.* 1998;102:616–620.
67. Goodwin JL, Kaemingk KL, Fregosi RF, et al. Clinical outcomes associated with sleep-disordered breathing in caucasian and hispanic children—the tucson children's assessment of sleep apnea study (tucasa). *Sleep.* 2003;26:587–591.
68. Suratt PM, Peruggia M, D'Andrea L, et al. Cognitive function and behavior of children with adenotonsillar hypertrophy suspected of having obstructive sleep-disordered breathing. *Pediatrics.* 2006;118:e771–e781.
69. Kurnatowski P, Putynski L, Lapienis M, Kowalska B. Neurocognitive abilities in children with adenotonsillar hypertrophy. *Int J Pediatr Otorhinolaryngol.* 2006;70:419–424.
70. Gozal D, Pope DW Jr. Snoring during early childhood and academic performance at ages thirteen to fourteen years. *Pediatrics.* 2001;107: 1394–1399.
71. Urschitz MS, Eitner S, Guenther A, et al. Habitual snoring, intermittent hypoxia, and impaired behavior in primary school children. *Pediatrics.* 2004;114:1041–1048.
72. Ali NJ, Pitson D, Stradling Jr. Sleep disordered breathing: effects of adenotonsillectomy on behaviour and psychological functioning. *Eur J Pediatr.* 1996;155(1):56–62.
73. Friedman BC, Hendeles-Amitai A, Kozminsky E, et al. Adenotonsillectomy improves neurocognitive function in children with obstructive sleep apnea syndrome. *Sleep.* 2003;26(8):999–1005.
74. Goldman AM, Potocki L, Walz K, et al. Epilepsy and chromosomal rearrangements in Smith-Magenis Syndrome [del(17)(p11.2p11.2)]. *J Child Neurol.* 2006;21(2):93–98.
75. Dinner DS. Effect of sleep on epilepsy. *J Clin Neurophysiol.* 2002;19(6):504–513.
76. Capdevila OS, Dayyat E, Kheirandish-Gozal L, Gozal D. Prevalence of epileptiform activity in healthy children during sleep. *Sleep Med.* 2008;9(3):303–309.
77. Silvestri R, Gagliano A, Calarese T, et al. Ictal and interictal EEG abnormalities in ADHD children recorded over night by video-polysomnography. *Epilepsy Res.* 2007;75(2–3):130–137.
78. Gunderson CH, Dunne PB, Feyer TL. Sleep deprivation seizures. *Neurology.* 1973;23(7): 678–686.
79. Bourgeois B. The relationship between sleep and epilepsy in children. *Semin Pediatr Neurol.* 1996;3(1):29–35.
80. Fang PC, Chen YJ, Lee IC. Seizure precipitants in children with intractable epilepsy. *Brain Dev.* 2008;30(8):527–532.

81. Nakken KO, Solaas MH, Kjeldsen MJ, Friis ML, Pellock JM, Corey LA. Which seizure-precipitating factors do patients with epilepsy most frequently report? *Epilepsy Behav.* 2005;6(1):85–89.
82. Kotagal S, Gibbons VP, Stith JA. Sleep abnormalities in patients with severe cerebral palsy. *Dev Med Child Neurol.* 1994;36(4):304–311.
83. Palm L, Anderson H, Elmqvist D, Blennow G. Daytime sleep tendency before and after discontinuation of antiepileptic drugs in preadolescent children with epilepsy. *Epilepsia.* 1992;33(4): 687–691.
84. Newman CJ, O'Regan M, Hensey O. Sleep disorders in children with cerebral palsy. *Dev Med Child Neurol.* 2006;48(7): 564–568.
85. Earley CJ, Allen RP, Chokroverty S, Hening WA. *Restless Legs Syndrome.* W.B. Saunders Co; 2009. Philadelphia.
86. Mikkelsson M, El-Metwally A, Kautiainen H, Auvinen A, Macfarlane GJ, Salminen JJ. Onset, prognosis and risk factors for widespread pain in schoolchildren: a prospective 4-year follow-up study. *Pain.* 2008;138(3):681–687.

CHAPTER 9

Autism and Other Neurodevelopmental Disorders

Suzanne E. Goldman and Beth A. Malow

Autism and Other Neurodevelopmental Disorders

Sleep is an essential component of health, and daytime function and disturbances can have a profound impact on a variety of neurologic and psychiatric conditions. Sleep disorders are a pervasive problem in children with developmental disorders, with prevalence rates as high as 88% dependent on the population of individuals studied [1]. Rates will also vary within a disorder on the basis of the heterogeneity of the group sampled. Sleep disturbances in these disorders have been found to be significantly higher than in age-matched typically developing (TD) individuals [2].

Sleep disturbances are included in the diagnostic criteria for many neurodevelopmental disorders including Angelman syndrome (AS), Prader-Willi syndrome (PWS), and Williams syndrome (WS), or else are known to have a high prevalence in conditions such as in autism spectrum disorders (ASD) (Stores G 2001). Although the specific type of neurodevelopmental disorder may be differentiated by a specific type of sleep problem [3], common symptomatology often occurs (Table 9.1). Sleep initiation, maintenance, and short sleep duration are the most commonly reported sleep disturbances in ASD, AS, PWS, and WS; these symptoms are consistent with *The International Classification of Sleep Disorders* definition of insomnia [4]. Other sleep disorders, such as sleep apnea, are also prevalent in children with PWS. In general, sleep problems are more severe in childhood, between the ages of 2 and 6 years [Stores G 2001; 5] with a decline after childhood. Reasons for the decline in sleep problems after childhood are multiple and include improvement in sleep behaviors or sleep consolidation, changes in parental perception, or maturation of sleep activity. However, in some individuals with neurodevelopmental

Key Points

1. Sleep disturbance is highly prevalent in individuals with neurodevelopmental disorders.
2. The sleep disturbance, in turn, may affect the underlying disorder and worsen associated features (eg, seizures, anxiety) as well as contribute to familial stress.
3. Treatment of sleep disturbance in neurodevelopmental disorders may impact favorably on the underlying disorder and also on the family. Additional research is needed in this area.

Clinical Pearl

Remember to look for medical, neurologic, and psychiatric causes in approaching sleep disorders in children with neurodevelopmental disorders.

Table 9.1 Sleep disturbances associated with neurodevelopmental disorders

	Autism	Angelman syndrome	Prader-Willi syndrome	Williams syndrome
Sleep onset insomnia	++			
Sleep maintenance insomnia	+	++	+	
Obstructive sleep apnea			+	
Daytime sleepiness			++	+
Nocturnal seizures	+	++		

disorders, sleep problems may persist in adolescence and young adulthood. These individuals may take longer to fall asleep, have a poor sleep efficiency, and spend more time awake after sleep onset than those without neurodevelopmental disorders [6,7].

Causes of insomnia in these neurodevelopmental disorders are multifactorial. These factors can both contribute to insomnia and be exacerbated by insomnia, and are therefore represented as bidirectional in Figure 9.1. Factors include neurobiological aspects such as aberrations in neurotransmitter systems that promote sleep and a regular sleep-wake cycle (eg, melatonin), medical disorders that disrupt sleep continuity (eg, neurological conditions such as epilepsy, gastrointestinal disorders such as reflux, and primary sleep disorders such as sleep apnea), and the medications used to treat these conditions. Additionally, psychiatric comorbidities, including anxiety, depression, attention deficit disorder/hyperactivity, and obsessive behavior can also contribute to insomnia as well as be exacerbated by insomnia. Sleep habits can impact negatively on neurobiological factors (eg, too much light at night can suppress melatonin levels) as well as on medical disorders (eg, sleep deprivation can exacerbate epileptic seizures). The core behavioral deficits associated with the disorders may impede the establishment of sound bedtime behaviors and routines. For example, children with ASD may have difficulty with emotional regulation (eg, ability to calm self) or with transitioning from preferred or stimulating activities to sleep. Children with AS or ASD may have difficulty with settling without the presence of a parent or other caregiver. Because of the deficits in communication skills, children may not readily understand the expectations of parents related to going to bed or staying in bed. The causes of sleep disturbances in children with neurodevelopmental disorders and the approach to treatment are summarized in Table 9.2 and 9.3.

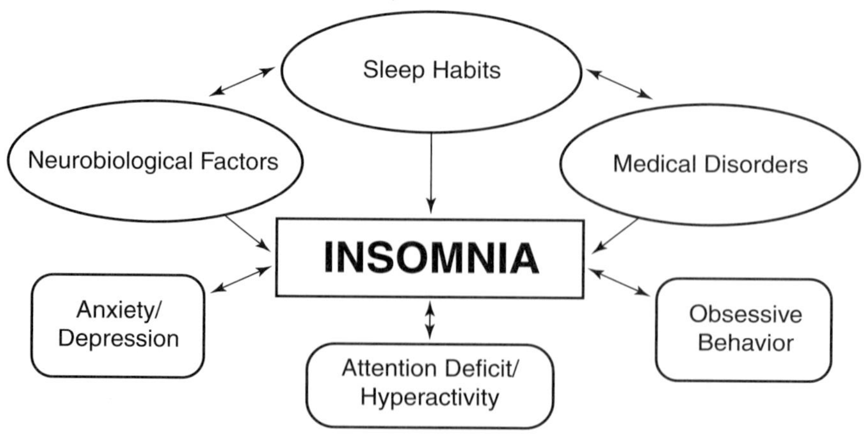

Figure 9.1 Causes and correlates of insomnia in children with neurodevelopmental disorders.

Table 9.2 Causes of sleep disturbances in neurodevelopmental disorders

- Medical or neurological disorder (eg, seizures, gastrointestinal reflux disease, nocturia)
- Sleep disorder (sleep apnea, restless legs syndrome, periodic limb movement disorder, circadian rhythm disorder)
- Psychiatric disorder (eg, anxiety, attention-deficit hyperactivity disorder)
- Medication use (eg, antidepressants, stimulants)
- Behavioral factors (eg, difficulty understanding parental expectations secondary to communication problems related to the neurodevelopmental disorder)
- Because of other factors associated with neurodevelopmental disorders (eg, neurotransmitter abnormalities, increased sensitivity to the environment)
- Sleep-related seizures
- Sleep-related movements (eg, periodic limb movements of sleep)
- Rapid eye movement sleep behavior disorder

Table 9.3 Approach to treating sleep disturbances in neurodevelopmental disorders

- Identify underlying causes of sleep disorder (listed in Table 9.2)
- Treat underlying medical conditions
- Initiate behavioral treatments
- Trial of melatonin or other sleep-promoting medications
- Maximize sleep promoting properties of child's other medications where possible (eg, antiepileptic drugs or antidepressants)

Disturbed sleep in children with neurodevelopmental disorders is associated with poorer daytime function and behavior. Disrupted sleep often manifests itself in children through behavioral symptoms such as hyperactivity, inattention, and aggression [8], and is likely to adversely impact behavior, mood, cognition, and family functioning (Stores G 2001). Disturbed nighttime sleep also impacts caregiver and familial burden [1], an often unrecognized and unaddressed challenge. Treatment of sleep problems in children with intellectual disabilities and challenging daytime behavior reduces parental stress, increases perceived control, and improves parental satisfaction with their own sleep, their child's sleep, and their ability to cope with their child's sleep [9].

Recognition of sleep problems in individuals with neurodevelopmental disorders is an emerging discipline achieving more prominence, especially as these disorders are better understood. This chapter will focus on sleep in children with neurodevelopmental disorders focusing on ASD, AS, and PWS—disorders associated at least in part with chromosomal aberrations in the 15q11–13 region, and WS, a disorder of chromosome 7q11–23.

Autism Spectrum Disorders

Autism, a disorder of neurodevelopment, is characterized by core deficits in social interaction, communication, and restricted interests. The *Diagnostic and Statistical Manual of Mental Disorders, Fourth Edition* (DSM-IV), defines autism as a spectrum disorder, encompassing Autistic Disorder, Pervasive Developmental Disorder Not Otherwise Specified (PDD-NOS), Asperger's syndrome, Childhood Disintegrative Disorder, and Rett syndrome [10]. Although the etiology of the disease is unknown, it is recognized that the incidence is increasing, to where an average of 1 in 110 children are being diagnosed as being on the autism spectrum [11–13]. In the United States the average prevalence rate of ASD in 2006 was estimated at 9.0 per 1000 (95% confidence interval = 8.6–9.3) [12].

Sleep problems are recognized as a coexisting symptom with ASD and can influence the course and severity of the disorder. Children with ASD have a higher prevalence of sleep problems than TD children with prevalence rates ranging from 44% to 83% [3,15] compared with a prevalence of 11% to 37% in TD children [16]. Research has shown that insomnia is the major sleep concern in children with ASD with prolonged sleep latency (time to fall asleep), decreased sleep efficiency (decreased time asleep/time in bed), decreased total sleep time, decreased sleep duration and continuity, and increased awakenings [17] when compared with TD children. In general, sleep-onset insomnia (difficulty falling asleep) is highly prevalent, as compared with sleep maintenance insomnia (difficulty staying asleep) [Williams, Sears et al 2004; 14]. Insomnia occurs regardless of age [17, Williams, Sears et al 2004] and gender has not been reported to influence sleep problems in these individuals. Few studies have investigated sleep complaints in adolescents or adults with ASD. It has been suggested that individuals adapt to their sleep problems rather than experiencing an actual decrease in problems [5]. Goudbout and colleagues [18] found decreased sleep time in the first two-thirds of the night, increased number of shifts into rapid eye movement (REM) sleep from a waking epoch, and REM sleep disruptions in individuals with ASD compared with those without ASD.

Daytime behaviors often displayed in ASD individuals, such as inattention, hyperactivity, and restricted behaviors, are affected by insomnia and other facets of disturbed sleep. Studies using objective measurements of sleep, such as polysomnography and actigraphy, and subjective parental reports showed 2 subsets of sleepers in ASD—good sleepers and poor sleepers [19,20]. Poor sleepers showed more hyperactivity and compulsive and ritualistic behavior than good sleepers. Fragmentation, an actigraphic measure of sleep disruption, was associated with more restricted/repetitive behaviors [20]. In small studies, severity of sleep problems in ASD does not appear influenced by communicative status [19], cognitive level [15], or adaptive function [19]. In ASD, short sleep duration has been associated with stereotypic behavior, with overall autism scores and social skills deficits [21], as well as with repetitive behaviors [22].

Angelman Syndrome

Angelman syndrome (AS) is a neurodevelopmental disorder caused by the absence or nonfunctioning of the maternal allele at the 15q11–q13 domain that occurs in an estimated 1 in 12,000 to 1 in 20,000 individuals [23]. There are 4 main genetic mechanisms underlying this disorder: (1) deletions of the 15q11–q13 on the maternal chromosome (approximately 70% of the cases); (2) parental uniparental disomy (UPD) (2%–3% of the cases); (3) mutation in the UBE3A gene on the maternal chromosome 15 (5%–10% of the cases); and (4) an imprinting defect where the chromosome 15 inherited from the mother has the paternal pattern for gene functioning so the UBE3A function is turned off (3%–5% of the cases). An additional 10% to 15% of the cases result from unknown causes [23,24]. Characteristics include developmental delay, intellectual disability, recurrent seizures, lack of speech, and walking and balance disorders [23,24].

Sleep disturbances are common in AS and are included in the diagnostic criteria established in 1995 and in the updated criteria in 2005 [25,26]. Although prevalence rates of sleep disturbances as high as 100% have been cited [26], there is also a subgroup of children with no problems [23]. In general, the prevalence of sleep problems in AS ranges from 20% to 80% [26]; this variation in prevalence may relate to how sleep problems are defined [5]. Sleep problems appear more prevalent, and severe, in childhood [27]. Although in some individuals sleep problems persist, they generally diminish or disappear by late childhood [5,28,29].

Symptoms of insomnia, in particular difficulty initiating or maintaining sleep, are primary concerns [27,28,30–32]. Related sleep problems, including dependence on medication or pacifiers to promote sleep, awakening from loud noises, disorientation when aroused, and bruxism have been cited [32]. Although symptoms of insomnia are primary concerns, children with AS may need less sleep than TD children [27,28,30,31]. Few studies have objectively investigated the specific sleep abnormalities present in this disorder [33,34] and additional research is needed in this area.

Types of Sleep Problems in AS

Similar to other neurodevelopmental disorders, the etiology of insomnia in AS is most likely multifactorial rather than because of one specific component. In AS, biological abnormalities in the circadian control of sleep are a plausible cause of insomnia. The possibility of disturbed melatonin metabolism has been suggested on the basis of the response to melatonin treatment in small trials [35]. Psychological factors, such as reliance on parents to promote sleep [32] or associating the bedroom with activities other than sleep, are also likely to be involved. Other causes or contributing factors to insomnia in AS may include primary sleep disorders such as nightmares [32] or epileptic seizures [27]. Independent of epileptic seizures, sleep continuity and architecture may be disrupted by frequent interictal epileptiform activity or by abnormal high-amplitude rhythmic slow-wave discharges that are characteristic findings in the waking electroencephalograms of AS patients [36].

Although evidence of the behavioral consequences of poor nighttime sleep can be seen in other populations with developmental disabilities, minimal information is available on the association of disturbed sleep and behavior in children with AS or the impact of disturbed sleep on the caregiver and family. Additional research is needed in this area.

Prader-Willi Syndrome

Prader-Willi syndrome (PWS) is a neurodevelopmental disorder that arises from failure to express paternal genes in the 15q11–q13 domain [37] with an estimated prevalence of between 1 in 12,000 to 1 in 15,000 births [38]. Three main genetic errors occur: (1) a noninherited deletion in the paternal contributed chromosome 15 (approximately 70%); (2) a maternal UPD—2 maternal chromosome 15's and no paternal chromosome 15 (25%); and (3) an error in the "imprinting" process rendering the paternal contribution nonfunctional (2%–5%) [38]. PWS is characterized by hypotonia, hypogonadism, hyperphagia, cognitive impairment, difficult behaviors, and morbid obesity.

Sleep disturbances are included in the diagnostic criteria for PWS with the most commonly reported disturbances being sleep apnea, nighttime awakenings, and hypersomnolence [39–41]. Hypoventilation and desaturation, daytime sleepiness with or without obesity, and nighttime enuresis occur at all ages [38]. Sleep-disordered breathing abnormalities include increased apnea events, decreased oxygen saturation, increased maximum heart rate, as well as abnormal arousal response to hypoxia and hypercapnia [42]. Patterns of apnea have been documented to be obstructive, central, mixed, and complex [43]. Prevalence of obstructive sleep apnea has been reported to be between 0% and 100%, although it is difficult to ascertain because of variability in sample size and inclusionary criteria [44]. Association of obstructive sleep apnea has been found with increased body mass, daytime sleepiness and inactivity, and behavioral disturbance [45]. Although obesity might play a role, most studies conclude that sleep apnea does not seem closely associated with the degree of obesity. The lack of association between sleep apnea and obesity most likely reflects the type of obesity. In PWS, obesity is usually central rather than truncal in distribution; truncal obesity is associated with sleep apnea [44].

REM sleep abnormalities have been reported in PWS, with sleep-onset REM periods and reductions of REM sleep latency, as well as abnormal arousal thresholds to hypoxia and hypocretin [44,46,47]. Possible associations between PWS and narcolepsy have been raised because both exhibit cases of REM sleep occurrence at sleep onset [44].

Sleep-Disordered Breathing and Genetic Type

Several clinical features displayed in individuals with PWS have been correlated with specific genotypes [48]. However, the association of genetic mutation and sleep problems is still uncertain. Subjectively reported sleep disturbances and central sleep apnea with a greater than 10% oxygen desaturation have been reported to occur more in PWS individuals with chromosome-15 paternal deletion [48], whereas another study reports more subjective sleep disturbances in the UPD subtype [49]. However, other studies report similar frequencies of sleep disturbance per apnea in chromosome-15 paternal deletion and maternal UPD [49–51].

Excessive Daytime Sleepiness

Excessive daytime sleepiness (EDS) is manifested by individuals with PWS, which tends to distinguish it from the other intellectual disorders [52]. Caregivers, as well individuals with PWS, have reported EDS. A review of EDS measured objectively with Multiple Sleep Latency Tests (MSLT) found that 29 of 72 cases had a sleep latency less than 5 minutes on MSLT. In other studies of PWS, including those with a history of both sleep apnea and EDS, 52% of patients with known EDS and sleep apnea and 48% of randomly selected patients with PWS had sleep latencies less than 5 minutes [52]. Unlike the general population where EDS is associated with sleep apnea, the relationship between EDS and degree of sleep-disordered breathing, or obesity, has not been demonstrated [44]. This suggests that in PWS, hypothalamic dysfunction is a primary contributor [52]. Results of 2 studies examining the association of a particular genotype with EDS suggested no specific association between EDS and genotype [53,54].

Behavioral disturbance was found associated with EDS in children and adolescents with PWS [55]. The association of age, body mass index (BMI), and sleep apnea with EDS appears mixed, varying by study and limited by small sample sizes. The reader is referred to a review on this for more detailed information [52].

Treatment of Sleep Disturbances in PWS

The association between sleep apnea and neurocognitive behavior, as well as sleep apnea and obesity, has been demonstrated in TD individuals. Camfferman et al [56] posit that sleep apnea may be a contributing factor to reduced psychosocial and neurocognitive performance in individuals with PWS and treatment may help improve behavior.

Continuous positive airway pressure (CPAP) is the gold standard of treatment for sleep apnea; however, there is minimal information on its effectiveness in PWS. Small studies and case reports have shown improvements in sleep structure and respiratory pattern, daytime somnolence, daytime somnolence, and improved daytime behavior [53,57,58].

Case reports, or small studies, have reported on alternative treatments to CPAP for control of sleep disturbances and/or apnea. Biliopancreatic diversion with duodenal switch performed in one patient resulted in disappearance of her sleep disturbances and sleep apnea [59]. Adenotonsillectomy in 3 patients had mixed results, with the highest body mass child having the most apnea resolution [60]. Additionally, although the leading threat to life expectancy and quality of life in individuals with PWS is obesity [59], the associations between sleep architecture and weight remains understudied.

Growth hormone therapy is controversial because of case reports of sudden death, primarily during sleep, on initiation of treatment, although a causal association cannot be demonstrated. Stafler and Wallis [61] provide a review of this controversy. Growth hormone therapy in a study of 12 children showed a trend toward reduction in apneic and hypopneic events and duration of event independent of BMI [62]. Further, administration of growth hormone has been associated with lower ghrelin levels and improvement in AHI [62].

Williams Syndrome

Williams syndrome (WS), a developmental disorder resulting from a microdeletion of several genes on chromosome 7q11.23, results in cardiovascular, endocrine, and neurological problems [63]. WS is associated with a distinctive cognitive-linguistic profile, marked by visual-spatial deficits and relative strengths in expressive language. Individuals with WS also have high levels of nonsocial anxiety, worries, and fears, as compared with others with intellectual disabilities [64,65,66], even though they show marked sociability and interests in interacting with others. In addition, children with WS may exhibit overactivity and short attention spans. Approximately 65% are diagnosed with attention deficit hyperactivity disorder (ADHD) or other behavioral disorders [63,64,66,67]. Both mental health and medical problems persist into adulthood and may reduce adult quality of life [65,68].

Given their behavioral phenotype of high anxiety and behavioral disorders, one could expect to find a high level of sleep problems. Sleep disorders may play a role in the overall phenotypical presentation of WS [69]. Disturbed sleep may complicate coexistent psychiatric disorders in WS such as ADHD, stress, and anxiety (Stores G 2001). However, sleep in WS has been relatively understudied. In a study of 28 children, parents reported symptoms consistent of a sleep disorder in 16 children with symptoms of restless sleep, sleep initiation, and nighttime awakenings [70]. Polysomnography performed on 7 of these children showed periodic limb movements 5-fold greater than control subjects. This was extrapolated based on TD children, and it was suggested that children with WS may be at a higher risk for sleep disturbances because of limb movements, restless leg syndrome, or sleep-disordered breathing [69].

Symptoms of periodic limb movements have been reported in adults [65,69] and sleep complaints in WS were believed to persist into adulthood [69], although until recently this had not been examined. Goldman et al [71] studied sleep-wake patterns of 23 adolescents and adults (mean [SD] age, 25.5[8.0] years) using wrist actigraphy, sleep-wake diaries, and questionnaires. They found that the majority of the participants acknowledged sleep problems and daytime tiredness. This was true even though they spent an average of 9 hours per night in bed and averaged 7.5 hours of sleep. The authors postulated that sleep disruption from multiple factors, including restless leg syndrome/periodic limb movements of sleep, sleep apnea, or factors intrinsic to WS, might be associated with the daytime sleepiness.

Further research is needed to refine the sleep phenotype in WS and to examine its impact on daytime behavior.

Rett Syndrome

Rett syndrome is a severe neurodevelopmental disorder, mainly affecting females. The overall incidence of this disorder is 1 per 10,000 females [72]. Classical Rett syndrome follows a distinctive developmental course, with the achievement of normal early milestones, followed by developmental regression, deceleration of head growth, the onset of stereotypic hand movements, and gait abnormalities.

The association between Rett syndrome and mutations in the methyl-CpG binding protein 2 (MECP2) gene was first identified in 1999 [73]. To date, more than 200 mutations have been identified and there appears to be considerable variation in phenotype [74].

Girls with Rett syndrome often show periods of hyperventilation followed by apneas during wakefulness, yet sleep-disordered breathing has not been observed at night [75]. They do, however, show specific sleep-related problems. An Australian study using a Rett syndrome database identified sleep problems in more than 80% of the cases [76]. Daytime napping, nighttime laughter, teeth grinding, night screaming, and seizures were the problems most frequently reported. These were identified more frequently in the younger age groups. Nighttime laughing reduced with age, whereas daytime napping and nighttime seizures worsened with age. The prevalence of sleep problems was highest in cases with a large deletion of the MECP2 gene and in those with the p.R294X and p.R306C mutation, and less common with the p.R270X and p.T158M mutations. In an attempt to improve sleep, melatonin, bromocriptine, and naltrexone have been used in this population, with variable success [77–79]. Further research is needed to identify treatment strategies in improving sleep at night and daytime alertness.

Summary

Sleep disturbance is highly prevalent in individuals with neurodevelopmental disorders. Existing research has focused primarily on children with few studies extending to adolescents and adults. Although sleep problems may improve with the transition to adulthood, acceptance of abnormal sleep patterns within the family setting might also exist. Future research needs to address this age-related transition. Additionally, outcome studies to determine the effects of treating sleep on quality of life and family function are warranted.

References

1. Lancioni GE, O'Reilly MF, Basii G. Review of strategies for treating sleep problems in persons with severe or profound mental retardation or multiple handicaps. *Am J Ment Retard.* 1999;104:170–186.
2. Cotton S, Richdale A. Brief report: parental descriptions of sleep problems in children with autism, Down syndrome, and Prader-Willi syndrome. *Res Dev Disabil.* 2006;27(2):151–161.
3. Richdale AL, Schreck KA. Sleep problems in autism spectrum disorders: prevalence, nature and possible biopsycosocial aetiologies. *Sleep Med Rev.* 2009;13:403–411.

4. American Academy of Sleep Medicine. *The International Classifications of Sleep Disorders.* West Chester, OH: American Academy of Sleep Medicine; 2005;4.
5. Pelc K, Cheron G, Boyd SG, Dan B. Are there distinctive sleep problems in angelman syndrome? *Sleep Med.* 2008;9:434–441.
6. Oyane NM, Bjorvatn B. Sleep disturbances in adolescents and young adults with autism and asperger syndrome. *Autism.* 2005;9(1):83–94.
7. Hare DJ, Jones S, Evershed K. Objective investigation of the sleep-wake cycle in adults with intellectual disabilities and autistic spectrum disorders. *J Intellect Disabil Res.* 2006;50(pt 10):701–710.
8. Veasey S, Rosen R, Barzansky B, Rosen I, Owens J. Sleep loss and fatigue in residency training: a reappraisal. *JAMA.* 2002;288(9):1116–1124.
9. Wiggs L, Stores G. Behavioral treatment for sleep problems in children with severe intellectual disabilites and daytime challenging behavior: effects on mothers and fathers. *Br J Health Psychol.* 2001;6:257–269.
10. American Psychiatric Association. *Diagnostic and Statistical Manual of Mental Disorders.* Washington, DC: American Psychiatric Association; 2000; section 299.00 AUTISTIC DISORDER.
11. Center for Disease Control. Parental report of diagnosed autism in children ages 4–17 years—United States 2003–2004. *MMWR.* 2006;55: 481–486.
12. Center for Disease Control. Prevalence of autism spectrum disorders—autism and developmental disabilities monitoring netword, United States, 2006. *MMWR Surveill Summ.* 2009;58:1–20.
13. Centers for Disease Control and Prevention. Autism Spectrum Disorders (ASDs). http://www.cdc.gov/ncbddd/autism/index.html. Updated January 4, 2009. Accessed December 18, 2009.
14. Williams PG, Sears L, Allard A. 2004. Sleep Problems in children with autism. 13: 265–269.
15. Krakowiak P, Goodlin-Jones B, Hertz-Picciotto I, Croen LA, Hansen RL. Sleep problems in children with autism spectrum disorders, developmental delays, and typical development: a population-based study. *J Sleep Res.* 2008;17(2):197–206.
16. Owens JA, Spirito A, McGuinn M. The Children's Sleep Habits Questionnaire (CSHQ): psychometric properties of a survey instrument for school-aged children. *Sleep.* 2000;23(8):1043–1051.
17. Richdale AL. Sleep problems in autism: prevalence, cause, and intervention. *Child Neurol.* 1999;41:60–66.
18. Godbout R, Bergeron C, Limoges E, Stip E, Mottron L. A laboratory study of sleep in Asperger's syndrome. *Neuroreport.* 2000;11(1):127–130.
19. Malow BA, Marzec ML, McGrew SG, Wang L, Henderson LM, Stone WL. Characterizing sleep in children with autism spectrum disorders: a multidimensional approach. *Sleep.* 2006;29(1):8.
20. Goldman SE, Surdyka K, Cuevas R, Adkins K, Wang L, Malow BA. Defining the sleep phenotype in children with autism. *Dev Neuropsychol.* 2009;34(5):560–573.
21. Schreck KA, Mulick JA, Smith AF. Sleep problems as possible predictors of intensified symptoms of autism. *Res Dev Disabil.* 2004;24:57–56.
22. Gabriels RL, Cuccaro ML, Hill DE, Ivers BJ, Goldson E. Repetitive behaviors in autism: relationships with associated clinical features. *Res Dev Disabil.* 2005;26:169–181.
23. National Institute of Health. Genetics Home Reference Angelman syndrome. http://ghr.nlm.nih.gov/condition=angelmansyndrome. Updated January 11, 2010. Accessed 2010, January 12, 2010.
24. Angelman Syndrome Foundation. http://www.angelman.org. 2009.
25. Williams CA, Beaudet AL, Clayton-Smith J, et al. Angelman syndrome: consensus for diagnostic criteria. *Am J Med Genet.* 1995;56(2):237–238.
26. Williams CA, Beaudet A, Clayton-Smith J, et al. Angelman Syndrome 2005: updated consensus for diagnostic criteria. *Am J Med Genet A.* 2006;140A(5):413–418.
27. Clayton-Smith J. Clinical research on Angelman syndrome in the United Kingdom: observations on 82 affected individuals. *Am J Med Genet.* 1993;46(1):12–15.
28. Bruni O, Ferri R, D'Agostino G, Miano S, Roccella M, Elia M. Sleep disturbances in Angelman syndrome: a questionnaire study. *Brain Dev.* 2004;26(4):233–240.
29. Didden R, Korzilius H, Smits MG, Curfs LM. Sleep problems in individuals with Angelman syndrome. *Am J Ment Retard.* 2004;109:275–284.
30. Zhadanova IV, Wurtman RJ, Wagstaff J. Effects of a low dose of melatonin on sleep in children with Angelman syndrome. *J Pediatr Endocrinol Metab.* 1999;12:57–67.
31. Berry RJ, Leitner RP, Clarke AR, Einfeld SL. Behavioral aspects of Angelman syndrome: a case control study. *Am J Med Genet A.* 2005;132A(1): 8–12.
32. Walz NC, Beebe D, Byars K. Sleep in individuals with Angelman syndrome: parent perceptions of patterns and problems. *Am J Ment Retard.* 2005;110(4):243–252.
33. Miano S, Bruni O, Leuzzi V, Elia M, Verrillo E, Ferri R. Sleep polygraphy in Angelman Syndrome. *Clin Neurophysiol.* 2004;115(4):938–945.
34. Miano S, Bruni O, Elia M, Musumeci SA, Verrillo E, Ferri R. Sleep breathing and periodic leg movement pattern in Angelman syndrome: a polysomnographic study. *Clin Neurophysiol.* 2005;116(11):2685–2692.
35. Braam W, Didden R, Smits MG, Curfs LM. Melatonin for chronic insomnia in Angelman syndrome: a randomized placebo-controlled trial. *J Child Neurol.* 2008;23:649–654.
36. Dan B, Boyd SG. Angelman syndrome reviewed from a neurophysiological perspective, the ube3a-gabrb3 hypothesis. *Neuropediatrics.* 2003;34: 169–176.
37. Nichols RD. Genomic imprinting and candidate genes in the Prader-Willi and Angelman syndromes. *Curr Opin Genet Dev.* 1993;3:445–456.

38. Prader-Willi Syndrome Association. Basic Facts About PWS: A Diagnosis and Reference Guide for Physicians and Other Health Professionals. http://www.pwsausa.org/syndrome/basicfac.htm. Updated January 9, 2010. Accessed June 10, 2009.
39. Gunay-Aygun M, Schwartz S, Heeger S, O'Riordan MA, Cassidy SB. The changing purpose of Prader-Willi Syndrome clinical diagnostic criteria and proposed revised criteria. *Pediatrics.* 2001;108(5):e92.
40. Burrow C, Oliver C, Shaw R, Strachan R. An investigation of sleep disturbance experienced by children with Angelman and Prader-Willi syndromes and their parents. *J Intellect Disabil Res.* 2007;51:664.
41. Heussler H, Harris M, Cooper D, et al. Sleep disruption in Prader Willi syndrome. *J Intellect Disabil Res.* 2007;51:660–660.
42. Arens R, Gozal D, Burrell BC. Arousal and cardiorespiratory responses to hypoxia in Prader-Willi Syndrome. *Am J Respir Crit Care Med.* 1996;153:283–287.
43. Lin HY, Lin SP, Lin CC, et al. Polysomnographic characteristics in patients with Prader-Willi syndrome. *Pediatr Pulmonol.* 2007;42(10):881–887.
44. Nixon GM, Brouillette RT. Sleep and breathing in Prader-Willi syndrome. *Pediatr Pulmonol.* 2002;34:209–217.
45. O'Donoghue FJ, Camfferman D, Kennedy JD, et al. Sleep-disordered breathing in Prader-Willi syndrome and its association with neurobehavioral abnormalities. *J Pediatr.* 2005;147(6):823–829.
46. Vgontzas AN, Bixler EO, Kales A, et al. Daytime sleepiness and REM abnormalities in Prader-Willi syndrome: evidence of generalized hypoarousal. *Int J Neurosci.* 1996;87:127–139.
47. Manni R, Politini L, Nobili L, et al. Hypersomnia in the Prader Willi syndrome: clinical-electrophysiological features and underlying factors. *Clin Neurophysiol.* 2001;112:800–805.
48. Torrado M, Araoz V, Baialardo E. Clinical-etiologic correlation in children with Prader-Willi syndrome (PWS): an interdisciplinary study. *Am J Med Genet A.* 2007; 143A(5):460–468.
49. Webb T, Whittington J. A study of the influence of different genotypes on the physical and behavioral phenotypes of children and adults ascertained clinically as having PWS. *Clin Genet.* 2002;62(4):273–281.
50. Cassidy SB, Forsythe M, Heeger S. Comparison of phenotype between patients with Prader-Willi syndrome due to deletion 15q and uniparental disomy 15. *Am J Med Gen.* 1997;68(4):433–440.
51. Lin HY, Lin SP, Lin CC. Polysomnographic characteristics in patients with Prader-Willi syndrome. *Pediatr Pulmonol.* 2007;42(10):881–887.
52. Camfferman D, McEvoy RD, O'Donoghue F, Lushington K. Prader Willi syndrome and excessive daytime sleepiness. *Sleep Med Rev.* 2008;12(1):65–75.
53. Clift S, Dahlitz M, Parkes JD. Sleep apnoea in the Prader-Willi syndrome. *J Sleep Res.* 1994;3(2): 121–126.
54. Vgontzas AN, Kales A, Seip J, et al. Relationship of sleep abnormalities to patient genotypes in Prader-Willi syndrome. *Am J Med Genet.* 1996;67(5):478–482.
55. Richdale AL, Cotton S, Hibbit K. Sleep and behaviour disturbance in Prader-Willi syndrome: a questionnaire study. *J Intellect Disabil Res.* 1999;43:380–390.
56. Camfferman D, Lushington K, O'Donoghue F, Doug McEvoy R. Obstructive sleep apnea syndrome in Prader-Willi syndrome: an unrecognized and untreated cause of cognitive and behavioral deficits? *Neuropsychol Rev.* 2006;16(3): 123–129.
57. Sforza E, Krieger J, Geisert J, Kurtz D. Sleep and breathing abnormalities in a case of Prader-Willi syndrome—the effects of acute continuous positive airway pressure treatment. *Acta Paediatr Scand.* 1991;80(1):80–85.
58. Doshi A, Udwadia Z. Prader-Willi syndrome with sleep disordered breathing: effect of two years nocturnal CPAP. *Indian J Chest Dis Allied Sci.* 2001;43:51–53.
59. Papavramidis ST, Kotidis EV, Gamvros O. Prader-Willi syndrome-associated obesity treated by biliopancreatic diversion with duodenal switch. Case report and literature review. *J Pediatr Surg.* 2006;41(6): 153–1158.
60. Tanna N, Choi SS. Efficacy and safety of adenotonsillectomy for pediatric obstructive sleep apnea in Prader-Willi syndrome. *Ann Otol Rhinol Laryngol.* 2009;118(4):267–269.
61. Stafler P, Wallis C. Prader-Willi syndrome: who can have growth hormone? *Arch Dis Child.* 2008;93(4):341–345.
62. Haqq AM, Stadler DD, Jackson RH, Rosenfeld RG, Purnell JQ, LaFranchi SH. Effects of growth hormone on pulmonary function, sleep quality, behavior, cognition, growth velocity, body composition, and resting energy expenditure in Prader-Willi syndrome. *J Clin Endocrinol Metab.* 2003;88(5):2206–2212.
63. Pober BR, Morris CA. Diagnosis and management of medical problems in adults with Williams-Beuren syndrome. *Am J Med Genet Part C: Semin Med Genet.* 2007;145C(3):280–290.
64. Einfeld SL, Tonge BJ, Florio T. Behavioral and emotional disturbance in individuals with Williams syndrome. *Am J Ment Retard.* 1997;102:45–53.
65. Davies M, Udwin O. Adults with Williams syndrome. *Br J Psychiatry.* 1998;172: 273–276.
66. Dykens EM. Anxiety, fears, and phobias in persons with Williams syndrome. *Dev Neuropsychol.* 2003;23(1–2):291–316.
67. Leyfer OT, Woodruff-Borden J, Klein-Tasman BP, Fricke JS, Mervis CB. Prevalence of psychiatric disorders in 4 to 16-year-olds with Williams syndrome. *Am J Med Genet B Neuropsychiatr Genet.* 2006;141B:615–622.
68. Howlin P, Udwin O. Outcome in adult life for people with Williams syndrome—results from a survey of 239 families. *J Intellect Disabil Res.* 2006;50(2):151–160.

69. Mason TB, Arens R. Sleep patterns in Williams–Beuren syndrome. In: Morris CA, Lenhoff HM, Wang PP, eds. *Williams-Beuren Syndrome: Research, Evaluation, and Treatment.* Baltimore, MD: The Johns Hopkins University Press; 2006.
70. Arens R, Wright B, Elliott J. Periodic limb movement in sleep in children with Williams syndrome. *J Pediatr.* 1998;133:670–674.
71. Goldman SE, Malow BA, Newman KD, Roof E, Dykens EM. Sleep patterns and daytime sleepiness in adolescents and young adults with Williams syndrome. *J Intellect Disabil Res.* 2009;53(2):182-188.
72. Laurvick CL, de Klerk N, Bower C., et al. Rett syndrome in Australia: a review of the epidemiology. *J Pediatr.* 2006;148:347–352.
73. Amir RE, Van den Veyver IB, Wan M, Tran CQ, Francke U, Zoghbi HY. Rett syndrome is caused by mutations in X-linked MECP2, encoding methyl-CpG-binding protein 2. *Nat Genet.* 1999;23:185–188.
74. Ham Al, Kumar A, Deeter R, Schanen NC. Does genotype predict phenotype in Rett syndrome? *J Child Neurol.* 2005;20:768–778.
75. Marcus Cl, Carroll JL, McColley SA, et al. Polysomnographic characteristics of patiens with Rett syndrome. *J Pediatr.* 1994;125:218–224.
76. Young D, Nagarajan L, de Klerk N, Jacoby P, Ellaway C, Leonard H. Sleep problems in Rett syndrome. *Brain Dev.* 2007;29:609–616.
77. McArthur AJ, Budden SS. Sleep dysfunction in Rett syndrome: a trial of melatonin treatment. *Dev Med Child Neurol.* 1998;40:186–192.
78. Percy AK, Glaze DG, Schultz RJ, et al. Rett syndrome: controlled study of an oral opiate antagonist, naltrexone. *Ann Neurol.* 1994;35:464–470.
79. Zapella M, Genazzani A, Facchinetti F, Hayek G. Bromocriptine in the Rett syndrome. *Brain Dev.* 1990;12:221–225.
80. Stores G. *Sleep Disturbance in Children and Adolescents With Disorders of Development: Its Significance and Management.* Cambridge, UK: Cambridge University Press on behalf of Mac Keith Press; 2001.
81. Stores G. Sleep-wake function in children with neurodevelopmental and psychiatric disorders. *Semin Pediatr Neurol.* 2001;8(4): 188–197.

CHAPTER 10

Psychiatric Disorders and Sleep

Oliviero Bruni, Luana Novelli, Valeria Savoja, and Raffaele Ferri

Introduction

The literature on sleep disruption in adults with psychiatric disorders is extensive, and several features seem to be well defined. In children, the research is growing with very interesting studies that throw light on the crucial role of sleep psychiatric disorders in childhood and adolescence.

There is a bidirectional relationship between sleep and emotional and behavioral functioning: Sleep predicts the development of mood and anxiety disorders as well as neurobehavioral dysfunction [1–4] and sleep deprivation is known to be a worsening factor for mood and anxiety disorders [5–7]. On the other hand, children with insomnia often meet the criteria for a *Diagnostic and Statistical Manual of Mental Disorders, Fourth Edition* (DSM-IV) diagnosis [8].

Because of this bidirectional connection, sleep clinicians should always screen children and adolescents for a mental/behavioral disorder and psychiatrists should always be aware of sleep disturbance as a predictive symptom of a mental disorder and as a modulating factor of improvement or worsening of a psychiatric illness. Additionally, early sleep problems have been identified as predictors of headache, in association with anxiety and depression [9] and may be a prognostic indicator for emotion and behavioral problems in adolescence and adulthood; in fact, the presence of sleep problems at preschool age significantly predicts internalizing symptoms in prepubertal/pubertal ages [2,3].

In general, findings reported in the literature suggested that early childhood sleep disturbance is more closely associated with anxiety, whereas adolescent sleep problems are closely linked to depression [10,11]. The magnitude of depressive symptoms in adolescents is related to the likelihood of experiencing sleep problems, and depression accounted for 15% of the variance in sleep problems after controlling for anxiety; on the contrary, in prepubertal children, anxiety was a stronger predictor of sleep disturbance; however, it should be considered that anxiety and fears are common in young children and decline with age [11]. An age-related susceptibility, depending on the stage of affective development, could be hypothesized to explain these data.

The biological systems regulating sleep, affectivity, emotion, and behavior are strictly associated during development as shown by the majority of sleep-disordered children that meet criteria for an internalizing disorder and/or exhibit other emotional and behavioral problems [12]. The trajectories leading to a psychiatric disorder might start with persistent sleep problems that exacerbate inter-nalizing symptoms and then lead to the development of affective disorders [13].

Based on the above studies, the reciprocal interactions between sleep and emotion/behavior can be summarized as follows: (a) childhood psychiatric disorders may lead to or exacerbate sleep problems; (b) insufficient or disturbed sleep may interfere with a child's ability to regulate emotion and behavior and lead to mental health problems and disorders; and (c) these problems may persist in a cyclic fashion for extended periods of time, impairing a child's functioning across numerous areas [11].

Sleep Problems as Predictors of Psychiatric Disturbances

Children with psychiatric illness have a greater risk for the endurance of sleep disorders and the presence of early sleep disturbances is predictive for the development of depressive disorders in adults [14].

In a longitudinal study, Saarenpää-Heikkilä et al [15] found that almost two-thirds of children with sleep problems at the age of 3 years developed a psychiatric disorder 5 years later. In addition, other reports showed that sleep problems during early childhood predicted an increase in depression/anxiety, inattention/hyperactivity, and aggression at mid-adolescence [2,4] and insomnia predicted depression and low self-esteem in a group of 11- to 17-year-old U.S. adolescents [16].

Insomnia in children and adolescents is either a predictor or acts as a modulating factor for the severity of psychiatric symptoms. Conflicting data have been published on the role of sleep as a predictor of anxiety or depressive disorders: Gregory et al [13] showed an association with adult anxiety disorders but not with adult depressive disorders, and the same authors [17] reported a more robust association between sleep problems and depression than between sleep and anxiety in 300 twin pairs, at 8 years of age. Another study based on parental reports showed that irregularity in childhood sleeping and eating schedules was associated with both adolescent-onset major depressive disorders (MDD) and childhood-adolescent anxiety disorder [4]. Further, the presence of insomnia in adolescence was a worsening factor for depression and a predictor of suicide attempt [18].

More recently, a study on monozygotic and dizygotic twins, aimed at establishing the direction and etiology of longitudinal associations between sleep problems and depression symptoms in children, confirmed that only sleep problems at age 8 predicted depression at age 10, whereas depression symptoms did not predict later sleep problems. This study also demonstrated a stability of both sleep problems and depression from ages 8 to 10 years, which partially accounted for the longitudinal association with phenotype and showed that the cross-lagged association between sleep problems at 8 and depression at 10 years was largely because of genetic factors [17].

In summary, it seems that insomnia precedes the onset of depressive disorders, whereas previous anxiety is associated with future insomnia, but data do not support the reverse for both [19].

Anxiety Disorder

Anxiety disorder (AD) is one of the most common childhood psychiatric problems, with a prevalence of approximately 20% [20]. ADs in the DSM-IV [21] include separation anxiety disorder (SAD), generalized anxiety disorder (GAD), social and specific phobias, obsessive compulsive disorder (OCD), posttraumatic stress disorder (PTSD), and panic disorder.

A large body of literature supports the strong relationship between anxiety and sleep disturbances during childhood. In the DSM-IV-TR [21], sleep-related problems (SRPs) are listed among the symptoms of several anxiety disorders, such as difficulty initiating sleep in GAD and nightmares in SAD.

Parents reported that 88% of children with AD experienced at least 1 sleep problem, and 55% 3 or more [22,23], mainly represented by sleep terrors and sleepwalking [24], nightmares, and refusal to sleep alone or away from home [23]. A recent study on 37 children with clinically diagnosed anxiety disorders and 26 nonclinical children aged 7 to 12 years showed that anxious children reported going to bed significantly later and had a shorter sleep duration on school nights, compared with nonanxious children, whereas no significant differences in sleep onset latency, number of awakenings or time awake during the night, daytime sleepiness, or fatigue were found between the 2 groups.

School-aged children with anxiety disorder showed a different sleep pattern from their nonanxious peers only during the school week, mainly represented by a later bedtime and refusal to sleep alone, which could result in bedtime resistance [22]. Apart from the reduced nocturnal sleep duration during the school week, anxious children did not experience significantly different levels of daytime sleepiness from nonanxious children, probably because of the hyperarousal condition intrinsic to anxiety [25], which is able to override any excessive daytime sleepiness experienced by reduced nocturnal sleep [26].

Bedtime behaviours are influenced by anxiety in children: sleeping with the lights on, requiring a toy/object for sleep onset, sensitivity to noises, fear of the dark or of being alone, requiring bedtime rituals, nightmares, and crying during sleep are frequent [27].

A recent study examined sleep problems and presleep arousal among 52 anxious youth aged 7 to 14 years in relation to age, sex, ethnicity, and primary anxiety disorder, including GAD, SAD, SP, and OCD. It has been shown that 85% of parents of anxious children reported clinically significant child sleep problems with few differences based on their primary anxiety diagnosis. Although only 54% of anxious youth reported sleep problems, close to 90% with primary GAD endorsed trouble sleeping. Young children and Latino youth experience more sleep problems than older children and Caucasian youth, respectively. Moreover, anxious children had greater levels of cognitive than somatic arousal and pre-sleep cognitive arousal was associated with sleep onset problems and decreased total sleep duration [28].

The specific anxiety diagnosis is associated with different sleep problems: insomnia, refusal to sleep alone, and nightmares were more common in children with SAD and GAD than in children with social phobia [22].

Posttraumatic Stress Disorder

Children with PTSD show signs of disturbed sleep and poor sleep efficiency [29,30] and generally present recurrent nightmares, fearfulness at bedtime, avoidance of going to bed or staying in the dark alone [31], or parasomnias such as sleep terrors, sleep talking, and enuresis [32]. Different symptoms were described between the acute and chronic types of PTSD: If the trauma is recent, the predominant disturbances are related to the hyperarousal state, whereas, in chronic conditions, the symptoms are mainly related to sadness, numbing, disassociation, and even increased sleep [33].

Obsessive Compulsive Disorders

Sleep disturbances are present in more than 50% of children and adolescents with OCD and their co-occurrence usually characterizes the most severe forms.

Although sleep complaints in children and adolescents with OCD have not been studied systematically, Storch et al [34] reported that 92% of subjects with OCD experienced at least 1 sleep problem, and 27.3% experienced 5 or more of them. The total number of SRPs was positively and significantly correlated with the Children's Yale-Brown Obsessive Compulsive Scale, the Multidimensional Anxiety Scale for Children, and the Child Behavior Checklist (CBCL) internalizing and externalizing scores, but was not correlated with measures of depression or OCD-related functional impairment.

In agreement with Alfano et al [22], the most commonly reported SRPs were nightmares, being overtired, sleeping next to someone in the family, and parent and child reports of having trouble sleeping. Younger children had more nightmares and overall SRPs than older youth, but older youth were more frequently rated as sleeping more than other kids. Remarkably, the amount and severity of sleep problem were reduced following cognitive-behavioral treatment.

Polysomnographic Studies in Anxiety Disorders

Although there is strong evidence of a high prevalence of sleep disturbances in children with anxiety disorders, only few studies have investigated sleep characteristics in these children using objective measures such as polysomnography (PSG) or actigraphy.

Forbes et al [35] evaluated sleep parameters in anxious children compared with depressed and healthy children revealing more awakenings, longer sleep onset latencies, and decreased slow-wave sleep (SWS). Rapoport et al [36] reported significant sleep alterations in adolescents with OCD: compared with healthy controls, they revealed significantly reduced sleep efficiency, increased sleep onset latency, reduced NREM sleep, and decreased REM sleep latency [36]. This sleep pattern is similar to that seen in patients with depression, which suggests a possible link between these 2 disorders.

Another interesting finding is that sleep difficulties were generally underreported by this group, as compared with objective measures. Sadeh et al [30] used actigraphy to evaluate sleep patterns in children with a history of physical and sexual abuse. Lower sleep efficiency was found in abused children compared with nonabused controls. Another study that used actigraphic sleep assessment indicated similar findings with lower sleep efficiency, increased nocturnal activity, and longer sleep-onset latencies in abused children [29].

Treatment of AD and Sleep

Children with AD should be referred to a psychotherapist to treat their primary psychiatric disorder. Cognitive-behavioral therapy (CBT) has been shown to be an effective treatment option for school-age children and younger with GAD, SAD, OCD, and PTSD, and in many cases, a successful treatment of anxiety disorder results in improvement of sleep-related symptoms. In children, CBT can be integrated into a play therapy focused on the anxiety-provoking situations or thoughts [37]. Other types of therapeutic interventions such as systemic desensitization to fear with emotional imagery have been shown to be helpful in reducing the frequency and intensity of nighttime fears in children [38]. Pharmacologic interventions may be necessary in cases of more severe AD that do not react to nonpharmacologic interventions; more specifically, antidepressants, anxiolytics, and atypical antipsychotics have been successfully applied.

Mood Disorders

Depression occurs approximately in 1% of children and up to 8% of adolescents [39,40] and is classified into 3 main DSM-IV categories including MDD, dysthymic disorder (DD), and depressive disorder not otherwise specified.

Sleep problems associated with depressive disorders include insomnia (ie, difficulty falling and staying asleep) and/or hypersomnia (ie, excessive daytime sleepiness).

Sleep-onset and sleep-maintenance problems were common complaints reported in 66% of children with MDD, whereas 50% reported terminal insomnia; sleep problems follow the course of depressive symptoms with only 10% of patients showing insomnia after recovery from depression. After remission, children reported going to bed and falling asleep 30 minutes later than during their depression with a decreased sleep duration [41].

Different studies consistently reported insomnia in outpatients with DD ranging from 44% to 65% and hypersomnia ranging from 6% to 14% [42–44].

Sleep problems, again, act as modulating factors for the severity of the depressive disorder: MDD children with sleep problems were more severely depressed, had more depressive symptoms and comorbid anxiety disorders, and were more likely to have taken selective serotonin reuptake inhibitors (SSRIs) [44].

In adolescence, sleep complaints are the most prevalent symptoms of major depression and 88% of individuals who met diagnostic criteria for a major depressive episode reported sleep disturbances [45]. Sleep-onset and sleep maintenance insomnia are typical symptoms of children with depression, but also terminal insomnia has been reported, associated with endogenous depression [46].

In adolescents with a depressive disorder, sleep disturbances were the second most frequently reported symptoms of depression (89%) divided into insomnia (initial 55%; middle 39%; and terminal 21%) and hypersomnia (46%) [45,47]. Other studies showed that 12- to 18-year-old subjects reported rates of 45% for insomnia and 13% for hypersomnia [42] and 13- to 18-year-old outpatients with MDD complained of insomnia in 68% and of hypersomnia in 36% of cases [43].

Population-based studies also demonstrated that adolescents with poor sleep had more mild depression, more depressive symptoms, and lower self-esteem than "good sleepers" [48,49], with a higher prevalence in girls [50,51] and the presence of sleep problems was associated with an increased incidence of depressive symptoms (54%) and suicidal ideation (26%) and attempts (10%) [18].

Liu et al [44] reported in 500 children with MDD that 72.7% of them had sleep disturbance, and specifically 53.5% had insomnia alone, 9.0% had hypersomnia alone, and 10.1% had both disturbances; they also found that depressed girls were more likely to have sleep disturbance than boys (77.0% vs 69.2%), but age had no significant effects. Compared with children without sleep disturbances, sleep-disturbed children were more severely depressed and had more depressive symptoms and comorbidity anxiety disorders.

The comparison of sleep complaints in prepubertal children and adolescents with depression has shown that insomnia was similarly reported across age (74%), and hypersomnia was significantly more prevalent in adolescents (34%) than in children with major depression (16%) [52].

Hypersomnia is a less frequent complaint, ranging from 6% to 14% [41–44] in children and in 25% to 46% of adolescents [47,52].

In general, the presence of both insomnia and hypersomnia has a worse prognostic value: Children and adolescents with both complaints have more severe depression, anhedonia, weight loss, psychomotor retardation, and fatigue than those with either insomnia or hypersomnia alone. Moreover, the persistence of hypersomnia was consistently associated with depressed mood, anhedonia, psychomotor retardation, social withdrawal, fatigue, decreased appetite and weight, hopelessness, and helplessness [44]. An additional evidence for this association comes from an older study in 10- to 17-year-old schoolchildren, which reported that insomnia and hypersomnia were independently associated with depression and that this relationship was even stronger when both sleep problems were present [53].

Polysomnographic Studies in Depressive Disorders

Objective neurophysiological studies in adults with depression reported sleep abnormalities such as prolonged sleep latency, decreased REM latency, decreased SWS, and increased sleep fragmentation [54]. Despite the presence of sleep complaints in most of the youth with depression, several studies failed to show objective evidence of sleep disruption [41,55], whereas others provided evidence of sleep abnormalities such as shortened REM sleep latency [56–58] and longer sleep onset latency [59,60] in children with MDD compared with normal controls [61]. Another study showed that sleep alterations only in preadolescent and adolescent boys represented by an increa- sed stage-1 sleep, short REM latency, and reduced SWS during the first non-REM period, whereas the sleep of preadolescent and adolescent girls did not differ from that of healthy controls [62].

In 2008, 3 studies were published showing only minor differences in PSG parameters between children with DD and controls. It has been reported that 7- to 17-year-old subjects with MDD or anxiety disorders do not have differences in sleep parameters compared with healthy controls and the MDD group only exhibits less wakefulness after sleep onset than controls and less stage 1 sleep than anxiety or control group [35]. Consistent with the findings in adults Arana-Lechuga et al [63] found that children with depressive symptoms showed a significant reduction in REM sleep latency associated with an increase in sleep latency, REM sleep duration and number of awakenings. Finally, in 2008 Rao et al [64] correlated sleep EEG and hypothalamic-pituitary-adrenal changes during a depressive episode and during recovery in 15- to 17-year-old subjects with MDD and healthy controls. During the MDD episode, nocturnal urinary–free cortisol (NUFC) increased in parallel to REM density and sleep efficiency and to REM latency decrease; during recovery, NUFC concentration normalized, whereas EEG sleep disturbances did not change.

At the time of this review, a literature analysis revealed a total of 32 sleep PSG publications on depressed children and adolescents; showing only 2 main PSG differences from controls:

1. reduced REM-latency, which was present in 86%, 63%, and 44% of the child, adolescent, and mixed-age studies, respectively.
2. increased sleep latency in only 3%, 13%, and 6% of studies, respectively [19].

In conclusion, the most compelling evidence from the these studies in children and adolescents is that, despite the presence of subjectively reported sleep disturbances, very few PSG differences were found and paradoxically, youth subjectively reporting the greatest number of sleep problems showed better sleep in terms of the number of awakenings identified by EEG and objective disturbances [19]. This paradoxical finding might be explained by maturational factors and it is possible to hypothesize that children with MDD have normal sleep parameters because of the enhanced delta-sleep density and a more robust homeostatic drive [65] and disruption in sleep architecture may only appear in extremes of childhood depression [55] or if a genetic predisposition is present, as witnessed by evident family history of depression and sleep abnormalities [66]. It is possible that the most commonly used EEG measures are not sensitive enough to pick up sleep alterations induced by the depressive disorder.

EEG Spectral Analysis Studies in Depressive Disorders

Several studies used spectral analysis of sleep EEG to detect eventual abnormailities in sleep microstructure and frequency bands in depressed patients. Spectral EEG analysis in adults with MDD showed high beta activity and either a reduction in the amplitude or timing of delta activity during sleep [67–76].

In children and adolescents with MDD, few studies have so far been published. Because it has been suggested that a primary ultradian (80–120 minute) rhythm disturbance in EEG underlies sleep abnormalities in adults with depression, Armitage et al [77] evaluated ultradian rhythm disturbances in childhood and adolescent depression by investigating temporal coherence in quantitative EEG rhythms of 50 children/adolescents with major depression and 15 healthy normal controls (8–16 years old). Both depressed children and adolescents had decreased intrahemispheric coherence, whereas interhemispheric coherence was lower than controls only in depressed adolescents. Gender differences were evident in adolescents with MDD, but not children, with the lowest interhemispheric coherence in adolescent girls. These findings demonstrated that low temporal coherence in depression reflects a disruption in the fundamental basic rest-activity cycle of arousal and organization in the brain that is strongly influenced by gender.

The same research group [78] examined delta activity during non-REM sleep in adolescent females with MDD. Compared with healthy controls, the depressed group showed significantly lower delta amplitude and power in the first non-REM period. By contrast, standard sleep architecture did not differentiate between groups. These results are in contrast with the reports in adults with MDD, in whom delta abnormalities are more prevalent in men. The authors suggested that early emergence of delta abnormalities in depression may be of relevance to clinical course of illness.

Armitage et al [79] hypothesized that polysomnographic measures may be of predictive value in assessing the course of MDD illness and analyzed the temporal coherence of sleep EEG rhythms to predict recovery and recurrence in a 1-year naturalistic follow-up in 47 children and adolescents with MDD, aged 8 to 18 years. They found that standard sleep measures did not predict clinical course, whereas temporal coherence measures discriminated between those who recovered, recovered but recurred, and those who did not recover from the index episode: coherence between beta, theta and delta recorded in the right hemisphere was significantly lower in the no-recovery group. Coherence was also associated with time to recovery and recurrence, with the lowest coherence being less likely to recover or recur sooner. Finally, the relationship between coherence and clinical course was stronger in boys.

The same predictive finding of temporal coherence was found in a subsequent study [80] evaluating sleep electroencephalographic rhythms in 41 adolescent girls with a maternal history of depression (high risk) and 40 healthy controls (low risk). Temporal coherence was significantly lower among the high-risk girls than in controls and correctly classified 70% of the high-risk group with a false-positive rate of 5% among controls. Moreover, 54% of the high-risk girls were identified with extreme low coherence. At clinical follow-up, 14 girls showed depressive symptoms, 9 in the high-risk group (22.5%) and 5 controls (12.2%). The authors concluded that more abnormal the coherence, the greater the risk of a first episode of MDD within 2 years from sleep study, approximately 10 times greater than in controls.

A subsequent analysis of temporal coherence of ultradian sleep EEG rhythms involved a larger sample of 173 children and adolescents (8–17 years of age), including 97 who met criteria for MDD and were symptomatic but unmedicated at the time of the study and 76 healthy controls. The study corroborated the previous findings showing a lower temporal coherence in adolescents with MDD (more pronounced in girls), compared with healthy controls, and demonstrating that early onset depression is associated with a reduction in synchronization of sleep EEG rhythms that shows a differential maturational course in boys and girls [81].

A recent research evaluated the combined effects of depression and body mass index (BMI) on polysomnographic parameters in 104 children with MDD, compared with 32 healthy controls. In the MDD group only, higher BMI was significantly correlated with decreased sleep efficiency, decreased percentage of REM, and higher percentage of time spent awake and moving (TSPAM). Healthy control and MDD groups with higher BMI had increases and decreases in REM sleep, respectively, and TSPAM increased in the high-weight MDD group, but decreased in the high-weight HC group [82].

Actigraphic Studies in Depressive Disorders

The first actigraphic study by Sadeh et al [30] found that wake time after sleep onset was associated with ratings of depression, hopelessness, and low self-esteem; shorter sleep periods with depression; longer-sleep onset time with hopelessness; and less time spent in quiet sleep with lower self-esteem. A subsequent study failed to confirm these results [29] and another study found that longer sleep latency was associated with teacher-reported but not with parent-reported internalizing problems [83]. Teicher et al [84] demonstrated an abnormal circadian rhythm in depressed children with diurnal variation of activity level that did not peak until early evening. Aronen et al [83] showed that children with shorter duration of sleep had teacher-reported externalizing and internalizing behaviors, but no relationship existed between parental reports of depressive symptoms and sleep latency.

Effects of Treatment of Depression and Sleep

The treatment of depression with drugs in children and adolescents affects both sleep and psychiatric symptoms. In cases of severe depression, the therapeutic approach includes a trial of CBT with or without the use of an antidepressant [85]. The effects of different antidepressants on sleep have been studied; the administration of imipramine showed a decrease of REM sleep and of sleep stage 4 and an increase in sleep stage 2 [86,87]. The only study on fluoxetine in childhood depression showed an increase of sleep stage 1, number of arousals, and periodic limb movements [88]. Lofthouse et al [89] recently revealed that the combination of fluoxetine and CBT showed better efficacy than the CBT treatment alone.

Although limited research has been conducted in this area for youth, one commonly used approach is to treat depression and insomnia concurrently [37]. Studies in the adult population showed that treatment of insomnia is necessary for the remission of depressive symptoms [90]. Therefore sleep hygiene and CBT are recommended first-line treatments also for primary insomnia in youth with MDD [91], before turning to pharmacologic interventions [37].

Pediatric Bipolar Disorders

The predominant features of the pediatric bipolar disorder (PBD) are elation, grandiosity, flight of ideas or racing thoughts, decreased need for sleep, and hypersexuality during manic states, severe irritability and high levels of hyperactivity [92]. PBD is a severe and chronic disorder that, although rare in childhood has a particularly severe course, including high frequency of suicide attempts and comorbidity, especially sleep disturbances, that may be considered to be early markers for PBD, distinguishing features of PBD and contributors to relapse [93].

Numerous studies have reported decreased need for sleep associated with DSM-IV pediatric mania [94,95]; but only 5 publications have examined pediatric bipolar sleep per se [96–99]. In addition to decreased need for sleep, pediatric bipolar spectrum subjects are reported to exhibit "insomnia" [96] and "initial insomnia" [97] or difficulty in initiating sleep [98].

A small number of studies have examined the sleep characteristics of pediatric bipolar depression [97,99]. Parker et al [100] reported that depressed bipolar patients under age 25 (presumably including a number of older adolescents) exhibit a very high prevalence of hypersomnia, manifested in part by difficulty awakening in the morning.

Subjective Reports of Sleep in PBD

A 2005 review of 6 studies on PBD found a weighted average of 72% of subjects reporting decreased need for sleep [95]; the prevalence values reported ranged from 43% in a 2004 community-based sample of 7- to 16- year-olds with BP-I [101], to 61% in a 1995 community-based prospective study of 14- to 18-year-olds with BP-I, BP-II, or cyclothymia [102], to 67% in 21-year-old patients with BP-I [103], to 72% in 5- to 17-year-old outpatients with BP-I [104], to 76% in 6- to 17-year-old outpatients with BPI and BP-II [105], and to 95% in 3- to 17-year-old outpatients with BP-I, BP-II, or cyclothymia [96].

The reduced need for sleep was used to differentiate 7- to 16-year-old subjects with BP-I from those with ADHD and controls (rates of 40%, 6%, and 1%, respectively) [94].

Lofthouse et al [97] reported that 96.2% of children suffered from sleep problems related to manic, depressive, or comorbid symptoms, with 82% having depressive-related and 58% having manic-related sleep problems. Initial insomnia was the most pervasive problem, followed by middle insomnia, then terminal insomnia. Another support of the high comorbidity of sleep problems with BPD came from a large exploratory Web-based survey completed by parents of 4- to 12-year-old children with BPD: nearly all (99%) parents identified mood-related sleep problems during their child's current, worst, or other mood periods. Sleep difficulties were most commonly reported in mixed (89%), manic-only (56%), and depressive-only (31%) states. Sleep problems included daytime sleepiness (99%), parasomnias (97%), nighttime awakenings (96%), bedtime resistance (94%), anxiety (91%), sleep duration (90%), sleep onset delay (87%), and sleep disordered breathing (47%) [106].

In a study aimed at determining whether the frequency and severity of sleep problems were greater in children of mothers with a diagnosis of unipolar and bipolar affective illness than in children of control mothers, Stoleru et al [107] found that sleep problems, as assessed by the CBCL, were more frequent and severe in children of effectively ill mothers. In younger siblings, the persistence of sleep problems was more frequent in children of affectively ill mothers.

Staton et al [108] studied 130 outpatient pediatric bipolar subjects (aged 3–17 years) and observed that: (1) 85.4% displayed disturbed sleep, typically evening acceleration and significant delay of sleep onset, with or without decreased need for sleep; (2) most subjects had difficulty awakening; and (3) decreased need for sleep was most prevalent among subjects who exhibited days-long manic cycles (pediatric bipolar type I) or chronic mania (pediatric bipolar type IIIA).

Another study used subjective (self-ratings) and objective (actigraph) assessments to compare 13- to 19-year-old offspring of BP parents and adolescents of healthy controls: children of bipolar parents did reveal higher rates of subjective sleep disturbance but actigraphic sleep data seemed to indicate that they went to sleep more quickly, with a trend towards longer sleep and a better sleep continuity [109].

A recent research paper analyzed the evolution of psychopathology in offspring of bipolar parents showing that high-risk offspring manifest higher rates of anxiety and sleep disorders, as well as major mood and substance use disorders, compared with controls [110].

Polysomnographic and Actigraphic Studies in PBD

Few and controversial studies focused on the polysomnographic characteristics of children with PBD. Rao et al [99] reported increased sleep stage 1 and reduced sleep stage 4 in PBD children; persons with depression and unipolar course showed reduced REM latency, higher REM density, and increased REM sleep (specifically in the early part of the night), whereas adolescents with depression who converted to bipolar disorder and controls who remained free from psychopathology at follow-up showed a normal REM sleep profile.

To determine if the children with PBD exhibited alterations in their sleep characteristics, Mehl et al [98] compared PSG findings and results of a parent-report sleep questionnaire for a group of 6- to 7-year-old children with a PBD profile with those of a matched group of controls. Results of the PSG analysis indicated significant differences for the PBD profile group with less efficient sleep, less percentage time in REM sleep, and more time in sleep stage 3 than the comparison group. The PBD profile group also displayed a trend toward more numerous awakenings after sleep onset than the comparison group. The analysis of the parent-report data indicated that the PBD profile group had significantly more remembered and unremembered nightmares, significantly more difficulties initiating sleep, and significantly more morning headaches.

Only 2 actigraphic studies have been conducted in children with PBD; Faedda et al [96] obtained 5- to 7-day actigraphic recordings in bipolar children and observed increased sleep latency, decreased sleep continuity and efficiency, and variable duration of total sleep time.

Finally, Faedda and Teicher [111] described a 6-year-old bipolar girl with an actigraphy-demonstrated circadian phase delay of 2.5 hour.

Treatment of PBD and Sleep

Pharmacological treatment of PBD in children showed a parallel improvement of manic symptoms and sleep disturbances: the drugs used were olanzapine or risperidone that determined mainly asignificant reduction in decreased need for sleep and a better sleep continuity [112,113].

A recent Web-based parent survey to explore the use of pharmacologic and nonpharmacologic interventions for 4- to 12-year-old children with PBD showed that most parents (95%) reported seeing at least 1 medical, mental health, or school professional for their child's sleep problems [89]. Over half of the parents (60%) reported various medications or supplements worsened sleep problems, whereas 87% reported that non-pharmacologic treatments were helpful in alleviating sleep problems (identifying maintaining a sleep routine with a set bedtime, a nightlight/cuddly toy/blanket or staying with their child until the child fell asleep) [19].

Based on the published clinical, polysomnographic, or actigraphic studies, Staton [108] hypothesized that the core defect of pediatric bipolar sleep is represented by a significant delay of the circadian sleep-wake cycle, a form of the delayed sleep-phase syndrome. Children and adolescents with part-day manic cycles and chronic mixed conditions typically will manifest delayed sleep onset, but not decreased need for sleep. Pediatric individuals with days-long manic cycles or chronic mania typically will manifest decreased need for sleep, produced by interaction between the sleep-onset phase delay and bedtime and early morning manic psychomotor acceleration. The sleep-onset phase delay, when expressed, is hypothesized to be a trait marker of bipolar spectrum illness.

Sleep Disturbances and Suicide

Sleep disturbances have been linked to an increased risk of attempted or ideation of suicide as revealed by several studies. Choquet and Menke [50] found that adolescents with suicidal ideation reported more insomnia as well as more nightmares than adolescents who denied suicidal ideation. In a following study, Choquet et al [114] confirmed that suicidal ideation was linked to more sleep difficulties and frequent feelings of daytime tiredness. Similarly, Vignau et al [115] in an epidemiological study found that "poor sleepers" experienced more suicidal ideation and attempts than "good sleepers." Regarding suicide attempt, Tishler et al [116] reported that 81% of adolescents presenting to the emergency room following a suicide attempt, presented difficulty falling asleep or early morning waking immediately before the attempt. In a recent study, Liu [117] reported that insomnia (16.9%) and nightmares (48.9%) were associated with increased risk for suicidal ideation and attempt. Furthermore, those who slept less than 8 hour per night were 3 times more likely to attempt suicide, even after adjusting for overall depressive symptoms. Insomnia also emerged as a significant predictor of attempted suicide in this sample but was no longer significant when accounting for depressive severity. These results confirm the association between sleep disturbance, poor sleep quality, and suicidal behavior and highlight the potential role of sleep intervention in the prevention of adolescence suicide. Goldstein et al [118] recently examined sleep difficulties preceding death in a sample of adolescent suicide completers in comparison to control adolescents. They found that suicide completers had higher rates of overall sleep disturbance (31% vs 4%), insomnia (30% vs 3%), and hypersomnia (15% vs 1%) than controls within the preceding week. Only a small percentage of the sample exhibited changes in sleep symptom severity in the week preceding the suicide attempt, but of these, a higher proportion were completers. These findings support a significant and temporal relationship between sleep problems and completed suicide in adolescents; therefore sleep difficulties should be carefully considered in prevention and intervention efforts for adolescents at risk for suicide.

Sleep in Eating Disorders

Anorexia is the most serious eating disorders in terms of morbidity and mortality. Generally, eating disorders onset is during adolescence, with 85% of eating disorders starting before 20 years of age [119]. Although eating disorders begin mainly during adolescence, only few studies have evaluated sleep architecture in adolescents with these problems.

Delvenne et al [120], in a first attempt to evaluate sleep architecture in adolescents with eating disorders, compared anorectic girls with depressed and healthy youth. They found that anorectic differed from depressed patients in a greater number of awakenings. In respect to controls, anorectic adolescents showed lower sleep efficiency, longer awakenings and decreased REM sleep. Subsequently, they divided anorectic patients in restricting and bulimic subtypes, showing that bulimic anorectics had an increase in sleep stage 3 in respect to restricting; furthermore, sleep EEG variables were not significantly correlated to BMI.

Nobili et al [121] in a successive study confirmed a reduction of sleep efficiency and an increased number of awakenings; in addiction they performed power spectral analysis that revealed a significant reduction of slow-wave activity (SWA; 0.5–4.5 Hz) in all NREM-REM cycles of sleep and found a positive correlation between BMI and amount of SWA.

Subsequently the same group of resear-chers tried to assess if the reduced SWA is the result of increased sleep fragmentation or if it is dependent on an intrinsic weakness of the SWA producing mechanisms [122]. They found no relationship between the reduction of SWA and duration of disorder, whereas there is a relationship between SWA decrease and BMI. They conclude that SWA reduction is independent of the increased sleep fragmentation and probably is related to the primary pathophysiologic characteristics of anorexia.

Sleep in Psychosis

Most studies on sleep in psychotic disorders focus on adults and data available for children or adolescents are essentially retrospective in nature. To our knowledge, there is only 1 study that examined sleep in childhood onset-schizophrenia (COS) [123]. The majority of COS subjects suffered from clear sleep disturbances: the average duration of sleep for COS good sleepers was 7.44 hour and that for COS poor sleepers was 4.10 hour. A poor average sleep score was associated with an increased severity of psychotic symptoms on admission and during the medication washout period.

Few recent studies dealt with sleep in children or adolescents with schizophrenia or bipolar disorder, but sleep disturbances are part of the prodromal syndrome and precede the development of psychosis in more than two-thirds of cases [124,125].

Sleep onset and maintenance insomnia is a feature of schizophrenic subjects regardless of their medication status or the phase of the disorder: Objective sleep measures show decreased duration of SWS and reduced REM latency, whereas REM duration remains unchanged. The presence of insomnia in schizophrenic patients may be related to a putative mesolimbic dopaminergic overactivity and to the reduced GABA concentrations that were found in postmortem human brain studies [126].

Sleep disturbances were found to constitute a significant predictor of psychotic evolution in a study of 245 adolescents and young adults of the European Prediction of Psychosis Study who were at putative high risk for transition to psychosis, if entered in a predictive model along with positive symptoms, bizarre thinking, sleep disturbances, presence of schizotypal disorder, level of functioning in the last 12 months, and years of education [127].

Drugs for Psychiatric Disorders and Sleep

Few studies focused on the effects of drugs for psychiatric conditions on sleep of children and adolescents; thus, most data are derived from adult studies. The drugs commonly used for psychiatric disorders exert specific effects on sleep behavior and sleep architecture (Table 10.1). We concisely summarize the effects on sleep patterns and parameters of the most commonly used substances, either in adults or in children and adolescents [128].

Tricyclic Antidepressants

The main action of tricyclic antidepressants (TCAs) in their therapeutic effects is consid-ered to be the blockade of the presynaptic reuptake of norepinephrine (NE) and serotonin (5-HT). It is held that the noradrenergic effect of TCAs determines an increase of sleep latency, awakenings, and arousals and a reduction in total sleep time [129], whereas the serotoninergic effect of some TCAs (eg, chlomipramine, amitriptyline and doxepin) induces sleep and daytime somnolence [130–132], as well as the REM-suppressive effect. However, REM sleep latency, which is abnormally short in depressive disorders, is increased by most antidepressants, along with REM suppression, and this has been linked with their therapeutic action. The most potent drug in this respect is clomipramine. All TCA

Table 10.1 Effects on sleep parameters of the drugs commonly used for psychiatric disorders

First author, year [Ref.]	Drug Antidepressants	Effects on sleep
	TCAs	
Hajak et al, 2001 [135]:	Doxepin	↑ SE, ↑ TST, ↓ WASO
Riemaann et al, 2002 [160]	Trimipramine	↑ SE
Lacey et al, 1977 [161]	Clomipramine	↓ REM
Volkers et al, 2002 [162]	Imipramine	↑ Fragmentation of motor activity during sleep
	SSRIs	
Mendels et al, 1999 [163]	Citalopram	No effect on sleep
Vasar et al, 1994 [164]; Gillin et al, 1997 [139]	Fluoxetine	↑ SL, ↓ SE, ↑REML, ↓ REM, ↑ S2, ↑ S3, ↑ WASO
Nowell et al, 1999 [148]:		↓ SL, ↑ TST, ↓ WASO;
Sharpley et al, 1996 [147]	Paroxetine	↓ REM, ↑ REML and WASO, ↓ TST and SE
Silvestri et al, 2001 [165]	Paroxetine	↓ REM, ↑ REML; REM sleep suppressed
	Serotonin receptor/transporter inhibitors	
Sharpley et al, 1996 [147]; Gillin et al, 1997 [139]	Nefazodone	No effect on sleep
Walsh et al, 1998 [166]	Trazodone	↓ SL, ↑ TST, ↓ WASO
	NaSSAs	
Winokur et al, 2000 [148]; Winokur et al, 2003 [149]	Mirtazapine	↓ SL, ↑ TST
	Mood stabilizers	
Campbell et al, 1989 [149]; Hudson et al, 1989 [150]	Lithium	↑ REML, ↓ REM
	Antipsychotics	
	Classical	
Kaplan et al, 1974 [167]	Chlorpromazine	↑ S2, ↑ SWS, ↑ REML
Maixner et al, 1998 [168]	Haloperidol	↓ SL, ↑ TST, ↓WASO, ↑ REML
Gillin et al, 1997 [169]	Pimozide	↑ TST, ↑ SE
Brannen and Jewett, 1969 [170]	Promethazine	↑ TST, ↓ REM
	Atypical	
Lee et al, 2001 [171]	Clozapine	↑ TST, ↑ SE
Salin Pascual et al, 2004 [172]	Olanzapine	↓ SL, ↑ TST, ↑ SWS
Luthirnger et al, 2007 [173]	Paliperidone	↓ SL, ↑ TST, ↑ SE, ↑ S2, ↑ REM
Tandon, 1997 [174]	Risperidone	↓ SL

Abbreviations: REM, rapid eye movement; REML, REM latency; S2, stage 2 NREM; S3, stage 3 NREM; SE, sleep efficiency; SL, sleep latency; SWS, slow-wave sleep; TST, total sleep time; WASO, wake after sleep onset; TCAs, tricyclic antidepressants; SSRIs, selective serotonin reuptake inhibitors; NaSSAs, noradrenergic and specific serotonergic antidepressants.

effects and REM suppression are also mediated by the blockade of other neurotransmitter receptors, including histamine H1 and alpha1 adrenergic and muscarinic cholinergic receptors [133,134].

Specific studies on single drugs showed that doxepin improves quality of sleep and daytime alertness, as well as sleep efficiency, total sleep time, and amount of wakefulness after sleep onset [135], whereas trimipramine showed no effects on sleep latency or on the number of wake periods [136]. Rebound insomnia and tolerance were reported in the short-term.

Selective Serotonin Reuptake Inhibitors

The main action of the SSRIs consists in the inhibition of the serotonin transporter; this action ensues in the increase of the content of intrasynaptic serotonin. In sleep-related brain areas this may result in various effects on sleep according to the different 5-HT receptor subtypes present in these areas: (a) 5-HT1A receptor agonists produce a decrease in REM sleep as well as an increase in wakefulness; (b) agonists at the 5-HT1D receptor inhibit REM sleep and increase wakefulness; (c) 5-HT2 receptor agonists inhibit SWS; (d) 5-HT2 antagonists markedly increase SWS; and (e) 5-HT3 receptor agonists reduce both REM sleep and SWS [137–140].

Specifically, most SSRIs tend to disrupt normal sleep, but they are all endowed with REM suppression and REM latency increase, which are effects common also to TCAs [141].

Fluoxetine determines lengthening of sleep onset latency and/or disruption of sleep continuity measures, including increases in wake time after sleep onset and number of awakenings or arousals, and a decrease in total sleep time with suppression of REM sleep [142,143]. Paroxetine improves sleep continuity and suppresses REM sleep in depressed patients and determines an increase of sleep onset latency, but improves wake time after sleep onset and total sleep time [144,145]. The studies on sertraline, citalopram, or escitalopram showed that these substances have fewer effects in disrupting sleep continuity.

Other Second-Generation Antidepressant Drugs

Trazodone exerts inhibitory effects on 5-HT1A, 5-HT2A/2C, alpha1 and 2 adrenoceptors, and histamine H1 receptors and moderately inhibits the serotonin transporter, contributing to sleep promotion [137]. Nefazodone, another phenylpiperazine chemically related to trazodone, does not seem to have specific effects on sleep parameters and especially on REM sleep [146]. Bupropion increases REM sleep, probably because of its selective action in blocking presynaptic reuptake of the catecholamines dopamine (DA) and NE [147]. Mirtazapine, a noradrenaline-specific serotonin antagonist chemically related to mianserin, has been reported to produce pronounced improvement in both sleep latency and total sleep time, probably related to the blockade of 5-HT2 receptors and, possibly, of 5-HT3 receptors and histamine H1 receptors [148,149].

Lithium

Lithium is a mood-stabilizing agent with some antidepressant properties and is used mainly in patients with bipolar disorder. It induces a decrease of REM latency, as well as a global reduction of REM duration [150,151]

Monoamine Oxidase Inhibitors

Monoamine oxidase (MAO) inhibitors enhance monoamine neurotransmission by increasing presynaptic concentrations of NE, DA, and 5-HT following inhibition of the enzyme MAO and disrupt sleep continuity, most likely secondary to its pronounced catecholaminergic stimulation [152].

Antipsychotic Drugs

All antipsychotic drugs determine potent inhibition of DA D2, D1, and D4 receptors, and also inhibition of 5-HT2, alpha-1 adrenergic, histamine H-1, and muscarinic cholinergic receptors [153,154], all inducing sedation and sleep. The 5-HT2 receptor blockade may be responsible for the beneficial effects on sleep patterns, including increased sleep efficiency and total sleep time, decreased awakenings and wake time, and increased SWS.

Typical neuroleptics such as the phenothiazines (eg, chlorpromazine, promazine, mesoridazine, and thioridazine) or the dibenzoazepines (eg, clotiapine and loxapine) exert important effects on sleep; their sleep-inducing effect is often used to induce sedation and sleep in agitated patients. Another class of typical neuroleptics, the butyrophenones (eg, haloperidol, and droperidol), do not disrupt sleep architecture, whereas the atypical antipsychotics (clozapine, olanzapine, quetiapine, risperidone, ziprasidone, and paliperidone) demonstrate a positive effect on sleep continuity, with an increase in total sleep time or sleep efficiency, and individually varying effects on other sleep parameters, such as an increase in REM latency observed for olanzepine, quetiapine, and ziprasidone, and an increase in SWS documented for olanzepine and ziprasidone in healthy subjects [155].

Olanzapine and clozapine have high affinities for the histamine H1 receptor that is responsible for the clinically observed sedation [128]; they also have similar effects on PSG sleep parameters: reduced sleep latency, decreased wake time after sleep onset and increased total sleep time, stage 2 sleep, and SWS [156,157]. Risperidone has low affinity for the H1 receptor and determines only mild clinical sedation but induces great improvement in sleep maintenance and number of awakenings, and an increase in stage 3 sleep [158]. Ritanserin, a 5-HT2 receptor antagonist that has not shown clear-cut antipsychotic properties and has not been developed as an antipsychotic, has been shown to increase SWS in healthy subjects [159].

In summary, atypical antipsychotics exert sleep-inducing effects, with a prolongation of total sleep time and an increase of sleep efficiency, in healthy subjects and schizophrenic patients, with the exception of risperidone, which lacks this effect. The influence on sleep stages 1 and 2 appears to be variable, whereas, olanzapine and ziprasidone demonstrate SWS-increasing properties and clozapine demonstrates SWS-decreasing properties [155].

Conclusions

The literature on sleep in children with psychiatric disorders is scarce and relatively little is known about the association between regulation of sleep, emotion, and behavior during early development. Available data suggest that child and adolescent psychiatric disorders are associated with sleep problems and early sleep disruption is considered to be a negative prognostic indicator for emotion and behavioral problems in adolescence and adulthood; moreover, there is a strong link between sleep alterations and psychosis and between suicidality and insomnia.

The bidirectional connection between sleep and emotional and behavioral functioning provides explanations as to why the treatment of psychiatric disturbances improves sleep and why sleep normalization is determinant for reducing the risk of relapse of psychiatric symptoms.

Both psychiatrists and sleep clinicians should always be aware of this strict linkage to improve the treatment and prognosis of psychiatric disturbances during development.

References

1. Gregory AM, Eley TC, O'Conner TG, Plomin R. Etiologies of associations between childhood sleep and behavioral problems in a large twin sample. *J Am Acad Child Adolesc Psychiatry.* 2004;43:744–751.
2. Gregory AM, O'Connor TG. Sleep problems in childhood: a longitudinal study of developmental change and association with behavioral problems. *J Am Acad Child Adolesc Psychiatry.* 2002;41:964–971.
3. Johnson EO, Chilcoat HD, Breslau N. Trouble sleeping and anxiety/depression in childhood. *Psychiatry Res.* 2000;94:93–102.
4. Ong SH, Wickramaratne P, Tang M, Weissman MM. Early childhood sleep and eating problems as predictors of adolescent and adult mood and anxiety disorders. *J Affect Disord.* 2006;96:1–8.
5. Dinges DF, Pack F, Williams K, et al. Cumulative sleepiness, mood disturbance and psychomotor vigilance performance decrements during a week of sleep restricted to 4–5 hours per night. *Sleep.* 1997;20:267–277.
6. Leotta C, Carskadon MA, Acebo C, et al. Effects of acute sleep restriction on affective response in adolescents: preliminary results. *Sleep Res.* 1997;26:201.
7. Sagaspe P, Sanchez-Ortuno M, Charles A, et al. Effects of sleep deprivation on color-word, emotional, and specific stroop interference and on self-reported anxiety. *Brain Cogn.* 2006;60:76–87.
8. Ivanenko A, Barnes ME, Crabtree VM, Gozal D. Psychiatric symptoms in children with insomnia referred to a pediatric sleep medicine center. *Sleep Med.* 2004;5:253–259.
9. Guidetti V, Galli F, Fabrizi P, et al. Headache and psychiatric comorbidity: clinical aspects and outcome in an 8-year follow-up study. *Cephalalgia.* 1998;18:455–462.
10. Dahl RE. The regulation of sleep and arousal: development and psychopathology. *Dev Psychopathol.* 1996;8:3–27.
11. Alfano CA, Zakem AH, Costa NM, Taylor LK, Weems, CF. Sleep problems and their relation to cognitive factors, anxiety, and depressive symptoms in children and adolescents. *Depress Anxiety.* 2009;26:503–512.
12. Ivanenko A, Crabtree VM, Gozal D. Sleep in children with psychiatric disorders. *Pediatr Clin North Am.* 2004;51:51–68.
13. Gregory AM, Caspi A, Eley TC, Moffitt TE, Oconnor TG, Poulton R. Prospective longitudinal associations between persistent sleep problems

in childhood and anxiety and depression disorders in adulthood. *J Abnorm Child Psychol.* 2005;33:157–163.
14. Riemann D, Voderholzer U. Primary insomnia: a risk factor to develop depression? *J Affect Disord.* 2003;76:255–259.
15. Saarenpaa-Heikkila O, Laippala P, Koivikko M. Subjective daytime sleepiness and its predictors in Finnish adolescents in an interview study. *Acta Paediatr.* 2001;90: 552–557.
16. Roberts RE, Roberts CR, Chen IG. Impact of insomnia on future functioning of adolescents. *J Psychosom Res.* 2002;53:561–569.
17. Gregory AM, Rijsdijk FV, Lau JYF, Dahl RE, Eley TC. The direction of longitudinal associations between sleep problems and depression symptoms: a study of twins aged 8 and 10 years. *Sleep.* 2009;32:189–199.
18. Roane BM, Taylor DJ. Adolescent insomnia as a risk factor for early adult depression and substance abuse. *Sleep.* 2008;31: 1351–1356.
19. Lofthouse N, Gilchrist R, Splaingard M. Mood-related Sleep Problems in Children and Adolescents. *Child Adolesc Psychiatric Clin N Am.* 2009;18:893–916.
20. Costello EJ, Egger H, Angold A. 10-year research update review: the epidemiology of child and adolescent psychiatric disorders: I. Methods and public health burden. *J Am Acad Child Adolesc Psychiatry.* 2005;44:972–986.
21. *Diagnostic and Statistical Manual of Mental Disorders.* 4th ed. Washington, DC: American Psychiatric Association; 2000.
22. Alfano CA, Ginsburg GS, Kingery J. Sleep-related problems among children and adolescents with anxiety disorders. *J Am Acad Child Adolesc Psychiatry.* 2007;46:224–232.
23. Alfano CA, Beidel DC, Turner SM, Lewin DS. Preliminary evidence for sleep complaints among children referred for anxiety. *Sleep Med.* 2006;7:467–473.
24. Gau SF, Soong WT. Psychiatric comorbidity of adolescents with sleep terrors or sleepwalking: a case-control study. *Aust N Z J Psychiatry.* 1999;33:734–739.
25. Hossain JL, Ahmad P, Reinish LW, Kayumov L, Hossain NK, Shapiro CM. Subjective fatigue and subjective sleepiness: two independent consequences of sleep disorders? *J Sleep Res.* 2005;14:245–253.
26. Hudson JL, Gradisar M, Gamble A, Schniering CA, Rebelo I. The sleep patterns and problems of clinically anxious children. *Behaviour Res Ther.* 2009;47:339–344.
27. Ivanenko A, Crabtree VM, O'Brien LM, Gozal D. Sleep complaints and psychiatric symptoms in children evaluated at the pediatric mental health clinic. *J Clin Sleep Med.* 2006;2:42–48.
28. Alfano CA, Pina AA, Zerr AA, Villalta IK. Presleep arousal and sleep problems of anxiety-disordered youth. *Child Psychiatry Hum Dev.* 2010;41:156–167.
29. Glod CA, Teicher MH, Hartman CR, Harakal T. Increased nocturnal activity and impaired sleep maintenance in abused children. *J Am Acad Child Adolesc Psychiatry.* 1997;36:1236–1243.
30. Sadeh A, McGuire JP, Sachs H, et al. Sleep and psychological characteristics of children on a psychiatric inpatient unit. *J Am Acad Child Adolesc Psychiatry.* 1995;34:813–819.
31. Sadeh A. Stress, trauma and sleep in children. *Child Adolesc Clin North Am.* 1996;5:685–700.
32. Kravitz M, McCoy BJ, Tompkins DM, et al. Sleep disorders in children after burn injury. *J Burn Care Rehabil.* 1993;14:83–90.
33. Famularo R, Fenton T, Augustyn M, Zuckerman B. Persistence of pediatric postrtraumatic stress after two years. *Child Abuse Negl.* 1996;20:1245–1248.
34. Storch EA, Murphy TK, Lack CW, et al. Sleep-related problems in pediatric obsessive compulsive disorder. *J Anxiety Dis.* 2008;22:877–885.
35. Forbes EE, Bertocci MA, Gregory AM, et al. Objective sleep in pediatric anxiety disorders and major depressive disorder. *J Am Acad Child Adolesc Psychiatry.* 2008;47:148–155.
36. Rapoport J, Elkins R, Langer DH, et al. Childhood obsessive-compulsive disorder. *Am J Psychiatry.* 1981;138:1545–1554.
37. Ivanenko A, Johnson K. Sleep disturbances in children with psychiatric disorders. *Semin Pediatr Neurol.* 2008;15:70–78.
38. Ollendick TH, Hagopian LP, Huntzinger RM. Cognitive-behavior therapy with nighttime fearful children. *J Behav Ther Exp Psychiatry.* 1991;22:113–121.
39. Birmaher B, Ryan ND, Williamson DE, et al. Childhood and adolescent depression: a review of the past 10 years. Part I. *J Am Acad Child Adolesc Psychiatry.* 1996;35:1427–1439.
40. Lewinsohn PM, Hops H, Roberts RE, Seeley JR, Andrews JA. Adolescent psychopathology I: prevalence and incidence of depression and other DSM-III-R disorders in high school students. *J Abnorm Psychol.* 1993;102:133–144.
41. Puig-Antich J, Goetz R, Hanlon C, et al. Sleep architecture and REM sleep measures in prepubertal children with major depression: a controlled study. *Arch Gen Psychiatry.* 1982;39:932–939.
42. Masi G, Millepiedi S, Mucci M, Pascale RR, Perugi G, Akiskal HS. Phenomenology and comorbidity of dysthymic disorder in 100 consecutively referred child and adolescents: beyond DSMIV. *Can J Psychiatry.* 2003;48:99–105.
43. Yorbik O, Birmaher B, Axelson D, Williamson DE, Ryan ND. Clinical characteristics of depressive symptoms in children and adolescents with major depressive disorder. *J Clin Psychiatry.* 2004;65:1654–1659.
44. Liu X, Buysse DJ, Gentzler AL, et al. Insomnia and hypersomnia associated with depressive phenomenology and comorbidity in childhood depression. *Sleep.* 2007;30:83–90.
45. Roberts RE, Lewinsohn PM, Seeley JR. Symptoms of DSM-III-R major depression in adolescence: evidence from an epidemiological survey. *J Am Acad Child Adolesc Psychiatry.* 1995;34: 1608–1617.

46. Puig-Antich J, Goetz R, Hanlon C, Tabrizi MA, Davies M, Weitzman ED. Sleep architecture and REM sleep measures in prepubertal children with major depression: studies during recovery from the depressive episode in a drug-free state. *Arch Gen Psychiatry*. 1983;40:187–192.
47. Morrison DN, McGee R, Stanton WR. Sleep problems in adolescence. *J Am Acad Child Adolesc Psychiatry.* 1992;31:94–99.
48. Price VA, Coates TJ, Thoresen CE, Grinstead OA. Prevalence and correlates of poor sleep among adolescents. *Am J Dis Child*. 1978;132:583–586.
49. Kirmil-Gray K, Eagleston JR, Gibson E. Sleep disturbance in adolescents: sleep quality, sleep habits, beliefs about sleep, and daytime functioning. *J Youth Adolesc*. 1984;13:375–384.
50. Choquet M, Menke H. Development of self-perceived risk behavior and psychosomatic symptoms in adolescents: a longitudinal approach. *J Adolesc*. 1987;10:291–308.
51. Manni R, Ratti MT, Marchioni E, et al. Poor sleep in adolescents: a study of 869 17-year-old Italian secondary school students. *J Sleep Res*. 1997;6:44–49.
52. Ryan ND, Puig-Antich J, Ambrosini P, et al. The clinical picture of major depression in children and adolescents. *Arch Gen Psychiatry.* 1987;44:854–861.
53. Roberts RE, Roberts CR, Chen IG. Functioning of adolescents with symptoms of disturbed sleep. *J Youth Adolesc*. 2001;30:1–18.
54. Benca RM. Mood disorders. In: Kryger MH, Roth T, Dement WC, eds. *Principles and Practice of Sleep Medicine*. 3rd ed. Philadelphia, PA: WB Saunders; 2000:1140–1157.
55. Dahl RE, Pelham WE, Wierson M. The role of sleep disturbances in attention deficit disorder symptoms: a case study. *J Pediatr Psychol.* 1991;16:229–239.
56. Kane J, Coble P, Conners CK, Kupfer DJ. EEG sleep in a child with severe depression. *Am J Psychiatry.* 1977;134:813–814.
57. Dahl RE, Ryan ND, Birmaher B, et al. Electroencephalographic sleep measures in prepubertal depression. *Psychiatry Res*. 1991;38: 201–214.
58. Young W, Knowles JB, MacLean AW, Boag L, McConville BJ. The sleep of childhood depressives: comparison with age-matched controls. *Biol Psychiatry.* 1982;17:1163–1168.
59. Emslie GJ, Rush AJ, Weinberg WA, Rintelmann JW, Roffwarg HP. Children with major depression show reduced rapid eye movement latencies. *Arch Gen Psychiatry.* 1990;47:119–124.
60. Lahmeyer HW, Poznanski EO, Bellu SN. EEG sleep in depressed adolescents. *Am J Psychiatr.* 1983;40:1150–1153.
61. Ivanenko A, Crabtree VM, Gozal D. Sleep and depression in children and adolescents. *Sleep Med Rev.* 2005;9:115–129.
62. Robert JJ, Hoffmann RF, Emslie GJ, et al. Sex and age differences in sleep macroarchitecture in childhood and adolescent depression. *Sleep*. 2006;29:351–358.
63. Arana-Lechuga Y, Nunez-Ortiz R, Teran-Pérez G, et al. Sleep-EEG patterns of school children suffering from symptoms of depression compared to healthy controls. *World J Biol Psychiatry.* 2008;9:115–120.
64. Rao U, Poland RE. Electroencephalographic sleep and hypothalamic-pituitary-adrenal changes from episode to recovery in depressed adolescents. *J Child Adolesc Psychopharmacol*. 2008;18: 607–613.
65. Gruber R, Brouillette RT. Towards an understanding of sleep problems in childhood depression: comment. *Sleep*. 2006;29:418–420.
66. Giles DE, Roffwarg HP, Dahl RE, Kupfer DJ. Electroencephalographic sleep abnormalities in depressed children: a hypothesis. *Psychiatry Res*. 1992;41:53–63.
67. Armitage R. Microarchitectural findings in sleep EEG in depression: diagnostic implications. *Biol Psychiatry*. 1995;37:72–84.
68. Armitage R, Roffwarg HP, Rush AJ, Calhoun JS, Purdy DG, Giles DE. Digital period analysis of sleep EEG in depression. *Biol Psychiatry.* 1992;31:52–68.
69. Armitage R, Calhoun JS, Rush AJ, Roffwarg HP. Comparison of the delta EEG in the first and second non-REM periods in depressed adults and normal controls. *Psychiatry Res*. 1992;41:65–72.
70. Armitage R, Hoffmann R, Fitch T, et al. A comparison of period amplitude and power spectral analysis of sleep EEG in normal adults and depressed out-patients. *Psychiatry Res*. 1995;56:245–256.
71. Borbely AA, Tobler I, Loepfe M, et al. All-night spectral analysis of the sleep EEG in untreated depressives and normal controls. *Psychiatry Res*. 1984;12:27–33.
72. Beersma DGM, Daan S, Van den Hoofdakker RH. The timing of sleep in depression: theoretical considerations. *Psychiatry Res*. 1985;16:253–262.
73. Kupfer DJ, Ulrich RF, Coble PA, et al. Application of an automated REM and slow wave sleep analysis: I. Normal and depressed subjects. *Psychiatry Res*. 1984;13:325–334.
74. Kupfer DJ, Ulrich RF, Coble PA, et al. Application of an automated REM and slow wave sleep analysis: II. Testing the assumptions of the two-process model of sleep regulation in normal and depressed subjects. *Psychiatry Res*. 1984;13:335–343.
75. Kupfer DJ, Grochocinski VJ, McEachran AB. Relationship of awakening and delta sleep in depression. *Psychiatry Res*. 1986;19:297–304.
76. Van den Hoofdakker RH, Beersma DG. On the contribution of sleep wake physiology to the explanation and treatment of depression. *Psychiatry Res*. 1986;16:155–163.
77. Armitage R, Emslie GJ, Hoffmann RF, et al. Ultradian rhythms and temporal coherence in sleep EEG in depressed children and adolescents. *Biol Psychiatry.* 2000;47:338–350.
78. Armitage R, Hoffmann RF. Sleep EEG, depression and gender. *Sleep Med Rev.* 2001;5:237–246.
79. Armitage R, Hoffmann RF, Emslie GJ, Weinberg WA, Mayes TL, Rush AJ. Sleep microarchitecture as

a predictor of recurrence in children and adolescents with depression. *Int J Neuropsychopharmacol.* 2002;5:217–228.
80. Morehouse RL, Kusumakar V, Kutcher SP, LeBlanc J, Armitage R. Temporal coherence in ultradian sleep EEG rhythms in a never-depressed, high-risk cohort of female adolescents. *Biol Psychiatry.* 2002;51:446–456.
81. Armitage R, Hoffmann R, Emslie G, Rintelmann J, Robert J. Sleep microarchitecture in childhood and adolescent depression: temporal coherence. *Clin EEG Neurosci.* 2006;37:1–9.
82. Wojnar J, Brower KJ, Dopp R, et al. Sleep and body mass index in depressed children and healthy controls. *Sleep Med.* 2010;11:295–301.
83. Aronen ET, Paavonen EJ, Fjallberg M, Soininen M, Törrönen J. Sleep and psychiatric symptoms in school-age children. *J Am Acad Child Adolesc Psychiatry.* 2000;39:502–508.
84. Teicher MH, Glod CA, Harper D, et al. Locomotor activity in depressed children and adolescents: I. Circadian dysregulation. *J Am Acad Child Adolesc Psychiatry.* 1993;32:760–769.
85. Birmaher B, Brent D, Bernet W, et al. Practice parameter for the assessment and treatment of children and adolescents with depressive disorders. *J Am Acad Child Adolesc Psychiatry.* 2007;46:1503–1526.
86. Kupfer DJ, Coble P, Kane J, Petti T, Conners CK. Imipramine and EEG sleep in children with depressive symptoms. *Psychopharmacology.* 1979;60: 117–123.
87. Shain BN, Naylor M, Shipley JE, Alessi N. Imipramine effects on sleep in depressed adolescents: a preliminary report. *Biol Psychiatry.* 1990;28:459–462.
88. Armitage R, Emslie G, Rintelmann J. The effect of fluoxetine on sleep EEG in childhood depression: a preliminary report. *Neuropharmacology.* 1997;17:241–245.
89. Lofthouse N, Fristad MA, Splaingard M, Kelleher K, Hayes J, Resko S. Web-survey of pharmacological and nonpharmacological sleep interventions for children with early-onset bipolar spectrum disorder. *J Affect Disord.* 2010;120:267–271.
90. Kupfer DJ. Pathophysiology and management of insomnia during depression. *Ann Clin Psychiatry.* 1999;11:267–276.
91. Mindell JA, Emslie G, Blumer J, et al. Pharmacologic management of insomnia in children and adolescents: consensus statement. *Pediatrics.* 2006;117: e1223–e1232.
92. Geller B, Zimerman B, Williams M, et al. DSM-IV mania symptoms in a prepubertal and early adolescent bipolar phenotype compared to attention-deficit/hyper-active and normal controls. *J Child Adolesc Psychopharmacol.* 2002;12: 11–25.
93. Harvey AG. The adverse consequences of sleep disturbance in pediatric bipolar disorder: implications for intervention. *Child Adolesc Psychiatr Clin N Am.* 2009;18:321–338.
94. Geller B, Zimerman B, Williams M, Delbello MP, Frazier J, Beringer L. Phenome- nology of prepubertal and early adolescent bipolar disorder: examples of elated mood, grandiose behaviors, decreased need for sleep, racing thoughts and hypersexuality. *J Child Adolesc Psychopharmacol.* 2002;12:3–9.
95. Kowatch RA, Youngstrom EA, Danielyan A, Findling RL. Review and meta-analysis of the phenomenology and clinical characteristics of mania in children and adolescents. *Bipolar Disord.* 2005;7:483–496.
96. Faedda GL, Baldessarini RJ, Glovinsky IP, Austin NB. Pediatric bipolar disorder: phenomenology and course of illness. *Bipolar Disord.* 2004;6(4):305–313.
97. Lofthouse N, Fristad M, Splaingard M, Kelleher K. Parent and child reports of sleep problems associated with early-onset bipolar spectrum disorders. *J Fam Psychol.* 2007;21(1):114–123.
98. Mehl RC, O'Brien LM, Jones JH, Jones JH, Dreisbach JK, Mervis CB, Gozal D. Correlates of sleep and pediatric bipolar disorder. *Sleep.* 2006;29:193–197.
99. Rao U, Dahl RE, Ryan ND, et al. Heterogeneity in EEG sleep findings in adolescent depression: unipolar versus bipolar clinical course. *J Affect Disord.* 2002;70:273–280.
100. Parker G, Malhi G, Hadzi-Pavlovic D, Parker K. Sleeping in? The impact of age and depressive sub-type on hypersomnia. *J Affect Disord.* 2006;90:73–76.
101. Geller B, Tillman R, Craney JL, Bolhofner K. Four-year prospective outcome and natural history of mania in children with a prepubertal and early adolescent bipolar disorder phenotype. *Arch Gen Psychiatry.* 2004;61:459–467.
102. Lewinsohn PM, Klein DN, Seeley JR. Bipolar disorders in a community sample of older adolescents: prevalence, phenomenology, comorbidity, and course. *J Am Acad Child Adolesc Psychiatry.* 1995;34:454–463.
103. Ballenger JC, Reus VI, Post RM. The "atypical" clinical picture of adolescent mania. *Am J Psychiatry.* 1982;139:602–606.
104. Findling RL, Gracious BL, McNamara NK, et al. Rapid, continuous cycling and psychiatric comorbidity in pediatric bipolar I disorder. *Bipolar Disord.* 2001;3:202–210.
105. Bhangoo RK, Dell ML, Towbin K, et al. Clinical correlates of episodicity in juvenile mania. *J Child Adolesc Psychopharmacol.* 2003;13:507–514.
106. Lofthouse N, Fristad M, Splaingard M, Kelleher K, Hayes J, Resko S. Web survey of sleep problems associated with early-onset bipolar spectrum disorders. *J Pediatr Psychol.* 2008;33:349-357.
107. Stoleru S, Nottelmann ED, Belmont B, Ronsaville D. Sleep problems in children of affectively ill mothers. *J Child Psychol Psychiatry.* 1997;38:831–841.
108. Staton D, Volness LJ, Beatty WW. Diagnosis and classification of pediatric bipolar disorder. *J Affect Disord.* 2008;105:205–212.

109. Jones SH, Tai S, Evershed K, Knowles R, Bentall R. Early detection of bipolar disorder: a pilot familial high-risk study of parents with bipolar disorder and their adolescent children. *Bipolar Disord.* 2006;8:362–372.
110. Duffy A, Alda M, Hajek T, Sherry SB, Grof P. Early stages in the development of bipolar disorder. *J Affect Disord.* 2010;121:127–135.
111. Faedda GL, Teicher MH. Objective measures of activity and attention in the differential diagnosis of psychiatric disorders of childhood. *Essent Psychopharmacol.* 2005;6:239–249.
112. Biederman J, Mick E, Hammerness P, et al. Open-label, 8-week trial of olanzapine and risperidone for the treatment of bipolar disorder in preschool-age children. *Biol Psychiatry.* 2005;58:589–594.
113. Tohen M, Kryzhanovskaya L, Carlson G, et al. Olanzapine versus placebo in the treatment of adolescents with bipolar mania. *Am J Psychiatry.* 2007;164:1547–1556.
114. Choquet M, Kovess V, Poutignat N. Suicidal thoughts among adolescents: an intercultural approach. *Adolescence.* 1993;28:649–659.
115. Vignau J, Bailly D, Duhamel A, Vervaecke P, Beuscart R, Collinet C. Epidemiologic study of sleep quality and troubles in French secondary school adolescents. *J Adolesc Health.* 1997;21: 343–350.
116. Tishler CL, McKenry PC, Morgan KC. Adolescent suicide attempts: some significant factors. *Suicide Life-Threat Behav.* 1981;11:86–92.
117. Liu X. Sleep and adolescent suicidal behavior. *Sleep.* 2004;27:1351–1358.
118. Goldstein T, Bridge J, Brent D. Sleep disturbance preceding completed suicide in adolescents. *J Consult Clin Psychol.* 2008;76:84.
119. Lucas AR. The eating disorder "epidemic": more apparent than real? *Pediatr Ann.* 1992;21: 746–751.
120. Delvenne V, Kerkhofs M, Appelboom-Fondu J, Lucas F, Mendlewicz J. Sleep polygraphic variables in anorexia nervosa and depression: a comparative study in adolescents. *J Affect Disord.* 1992;25:167–172.
121. Nobili L, Baglietto MG, De Carli F, et al. A quantified analysis of sleep electroencephalography in anorectic adolescents. *Biol Psychiatry.* 1999;45:771–775.
122. Nobili L, Baglietto MG, Beelke M, et al. Impairment of the production of delta sleep in anorectic adolescents. *Sleep.* 2004;27:1553–1559.
123. Mattai AA, Tossell J, Greenstein DK, et al. Sleep disturbances in childhood-onset schizophrenia. *Schizophr Res.* 2006;86:123–129.
124. Yung AR, McGorry PD. The initial prodrome in psychosis: descriptive and qualitative aspects. *Aust N Z J Psychiatry.* 1996;30:587–599.
125. Tan HY, Ang YG. First-episode psychosis in the military: a comparative study of prodromal symptoms. *Aust N Z J Psychiatry.* 2001;35:512–519.
126. Monti JM, Monti D. Sleep disturbance in schizophrenia. *Int Rev Psychiatry.* 2005;17:247–253.
127. Ruhrmann S, Schultze-Lutter F, Salokangas RK, et al. Prediction of psychosis in adolescents and young adults at high risk: results from the prospective European prediction of psychosis study. *Arch Gen Psychiatry.* 2010;67:241–251.
128. DeMartinis NA, Winokur A. Effects of psychiatric medications on sleep and sleep disorders. *CNS & Neurological Disorders Drug Targets.* 2007;6: 17–29.
129. Kupfer DJ, Perel JM, Pollack BG, et al. EEG sleep profiles and recurrent depression. *Biol Psychiatry.* 1991;30:641–655.
130. Saletu B. Pharmaco-EEG profiles of typical and atypical antidepressants. In: Costa E, Racagni G, eds. Typical and Atypical Antidepressants: Clinical Practice, New York: Raven Press, 1982: 257–268.
131. Shipley JE, Kupfer DJ, Dealy RS, et al. Differential effects of amitriptyline and of zimelidine on the sleep electroencephalogram of depressed patients. *J Clin Pharmacol Ther.* 1984;36:251–259.
132. Ware JC, Brown FW, Moorad PJ Jr, Pittard JT, Cobert B. Effects on sleep: a double-blind study comparing trimipramine to imipramine in depressed insomniac patients. *Sleep.* 1989;6:537–549.
133. Nofzinger EA, Schwartz RM, Reynolds CF Jr, et al. Affect intensity and phasic REM sleep in depressed men before and after treatment with cognitive-behavioral therapy. *J Consult Clin Psychol.* 1994;62:83–91.
134. Richelson E. Synaptic effects of antidepressants. *J Clin Psychopharmacol.* 1996;16(suppl 2):1s–7s.
135. Hajak G, Rodenbeck A, Voderholzer U, et al. Doxepin in the treatment of primary insomnia: a placebo-controlled, double-blind, polysomnographic study. *J Clin Psychiatry.* 2001;62: 453–463.
136. Riemann D, Voderholzer U, Cohrs S, et al. Trimipramine in primary insomnia: results of a polysomnographic double-blind controlled study. *Pharmacopsychiatry.* 2002;35:165–174.
137. Adrien J. The serotoninergic system and sleep-wakefulness regulation. In: Kales A, ed. *The Pharmacology of Sleep.* New York, NY: Springer; 1995:91–116.
138. Landolt HP, Meier V, Burgess HJ, et al. Serotonin-2 receptors and human sleep: effect of a selective antagonist on EEG power spectra. *Neuropsychopharmacology.* 1999;21:455–466.
139. Gillin JC, Rapaport M, Erman MK, Winokur A, Albala BJ. A comparison of nefazodone and fluoxetine on mood and on objective, subjective, and clinician-rated measures of sleep in depressed patients: a double-blind, 8-week clinical trial. *J Clin Psychiatry.* 1997;58:185–192.
140. Gillin JC, Sohn JW, Stahl SM, et al. Ipsapirone, a 5-HT1A agonist, suppresses REM sleep equally in unmedicated depressed patients and normal controls. *Neuropsychopharmacology.* 1996;15: 109–115.
141. Holshoe JM. Antidepressants and sleep: a review. *Perspectives in Psychiatric Care.* 2009;45:191–197.

142. Trivedi MH, Rush AJ, Armitage R, et al. Effects of fluoxetine on the polysomnogram in outpatients with major depression. *Neuropsychopharmacology*. 1999;20: 447–459.
143. Hendrickse WA, Roffwarg HP, Grannemann BD, et al. The effects of fluoxetine on the polysomnogram of depressed outpatients: a pilot study. *Neuropsychopharmacol*. 1994;10:85–91.
144. Sharpley AL, Williamson DJ, Attenburrow ME, Pearson G, Sargent P, Cowen PJ. The effects of paroxetine and nefazodone on sleep: a placebo controlled trial. *Psychopharmacology*. 1996;126:50–54.
145. Nowell PD, Reynolds CF, Buysse DJ, Dew MA, Kupfer DJ. Paroxetine in the treatment of primary insomnia: preliminary clinical and electroencephalogram sleep data. *J Clin Psychiatry*. 1999;60: 89–95.
146. Rush AJ, Armitage R, Gillin J, et al. Comparative effects of nefazodone and fluoxetine on sleep in outpatients with major depressive disorder. *Biol Psychiatry*. 1998;44:3–14.
147. Nofzinger EA, Reynolds CF, Thase ME, et al. REM sleep enhancement by bupropion in depressed men. *Am J Psychiatry*. 1995;152:274–276.
148. Winokur A, Sateia MJ, Hayes JB. Acute effects of mirtazapine on sleep continuity and sleep architecture in depressed patients: a pilot study. *Biol Psychiatry*. 2000;48:75–78.
149. Winokur A, DeMartinis NA, McNally DP, Gary EM, Cormier JL, Gary KA. Comparative effects of mirtazapine and fluoxetine on sleep physiology measures in patients with major depression and insomnia. *J Clin Psychiatry*. 2003;64:1224–1229.
150. Campbell SS, Gillin JC, Kripke DF, Janowsky DS, Risch SC. Lithium delays circadian phase of temperature and REM sleep in a bipolar depressive: a case report. *Psychiatry Res*. 1989;27:23–29.
151. Hudson JI, Lipinski JF, Frankenburg FR, Tohen M, Kupfer DJ. Effects of lithium on sleep in mania. *Biol Psychiatry*. 1989;25:665–668.
152. Kupfer DJ, Bowers MB. REM sleep and central monoamine oxidase inhibition. *Jr Psychopharmacologia*. 1972;27:183–190.
153. Kapur S, Mamo D. Half a century of antipsychotics and still a central role for dopamine D2 receptors. *Prog Neuropschopharm Biol Psychiatry*. 2003;27:1081–1090.
154. Wong AH, Van Tol HH. The dopamine D4 receptors and mechanisms of antipsychotic atypicality. *Prog Neuropsychopharmacol Biol Psychiatry*. 2003;27:1091–1099.
155. Cohrs S. Sleep disturbances in patients with schizophrenia: impact and effect of antipsychotics. *CNS Drugs*. 2008;22:939–962.
156. Hinze-Selch D, Mullington J, Orth A, Lauer CJ, Pollmächer T. Effects of clozapine on sleep: a longitudinal study. *Biol Psychiatry*. 1997;42: 260–266.
157. Salin-Pascual RJ, Herrera-Estrella M, Galicia-Polo L, Laurrabaquio MR. Olanzapine acute administration in schizophrenic patients increases delta sleep and sleep efficiency. *Biol Psychiatry*. 1999;46:141–143.
158. Yamashita H, Morinobu S, Yamawaki S, Horiguchi J, Nagao M. Effect of risperidone on sleep in schizophrenia: a comparison with haloperidol. *Psychiatry Res*. 2002;109:137–142.
159. Idzikowski C, Mills FJ, Glennard R. 5-Hydroxytryptamine-2 antagonist increases human slow wave sleep. *Brain Res*. 1986;16;378: 164–168.
160. Riemann D, Voderholzer U, Cohrs S, et al. Trimipramine in primary insomnia: results of a polysomnographic double-blind controlled study. *Pharmacopsychiatry*. 2002;35:165–174.
161. Lacey JH, Crisp AH, Crutchfield M, Hawkins C, Hartmann M. Clomipramine and sleep: a preliminary communication. *Postgrad Med J*. 1977; 53:35–40.
162. Volkers AC, Tulen JHM, van den Broek WW, Bruijn JA, Passchier J, Pepplinkhuizen L. 24-Hour motor activity after treatment with imipramine or fluvoxamine in major depressive disorder. *Eur Neuropsychopharmacol*. 2002;12:273–278.
163. Mendels J, Kiev A, Fabre LF. Double-blind comparison of citalopram and placebo in depressed outpatients with melancholia. *Depress Anxiety*. 1999;9:54–60.
164. Vasar V, Appelberg B, Rimon R, Selvaratnam J. The effect of fluoxetine on sleep: a longitudinal, double-blind polysomnographic study of healthy volunteers. *Int Clin Psychopharmacol*. 1994;9:203–206.
165. Silvestri R, Pace-Schott EF, Gersh T, Stickgold R, Salzman C, Hobson JA. Effects of fluvoxamine and paroxetine on sleep structure in normal subjects: a home-based nightcap evaluation during drug administration and withdrawal. *J Clin Psychiatry*. 2001;62:642–652.
166. Walsh JK, Erman M, Erwin CW, et al. Subjective hypnotic efficacy of trazodone and zolpidem in DSMIII-R primary insomnia. *Hum Psychopharmacol Clin Exp*. 1998;13:191–198.
167. Kaplan J, Dawson S, Vaughan T, Green R, Wyatt RJ. Effect of prolonged chlorpromazine administration on the sleep of chronic schizophrenics. *Arch Gen Psychiatry*. 1974;31:62–66.
168. Maixner S, Tandon R, Eiser A, Taylor S, DeQuardo JR, Shipley J. Effects of antipsychotic treatment on polysomnographic measures in schizophrenia: a replication and extension. *Am J Psychiatry*. 1998;155:1600–1602.
169. Gillin JC, van Kammen DP, Post R, Bunney WE Jr. Effects of prolonged administration of pimozide on sleep-EEG patterns in psychiatric patients. *Commun Psychopharmacol*. 1977;1:225–232.
170. Brannen JO, Jewett RE. Effects of selected phenothiazines on REM sleep in schizophrenics. *Arch Gen Psychiatry*. 1969;21:284–290.
171. Lee JH, Woo JI, Meltzer HY. Effects of clozapine on sleep measures and sleep-associated changes in growth hormone and cortisol in patients with schizophrenia. *Psychiatry Res*. 2001;103:157–166.

172. Salin Pascual RJ, Herrera Estrella M, Galicia Polo L, Laurrabaquio MR. Olanzapine acute administration in schizophrenic patients increases delta sleep and sleep efficiency. *Biol Psychiatry.* 1999;46:141–143.
173. Luthringer R, Staner L, Noel N, et al. A double-blind, placebo-controlled, randomized study evaluating the effect of paliperidone extended-release tablets on sleep architecture in patients with schizophrenia. *Int Clin Psychopharmacol.* 2007;22:299–308.
174. Tandon R. Effects of atypical antipsychotics on polysomnographic measures in schizophrenia. In: Judd LL, Saletu B, Filip V, eds. *Basic and Clinical Science of Mental and Addictive Disorders.* Vol. 167. Basel: Karger; 1997:219–222.

CHAPTER 11

Sleep and Wakefulness in Children With Brain Tumors

Gerald Rosen and Audrey Shore

Introduction

The relationship between brain tumors and sleep is complex because sleep and wakefulness are regulated by the brain. Most of the biological machinery controlling the various facets of sleep is located in the nuclei in the hypothalamus, brainstem, and basal forebrain [1,2]. Injury to these nuclei from brain tumors, neurosurgery, chemotherapy, or cranial radiation therapy (CRT) may disrupt the delicate neurologic balance required to support and sustain normal sleep/wake. Sleep also occurs in a psychological context and can be impacted by stress, anxiety, depression, or posttraumatic stress disorder (PTSD), all of which occur in children with cancer or adult survivors of childhood cancer.

The sleep problems in children with brain tumors can be understood as the results of 3 distinct processes:

1. Children with brain tumors are expected to have the same background prevalence of sleep problems seen in all children.
2. Sleep problems that result from the stress on the child and family resulting from the child having a life-threatening disease.
3. Sleep problems are the direct result of brain injury from brain tumors, neurosurgery, and CRT or the indirect result of chemotherapy and the many medical complications of cancer including cancer-related fatigue (CRF), pain, seizures, obesity, endocrinopathies, heart failure, blindness, and medication [3,4].

There have been no prospective studies of sleep problems in children with cancer, so that the true prevalence and range of sleep disorders in children with brain tumors is not known. However, a large case series of children with cancer seen at a pediatric sleep center over a 15-year period does provide descriptive data as shown in Table 11.1 [5]. This chapter will provide an overview of brain tumors in children, explore the 3 processes that underpin the sleep problems of children with brain tumors, and suggest an approach to the evaluation of sleep problems in children with brain tumors.

Overview of Cancer/Brain Tumors in Children

Cancer is caused by a breakdown of the existing biological balance of cellular renewal and cellular apoptosis/elimination within the body. This disruption is the result of an imbalance of the signaling pathways that control essential cellular functions including cell growth, differentiation, and survival [6]. The majority of cancers are caused by random mutations or alterations to molecular pathways, which increase cancer susceptibility, though some may be the result of hereditary and/or environmental factors [7]. Childhood cancers comprise a wide spectrum of markedly different malignancies, which vary by histology, gender, age, site of origin, and race. The most commonly diagnosed childhood cancers are

Table 11.1 Common pediatric brain tumors, treatment prognosis

Tumor	%	Treatment	Prognosis (5-year tumor free)
Medulloblastoma	10–20	Surgery, Radiation, and Chemotherapy	Average risk 80% High risk 60%–80% Infant 30%–60%
Glioma	40–60		
Low grade	25–35		
Cerebellum	10–20	Surgery often curative	95%
Cerebrum	10–20	Surgery often curative	80%
High grade	15–25		
Cerebral	10–15	Surgery	30%
Brainstem	5–10	Not resectable, radiation and chemotherapy	<5%
Craniopharyngiomas	6–9	Surgery and/or radiation	>60%

Reprinted with permission from Ref. [5].

acute lymphoblastic leukemia and brain/central nervous system (CNS) malignancies, which comprise 27% and 22% of all childhood cancers, respectively [8,9]. Brain tumors are the most commonly diagnosed solid tumors in children.

Data on brain tumors in the United States are systematically collected and analyzed in 2 slightly different databases. The Central Brain Tumor Registry of the United States (CBTRUS) [8] includes all primary malignant and nonmalignant tumors of the brain and CNS prior to 2004. The National Cancer Institute's Surveillance, Epidemiology and End Results program [9] only includes data on primary malignant tumors of the brain and CNS, excluding tumors of the pituitary and pineal, 2 areas that are important in sleep regulation. Both data sets rely on data collected from cancer registries from a defined group of states and then extrapolate from these populations to derive rate estimates for the entire United States. The most important differences between the 2 data sets are the inclusion of nonmalignant pituitary tumors such as craniopharyngiomas and pineal tumors such as pinealoblastomas in the CBTRUS data. Because these tumors are often associated with sleep problems, the CBTRUS data are used in the description of brain tumor in this chapter. The CBTRUS incidence rates for all pediatric (ages 0–19) primary brain and CNS tumors is 4.74/100,000 person years. Brain tumors are classified both by histology and location. The most widely used classification schema was the result of a World Health Organization consensus conference and is based on histopathology. This schema was revised by Rorke et al [10] to include a designation for location. Though there is still considerable controversy in the oncology community regarding the proper histopathologic classification of some brain tumors, in regard to the association of brain tumors with sleep problems, location of the tumor in the brain and the treatments are far more important determinants than cell histology in the development of sleep problems. This is best illustrated by considering craniopharyngiomas, a tumor that usually arises in the pituitary stalk in the suprasellar region of the hypothalamus, which histopathologically is benign, but because of its location, commonly results in severe excessive daytime sleepiness (EDS) and morbid obesity [11,12].

The distribution of all childhood brain and CNS tumors by histology is shown in Figure 11.1 and by age and anatomic site in Figure 11.2, both from the CBTRUS data [8]. Surgery is the initial treatment for the majority of children with brain tumors, with the exception of infiltrative brainstem tumors, which are often unresectable. Surgery provides tissue for a histologic diagnosis, which is important for planning treatment and decreases the tumor burden. Because of the difficulty in resecting the entire tumor, and the frequency of metastases, many brain tumors also require

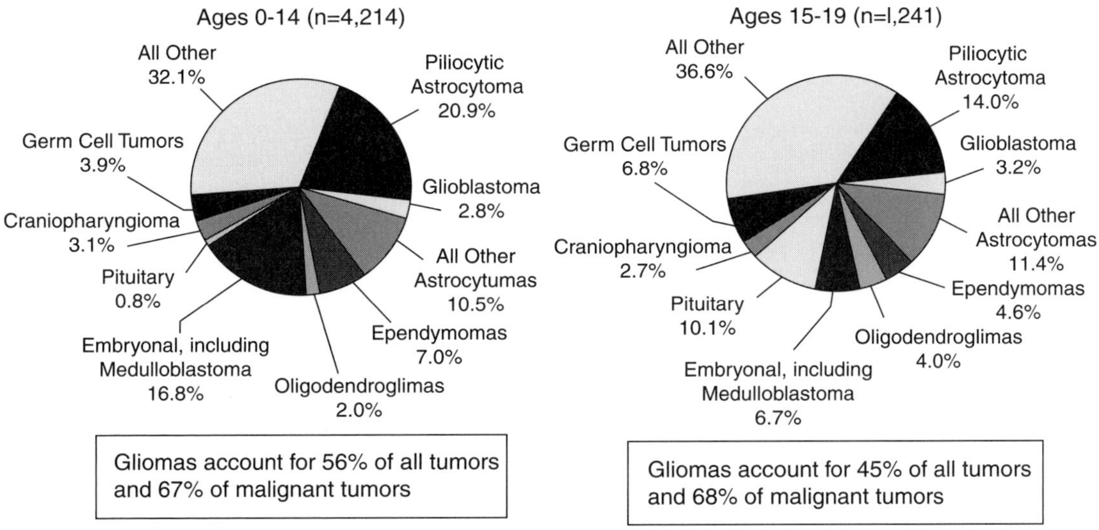

Figure 11.1 Distribution of childhood brain tumors by histology. Reprinted with permission from Ref. [8].

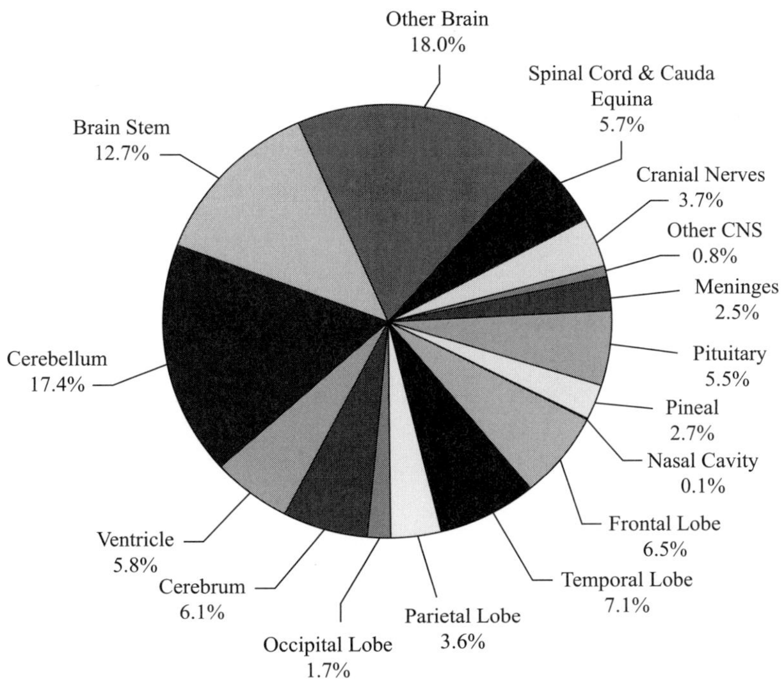

Figure 11.2 Distribution of childhood brain tumors by site. Reprinted with permission from Ref. [8].

CRT and/or chemotherapy to improve long-term prognosis. Cranial radiation is a mainstay in the treatment of many brain tumors because it is highly effective in the treatment of brain tumors and can be used for tumors that involve areas of the brain that are not amenable to neurosurgery. Even with combined therapies, the overall 5-year survival rates for pediatric brain tumors is approximately 65% [8,9], with astrocytomas having the best prognosis of nearly 76% (Table 11.1).

Gliomas are the most common brain tumor in children. They are a heterogeneous group of tumors constituting 40%–60% of all brain and CNS tumors in children. They are predominantly low-grade astrocytomas involving the cerebrum or cerebellum, which can often be cured with surgery alone. However, about 10% involves the optic pathway or hypothalamus, may be infiltrative, and are not resectable, making CRT and chemotherapy the only treatment options. High-grade malignant pontine gliomas are rapidly progressive and have a very poor prognosis. Medulloblastomas, also described as infratentorial primitive neuroectodermal tumors (PNET), account for about 20% of all brain tumors and 40% of all cerebellar tumors in children. Medulloblastomas are the most common brain tumor in children 0 to 4 years of age. The tumor usually arises from the cerebellar vermis in the roof of the fourth ventricle. Supratentorial PNETs (sPNET) are much less common, accounting for 3% of all brain tumors and have a much poorer prognosis. There is some controversy within the oncology community as to whether sPNET and medulloblastomas are the same tumor, in a different location [13]. Both of these tumors commonly metastasize within the CNS, so their treatment usually involves surgery—CRT to the tumor bed and the entire craniospinal axis and chemotherapy.

Craniopharyngiomas are a histologically benign tumor accounting for 6% to 9% of pediatric brain tumors, which has a clinically malignant course because of its location and the morbidity associated with treatment. Craniopharyngiomas arise from the remnants from Rathke's pouch and are most commonly located in the suprasellar region. Because of the location, in close proximity to the pituitary in the hypothalamus, and treatments that often include both surgery and CRT, neuroendocrine deficiencies, hyperphagia, and obesity are commonly seen in children with craniopharyngiomas either as a result of the destructive effect of the tumor or the treatments.

As survival for pediatric brain tumors has improved, the incidence of neurologic, neurobehavioral, neuroendocrine, and other medical complications in cancer survivors has also risen [3,4]. The morbidities associated with pediatric brain tumors result from both the destructive effects of the tumor and collateral damage to normal brain tissues from neurosurgery, chemotherapy, and CRT. Morbidity associated with cancer treatment may occur immediately, as a result of the tumor or the toxic side effects of treatment, or as "late effects," which may not become apparent until months or years after the cancer has been cured. The other medical problems commonly associated with brain tumors and their treatment include cognitive and behavioral problems, obesity, neuropathies, seizures, and second tumors of the CNS, fatigue, growth hormone deficiency, hypothyroidism, cortisol deficiency, diabetes insipidus, stroke, severe visual loss, heart failure, kidney failure, liver dysfunction, anxiety, and depression, all of which can indirectly affect sleep. These nonsleep sequelae may play an indirect role in the development of sleep disorders in children with brain tumors mediated through sleep-disordered breathing, sleep fragmentation, depression, PTSD, or anxiety. When looked for, sleep problems have been recognized in children both during and after treatment for leukemia [14–18] and brain tumors [5,19,20], the 2 most common malignancies in children. However, there has been no systematic evaluation of sleep in children with cancer, so the overall prevalence of sleep problems in childhood brain tumors is unknown.

Neuroanatomy of Sleep and Wakefulness

Sleep and wake are complex neurologic processes that are actively generated by coordinated, overlapping mechanisms controlled by nuclei in the hypothalamus, thalamus, basal forebrain, and brainstem [1,2]. Each of these systems controls a different facet of sleep and/or wake, each has different roles, so the loss of any one system may be partially compensated by other systems. Figure 11.3 illustrates the neuroanatomy of the known CNS systems supporting wakefulness and

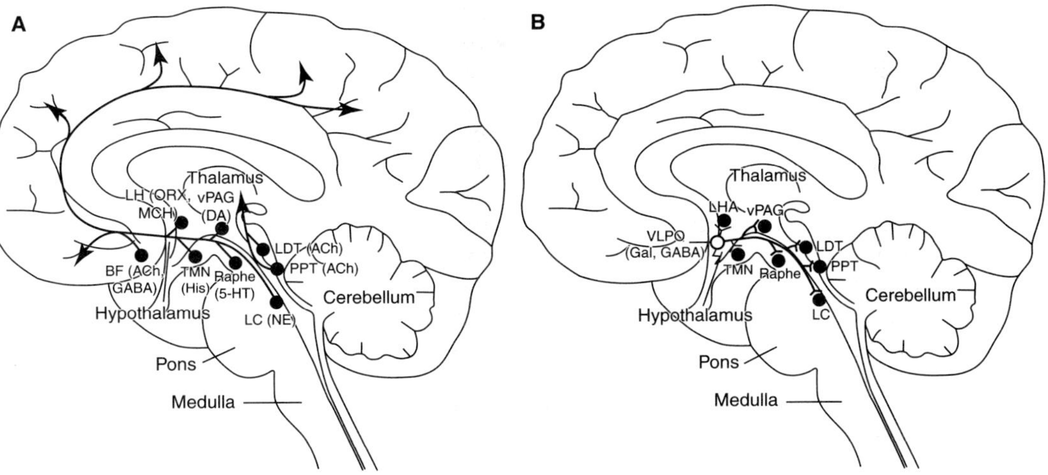

Figure 11.3 Neuroanatomy of the known central nervous systems supporting wakefulness and sleep. Reprinted with permission from Ref. [2].

sleep [2]. Brain tumors and/or their treatments may impact on sleep by a direct damage to these brain centers that are responsible for the regulation of sleep/wake by the tumor or neurosurgery, by the neurotoxic effects of CRT and chemotherapy, or by the indirect effects of cognitive and behavioral impairments, pain, or sleep fragmentation. The relationship between injury to the brain and the development of sleep problems was first described by Von Economo [21], based on his observations of patients with encephalitis. The majority of individuals with encephalitis lethargica slept excessively, often up to 20 hr/d. Postmortem examinations of their brains revealed inflammatory lesions at the junction of the brainstem and the forebrain in the diencephalon, in the posterior hypothalamus. A minority of patients, with lesions in the basal forebrain and anterior hypothalamus, experienced insomnia. The anatomical basis of these clinical observations has been explored and expanded by many neuroscientists since Von Economo. Moruzzi and Magoun [22] described the ascending reticular activating system, which originates in the pons and facilitates arousal. Sleep active neurons have been identified in the ventrolateral preoptic nucleus of the hypothalamus [1]. These cells have many projections to the various nuclei composing the reticular activating system. Saper et al [23] proposed a "sleep switch" in the hypothalamus that regulates the balance between sleep and wakefulness. A schematic representation of the key elements of the CNS structures supporting wakefulness and sleep are shown in Figure 11.3 [2]. Since Von Economo's original clinical observations, many other types of injuries to this critical area of the brain have been recognized as causing problems with sleep. The most commonly reported sleep problem after a CNS injury is EDS. Brain injuries that have resulted in EDS have been recently summarized in a comprehensive review of symptomatic narcolepsy by Nishino and Kanbayashi [24]. The 116 cases of symptomatic narcolepsy that have been reported in the literature were associated with inherited disorders (34%), brain tumors (29%), head trauma (16%), demyelinating disorders (9%), stroke (5%), infection (3%), and degenerative disorders (3%). In Nishino's series, many different types of brain tumors were associated with EDS including craniopharyngioma, adenomas, angioma, cerebral, sarcoid, glioma, germinoma, glioblastoma, histiocytosis, lymphoma, medulloblastoma, and subependyoma. Seventy percent of the tumors involved the hypothalamus or adjacent structures including pituitary, suprasellar, or optic chiasm, and 10% involved the brainstem. Some tumors involved multiple sites, but in only 12% were areas of the brain other than the brainstem or hypothalamus involved, and in many of these cases, CRT was one of the treatments. In 10 patients with brain tumors in Nishino's review, cerebrospinal fluid (CSF) hypocretin was measured. Hypocretin was found to be low in 3/10 and normal in 7/10, suggesting that in the majority of cases, EDS in patients with brain tumors is not simply caused by the destruction of the hypocretin-secreting cells in the lateral hypothalamus.

The complete loss of circadian rhythmicity has been reported [25], but is an uncommon sequelae of brain tumors involving the hypothalamus. The circadian rhythm disorders in children that are the direct result of brain injuries in children with brain tumors are more likely to be the result of severe visual impairment. This is consistent with the ablation experiments in animals where the entire suprachiasmatic nucleus must be destroyed before circadian rhythms are lost.

Cranial Radiation and Brain Tumors

Cranial radiation is a common treatment modality for pediatric brain tumors for 4 reasons: many brain tumors infiltrate into areas of the brain that cannot be totally resected without injuring vital brain centers, some tumors are very radiosensitive, some brain tumors (medulloblastomas) commonly metastasize throughout the CNS, and most brain tumors are not highly sensitive to chemotherapy. CRT is typically directed to the tumor bed, and in tumors likely to metastasize, also to the entire cranial-spinal axis. Though effective, CRT has substantial morbidity, which is related to the radiation dose and field, and is especially toxic to children younger than 3 years. Though no systematic survey has been done of sleep in children receiving radiotherapy, sleep problems do appear to be common in case reports of children with brain tumors treated with CRT. The most common sleep problem reported is EDS. The increase in daytime sleepiness after treatment with CRT can be transient or permanent. Radiation hypersomnia is a constellation of symptoms including EDS, increased total sleep time, irritability, anorexia, low-grade fever, nausea, vomiting, dysphagia, and headaches, which can be seen in up to 60% of children treated with 2400 cGy cranial radiation [26–28]. The syndrome typically appears 3 to 12 weeks postradiation and lasts for 3 to 14 days. These children become sleepier; increasing the amount of sleep they require on a daily basis and often, in spite of an increased total sleep time, they are fatigued and experience EDS. These findings were described in a long-term follow-up study of sleep in adult cancer survivors, who were treated as children with cranial radiation 5 to 15 years earlier for brain tumors [29]. Actigraphy was used to compare the sleep of the adult brain tumor survivors with that of normal controls. The radiation-treated group showed an increase in sleep duration, decreased sleep fragmentation, and decreased tolerance for alterations in the timing of sleep. There was a clear dose-effect relationship with higher doses of cranial radiation associated with longer sleep bouts and decreased tolerance for alterations in the timing of sleep. The underlying mechanism responsible for these changes is not understood.

Cancer-Related Fatigue

Cancer-related fatigue (CRF) is described as a near-universal experience of individuals with cancer, present in more than 70% of patients [30–35]. Fatigue, though typically present in an individual who has EDS, is different from sleepiness, a distinction that is often not made by parents and oncologists. Fatigue is a subjective complaint that is quantified by using standardized questionnaires. However, all standardized questionnaires in use to measure fatigue include questions regarding sleep, so the distinction between fatigue and sleepiness is often blurred. Children and their parents characterize CRF as multidimensional, with physical, emotional, and mental facets [33]. The multidimensional fatigue scale is a well-validated scale that distinguishes general fatigue, sleep/rest fatigue, and cognitive fatigue and has demonstrated an increasing level of fatigue in children with brain tumors, after they have completed therapy and have been "cured" of their cancer [34,36]. Children with brain tumors had more fatigue than children with leukemia, and 2/3 of children with brain tumors were >1 SD below the norms of fatigue of healthy control children (greater fatigue). Numerous causes and comorbidities for CRF have been proposed, including pain, depression, anxiety, anemia, poor nutrition, sleep disorders, physical deconditioning, infection, and organ system failure [30]. Fatigue from whatever cause often results in an increased time in bed, with an earlier bedtime and a later rise time. These schedule modifications are often accompanied by a decrease in daytime activity, which in turn may result in a decrease in morning light exposure. The net result of all these changes, many of which seem to make intuitive sense and are often recommended by physicians, who encourage their patients to get more "rest," is a loss of the normal synchronization between circadian rhythmicity and homeostatic sleep drive. This inevitably leads to a poorer quality sleep, with decreased sleep efficiency, a poorer quality of wakefulness as well as contributing to physical deconditioning, all of which leads to worsening fatigue. In surveys, children with cancer describe feeling impaired by fatigue and rate it as one of the most distressing treatment-related symptoms they experience [30]. Fatigue in children with cancer is often made worse during hospitalization because of frequent interruptions of the child's sleep by caregivers. This was described in a study of 29 children with cancer hospitalized for 2 to 3 days. The children were awakened 0 to 40 times per night (mean 14). The longest duration of uninterrupted sleep for 70% of the children was 1 hour [37].

Sleep-Disordered Breathing in Children With Brain Tumors

Snoring is a common pediatric symptom that is present in 12% of all children and obstructive sleep apnea (OSA) in about 2%, so either may be present before a child develops cancer [38]. OSA is always a multifactorial problem, the cumulative result of craniofacial, neuromuscular, and soft tissue factors. In children with brain tumors, the neurologic contributors to OSA may be secondary to (a) state-dependent change in pharyngeal tone during sleep, (b) hypotonia, (c) hypertonia, (d) injury to the medulla resulting in a loss of the synchronization of the pharyngeal dilators with the diaphragmatic contractions, or (e) peripherally mediated injury to the vagus, glossopharyngeal, or hypoglossal nerves, which control the pharyngeal dilators [39].

Two important nonrespiratory, nonneurologic contributors to OSA seen in children with brain tumors are obesity and hypothyroidism. In most children with OSA, the sleep-disordered breathing is present whenever the child is asleep, but in some children, the OSA is only present or is much worse when the child is asleep, sedated with drugs such as benzodiazepines or chloral hydrate or when treated for pain with narcotic analgesics. These dangers are especially important in children with brain tumors because these children frequently undergo conscious sedation for diagnostic procedures and are commonly treated with narcotics for pain control. Both conscious sedation and good pain control can be achieved in children with OSA, but it is important that appropriate precautions are taken.

Central Sleep Apnea

Clinically significant central sleep apnea (CSA) is uncommon in children older than 1 year, unless they have a brainstem malformation such as an Arnold-Chiari malformation or have sustained a severe brain injury from a tumor, infection, trauma, or stroke. CNS injury may result in CSA or centrally mediated OSA. CSA in children with brain tumors is most commonly caused by (1) an injury to the respiratory control center of the brain located in the medulla oblongata, (2) an unusual manifestation of a seizure, or (3) damage to the phrenic nerve. The symptoms of a child with CSA typically is nonobstructive hypoventilation during sleep, which leads to sleep-related hypoxemia and/or hypercarbia and if severe may cause waking hypercapnia and/or cor pulmonale.

Psychiatric/Behavioral

Though sleep is a neurologic process, it occurs in a psychological context. This is never so important than at the transition to sleep from wakefulness, which occurs at sleep onset and again at numerous times throughout the night after normal awakenings. For this transition to go smoothly, a child must feel safe and be free from anxiety. If for any reason the child is fearful, anxious, depressed, or angry at bedtime, it may result in an inability to transition easily to sleep at bedtime and/or after normal awakenings during the night [40,41]. Falling asleep is also a learned behavior that has clear associations. Ideally, the learned associations at sleep onset are conducive to sleep, but they may not be, in which case insomnia may occur.

Problems with sleep, particularly insomnia or hypersomnia are 2 of the most common symptoms seen in children and adolescents with psychiatric disease, particularly depression and anxiety [41] diagnoses, which may be comorbid conditions in children with cancer. Another sleep problem that is often seen in children with cancer, especially in a young child, is conditioned insomnia. This problem can easily be induced in a child, especially a young child who is ill. In the setting of cancer, this occurs because when a child is diagnosed with cancer, the child often becomes more dependent on their parents, with the parents often becoming more involved in the details of the child's life. If the parents become overinvolved in the child's sleep onset, this sets the stage for the development of a conditioned sleep-onset association disorder. The hallmark symptom of this problem is the parental presence as the child transitions to sleep at bedtime and the necessity of parental involvement after the child has a normal nighttime awakening. The symptom arises because the transition to sleep may be difficult for the child because of pain or fears and the parents want to help the child. If the parent is present at the beginning of the night at sleep onset, this often does help the child transition to sleep at bedtime, but it may also inadvertently create a learned association, resulting in the child's wanting and/or needing to have the parents present to facilitate the return to sleep after normal awakenings, which may occur 5 to 6 times throughout the night. When the parent responds to these awakenings by again helping the child return to sleep during the night, they are inadvertently reinforcing the sleep-onset association and perpetuating the arousals. In adolescents or young adults, the use or withdrawal from psychotropic drugs and/or alcohol may lead to insomnia or daytime sleepiness and should be assessed. Cancer is considered a model for the development of pediatric traumatic stress in children [42,43] and may lead to the development of clinical PTSD, which is seen in 12% of the adult survivors of pediatric cancer [43]. Sleep problems, particularly sleep onset and sleep maintenance insomnia, are common symptoms seen in patients with PTSD though these have not been specifically characterized in children with cancer.

Pain

Pain is common in children with cancer, particularly at the time of diagnosis, and when pain is present, sleep is often disrupted. In a study of pain in children with cancer [44], at the time of their diagnosis, 78% experienced significant pain and in almost three-fourths of them, the pain lead to sleep disruption, causing multiple awakenings from sleep. Nine percent had severe sleep disruption and were unable to return to sleep, even with analgesic medication, 32% had a moderate degree of sleep disruption and were able to return to sleep only after medication, and 20% had mild sleep disruption, returning to sleep without medication. In many clinical settings, acute and chronic pain leads to sleep fragmentation, which in turn has been associated with increased pain sensitivity [45] establishing a vicious spiral. In adults, pain has also been shown to play a mediating role in the development of CRF [46]. Medications used to treat pain, particularly the narcotic analgesics can also cause sleep problems or cause daytime sedation, which may lead to daytime napping, which in turn may impact on circadian rhythmicity and synchronization with the homeostatic sleep drive.

Other Medical Problems

Sleep disruption may occur in many other medical problems that may be present in a child with cancer including obesity, asthma, endocrinopathies, gastroesophageal reflux, heart failure, abdominal pain, arthritis, seizures, and atopic dermatitis. These medical problems may cause sleep fragmentation, which may contribute to the symptoms of insomnia, increase in pain sensitivity, and/or daytime sleepiness.

Medications

Sedation and/or insomnia are listed as a side effect of more than 500 prescriptions and over-the-counter drugs in the side-effect index of the physician's desk reference [47]. These drugs may affect sleep/wake directly by leading to either an increased level of arousal (causing insomnia) or a decreased level of arousal (causing sedation) or indirectly by causing sleep fragmentation. In many of the medications that affect the CNS neurotransmitters, the drugs may have a primary effect (often sedation or increased arousal) or the opposite effect, which may be secondary to withdrawal or to an idiosyncratic reaction to the drug. This has been most commonly described with diphenhydramine (H1 antagonist), which usually results in sedation; but may cause hyperactivity in some children. Opioid analgesics are an important part of the pain management of children with cancer. Good pain control is essential for good sleep in children. However, opioids may also be a factor that can negatively impact on sleep in a number of ways. Opioids may cause daytime sedation and fatigue, raise the arousal threshold for sleep apnea, and lead to respiratory depression. Many children with cancer are treated with high-dose corticosteroids. In case series studies of children with cancer treated with high-dose prednisone or dexamethasone [17] for leukemia, sleep problems are common: fatigue 56%, insomnia 38%, hyperinsomnia 31%, and an increase in total sleep time [5].

Sleep During the Terminal Phase of Childhood Cancer

Thirty-two percent of children with brain tumors die, and sleep problems are common in children during the terminal phase of the disease. Two studies detailed this from the perspective of palliative care providers [48] and parents [49]. In the last month of the child's life, parents and the doctors reported fatigue in 92%, daytime sleepiness in 60%, and insomnia present in 16% to 40% of children. The treatment of sleep problems may need to be addressed within the context of palliative care in these children.

Review of Clinical Problems of Children With Cancer

There have been no prospective studies of sleep problems in children with cancer, so the prevalence of sleep problems in children with cancer is unknown. However, a recent case series review of children with cancer referred to a pediatric sleep center for a comprehensive sleep evaluation provides some insight into the sleep problems children with cancer experience [5]. The limitations of a case series review of children referred for a specialty evaluation are numerous and obvious. However, this type of descriptive information does allow for the characterization of the problems. Of 70 children with cancer, 48 with CNS tumors were seen over a 15-year period. Twenty-five percent of the children were referred while they were still receiving treatment for cancer, and 75% had completed their cancer treatment. All the children had a comprehensive sleep interview, after which further objective sleep diagnostic testing was performed only when clinically indicated to better characterize a suspected sleep disorder. A polysomnogram (PSG) was performed in 53 children when there was a history suggestive of OSA, CSA, or EDS and was followed by a multiple sleep latency test (MSLT) in the 36 children who had a history of EDS. Seven children had 2 to 4 weeks of actigraphy. In this group of children, sleep disorders were defined using the pediatric guidelines as established by the American Academy of Sleep Medicine and published in the International Classification of Sleep Disorders [50], except for children with EDS, which was defined

1. Subjectively—based on the history of frequently falling asleep at inappropriate times during routine activities of daily living such as school or after-school activities and the resumption of daily naps which had previously been discontinued or
2. Objectively—based on either
   - A. MSLT—mean sleep latency less than 15 minutes with sleep present on at least 2 of the nap opportunities of the MSLT
   - B. Actigraphy—consistent daytime sleep greater than 30 minutes a day.

This more expansive definition was used because one third of the children with a history of EDS—which began after their brain tumor, resulted in an increase in the total duration of sleep per 24 hours, and was associated with the resumption of daytime naps that had previously been discontinued, an inability to awaken at the desired rise time, and/or the inability to remain awake during daytime activities—had mean latencies on the MSLT of greater than 15 minutes and would not be considered hypersomnolent. Table 11.2 describes the sleep problems and type of cancers in these children. EDS was the most common clinical sleep problem found in these children, present in 60% of the entire group and 80% of the children with CNS neoplasms involving the

Table 11.2 Children with cancer seen in sleep clinic type/location of cancer and sleep problems

Children with cancer seen in sleep clinic 1994–2009	Total no. of patients	EDS/Long sleepers	Apnea	Insomnia	Circadian	Parasomnia
Total	70	42/70(60%)	28/70(40%)	17/70(24%)	3/70(4%)	6/70(9%)
Tumors of central nervous system	48					
Hypothalamus/ brainstem	35	28/35(80%)	16/35(46%)	5/35(14%)	2/35(6%)	2/35(6%)
Posterior fossa	7	6	2	2	0	1
Cortex	6	4	2	1	0	2
Leukemia/other blood	18	4/18(22%)	6/18(33%)	7/18(39%)	1/18(6%)	1/18(6%)
Other solid tumors	4					
Upper airway	3	0	2	1	0	0
Kidney	1	0	0	1	0	0

Abbreviations: EDS, excessive daytime sleepiness.
Reprinted with permission from Ref. [5].

hypothalamus, thalamus, and brainstem. The parents of children with EDS did not describe sleepiness as one of the presenting symptoms of the cancer, but rather, that it developed after CNS-directed therapy was initiated. In 13 of 39 children with a history of EDS, a possible cause for their sleepiness was identified on the overnight PSG. Obstructive sleep apnea in 9, sleep-related seizures in 2, pain causing sleep fragmentation in 1, and drug abuse in 1. In the children with seizures and drug abuse, EDS improved after treatment. EDS persisted in 5 of the 9 children with OSA in whom the OSA was successfully corrected with continuous positive airway pressure (CPAP). In 66% there was no identifiable cause of the EDS.

Sleep-disordered breathing was found in 28 of the children with cancer (40%), 6 of 28 had CSA, 20 of 28 had OSA, and 2 of 28 had nocturnal hypoxemia. Of the 20 children with OSA, 7 had an apnea index (AI) less than 5 and did not require treatment, 4 were referred for an adenotonsillectomy, and in 9 children, in whom the OSA did not appear to be related to adenotonsillar hypertrophy, the OSA was treated with CPAP or bilevel PAP. One child with morbid obesity and severe OSA who was intolerant of CPAP required a tracheotomy. Of the 6 children with CSA, in 2, the event that lead to their referral was a respiratory arrest during conscious sedation for an elective procedure. In one other child, the CSA was a manifestation of a seizure disorder and was effectively treated with anticonvulsants. Three children with CSA required nocturnal ventilation, all of whom had tumors involving the medulla. Nocturnal ventilation was achieved with noninvasive mask ventilation using bilevel PAP with a rate or a tracheotomy with a ventilator in 2, both of whom also required daytime respiratory support as well. The 2 children with nocturnal hypoxemia without significant CO_2 retention were treated with supplemental oxygen during sleep.

As noted in Table 11.2, many of the children with cancer seen for the sleep evaluation had more than one sleep problem identified. EDS was the most common sleep problem identified in children with cancer, present in 60% of all the children evaluated, and 80% of the children with brain tumors. The parents did not describe EDS as present at the time of diagnosis of cancer, but rather that it developed after the treatment with neurotoxic therapies was instituted. Insomnia was present in 24% of the children, but in most cases was not of great concern to the parents, who did not describe it as a problem that needed to be addressed. The treatments used for the sleep problems identified are described in Table 11.3.

All the children diagnosed with EDS were provided with education regarding sleep hygiene to regularize and extend their sleep duration, but this alone did not correct their EDS and so stimulant medication was offered to them. Methylphenidate (10–56 mg/d), modafanil (200–400 mg/d), and amphetamine salts (20–40 mg/d) were all effective in correcting the EDS. The medication was titrated clinically with the primary goal to help the children remain awake during the school day and allowing them to participate in after-school activities. Once an effective dose was established, the hypersomnia continued to be well controlled without significant dose escalation. Side effects of medications were uncommon and included headaches and anorexia. In these children, the EDS has persisted long term, recurring whenever the stimulant medication is discontinued over a 15-year follow-up.

What is of interest in this large case series of sleep problems in children with cancer is not that these children have a wide range of sleep problems. What is noteworthy is the distribution of the types of sleep problems seen and the types of cancers in children who were referred for a diagnostic sleep evaluation. Neither the sleep problems seen nor the types of cancers were representative of the expected prevalence of either condition. Leukemia accounts for about half of all childhood cancers [8,9], but only 26% of the referrals; brain tumors, which account for 25% of childhood cancers [8], accounted for 68% of the referrals. Tumors of the hypothalamus, thalamus, and brainstem account for 25% of all brain tumors, but accounted for 73% of the children with brain tumors referred for sleep evaluation. Tumors of the brainstem, thalamus, and hypothalamus also accounted for the majority of the children with both EDS and OSA and for all of the children with severe CSA.

Table 11.3 Treatments of sleep problems in children with cancer

Sleep Problems	#	Treatments
Parasomnia, $N = 6$		
Seizures	3	Anticonvulsants
Confusional arousals	2	Clonazepam-1 No Tx-1
Sleep eating	1	Topiramate
Sleep-disordered breathing, $N = 28$		
Obstructive sleep apnea, $N = 20$	1	Trach
	8	CPAP/bilevel
	6	Success
	2	Fail
	4	T & A
	7	No Tx (snoring)
Central sleep apnea, $N = 6$		
	1	Bilevel + rate + O_2
	1	Trach + vent
	1	Diaphramatic pacers
	2	No Tx
	1	Tx seizures
Hypoxia, $N = 2$		
	2	O_2

Reprinted with permission from Ref. [5].

Evaluation and Treatment of Sleep Problems

The evaluation of sleep problems in children with cancer is challenging because sleep is the result of the interaction and synchronization of a number of different physiologic processes. The sleep process matrix (Figure 11.4) is a tool for organizing and analyzing the processes that regulate sleep and is particularly helpful when evaluating children with complex medical problems such as cancer [51]. The sleep history is the primary tool for evaluating sleep problems in children (Table 11.4). The history can be organized into the different domains important to sleep regulation: circadian, ultradian, homeostatic, developmental, radiation, cardiorespiratory, neurologic, behavioral-psychiatric, drugs/alcohol, and other medical. The hypotheses, which are developed within each domain, are confirmed or refuted as the history unfolds to best explain the sleep problems. This process leads to an analysis/synthesis that may require a diagnostic test such as a PSG, an actigraphy, or an MSLT to confirm a diagnosis.

Addendum—Paraneoplastic Syndromes

Neoplasms can sometimes cause symptoms that are not the direct result of local invasion or compression. These manifestations are termed paraneoplastic syndromes [52] and are usually characterized by endocrine or neurological dysfunction. Common paraneoplastic, endocrine disturbances include the syndrome of inappropriate secretion of antidiuretic hormone, hypercalcemia, Cushing syndrome, and hypoglycemia. Common paraneoplastic, neurological disturbances include the opsoclonus myoclonus syndrome, limbic encephalitis, and myasthenic syndrome.

The patient develops antibodies to the tumor cell that cross-react with elements of the nervous system. The onconeural antibodies may be characterized into 3 categories: (a) those that are strongly associated with an underlying cancer and well characterized at a molecular level, such as anti-amphiphysin, anti-Hu, and anti-Ma2 antibodies; (b) those that are partially characterized,

Sleep process matrix

Sleep Process	Circadian	Homeo-static	Ultradian	Devel-opmental	Cardio-pulm	Neuro	Radiation	Psychiatric/ Behavior	Drugs / Chemo	Other/ Medical problems
Hypothesis										
Data to Gather										
Analysis Synthesis										
Treatment										

Figure 11.4 Sleep process matrix is a tool for organizing and analyzing how the fundamental processes that regulate sleep interact with each other and lead to sleep symptoms. Generally, the sleep history provides the information necessary to develop hypotheses within each pathophysiologic domain. As the patient's history unfolds, the data gathered either confirm or refute these hypotheses. Diagnostic sleep studies may be necessary to establish the diagnosis. Reprinted with permission from Ref. [50].

Table 11.4 Sleep history in children with brain tumors

Chief complaint—insomnia, excessive daytime sleepiness, unusual awakenings of sleep, snoring/obstructive sleep apnea (maybe more than one complaint)

History of present illness:

brain tumor—tumor type, location, age of diagnosis, presenting symptoms of brain tumor initial treatment:

surgeries—dates, type (biopsy, partial resection, gross total research, shunt)

cranial radiation–dose _______ cGray field _______

Chemotherapy–protocol_________

Sleep history:

sleep before brain tumor diagnosis

age of child, bedtime, wake time, naps

problems with sleep—sleep onset, snore/obstructive sleep apnea, awakenings, circadian—regularity, timing

Current sleep history:

Sleep log—2 weeks,

Bedtime—weekday/weekend

Wake time—weekday/weekend

Preferred vacation sleep schedule—timing, duration

Sleep onset—restless legs, fears, pain, parents present or not, hypnogogic hallucinations, sleep-onset paralysis,

Sleep—snore/obstructive sleep apnea, central sleep apnea, choke, vomit, seizures, enuresis, sleepwalking, confusional arousals, night terrors, nightmares, sleep eating, awakenings, response to awakenings by parents cataplexy

Past medical history current medications—what medications have been used for sleep? With what success?

Caffeine use—type (pop, coffee, tea, energy drinks), amount

Recreational drugs—nicotine, alcohol, marijuana, other–use/abuse

Hospitalizations—

Allergies—

HEENT—eye-visual impairment, blindness

ENT—ear infections, enlarged tonsils and adenoids, strep infections, sinusitis, chronic mouth breathing, difficulty swallowing, aspiration/choking on food

Cardiopulmonary—asthma, pneumonia, heart disease, cardiotoxic chemotherapy

Gastrointestinal—reflux, vomiting, abdominal pain, constipation, diarrhea

Neuro—headaches, seizures, hypotonia, hypertonia, developmental/cognitive/behavioral problems, pain

School—grade, academic performance, behavior

Endocrine Deficiencies—thyroid, growth hormone, cortisol, sex hormones, diabetes insipidus, diabetes, replacement hormones, obesity

Caregivers involved—cancer long-term follow-up clinic, psychiatry/psychology, pediatrics, endocrinology, social work

such as the anti-mGluR1 antibody; and (c) those that havebeen found in both cancer and noncancer-associated syndromes, such as the anti-nicotinic acetylcholine receptor antibody, the anti-voltage gated calcium channel antibody and the anti-voltage gated potassium channel (VGKC) antibody [52]. The pathogenesis of neurological dysfunction in these syndromes is still unclear.

Disruption of sleep-wake function from paraneoplastic antibodies has been recognized only recently [53,54], with VGKC antibodies implicated in this process. Montiel et al have described a patient with limbic encephalitis related to VGKC antibodies, who presented with confusion, partial seizures, hyperintensity in one mesial temporal lobe and hippocampal atrophy in the other, along with insomnia, hypothermia, and absence of rapid eye movement (REM) sleep [53]. Treatment with intravenous immunoglobulin and methylprednisolone led to resolution of symptoms and the reappearance of REM sleep. REM sleep behavior disorder accompanying limbic encephalitis and voltage gated potassium channels has been described in another adult patient by Lin et al [54].

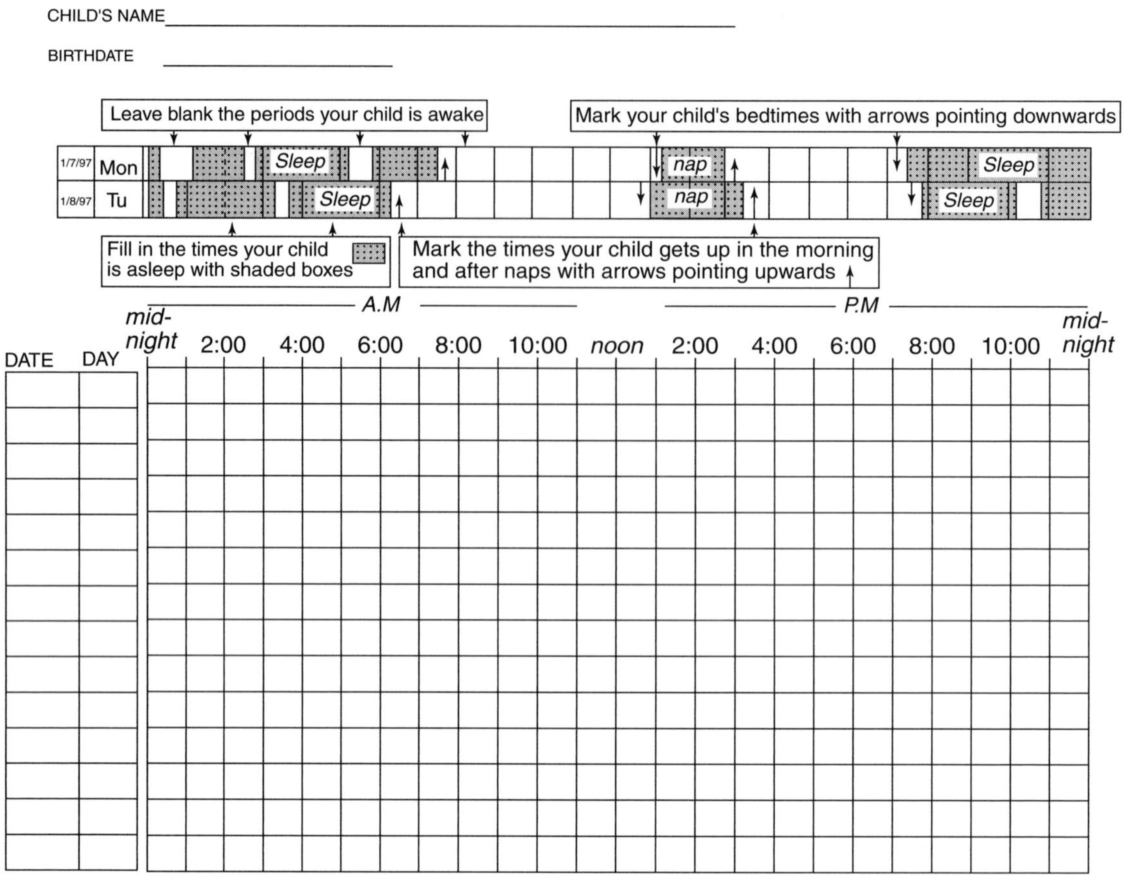

Figure 11.5 Sleep log.

References

1. Saper C, Scammell T, Lu J. Hypothalamic regulation of sleep and circadian rhythms. *Nature*. 2005; 437:1257–1263.
2. Fuller PM, Gooley JJ, Saper CB. Neurobiology of the sleep-wake cycle: sleep architecture, circadian regulation, and regulatory feedback. *J Biol Rhythms*. 2006;21(6):482–493.
3. Oeffinger K, Mertens A, Sklar C, et al. Chronic health conditions in adult survivors of childhood cancer. *N Engl J Med*. 2006;355(15):1572–1582.
4. Feig, SA, Gamis AS, Hord JD, et al. Long-term follow-up care for pediatric cancer survivors. *Pediatrics*. 2009;123:906–915.
5. Rosen G, Brand SR. Sleep in children with cancer: case series of 70 children evaluated in a comprehensive pediatric sleep center. *Support Care Cancer*. 2010;DOI 10.1007/s00520-010-0921-y.
6. Song Y, Smaulski T, Van Dyke T. Cancer: a conceptual framework. In: DeVita V, Lawrence T, Rosenberg S, eds. *Cancer: Principles & Practices of Oncology*. 8th ed. Philadelphia, PA: Lippincott Williams & Wilkins; 2008:3–12.
7. Weinberg RA. The Biology of Cancer. New York: Garland Science, Taylor & Francis Group, LLC; 2007:25–56.
8. Central CBTRUS (2005). Statistical Report: Primary Brain Tumors in the United States, 1998–2002. Published by the Central Brain Tumor Registry of the United States.
9. Reis L, Eisner M, Kosary C, et al. *SEER Cancer Statistics Review, 1975–2002*. Bethesda, MD: National Cancer Institute; 2005.
10. Rorke LB, Gilles FH, Davis RL, et al. Revision of the World Health Organization classification of brain tumors for childhood brain tumors. *Cancer*. 1985;56:1869–1886.
11. Muller H, Handwerker G, Gebhardt U, et al. Melatonin treatment in obese patients with craniopharyngioma and increased sleepiness. *Cancer Causes Control*. 2007;17:583–589.
12. Puget S, Garnett M, Wray A, et al. Pediatric craniopharyngiomas: classification and treatment according to the degree of hypothalamic involvement. *J Neurosurg: Pediatrics*. 2007;106:3–12.
13. Blaney SM, Kun LE, Hunter J, et al. Tumors of the central nervous system. In: Pizzo PA, Poplack DG,

eds. *Principles and Practice of Pediatric Oncology*. 5th ed. Philadelphia, PA: Lippincott; 2006: 786–865.
14. Hockenberry-Eaton M, Hinds P. Fatigue in children and adolescents with cancer: evolution of a program of study. *Semin Oncol Nurs*. 2000;16:261–272.
15. Hinds P, Hockenberry M, Gattuso J, et al. Dexamethasone alters sleep and fatigue in pediatric patients with acute lymphoblastic leukemia. *Cancer*. 2007;110:2321–2330.
16. Harris J, Carel C, Rosenberg L, Joshi P, Leventhal BG. Intermittent high dose corticosteroid treatment in childhood cancer: behavioral and emotional consequences. *J Am Acad Child Psychol*. 1986:25(1): 120–124.
17. Drigan R, Spirito A, Gelber R. Behavioral effects of corticosteroids with acute lymphoblastic leukemia. *Med Pediatr Oncol*. 1992;20:13–21.
18. Meeske K, Siegel S, Globe D, Mack WJ, Bernstein L. Prevalence and correlates of fatigue in long-term survivors of childhood leukemia. *Clin Oncol*. 2005;23(24):5501–5510.
19. Rosen GM, Bendel AE, Neglia JP, Moertel CL, Mahowald M. Sleep in children with neoplasms of the central nervous system: case review of 14 children. *Pediatrics*. 2003;112(1):e46-e54.
20. Rosen GM. Sleep in children with cancer. *Sleep Biol Rhythms*. 2007;5:A73.
21. Von Economo C. Sleep as a problem of localization. *J Nerv Ment Dis*. 1930;71:249–259.
22. Moruzzi G, Magoun H. Brainstem reticular formation and activation of the EEG. *Electroencephalogr Clin Neurol*. 1949;1:455–473.
23. Saper C, Scammell T, Lu J. Hypothalamic regulation of sleep and circadian rhythms. *Nature*. 2005;437:1257–1263.
24. Nishino S, Kanbayashi T. Symptomatic narcolepsy, cataplexy and hypersomnia, and their implications in the hypothalamic hypocretin/orexin system. *Sleep Med Rev*. 2005;9:269–310.
25. Filipski E, Li XM, Levi F. Disruption of circadian coordination and malignant growth. *Cancer Causes Control*. 2006;17:509–514.
26. Ryan J. Radiation somnolence syndrome. *J Pediatr Oncol Nurs*. 2000:17:50–53.
27. Faithful S, Brada M. Somnolence syndrome in adults following cranial irradiation for primary brain tumors. *Clin Oncol*. 1998;10:250–254.
28. Jereczek-Fossa BA, Marsiglia HR, Orecchia R. Radiotherapy-related fatigue. *Crit Rev Hemat/ Oncol*. 2002;41:317–325.
29. Someren E, Swart-Heikens J, Endert E, et al. Long term effect of cranial irradiation for childhood malignancy on sleep in adulthood. *Eur J Endocrinol*. 2004;150:503–510.
30. National Comprehensive Cancer Network Practice Guidelines. *Cancer-Related Fatigue Panel 2004 Guidelines*. 2004.
31. Kline N, DeSwarte J, McCarthy P. Mock V, Mosher RB, O'Neill JB. Consensus statements: research on fatigue in children with cancer. *Semin Oncol Nurs*. 2000;16:277–278.
32. Cella D, Davis K, Breibart W, Curt G, Fatigue Coalition. Cancer related fatigue: prevalence of proposed diagnostic criteria in a United States sample of cancer survivors. *J Clin Oncol*. 2001;19(14):3385–3391.
33. Hockenberry MJ, Hinds PS, Barrera P, et al. Three instruments to assess fatigue in children with cancer: the child, parent, and staff perspective. *J Pain Symptom Manage*. 2003;25:319–328.
34. Meeske K, Katz ER, Burwinkle T, Varni JW. Parent proxy-reported health related quality of life and fatigue in pediatric patients diagnosed with brain tumors and acute lymphoblastic leukemia. *Cancer*. 2004;101:2116–2125.
35. Morrow G, Shelke A, Roscoe J, Hickok JT, Mustian K. Management of cancer related fatigue. *Cancer Invest*. 2005;23(3):229–239.
36. Varni JW, Burwinkle TM, Katz ER, et al. The PEDS QL in pediatric cancer. *Cancer*. 2002;94:2090–2106.
37. Hinds PS, Hockenberry M, Rai SN, et al. Nocturnal awakenings, sleep environment interruptions, and fatigue in hospitalized children with cancer. *Oncol Nurs Forum*. 2007;34:393–402.
38. Brooks L. Obstructive sleep apnea syndrome in infants and children: clinical features and pathophysiology. In: Sheldon S, Ferber R, Kryger M, eds. *Principles and Practice of Pediatric Sleep Medicine*. Philadelphia, PA: Elsevier; 2005:223–231.
39. Woodson B. Physiology of sleep disordered breathing. In: Lee-Chiong T, ed. *Sleep: A Comprehensive Handbook*. Hoboken, NJ: Wiley; 2006:215.
40. Gregory A, Rijsdik F, Dahl R, McGuffin P, Eley TC. Associations between sleep problems, anxiety, and depression in twins at 8 years of age. *Pediatrics*. 2006;118(3):1124–1132.
41. Alfano C, Beidel D, Turner S, Lewin DS. Preliminary evidence for sleep complaints among children referred for anxiety. *Sleep Med*. 2006; 7:467–473.
42. Kazak A, Kassam-Adams N, Schneider S, Zelikovsky N, Alderfer MA, Rourke M. An integrative model of pediatric medical traumatic stress. *J Pediatr Clin Psychol*. 2006;31:343–355.
43. Langeveld N, Grootenhuis M, Voute P, de Haan RJ. Posttraumatic stress symptoms in adult survivors of childhood cancer. *Pediatr Blood Cancer*. 2004;42:604–610.
44. Miser A, McCalla J, Dothage JA, Wesley M, Miser JS. Pain as a presenting symptom in children and young adults with newly diagnosed malignancy. *Pain*. 1987;29:85–90.
45. Smith M, Haythornthwaite JA. How do sleep disturbance and chronic pain inter-relate? Insight's from the longitudinal and cognitive-behavioral clinical trials literature. *Sleep Med Rev*. 2004; 8:119–132.
46. Beck S, Dudley W, Barsevick A. Pain, sleep disturbance, and fatigue in patients with cancer: using a mediation model to test a symptom cluster. *Oncol Nurs Forum*. 2005;32:E48–E55.
47. Thompson Healthcare. *Physicians Desk Reference*. 57th ed. Montvale, NJ: Medical Economics Company; 2003.

48. Goldman A, Hewitt M, Collins GS, et al. Symptoms in children/young people with progressive malignant disease: United Kingdom Children's Cancer Study Group/Paediatric Oncology Nurses Forum Study. *Pediatrics*. 2006;117(6):e1179–e1186.
49. Jalmsell L, Kreicbergs U, Onelov E, Steineck G, Henter JI. Symptoms affecting children with malignancies during the last month of life: a nationwide follow-up. *Pediatrics*. 2006;117(4):1314–1320.
50. Hauri P, Sateia M. *The International Classification of Sleep Disorders Diagnostic and Coding Manual*. 2nd ed. Westchester, IL: AASM; 2005.
51. Rosen G. Evaluation of the patient who has sleep complaints: a case based method using the sleep process matrix. *Prim Care Clin Office Pract*. 2005; 32:319–328.
52. Pelosof MC, Gerber DE. Paraneoplastic syndromes: an approach to diagnosis and treatment. *Mayo Clin Proc*. 2010;85(9):838–854.
53. Montiel P, Sellal F, Cleric C, Richard P, Battailard M. Limbic encephalitis with severe sleep disorder associated with voltage gated potassium channel (VGKC) antibodies. *Rev Neurol (Paris)*. 2008;164(2):181–184.
54. Lin FC, Liu CK, Hsu CY. Rapid-eye-movement sleep behavior disorder secondary to acute, aseptic limbic encephalitis. *J Neurol*. 2009;256(7): 1174–1176.

CHAPTER 12

Narcolepsy

Marcin Zarowski, Suresh Kotagal, and Sanjeev V. Kothare

Introduction

Narcolepsy is a life-long neurological, rapid eye movement (REM) sleep disorder characterized by excessive daytime sleepiness (EDS) and abnormal sleep-wake cycle regulation. According to the *International Classification of Sleep Disorders*, second edition (ICSD-2), narcolepsy is typically associated with cataplexy and/or other REM sleep phenomena such as hypnagogic or hypnopompic hallucinations and sleep paralysis [1].

Cataplexy is characterized by sudden onset of bilateral muscle weakness of short duration and often precipitated by emotions, such as laughter, anger, or surprise. Consciousness typically remains intact with good recall memory [2].

Dreamlike visual, acoustic, and sensory hallucinations are characterized as hypnagogic when they occur at the sleep onset and hypnopompic when experienced at awakening from sleep. Sleep paralysis is the inability to move on waking for seconds to minutes. These symptoms occur at the sleep-wake transition and are because of intrusion of REM sleep onto wakefulness [2].

People with narcolepsy usually have a sudden onset of irresistible sleep attacks during the day [2]. These sleep attacks are usually longer in children than in adults [3].

Narcolepsy was first time described in 1880, by the French physician, Jean-Baptiste-Edouard Gélineau (1828–1906) as a syndrome of an imperative need to sleep suddenly and for brief periods, recurring at more or less close intervals. He first coined the term "narcolepsie" [4]. In 1934, Daniels published a review and emphasized the associations of EDS, cataplexy, hypnagogic hallucinations, and sleep paralysis [5]. This review is considered as one of the most insightful clinical masterpiece published to this date [6]. In 1957, Yoss and Daly called these symptoms "the clinical tetrad" [7]. In the 1950s and 1960s, the duality of sleep with REM and non-REM sleep was recognized in normal people and sleep-onset REM was described in patients with narcolepsy [8].

Epidemiology

Narcolepsy is not an uncommon disorder, but certainly underrecognized. There is variability in the estimations of the prevalence of narcolepsy in various countries. It has an estimated prevalence of 0.047%, based on representative sample of 5 European countries in the general population using the minimal set of criteria proposed by the ICSD [9]. According to other studies, the prevalence is from 0.02% to 0.067% in North America [10–13], and in the Western Europe-Italian cohort it is 0.03% [14]. In the Finnish twin cohort study, the prevalence was 0.026% [15], and in a Norway cohort, it was 0.022% [16]. The Jewish population is known for its low rate of HLA-DR2 and low prevalence of narcolepsy [17,18], and an Israeli study found a prevalence at 0.00023% [19]. A study performed in Korea set the prevalence of narcolepsy with cataplexy in that country at 0.015% [20]. In Saudi Arabia, the prevalence was estimated to be 0.04% [21], and in Southern (Hong Kong) China it was between 0.015% and 0.034% [22,23]. A study performed in Japan recorded the highest reported figure from 0.16% to 0.59% [24,25].

Age of Onset

Symptoms of narcolepsy typically start in childhood and young adults. Narcolepsy can begin in infancy or as late as old age, but most commonly before the age of 25 [26] and often in childhood [2,27]. Retrospective studies suggest that about half of the adults with narcolepsy had the onset of symptoms much earlier in their youth [3,28]. The clinical severity of narcolepsy on the other hand does not depend on the age at onset [29]. The Ohayon study confirmed peak frequency of the first symptom of narcolepsy between 15 and 19 years of age for daytime sleepiness and cataplexy [28]. A clinic-based study of narcoleptics in Quebec and France suggested a bimodal pattern of age of onset, with a larger peak in the second decade and a smaller peak in the fourth decade [30]. The Silber study from Minnesota has shown that narcolepsy commences most frequently in the second decade with incidence rates more than twice that seen in the third decade and more than 3 times that seen in the first and fourth decades [11,31].

Gender Differences

Most studies suggest that narcolepsy is more common in men as compared with women, independent of age of onset [9,15,32]. Other case-based series have also suggested a male predominance [5,30]. In 2002, Silber showed a male predominance (1.8:1) in the prevalence of narcolepsy in Olmsted County, Minnesota [11]. In a pediatric referral clinic in North China there was also a 3:1 male to female preponderance [33].

Genetic Factors

Both genetic and environmental factors are involved in the pathogenesis of narcolepsy. Contribution of environmental factors in the development of narcolepsy has been well documented [34,35].

The importance of genetic factors in narcolepsy has been addressed for more than 60 years [36]. The risk of narcolepsy in first-degree relatives is 1% to 2%, compared with 0.02% to 0.18% in the general population [34,35,37–39]. The results vary from 6% to 40% amongst narcoleptic individuals who have a close relative afflicted with the disease [34,35,37–39]. Genetic factors are only partially influential, however, as among monozygotic twins, involvement of both siblings in the pair by narcolepsy occurs only approximately 25% to 31% of the subjects [40–44].

According to some authors [30], the age at onset clearly differentiates patients with a positive family history of narcolepsy who have an earlier onset from those without a family history, in whom the disease becomes manifest at a later age.

Narcolepsy has the highest human leukocyte antigens (HLA) association among all medical diseases, with the link to haplotype DRB1*1501, DQA1*0102, and DQB1*0602 being the most prominent. This association varies with ethnicity. DR2 is found in 100% of Japanese, 90% to 95% of whites, and 60% of African American narcoleptic subjects with cataplexy [34,45]. High-resolution mapping of these regions has demonstrated the existence of numerous alleles. DQB1*0602, a DQ1 subtype allele, is strongly linked with narcolepsy. The extraordinarily high association (99.6% among 461 Japanese narcoleptic patients) of narcolepsy with HLA-DR2(15) and DQ1(6), or in terms of DNA, with DRB1*1501 and DQB1*0602 was reported by Honda [42]. DQB1*0602 is found in 88% to 98% of narcoleptic subjects with unambiguous cataplexy, whereas it is found in only 12% of white American and 38% of African American controls [46,47]. This allele is found in only 40% of narcolepsy without cataplexy [41].

Testing for DQB1*0602 can be helpful, especially in patients with questionable cataplexy, but this allele is hardly predictive of narcolepsy because greater than 99% of DQB1*0602–positive individuals do not have narcolepsy [48].

Watson et al. recently found a dose-response relationship between HLA-DQB1*0602 allele status and measures of narcolepsy symptom severity and suggest that HLA-DQ may function as a disease-modifying gene [49]. They observed a linear relationship between HLA-DQB1*0602 frequency and sleepiness as defined by the Epworth Sleepiness Scale (ESS), narcolepsy severity as defined by Ullanlinna Narcolepsy Scale (UNS), age of symptom onset, and sleep latency [49].

Family studies of narcolepsy have reported an increased prevalence of EDS with idiopathic central nervous system (CNS) hypersomnia, which suggested that a spectrum of phenotypes exists across narcolepsy with cataplexy, narcolepsy without cataplexy, and idiopathic hypersomnia [34,35,38,39,50,51].

Pathophysiology

Narcolepsy is a disorder of regulation of REM sleep. Both REM sleep and wakefulness share certain neurophysiological traits, including a low-voltage electroencephalogram (EEG), similar evoked responses to sensory stimuli, and activation of brain motor and autonomic control systems [52,53]. High-amplitude theta activity in the hippocampus, characteristic of REM sleep, is also present during cataplexy [54]. However, there are also striking differences between the 2 states. During REM sleep, central motor systems are highly active, whereas motoneurons are hyperpolarized, leading to a reduction of muscle tone [55]. Lesions in the ventrolateral periaqueductal gray matter and the dorsolateral pontine tegmentum (locus ceruleus) can lead to REM sleep without atonia as both regions contain cells that turn off REM sleep. A third area, lesions of which can also produce REM sleep without atonia is the nucleus reticularis gigantocellularis. This nucleus is responsible for the "stilling" phenomenon, and suppression of activity of the spinal motor neurons [56]. A recent study suggests that inhibition of motor output is accompanied by a neurochemically similar inhibition of sensory relays during REM sleep [57].

Neurotransmitter Dysfunction

The 2 systems of neurons normally continuously interact to produce the alteration between REM and non-REM sleep. Aminergic neurons (REM-off) located in the dorsal raphe nuclei (serotoninergic) and the locus coeruleus (noradrenergic) produce inhibitory postsynaptic potentials on cholinergic (REM-on) neurons located in the mesencephalic, medullary, and pontine gigantocellular tegmental regions. Muscle atonia is produced by direct stimulation of pontomedullary reticular formation neurons that produce inhibitory postsynaptic potentials at the level of the anterior horn cell [58].

The possible substrate for the differences between the behavioral and physiological conditions in waking and REM sleep is the activity of monoaminergic neurons. The histaminergic cells are continuously and maximally active in waking but are minimally active or silent in REM sleep [59]. Further evidence for links between narcolepsy and REM sleep comes from studies of neuronal activity during cataplexy. The cessation of activity of these monoaminergic neurons might underlie the loss of muscle tone and loss of environmental awareness characteristic of REM sleep [54]. Cells that are maximally active in REM sleep (REM-on cells) are present in the pontine inhibitory area and also in the region of the medial medulla, which receives pontine inhibitory area projections [60]. Many of the same cell populations in the pons and medulla that are tonically active only during REM sleep in normal individuals become active during cataplexy in narcoleptics [61,62]. Histamine-containing cells are localized to the tuberomammillary region of the posterior hypothalamus in rats, cats, and humans [63–66]. Histaminergic cells actually increase discharge in cataplexy relative to quiet waking levels [54]. Cells that cease discharge in REM sleep (REM-off) have been recorded in posterior hypothalamic regions that contain histamine-immunoreactive cells [65]. The maintained activity of histamine neurons is a likely substrate for the maintenance of consciousness during cataplexy that distinguishes cataplexy from REM sleep [56]. The role of reduced serotonin release in the suppression of muscle tone has been investigated in the hypoglossal nucleus of the rat [67–69]. Located in the hypothalamus, hypocretin (Hcrt) neurons contribute to the regulation of the activity of norepinephrine, serotonin, histamine, and acetylcholine cell groups and have potent effects on arousal and motor control [56]. Hypocretin-1 (Hcrt-1) neurons also project to noradrenergic "REM-off" cells of the locus coeruleus [70], thus loss of Hcrt can lead to both impaired arousal and loss of inhibition of REM sleep.

Hcrt Pathway

In 1998, 2 groups of investigators simultaneously discovered a pair of closely related neuropeptides that may provide a stabilizing influence needed to help regulation of sleep and waking [71–73]. One group named this peptide orexin for its presumed role in appetite, whereas another group named it Hcrt for its possible resemblance to secretin [72,73].

DeLecea et al identified the preprohypocretin transcript using a directional tagged polymerase chain reaction subtraction technique [73]. They also suggested a possible role in feeding regulation based on the neuroanatomical localization in the lateral hypothalamus. The existence of Hcrts was independently confirmed by Sakurai [72] who also identified and mapped 2 receptors for these peptides [6]. Sakurai et al called this 33–amino acid peptide orexin-A, whereas a second peptide (28 amino acid sharing 13/28 amino acids identical with orexin-A) was called orexin-B [72]. Preprohypocretin is produced as a precursor and is split into 2 different peptides, Hcrt-1 and Hcrt-2. Hcrts bind to 2 G-coupled Hcrt receptors, which have been mapped to human chromosomes 1p33 and 6cen [74].

In 1999, 2 independent groups of investigators again simultaneously found that a lack of Hcrts or their type 2 receptor can cause symptoms of narcolepsy in experimental animals [75,76]. Lin and colleagues found exon-skipping mutations in the ox2 receptor gene probably resulting in a nonfunctional receptor [75]. They thus reported for the first time canine narcolepsy, which being phenotypically similar to human narcolepsy, was linked to alterations in Hcrt function [75]. Furthermore, in Doberman dogs, intravenous administration of Hcrt-1 reduced cataplexy and normalized sleep and waking duration [77]. It was found that nasal administration of the peptide reversed sleepiness in monkeys [78]. Meanwhile, Yanagisawa's group found that preprohypocretin knockout mice or mice lacking the hyopocretin receptors have a phenotype strongly resembling human narcolepsy. These mice displayed behavioral symptoms and electroencephalographic features consistent with narcolepsy [76], with brief periods of wakefulness, frequent transitions into REM sleep, and behaviors resembling cataplexy [76,79,80].

In 2001, it was reported that humans who have narcolepsy with cataplexy have few Hcrt neurons in the posterolateral hypothalamus, and levels of Hcrt-1 were undetectable in the cerebrospinal fluid (CSF) in most patients with narcolepsy with cataplexy [71,81–84]. Nishino and colleagues very quickly confirmed that most narcoleptic subjects with cataplexy have impaired Hcrt signaling [85]. Low CSF Hcrt-1 has also been shown to be very specific for patients with HLA-DQB1*0602–positive narcolepsy with cataplexy and is noted from the very early stages of the disease [86,87]. Approximately 90% of narcolepsy subjects with cataplexy have no detectable Hcrt-1 in their CSF, even within a few months of symptom onset [84–86,88–90]. Low CSF Hcrt-1 is thus highly specific (99.1%) and sensitive (88.5%) for narcolepsy with cataplexy [89]. Hcrt deficiency is rare in HLA-DQB1*0602–negative patients [91]. Levels of Hcrt-1 lesser than 110 pg/mL have been shown to be diagnostic of narcolepsy-cataplexy, whereas levels above 200 pg/mL are considered normal. In healthy subjects, Hcrt-1 levels in the CSF are highly constant over a large age range [86] (Figure 12.1). In addition, an undetectable Hcrt-1 level in the CSF is one of the most important diagnostic features of narcolepsy-cataplexy in children as well [85, 92,93].

The Hcrts may be the major sleep-modulating neurotransmitters and could potentially provide a

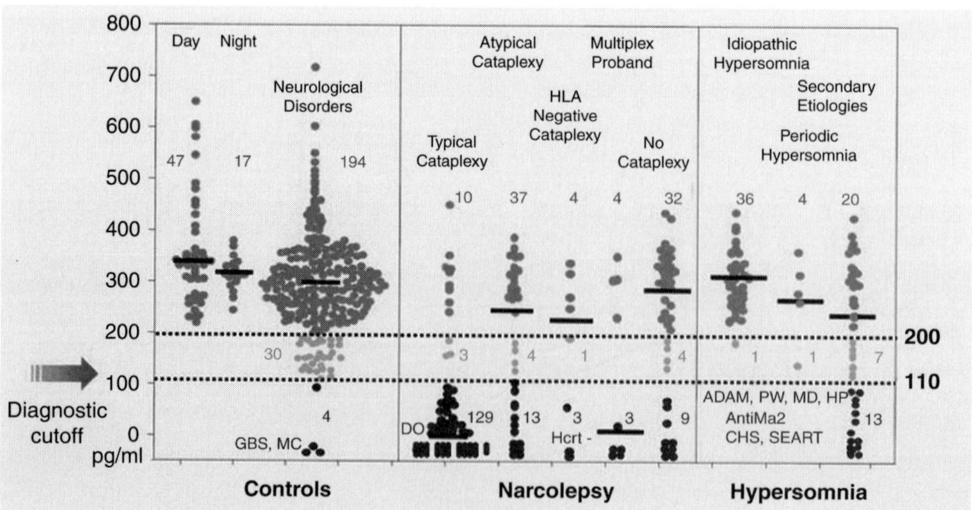

Figure 12.1 Cerebrospinal fluid hypocretin levels in diverse conditions [89].

novel therapeutic approach to the treatment of narcolepsy [26]. Wakefulness is promoted by aminergic brain regions such as the locus coeruleus, which diffusely activate the cortex, and by cholinergic regions that produce thalamic activation, allowing flow of information to and from the cortex. Hcrts are produced exclusively by a cluster of neurons only in the posterior half of the lateral hypothalamus [72,73,94]. They have ascending projections to the cerebral cortex, as well as descending projections to all the monoaminergic and cholinergic cell groups of the arousal systems, and Hcrt increases the firing rates of aminergic neurons in vitro [71,76,95–97] (Figure 12.2). In the absence of Hcrt-mediated facilitation of forebrain arousal centers, the waking periods are truncated, resulting in the sleepiness of narcolepsy [98]. Hcrt-containing neurons heavily innervate brain regions involved in the control of wakefulness, appetite, thermoregulation, and autonomic control [76,95], and Hcrts have excitatory effects on postsynaptic neurons [73,96]. Recent animal studies provide considerable evidence that orexin promotes wakefulness and inhibits REM sleep [48]. The Hcrt neurons are predominantly active during wakefulness and especially during motor activity when animals actively explore their environment [99–101]. The extracellular concentrations of Hcrt are higher during periods of wakefulness [102]. The injection of Hcrt-1 into the lateral ventricles increases wakefulness, food intake, body temperature, and sympathetic activity [72,96,103,104].

In a study in normal animals, it was identified that Hcrt neurons fire maximally during active waking [100]. Hcrt cells are silent in slow-wave sleep. Hcrt cells discharge in active waking and have maximal activity during exploratory behavior [100]. This discharge was reduced or absent during aversive waking situations, even if the EEG indicated high levels of alertness.

This is consistent with the hypothesis that these cells are activated during emotional and sensorimotor conditions similar to those

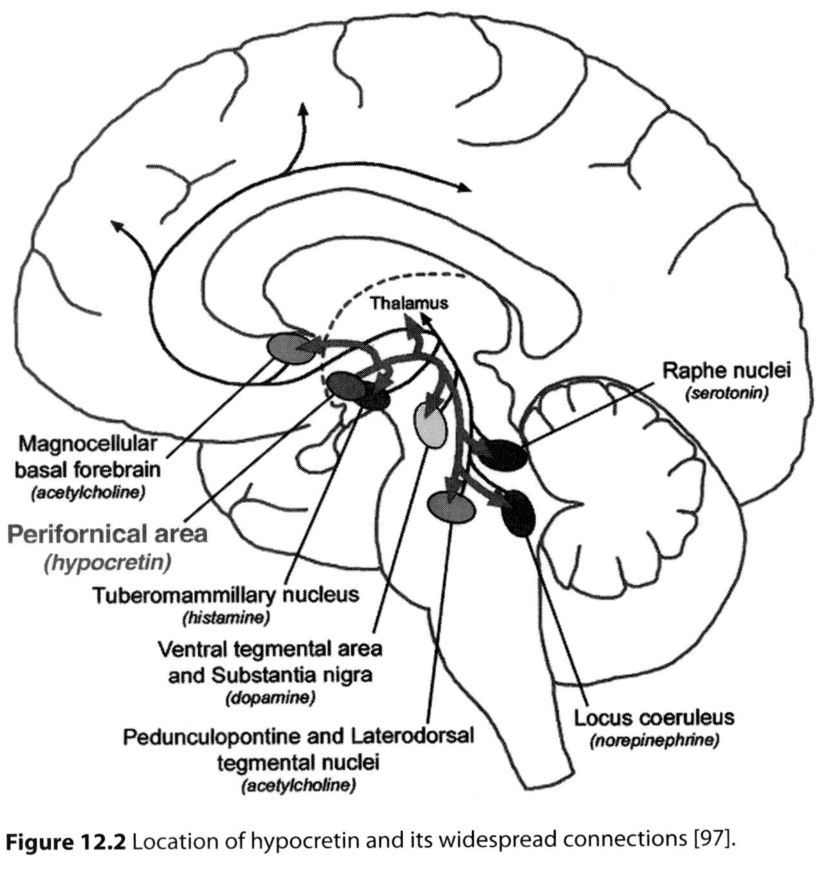

Figure 12.2 Location of hypocretin and its widespread connections [97].

that trigger cataplexy in narcoleptic animals [98,100,105,106]. Studies of Hcrt release are also consistent with this hypothesis [60,107]. In the absence of the Hcrt-mediated motor facilitation, muscle tone is lost at these times.

As yet, the etiology of the focal neurodegenerative process affecting Hcrt neurons in the lateral hypothalamus remains unknown. Impaired Hcrt signaling may produce insufficient activation of these wake-promoting areas, resulting in poorly sustained wakefulness. Autopsy studies of patients with narcolepsy have shown only about 10% of the normal number of Hcrt neurons in the lateral hypothalamus [82,83]. Peyron et al showed a complete disappearance of Hcrt mRNA in the perifornical hypothalamus of narcoleptic patients [83]. However, the number of astrocytes may be moderately increased in the Hcrt neuron region [82,108]. The presence of gliosis in this region is thought to imply a possible neurodegenerative or inflammatory process [82]. As follows from experimental studies [109], the decline of CSF Hcrt level in neurotoxically induced lesions of Hcrt neurons in rats starts very early (2–6 days) after neurotoxin, Hcrt-2 saporin is applied to the lateral hypothalamus, and this effect is permanent without any recovery [109]. A loss of 73% of Hcrt neurons causes a 50% decline in CSF Hcrt. On average, 90% of these cells are lost in narcoleptic patients with undetectable CSF [60]. Subsequently, it was discovered that a lesser reduction in the number of Hcrt cells was seen in Parkinson's disease, with a loss of up to 60% of Hcrt cells [110–112] (Figure 12.1).

Autoimmune Hypothesis

Very few disorders have been found in which CSF Hcrt-1 level less than 110 pg/mL can be present; 2 of these were autoimmune in nature. Two children with Guillain-Barre syndrome and 1 each with acute disseminated encephalomyelitis had low Hcrt levels [113–115]. Interestingly, the CSF of subjects with narcolepsy lacks increased protein or oligoclonal bands, and their serum lacks autoantibodies [116–118]. Recent studies have focused on the Hcrt system as possible autoantibody targets. Autoantibodies against the Hcrt were discovered; however, autoantibody-mediated dysfunction of the Hcrt system has not been demonstrated in patients with narcolepsy [119]. Black et al screened for IgG antibodies to preprohypocretin and Hcrt-1 and -2 [120,121] and found that their results did not support the hypothesis that narcolepsy is caused by autoantibodies directed against preprohypocretin or its peptide cleavage products. Several other studies have also not provided evidence for a humoral immune response against the Hcrt system in narcolepsy [122]. Microglia and TNF-alpha mRNA are not increased in the hypothalami of narcoleptic subjects examined decades after the onset of symptoms [83].

Streptococcal infections may initiate or catalyze an autoimmune response against Hcrt cells in narcolepsy [123]. Post-streptococcal diseases have also been linked to brain autoimmune diseases, most notably Sydenham chorea, obsessive-compulsive disorder, and tics [124]. Aran et al suggest that selective streptococcal infections may lead to the destruction of Hcrt neurons via molecular mimicry or superantigen interactions with the HLA-TCR complex [123]. A recent study by Tanaka and Honda show significant decrease in the total serum IgG levels observed in a subgroup of patients with narcolepsy. The HLA-DQB1*0602 allele contributes to the decrease in the serum total IgG levels. They also found IgG subclass alterations in narcolepsy, suggesting IgG3- and IgG4-related abnormal IgG maturation in narcolepsy [125].

Thus, the autoimmune hypothesis provides a rationale for the initiation of immunomodulating therapies near disease onset in an attempt to prevent the progression of cell loss and induce a long-lasting improvement [122,126–132]. If the autoimmune role in the development of narcolepsy is confirmed to be true, effective immunosuppressive therapy should be initiated at the earliest and continued in an ongoing manner to prevent recurrence, as done in other autoimmune diseases [3].

Clinical Features of Narcolepsy

The classic tetrad of narcolepsy consists of EDS, cataplexy, hypnagogic hallucinations, and sleep paralysis. However, this clear-cut, classic picture seems to be unusual in the early stages of the disorder [133]. The initial and sole manifestation of narcolepsy usually is hypersomnia followed by development of other symptoms months to years later [11,27,81,134–137]. In addition, sleep fragmentation has been recognized as a fifth but commonly present criterion in the diagnosis of narcolepsy [1].

Diagnostic criteria have been recently updated to define narcolepsy with cataplexy, narcolepsy without cataplexy, and narcolepsy caused by another underlying medical condition [1].

Diagnostic Criteria for Narcolepsy [1]

1. Narcolepsy with cataplexy
   - EDS (almost daily for at least 3 months)
   - Definite history of cataplexy
   - Multiple sleep latency test (MSLT; mean sleep latency [MSL] should be ≤8 minutes and at least 2 sleep-onset REM periods [SOREMPs]) or CSF Hcrt-1 level (≤110 pg/mL or 1/3 of mean normal controls) optional but advised
   - Hypersomnia not better explained by another disorder or medication
2. Narcolepsy without cataplexy
   - EDS (almost daily for at least 3 months)
   - Typical cataplexy is not present
   - Abnormal MSLT required (MSL should be ≤8 minutes and at least 2 SOREMPs)
   - Hypersomnia not better explained by another disorder or medication
3. Narcolepsy caused by medical condition
   - EDS (almost daily for at least 3 months)
   - Definite history of cataplexy, abnormal MSLT, or low CSF Hcrt-1 levels.
   - Underlying medical or neurological disorder accounts for daytime sleepiness
   - Hypersomnia not better explained by another disorder or medication.

Excessive Daytime Sleepiness

It is very important to consider narcolepsy in the differential diagnosis of hypersomnia, especially in younger patients, because it can take up to 20 years between the initial onset of the sleepiness and the subsequent development of the full clinical syndrome. Hypersomina usually begins with EDS and unintentional naps in the teens and early twenties [11,135]. Patients usually report dream content during these short naps [81]. The duration of the episode may vary from a few minutes to over an hour [2]. Such sleep attacks are refreshing on awakening [138]. Daytime naps, which are normal in younger children, compound the difficulty in recognizing the EDS in the pediatric population. Such naps should cease by age 3 to 4 years, after which time persistence or reappearance of napping is significant [139]. Sleepy behavior is more often recognized by teachers who may complain of apathy in the child, whereas the parents may misjudge the behavior as normal napping. During daytime, with "REM sleep intrusion," patients can suddenly feel overwhelmingly tired and appear transiently "unaware" of their surroundings [1,27]. It may be subtle and manifest simply as difficulty getting out of bed in the morning to sudden, usually brief (10–20 min) attacks of irresistible sleep during conversations, driving, and so on [81]. Sleepiness occurs regardless of the quantity of nocturnal sleep and is typically worse in sedentary and boring situations. The intensity of sleepiness varies across the day and between individuals. As a consequence of sleepiness, patients may report inattention, poor memory, irritability, blurry vision, diplopia, and automatic behaviors such as driving without awareness [48]. Unwanted episodes of sleep recur several times daily, not only under monotonous sedentary activity but also in situations in which the individual is fully involved in a task [2].

Disrupted nighttime sleep is common in narcolepsy and may partially contribute to chronic sleepiness [81]. Narcoleptic patients with the greatest sleep disturbance have more severe daytime sleepiness, but even those with good nighttime sleep still have substantial daytime sleepiness [140]. The inability to maintain sleep at night coupled with excessive sleepiness during the day can be very frustrating to patients and family members [81].

Recently, a newly recognized subgroup of narcoleptics have been described with long sleep requirements (total sleep time >11 hours) and less than 2 SOREMPs on their MSLT and are believed to comprise 18% of subjects with narcolepsy [141]. Their symptoms combine the disabilities of both narcolepsy (severe sleepiness) and idiopathic hypersomnia (long sleep time and unrefreshing naps) [141].

An important point to note is that in young children, sleepiness can take the form of an increase rather than a reduction in activity, with the presence of irritability, aggression, and symptoms of attention deficit and hyperactivity or social withdrawal and shyness [2,81,133,134].

Cataplexy

Cataplexy is a unique feature of narcolepsy [134,138,142]. Cataplexy is the sudden muscle weakness brought on by strong emotions, particularly joking, laughter, or anger [2,3,48].

The duration of each cataplectic attack usually ranges from a few seconds to 2 minutes and rarely up to 30 minutes [2]. "Status cataplecticus" refers to the rare occurrence of prolonged attacks that often occur with abrupt withdrawal of antidepressant medications [48,139]. The frequency of cataplexy ranges from only 1 or 2 episodes per year up to dozens of episodes per day. Cataplexy occurs in 60% to 90% of patients with narcolepsy, and its onset follows the onset of sleepiness by several months to 5 years [11,32,135,143]. Sometimes the 2 develop together and, in a minority, cataplexy is the initial symptom [133].

Most commonly, cataplexy is caused by laughter or humorous experiences, although sometimes even the memory of a humorous event can precipitate an attack [2,144–147]. Other emotions can also trigger cataplexy, including anger, embarrassment, surprise, or even arousal [146,147]. The frequency of cataplexy is highly variable, ranging from a few times a year to several per day [81]. Cataplexy is associated with an inhibition of monosynaptic H-reflexes and of the multi-synaptic tendon reflexes [2]. It may result from excessive activation of these descending motor inhibitory pathways that are active during strong emotions or REM sleep [62]. It is thought that cataplexy represents appearance of REM sleep atonia during wakefulness [81].

In early childhood, cataplexy attacks are more often the complete fall type. Attacks of cataplexy may be confused with atonic seizures (drop attacks), especially in children under the age of 5 years [2,138]. In rare cases, an isolated appearance of cataplexy preceding EDS may pose a diagnostic problem as it can be misdiagnosed as Doose syndrome: astatic myoclonic epileptic seizures [2,9,148].

More commonly, attacks of cataplexy are partial, affecting only certain muscle groups, namely the arms, neck, or face [145]. During partial cataplexy attacks, the jaw may sag, the head may drop forward, and speech becomes garbled [143]. "Cataplectic facies" appearing close to disease onset predated typical cataplexy triggered by emotions in some patients and in fact has been confused with sleepiness [142].

Severe episodes produce bilateral, generalized weakness sufficient to cause a fall, although usually without injury [48]. Cataplexy may involve only certain group of muscles or the entire voluntary musculature [138]. During an attack of cataplexy, the patient is unable to move, although the diaphragm and ocular muscles are spared. Recovery is rapid without post-ictal confusion, and only occasionally does sleep supervene [81]. Preservation of consciousness and intact memory are distinctive features, which differentiate them from atonic seizures [138].

Some patients also display unconscious behaviors such as touching and scratching themselves repetitively, or shaking their heads between attacks, interpretable as an effort of trying to "shake-off" droopy sensations and activate themselves [142]. The semipermanent state of facial muscle weakness with occasional exacerbations manifests with drooping eyelids, mouth opening, and/or sudden tongue protrusion [142]. This tongue protrusion almost had the appearance of a tic because it was often spontaneous, without any emotional link [142]. One patient in the Serra study presented with wide masticatory movements and odd stuttering speech, similar to Guilleminault's case [2,142]. These facial symptoms may be misdiagnosed as tics, but they respond positively to anti-cataplectic therapy [142]. The limb involvement, labeled with the acronym of "limp man syndrome," has also been described as a manifestation of continuous cataplexy [149,150].

In rare cases, symptoms of cataplexy can be seen during the course of some inherited diseases (such as Niemann-Pick disease, type C [NPC], Prader-Willi syndrome [PWS], myotonic dystrophy), Norrie disease, and Coffin Lowry syndrome. These are also known as examples of symptomatic cataplexy [151–153].

Sleep Paralysis and Hypnagogic/Hypnopompic Hallucinations

The prevalence of sleep paralysis in narcolepsy is around 25% (from 17% to 66%) [7,50,154]; however, in the general population is estimated to be between 2.3% and 40%, with 1% to 10% experiencing multiple episode [155].

Sleep paralysis occurs because of the persistence of REM atonia after awakening [81]. Sleep paralyses are brief episodes of an inability to move, generally occurring during awakening, on falling asleep, or both [2,138]. Usually the entire body is involved, but invariably respiratory and extraocular muscles are spared. Episodes are more common in the first 2 hours of sleep and tend to occur more often again in the morning hours [155]. These peaks coincide with SOREMPs and the longer REM observed in the morning hours. The child is fully aware of this state and able to recall the event that usually lasts seconds to minutes and end spontaneously or, sometimes, after sensory stimulation (being lightly touched or spoken to), or after intense effort of the patient to "break" the paralysis [81,154]. During episodes of sleep paralysis, particularly the first occurrence, the patient may have extreme anxiety associated with a fear of dying [2]. Children are often reluctant to talk about these events [156]. Fifty percent of the episodes can be associated with hypnagogic/hypnopompic hallucinations [154]. However, both these symptoms of sleep paralysis and hypnagogic/hypnopompic hallucinations can be unrecognized or misinterpreted by young children or their parents.

Hypnagogic and hypnopompic hallucinations occur in approximately 60% of patients with narcolepsy [32,157] and in up to 36% of healthy controls [158]. Hypnagogic/hypnopompic hallucinations tend to diminish with age [159].

These are typically vivid visual, auditory dreams or out-of-body experiences and are usually frightening [139,143]. These hallucinations are usually visual, consisting of simple forms (colored circles, parts of objects, and so forth) that are constant or changing in size sometimes with reports of seeing people or animals [34,48]. Auditory hallucinations are also common and can range from a simple sound to an elaborate melody [34]. Hypnagogic/hypnopompic hallucinations are exacerbated by fatigue and emotion, often associated with sleep paralysis or cataplexy. Hypnagogic hallucinations are more frequent (89%) than the hypnopompic ones (41%), and up to a third of narcoleptic patients can present with both types [50]. Though they may occur with any disorder in which there is significant sleep disruption, when these hallucinations occur during short daytime naps, narcolepsy should be strongly suspected [81]. Hypnopompic hallucinations may be a better indicator of narcolepsy in subjects reporting EDS [160,161] and can occur on awakening from night sleep in 22% cases, during naps in 18%, and during both in 59% cases [50].

Sleep paralysis and hypnagogic/hypnopompic hallucinations do not affect all patients with narcolepsy and can be transitory.

Other Symptoms

Narcolepsy patients have abnormal night sleep, with longer non-rapid eye movement (NREM)/REM cycles, longer intervals between REM episodes, and an attenuated progression of REM sleep (ie, long episodes of REM at the beginning of the night) [162]. Disrupted nighttime sleep may be seen in association with difficulty in falling asleep, and the patients may be misdiagnosed as having insomnia [136].

Sleep terrors, frequent nightmares, and bruxism can be seen in patients with narcolepsy [139,159]. Frequent awakenings are also described, possibly associated with periodic limb movements [133].

Abnormalities in REM sleep motor regulation have been described in narcolepsy, including persistence of muscle tone, excessive twitching, and movements during sleep [27,163].

Automatic behavior refers to a symptom complex of functioning (talking, putting things away, etc.) during sleep episodes, but awakening with no memory of performing such activities and is often seen in patients with narcolepsy [81,138].

Some studies in narcoleptic patients suggest abnormalities in REM sleep motor regulation, with an increased frequency of REM sleep without atonia, phasic EMG events, and PLMS, when compared with controls [163]. The presence of REM sleep without atonia associated with prominent motor behavioral manifestations associated with dreaming during REM sleep is the key feature of a condition called REM sleep behavior disorder (RBD) [1]. The prevalence of RBD in the narcoleptic population ranges from 12% to 36% [164–168]. PLMS and PLM-related arousals were also more prevalent in narcoleptics compared with age and body mass index (BMI)–matched normal controls [169]. The PLM index (number of PLM per hour of sleep) above 5 has been found in 25% to 70% of the population with narcolepsy [169,170].

The prevalence of migraine in patients with narcolepsy is also increased [171,172]. Children suffering from headaches were noted to have a higher prevalence of EDS, narcolepsy, and insomnia than children without headaches [173].

Depression has also been reported in 30% to 50% of patients with narcolepsy [159,174,175]. It must be borne in mind that mood disorders may also be masked by antidepressant therapy used to treat symptoms of the disease [176].

Patients with narcolepsy may experience symptoms of eating disorders, with an irresistible craving for food and binge eating as the most prominent features [177,178]. Eating disorders in this situation interferes with daily activities [177]. Changes in eating behavior (rather than in calorie intake), leptin modulation, and lower basal metabolism could explain the positive energy balance leading to observed obesity in narcolepsy [178,179]. Snacking is common, with up to 80% of patients indulging in bedtime snacks, and 32% having them in the middle of the night [180].

Obesity is very common in narcolepsy, but often overlooked [135,179]. In children, the weight gain occurs quickly and suddenly after the onset of other symptoms of narcolepsy [3,181]. These patients have been found to have significantly greater BMI across various ethnic groups and cultural backgrounds [135]. Changes in eating behavior, leptin modulation, and lower basal metabolism may explain the positive energy balance [178,179].

Because of the increased weight, obstructive sleep apnea is a frequent coexisting disorder with narcolepsy with prevalence ranging from 9.8% to 19% on polysomnographic studies [140,182].

Stores et al studied psychosocial problems in children with narcolepsy [183]. They found that as compared with age-matched healthy and other hypersomnolent controls, the patients with narcolepsy showed more behavioral difficulties, depressed mood, and impairment in the quality of life.

Laboratory Findings

Evaluation of children with narcolepsy may require assessment by a pediatric sleep physician in an accredited pediatric sleep disorder center. A detailed sleep history is crucial in evaluating patients with EDS. The history combined with polysomnography (PSG) and MSLT remain the current gold standard in the diagnosis of narcolepsy in adults as well as children [81,184]. If a patient is already receiving psychotropic medications such as antidepressants that cannot be safely stopped before the MSLT, one may need to resort to lumbar puncture for measurement of the CSF Hcrt-1 level.

Sleep logs give an estimate of the number, duration, and timing of daily episodes of nocturnal sleep, daytime naps, and wake periods. These can be used to evaluate sleep-wake habits over weeks to months, including weekdays and weekends [185]. They are frequently used before the PSG and MSLT and may reveal evidence of chronically insufficient sleep [186].

Subjective measures of EDS consist of validated scales for quantifying sleepiness. Three clinical sleep scales have been used to assess sleepiness: Stanford Sleepiness Scale (SSS) [187], Epworth Sleepiness Scale (ESS) [188], and Pediatric Daytime Sleepiness Scale (PDSS) [189]. PDSS is a recently introduced validated measure for assessing sleepiness in children [189]. SSS and ESS are 2 extensively used sleep scales used to assess sleepiness in adults.

Nocturnal Polysomnogram and MSLT

Nocturnal PSG is the only diagnostic technique shown to quantify the ventilatory and sleep abnormalities associated with sleep-disordered breathing, along with an objective measure of adequate sleep efficiency above 75% [190]. Overnight polygraphic sleep records also exclude parasomnias as a cause of fragmented and nonrestorative nocturnal sleep and/or verified REM behavior disorder as one of the possible symptoms of narcolepsy [3,191]. Nocturnal PSG is obtained to rule out other sleep disturbances such as sleep-disorder breathing and periodic limb movements of sleep [192]. Moreover, continuous polysomnography can also be performed for 24 hours or more to assess the degree of sleepiness, especially in younger children incapable of undergoing MSLTs. This also serves to evaluate circadian variations in sleepiness [192].

The polysomnogram may show a short REM sleep latency [2]. Frequent arousals, periodic limb movements, and increased wakefulness after sleep onset may also be seen [81].

This overnight study with a minimum sleep efficiency more than 75% is followed the next day by MSLT in which a patient is given 4 or 5 opportunities to nap every 2 hours to assess the degree of sleepiness and timing of REM sleep onset [193]. At least 2 weeks before these studies, all central nervous stimulants, sedative hypnotics, and antidepressants should be discontinued so as not to adversely affect the results [81,184]. Details of the protocol have been recently described [138,184]. On the basis of polygraphic recording, REM sleep, which occurs within 15 minutes of sleep onset, is defined as a SOREMP [184,194]. Sleep onset was originally defined as the occurrence of 3 consecutive epochs of stage 1 NREM sleep or the first epoch of another sleep stage [193]. However, the practice parameters for MSLT interpretation have been revised recently. The recently revised criteria recommend measuring the sleep latency at the MSLT as the occurrence of a single sleep epoch [184,194]. The MSL (arithmetic mean of sleep onset of all naps) is an index of severity of sleepiness [138].

MSL scores less than 8 minutes are generally considered to be in the pathological sleepiness range; those more than 10 minutes are considered normal in adults [2]. MSLTs in children are indicated in patients with suspected narcolepsy and idiopathic hypersomnia with long sleep time. Patients with narcolepsy usually have MSL of less than 8 minutes, whereas healthy children show an MSL of 15 to 20 minutes [184].

The naps of narcolepsy subjects often include REM sleep [22]. The occurrence of these SOREMPs in 2 or more naps is highly suggestive of narcolepsy [1,184,194,195]. The combination of 2 SOREMPs and an MSL of less than 5 minutes is estimated to have a sensitivity of 70% but a specificity of 97% for narcolepsy in adults [184,194,195]. However, 30% of patients with this combination did not have narcolepsy [196].

Based on the observation that the sensitivity for the identification of 2 or more SOREMPs in patients is 70%, the American Academy of Sleep Medicine (AASM) recommends repeating MSLT testing when the patient is suspected to have narcolepsy, when earlier MSLT evaluations did not provide polygraphic confirmation, so as to increase the likelihood of recording 2 or more SOREMPs [184]. However, the reliability of MSLT for the diagnosis of narcolepsy was called into question by recent evidence that similar results can occur in up to 15% of the normal population [194,196,197].

Comparable data are not available for children and adolescents. Test properties and available normative data have recently been extensively reviewed [194]. The validity of using the same criteria in children has been questioned [198]. Children have longer MSL, whereas adolescents and young adults have the shortest MSL. In prepubertal children, MSLs of 23.7 and 26.4 minutes were found [199,200]. For these reasons, 30-minute naps in MSLT in children have been proposed on a research basis [201]. A sleep latency of 5 to 10 minutes indicates moderate daytime sleepiness, whereas lower than 5 minutes indicates severe sleepiness [192].

Limitations of the MSLT in pediatric patients are the lack of normative data in this population, the last nap effect (increased arousal because of the anticipation of going home on completion of this extensive testing), and motivation (to remain awake or attempt to sleep) [192].

Maintenance of Wakefulness Test

The Maintenance of Wakefulness Test (MWT) is indicated to assess the efficacy of treatment in patients with narcolepsy. It is the mirror image of the MSLT and considered a validated, objective measure of the ability to stay awake for a defined time [202]. Motivation of the patient to stay awake is the key for the interpretation of the results [184]. The MWT consists of 4 trials performed at 2-hour intervals, with the first trial beginning about 1.5 to 3 hours after the patient's usual wakeup time [184]. Details of the protocol have been recently described [184]. Normal values of MWT are more than 30 minutes, whereas the test is considered abnormal when it is less than 12 minutes [184,194]. Pediatric normative values are not available.

CSF Hcrt-1 Analysis

Laboratory tests such as CSF Hcrt-1 analysis and HLA typing are useful but at present are not considered mandatory for a diagnosis of narcolepsy [138,203].

CSF Hcrt-1 testing should be considered in the following situations: (1) equivocal MSLT results; (2) children younger than 8 years; (3) individuals taking psychotropic medications (eg, anti-cataplexy agents or stimulants); (4) individuals who cannot afford formal sleep testing; and (5) individuals with severe or complex psychiatric, neurological, or medical disorders, which could compromise the validity of the MSLT results [81,204]. Kanbayashi et al [23] showed that the CSF level of Hcrt-1 remains stable from early infancy up to old age; hence, an undetectable level of Hcrt-1 in CSF is a very valuable diagnostic marker in children [3]. Lower CSF levels of Hcrt-1 (<110 pg/ml) in narcoleptic patients were found [88], especially in patients with human leukocyte B1_0602 antigen positivity [87,89] or signs of cataplexy [115].

A recently published Danish study showed that low CSF Hcrt-1 (<30% of the normal mean) is valid for diagnosing narcolepsy, but not narcolepsy without cataplexy. Hcrt-deficient narcoleptic patients seem to present a more severe phenotype than patients with normal CSF Hcrt-1 levels [91].

The situation is even more complicated in HLA-negative narcolepsy, where CSF Hcrt-1 level is usually normal [3]. CSF Hcrt-1 measurements may be especially useful when MSLT is difficult to conduct or to interpret in complex cases, and in children [138].

Histocompatibility (Human Leukocyte Antigen) Typing

HLA typing has been recommended as an adjuvant test for patients with narcolepsy [205]. Its sensitivity is highest in patients with narcolepsy and cataplexy [81]. The presence of the DQB1*0602 haplotype makes the diagnostic probability of narcolepsy much more likely, though DQB1*0602 negativity does not exclude it [206]. Twenty five percent of the normal population has a positive DQB1*0602 haplotype.

Differential Diagnosis

Chronic Sleep Deprivation with Erratic Sleep-Wake Schedule

Sleep deprivation and EDS are common in adolescents. EDS (ESS >10) was reported by 41% to 42% of the students in high schools [207]. EDS can be a symptom of delayed sleep phase syndrome or just poor hygiene combined with sleep deprivation [3]. The most common problem leading to EDS in adolescents is insufficient nocturnal sleep [138].

Idiopathic CNS Hypersomnia

Idiopathic CNS hypersomnia may be mistaken for narcolepsy, especially in cases without cataplexy. Similarities are the age of onset, the lifelong persistence (though remission has been reported in idiopathic CNS hypersomnia), sleepiness as the primary manifestation, and familial clustering in some cases [208–211]. Differences are the lack of cataplexy, lack of REM intrusion in sleep and wakefulness, and significant nocturnal sleep disruption. In addition, nocturnal sleep time tends to be long and naps are not refreshing [209].

Recently published data from the Bologna group suggest existence of different phenotypes of daytime sleep onset in idiopathic CNS hypersomnia versus narcolepsy patients. Patients with idiopathic CNS hypersomnia passed through a transitional state (mixture of sleep stage 1 NREM and wakefulness epochs) before reaching a sustained sleep condition, whereas patients' narcolepsy shifted abruptly into unequivocal sleep [212]. No amount of sleep ameliorates EDS in idiopathic hypersomnia [138]!

Recurrent Hypersomnia/Kleine-Levin Syndrome

Recurrent hypersomnia is characterized by recurrent episodes of sleep that typically occur weeks or months apart [1]. The best known form of recurrent hypersomnia is the Kleine-Levin syndrome [137]. This is a rare disorder characterized by relapsing-remitting episodes of hypersomnia, cognitive disturbances, and behavioral disturbances, such as hyperphagia and hypersexuality [213,214]. During episodes, the individual may sleep as long as 18 to 20 hours per 24-hour period, awakening only long enough to eat and void [137]. The episodes remit spontaneously. There may be a 2- to 10-pound weight gain during the sleep period. Between hypersomnia episodes (few days to several weeks), the individual is normal and exhibits normal sleep-wake behavior.

Menstrual-related periodic hypersomnia occurs in adolescents in association with the menstrual cycle, often within the first few months after menarche [1,215–217].

Primary Sleep Disorders

Obstructive sleep apnea, upper airway resistance syndrome, restless leg syndrome, and periodic limb movement disorder should first be excluded in evaluating EDS (or sleepiness camouflaged by hyperactivity) [2,3,218]. The clinical history of snoring and breathing pauses together with nocturnal polysomnographic examination should clarify this diagnosis [3]. It is not uncommon for narcolepsy to present with obesity and snoring, thus mimicking OSA.

Psychiatric Disorder/Depression

Hypersomnia can mask neuropsychiatric disturbances such as depression, autism, or attention-deficit hyperactivity disorder (ADHD) [219,220]. Pseudocataplexy, a phenomenon analogous to pseudoseizures, or simple malingering is rarely seen in adolescents [221,222]. Atypical hypnagogic hallucinations can be misdiagnosed as schizophrenia, whereas apathy and depressiveness accompanying narcolepsy may be mistaken for episodes of depression [3].

Atonic Drop Attacks Associated with Childhood Epilepsy Syndromes Such as Lennox Gastaut Syndrome

Cataplexy should be differentiated from atonic seizures, transient ischemic attacks, hypotension, vestibular disorders, and psychiatric disorders causing sudden loss of postural tone [1]. Very often, cataplectic attacks may be mistaken for seizures and atonic seizures may be misdiagnosed for cataplexy [2]. EDS can be a consequence of nocturnal seizures or, in coexisting epilepsy, because of an excessive dosage of antiepileptic drugs [3].

Medication Side Effects, Drug/Alcohol Abuse

Certain medical conditions and the use of medications or illicit drugs should also be taken into consideration in the evaluation of children and adolescents with daytime sleepiness [134]. The use of prescription drugs and over-the-counter sedatives such as antihistamines should also be considered as a possible cause of sleepiness. The abrupt cessation of REM sleep–suppressing medications, such as tricyclic antidepressants (TCAs) and selective serotonin reuptake inhibitors (SSRIs), may lead to a "REM rebound" phenomenon with multiple sleep-onset REM episodes on the MSLT [137].

Other Medical Condition

The complaint of sleepiness without cataplexy may be the sequel of head trauma [2]. However, many patients with hypersomnia following head trauma usually do not have narcolepsy [223,224].

Diagnosis such as Guillain-Barre syndrome, hepatitis, infectious mononucleosis, and atypical viral pneumonia may herald the onset of sleepiness in a subset of patients [225]. EDS occurs as part of acute illness but often persists after the other symptoms have subsided [138].

Secondary Narcolepsy

In rare situations, neurologic disorders may produce a narcolepsy-like picture called secondary narcolepsy [137].

There have been 5 cases with Mobius syndrome that had both EDS and laughter-provoked cataplexy and were diagnosed as symptomatic cases of narcolepsy [223].

Sleepiness, cataplexy, and SOREMPs can occur in uncommon diseases such as PWS and Norrie disease [151,226,227].

Isolated cataplexy has also been observed in NPC only [151,223,228]. Isolated stimulus–induced cataplexy has also been seen in Coffin-Lowry syndrome [151–153,223,226].

Although the majority of narcolepsy is idiopathic, structural lesions of the hypothalamus may on rare occasion precipitate secondary narcolepsy [223].

On infrequent occasions, narcolepsy occurs as a consequence of a focal CNS lesion, almost always involving the posterior hypothalamus, and tumors are the most common cause [229–232]. There are a number of reports of narcolepsy cases associated with tumors located mainly in the posterior thalamic region or the upper brainstem and 55% also exhibited cataplexy [223].

Hypothalamic sarcoidosis has caused narcolepsy in at least 2 cases, although neither had cataplexy [230,231].

Strokes or arteriovenous malformations of the hypothalamus are rare but can cause narcolepsy [231,233,234].

Treatment

Undoubtedly, narcolepsy is a lifelong disabling disorder [2]. At present, there is no cure for narcolepsy, with resultant significant impairment in the quality of life. For most patients, chronic sleepiness is the most disabling symptom [48]. Once symptoms of narcolepsy are established, treatment is generally required [137]. Individuals with EDS experience impaired alertness and decrements in performance across many areas of life [235–237]. Therefore, treatment should be individualized based on the severity of symptoms [26]. According to generally accepted opinion, there is no specific treatment for narcolepsy in children in comparison with adults [3,156,198]. Current management of narcolepsy involves a combination of behavioral and pharmacologic therapies [137].

Behavioral Approaches

Narcolepsy is a disorder often poorly understood by patients, family members, and peers, which can result in rejection from social entities, in the loss of self-esteem, and emergence of symptoms of depression [144,156]. Some nonpharmacological interventions can enhance the therapeutic effect such as regular sleep-wake schedules and planned naps [3]. The cornerstone of management is proper education of the patient and family regarding the nature of narcolepsy [137]. Good sleep habits, the avoidance of sleep deprivation and/or irregular sleep patterns, are important for many patients. Maintaining a consistent sleep-wake schedule and time for exercise in the morning can help control EDS [2,81,137]. Two 15-minute daytime naps can temporarily reduce sleepiness and improve alertness, especially in patients with more severe sleepiness; however, these attacks return after a few hours of remaining awake [81,238,239]. The combination of scheduled naps and regular nocturnal sleep times produced significant reduction in severity of sleepiness and duration of daytime sleep in patients treated with narcolepsy [240].

Obesity is very common in narcolepsy [135,179], and patients have been found to have significantly greater BMI across various ethnic groups and cultural backgrounds [135]. Foods high in refined sugars and carbohydrates tend to produce more EDS [81]. Dietary modification can also help in maintaining wakefulness [81]. Caffeine in sodas and coffee can serve as a stimulant. In older children and adults, 400 to 600 mg of caffeine (3–4 cups of coffee) is needed for an effect [81]. Meals at scheduled times and avoidance of alcohol and certain types of food is also recommended [241]. Lifestyle changes are, however, rarely sufficient to adequately control the symptoms of narcolepsy and, therefore, in most patients, must be combined with pharmacological management to optimally control the daytime sleepiness [26,81].

Pharmacological Treatment

The main goal of pharmacologic treatment for narcolepsy is to keep the patient alert during the day and reduce episodes of cataplexy while also minimizing the incidence of undesirable side effects and adverse events [26]. Recent practice parameters generated by the AASM and European Federation of Neurological Societies address the pharmacologic options available for treatment of sleepiness caused by narcolepsy using an evidence-based approach [242]. There are no double-blind placebo-controlled trials of medication specifically for children with narcolepsy [243]. Table 12.1 summarizes medications commonly used in current management of narcolepsy.

Daytime Sleepiness

Several medications are available for treating daytime sleepiness in narcolepsy patients. Some have been available for several decades, such as the psychostimulants [81]. The traditional stimulants are considered mainstays for treatment of sleepiness associated with narcolepsy [242].

Psychostimulants

Most clinical studies of stimulant medications report objective improvements in somnolence in 65% to 85% of subjects [244]. Amphetamines were first proposed in 1935 [245]. At low doses, the main effect of amphetamine is to release dopamine and to a lesser extent norepinephrine and serotonin [176]. This increased aminergic signaling may promote wakefulness through direct effects on the cortex or via activation of subcortical pathways [48]. Amphetamines also weakly inhibit monoamine oxidase (MAO) [26].

Table 12.1 Pharmacology of narcolepsy

Drug	Usual daily dosage	
Excessive daytime sleepiness		
	Pediatric	*Adult (mg)*
Modafinil	50–200 mg	100–600
Methylphenidate	10–30 mg	10–60
Dextroamphetamine	5–30 mg	5–50
Methamphetamine	5–40 mg	5–40
Amphetamine/dextroamphetamine mixture	10–30 mg	10–60
Selegiline	–	20–40
Cataplexy		
Imipramine	1.5–5 mg/kg/d	25–200
Clomipramine	3 mg/kg/d	10–200
Desipramine	25–200 mg	25–200
Fluoxetine	5–30 mg	20–60
Protriptiline	5–15 mg	5–30
Excessive daytime sleepiness + Cataplexy		
Sodium oxybate	3–9.0 g/d	4.5–9.0 g/d

Adapted from Refs. [26,176,240].

The D-isomer of amphetamine is more specific for dopaminergic transmission and is a better stimulant compound. Because of its sympathomimmetic effects, dextroamphetamine can also reduce the frequency of cataplexy [81]. Methamphetamine is more lipophilic than D-amphetamine and therefore has more central and fewer peripheral effects than D-amphetamine [176]. Many formulations of dextroamphetamine are available that allow greater flexibility in dosing [81]. The dextroamphetamine and methamphetamine are effective treatments of EDS in short-term use (up to 4 weeks) at starting doses of 15 to 20 mg increasing up to 60 mg/d [246–248]. There is no evidence of abuse and addiction in narcoleptic patients [249]. After a morning dose, many patients may experience some sleepiness in the afternoon or evening, and a combination of sustained-release drugs in the morning with additional short-acting drugs in the afternoon is often effective [48]. The development of drug tolerance is controversial, with some studies reporting tolerance in 30% to 40% of patients, others reporting no tolerance, and still others reporting tolerance only at high dosages [250]. Drug holidays of 1 ± 2 days per week with lower dosages or no medication are sometimes helpful for patients who develop tolerance, although their efficacy in preventing tolerance is uncertain [26,251,252]. Common adverse effects associated with these medications include nervousness, headaches, irritability, tremor, insomnia, anorexia, gastrointestinal upset, and heart palpitations [48,244]. There are conflicting views on the risk of developing hypertension with chronic administration [176,244]. Psychotic reactions occur in less than 1% of subjects [250]. Doses of amphetamine greater than 60 to 100 mg daily often cause serious toxic effects including "very fast thinking," "difficulty controlling burst of thoughts," and "bursts of verbal aggressiveness" [176]. The safety of dextroamphetamine in children below 6 years of age has not been established [81].

Methylphenidate is a dopamine and catecholamine reuptake inhibitor, thereby increasing the amount of these neurotransmitters in the synaptic cleft [81]. Similar to the action of amphetamine, methylphenidate induces dopamine release, but in contrast, it does not have any major effect on monoamine storage [176]. Methylphenidate may also enhance serotonin transmission, but this is a less significant effect [81]. Methylphenidate has similar efficacy to dextroamphetamine but probably has better therapeutic index because of a lower propensity to produce adverse effects [26]. There was a study showing significant improvement in dosages of 10, 30, and 60 mg/d compared with the baseline [253]. In children, the American Academy of Child and Adolescent Psychiatry recommends that treatment with methylphenidate be initiated with 5 mg dosed in the morning and a second dose at around noon because of its short half-life with upward titration by 5 to 10 mg/d at weekly intervals up to maximum total dose of 60 mg/d [176,254]. In adults, improvement in daytime sleepiness is seen with methylphenidate doses between 10 and 100 mg, with average effective doses being 20 to 30 mg/d [253]. In comparison with amphetamine, methylphenidate has a much shorter elimination half-life (2–7 hours) and the daily dose may be divided in 2 to 3 parts [176]. Because of catecholaminergic effects, methylphenidate may also reduce cataplexy attacks; however, this effect is usually mild [81]. Methylphenidate showed good to excellent response in 68% [30] of cases and mild to moderate improvement in 90% of cases [176]. On the MWT, the sleep latencies were increased to 80% of controls with a 60-mg daily dose [247]. Adverse effects are the same as with amphetamines with less reduction of appetite or increase in blood pressure [176]. Long-acting methylphenidate preparations are now available, thus allowing a single early morning dosing.

Pemoline, an oxazolidine derivative with long half-life (12 hours) and mild action, selectively blocks dopamine reuptake and only weakly stimulates dopamine release [176]. There was a moderate to marked improvement in sleepiness in 65% of subjects with narcolepsy [255]. Pemoline is usually better tolerated than dextroamphetamine or methamphetamine in terms of adverse effects (minimal sympathomimetic effects) and tolerance. However, because of a recent report in some cases of an acute liver failure, the U.S. Food and Drug Administration has recommended that pemoline should not be considered for use in narcolepsy [81,240,253].

Selegiline Hydrochloride

Selegiline is an irreversible MAO-B inhibitor (in dosages of up to 20 mg/d), which is metabolized to amphetamine and methylamphetamine; however, above this dosage, the drug starts to lose its selectivity [256]. Selegiline 10 ± 40 mg/d has produced statistically and clinically significant improvement in narcoleptic symptoms and polysomnographic measures in patients with narcolepsy [15,257–259]. The drug also reduced the number of cataplectic attacks by 89% [260]. The elimination half-life of the main metabolites is variable, 2.5 hours for desmethyl selegiline, 18 hours for amphetamine, and 21 hours for methamphetamine [176]. Selegiline has low abuse potential [260,261] and may be better tolerated than stimulants [262]. The adverse events associated with its use have included dry mouth, headache, insomnia, sweating, muscle twitching, dizziness, irritability, restlessness, and tremor [256,260,263]. Coadministration of triptans and serotonin-specific reuptake inhibitors is contraindicated [176]. The use of selegiline is limited by potential drug interactions and diet-induced interactions [240]. A diet low in tyramine is therefore recommended with higher dosages of selegiline to avoid the risk of hypertensive reactions [26].

Modafinil and Armodafinil

Modafinil is regarded as the first-line medication for the treatment of excessive sleepiness in narcolepsy [26]. Modafinil is a unique, nonamphetamine wake-promoting drug that effectively treats sleepiness with a minimum of side effects [48].

Modafinil is considered more as a "somnolytic" than a nonspecific stimulant. The mechanism of action of modafinil remains unknown; however, it does not appear to increase wakefulness by modulating the sympathomimmetic systems [81]. Involvement of adrenergic alpha-1 stimulation, indirect and direct interactions of dopamine systems, and involvement of serotonergic/GABAergic mechanisms have been suggested as possible mechanisms of action [264–266]. Selective activation of wake-generating sites in the hypothalamus may be a mechanism of action [26]. Functional imaging studies suggest that modafinil may exert its effect by acting on the thalamus, hypothalamus, and amygdale [81]. It reduces subjective sleepiness and clearly improves the ability of narcoleptic subjects to stay awake, although their latency to sleep is still shorter than normal [48,267,268]. Modafinil does not reduce cataplexy, and additional anticataplexy medications may be needed [48].

Modafinil was the first medication that underwent randomized clinical trial to demonstrate its effectiveness in improving sleepiness in adults with narcolepsy [267,268]. Starting dose of modafinil in adults is 200 mg in the morning [81]. Modafinil has an elimination half-life of 9 to 14 hours, permitting once-daily administration for most patients [26]. Second dose of 200 mg can be added either in the morning or around noon to extend the alerting effects [81]. Modafinil use has decreased sleep attacks in up to 71% of patients with narcolepsy in clinical trials [267–270]. Patients receiving modafinil stayed awake up to 75% longer than placebo-treated patients as measured by the MWT [26].

Little data are available for modafinil use in children with narcolepsy [100]. Some data in children are available from studies of modafinil in children and adolescents with ADHD [254, 271–273].

Tolerance or difficulties during withdrawal are very rare [268], and modafinil appears to have little potential for addiction [274,275]. Side effects of modafinil are generally mild and include headache, which can occur in 13%, and nervousness, nausea, insomnia, or dry mouth occurs in less than 10% [276], with fewer side effects if treatment is begun with a low dose [267,268]. Rare but more serious side effects include Stevens-Johnson syndrome, markedly elevated liver enzymes, suicidality, aggression, and psychosis [81]. The typical doses of modafinil do not produce hypertension, arrhythmias, restlessness, anorexia, or disruption of nighttime sleep [48,268].

Armodafinil is a combination of R-modafinil and S-modafinil. R-modafinil is a longer acting isomer of modafinil with a half-life of 10 to 14 hours, whereas S-modafinil has a half-life of 3 to 4 hours. Armodafinil has a T_{max} of 2 hours and a half-life of approximately 15 hours. This drug has been shown to be effective and produces longer wakefulness than modafinil in patients with sleepiness caused by acute sleep loss [26,277,278]. Most adverse effects appear to be mild or moderate in severity; headaches were described in 16% to 28%, nausea in 7% to 14%, dizziness in 2% to 8%, insomnia in 7%, and anorexia in 3% to 6% of patients [278,279]. Doses in the range of 250 to 600 mg have been used to treat the daytime sleepiness.

Sodium Oxybate

Sodium oxybate is the sodium salt of gamma-hydroxybutyrate (GHB) [26]. Pharma-ceutical interest in sodium oxybate (originally known only by its chemical name gamma-hydroxybutyrate) originated in the 1960s during a search for a peripherally acting GABA agonist [280]. Sodium oxybate induced sleep that closely resembled natural sleep and was initially used as an anaesthetic agent, as it induced a level of unconsciousness that was acceptable for some surgical procedures [281–283]. The drug is only available in liquid form and must be taken twice a night to induce sleep [81,176]. The administration of sodium oxybate at bedtime was found to reduce nocturnal awakenings, increase stage 3 and 4 (delta or slow wave) sleep, and consolidate REM sleep [284,285]. GHB reduced subjective daytime sleepiness and the number of hypnagogic hallucinations and daytime naps [286]. The extra delta sleep may in part be responsible for relieving daytime sleepiness [99,104,105]. Sodium oxybate is a rapidly acting sedative/hypnotic medication [240]. The results of several pharmacokinetic studies indicate that the average time to peak plasma concentration (T_{max}) ranges from 0.5 to 1.25 hours and the plasma half-life of the drug is 40 to 60 minutes [287–292]. It induces sleep within 15 to 25 minutes in most patients and maximal effect occurs after 45 to 90 minutes. Similar to modafinil, sodium oxybate has been shown in randomized controlled trials in adults to reduce daytime sleepiness [293–295]. One-half of a therapeutic dose of sodium oxybate is administered at bedtime and repeated 2.5 to 4.0 hours later, providing effective plasma concentrations throughout the night while ensuring that the majority of the drug has been eliminated when patients awaken in the morning [26,288–290]. Starting dose is 4.5 g per night, divided into 2 equal doses of 2.25 g per night. Full therapeutic benefit generally occurs at the 6- to 9-g-per-night doses [176,295–297]. The major elimination pathway is via the lungs [81].

The result of placebo-controlled trials indicate that adverse events occur with an incidence of 5% or greater including dizziness (23%), headache (20%), nausea (16%), pain (12%), somnolence (9%), sleep disorder (9%), confusion (7%) infection (7%), vomiting (6%), enuresis (5%), and night terrors (5%), with most described as mild to moderate in severity [298].

Most commonly reported adverse effects are nausea and dizziness, which usually recede after a few days, and nocturnal enuresis, which may persist intermittently, and may be dose related [176,298,299]. Overdose of sodium oxybate can result in respiratory depression, bradycardia, delirium, myoclonus, hypothermia, and coma [81].

The most improvement occurred when sodium oxybate was combined with modafinil; with this combination, patients' alertness improved to near-normal levels [300]. It is important to note that sodium oxybate improves both daytime sleepiness and cataplexy [81]. The exact mechanism by which sodium oxybate reduces cataplexy is unclear.

Reboxetine

Reboxetine is a new selective noradrenaline reuptake inhibitor with antidepressant efficacy not yet available in the United States [26,301]. It exerts stimulant and anti-cataplectic effects in narcolepsy patients [240]. In one study, the subjective (ESS) and objective (MSLT) measures of sleepiness were measured, following a 2-week treatment, with significant improvement in EDS observed as measured by a mean decrease of 48.6% on the ESS and a mean increase of 54.7% in sleep latency on the MSLT [301].

Ritanserin

Ritanserin is a 5-HT2 antagonist indicated for treatment of excessive sleepiness associated with narcolepsy, but is not available in the United States [240]. The study by Lammers et al [302] was a 4-week, double-blind, placebo-controlled trial involving 28 subjects with narcolepsy. There was improvement in subjective daytime sleepiness, but no significant change in MSL was demonstrated on the MSLT [302]. Another study by Mayer et al [303] reported results from a double-blind, placebo-controlled study in which 134 subjects with narcolepsy were enrolled. This study showed some improvement in subjective quality of sleep, but there was no significant improvement in daytime alertness as measured by a polygraphic recording [303].

Pemoline

Pemoline was identified as an effective option for treatment of sleepiness associated with narcolepsy [304]. However, the rare but potentially fatal hepatotoxcity associated with pemoline has severely limited clinical use of this medication and pemoline is no longer being manufactured in the United States [240].

Treatment of Cataplexy

Although EDS can often be managed with stimulants, these medications often do not provide significant relief from cataplexy [26]. Most patients with narcolepsy do not require treatment of their cataplexy because it is mild or infrequent, but in some patients, cataplexy occurs several times each day, producing embarrassment or even injury [48]. In these patients, the additional medications with anticataplectic activity must be used to reduce the frequency and severity of cataplexy [26].

TCAs have been used successfully to treat cataplexy for many years, but more recently, selective SSRIs, have been used [137]. Recently, sodium oxybate was approved for use in the United States and Europe for consolidating sleep in patients with narcolepsy and also improve cataplexy.

Tricyclic Antidepressants

Since the first report describing the anti-cataplectic effect of imipramine was published in 1960 [305], TCAs have been the most widely prescribed medications for the treatment of cataplexy but their effect on cataplexy has never been investigated in randomized clinical trials [204]. TCAs form the first line of medication widely available for the treatment of cataplexy [306]. Because of their anticholingeric activity, antidepressants also tend to suppress hypnogogic hallucinations and sleep paralysis [81]. Tricyclic medications include clomipramine, desipramine, imipramine, and protryptylin [143,145,307]. Because cataplexy is a REM phenomenon and REM is mediated by cholinergic activity, the anticholinergic activity of TCAs was thought to be mechanism by which they reduced cataplexy [81]. The anticataplectic effects of these drugs differ from their antidepressant effects in the rapid response to them (less than a week); however, rebound cataplexy typically occurs if intake is abruptly interrupted [308]. Imipramine is the original agent used for treatment of cataplexy. Protryptiline [309] and clomipramine [310] are probably the agents most widely used [306]. Clomipramine has the most REM-suppressing activity, which may be related to its greater ability to block serotonin reuptake [26]. Clomipramine doses of 10 to 75 mg daily are generally effective for cataplexy [311,312]. Common side effects of these antidepressants that limit their use include daytime sleepiness, orthostatic hypotension, weight gain, anorexia, diarrhea, dry mouth, tiredness, and decreased libido [305,309,310]. For many patients, clomipramine can remain effective for years, although, similar to all TCAs, tolerance may develop after a few months or even a few weeks of treatment [26]. Abrupt withdrawal of TCAs can lead to status cataplecticus [48,139].

Serotonin-specific reuptake inhibitors are effective, but higher doses than those for tricyclic drugs are often needed [48,143,145,307,313]. Fluoxetine is the most commonly prescribed of all SSRIs [313,314]. Headache, fatigue, anxiety, nervousness, and tremors can occur with use of fluoxetine [314]. The anticataplectic effect of this drug is less potent than that of the tricyclics, mainly because the affinity of the SSRIs is toward the serotonergic pathway [306]. Other SSRIs also used to treat cataplexy include sertraline, fluvoxamine, and citalopram [81].

More selective norepinephrine reuptake blocking agents are also effective against cataplexy with only minor adverse effects such as headache, dry mouth, hyperhydrosis, constipation, nausea, and dizziness [204]. These include viloxazine, reboxetine, and atomoxetine [204,301,315]. These compounds are often effective at lower doses than used for treatment of depression [204].

The dual norepinephrine and serotonin reuptake inhibitor venlafaxine is also effective against cataplexy, with nausea as the main adverse effect [307,316,317]. Doses lower than the ones used in depression are effective. It is increasingly used as a first-line therapy against cataplexy, and long-acting formulationsare ideal because they are effective for the entire day [204].

Finally, both mazindol and selegiline have combined anticataplectic and stimulant properties [204,318–320]. Although MAO inhibitors have been used for the treatment of cataplexy, the efficacy of these drugs is not supported by controlled clinical trials [26]. In one study, 1 to 3 mg/d of mazindol decreased cataplexy in 85% of patients [319].

Sodium Oxybate

It may be the drug of choice because of the opportunity to treat both symptoms (EDS and cataplexy) at the same time [306]. Sodium oxybate is the only approved treatment for cataplexy in the United States and Europe [204]. Its efficacy has been established in randomized controlled trials [293–296,321]. The drug decreased the number of cataplectic attacks in patients with increasing doses between 3 and 9 g nightly [293]. Sodium oxybate reduced the median frequency of weekly attacks by 49% and 69% at nightly doses of 6 and 9 g, respectively, and there was no rebound cataplexy noted on abrupt cessation of treatment at the end of the trial [296]. The benefit was significant after 4 weeks, at its highest after 8 weeks, and was maintained during long-term (7–44 months) therapy [294]. After 12 months of treatment, none of these patients displayed evidence of tolerance [293] and unlike for antidepressant-based therapies for cataplexy, interruption of sodium oxybate treatment did not result in a return of cataplexy [321].

Data in children are limited; however, one study with 8 children did show reduction of cataplexy in this age group as well [297]. Doses ranged from 3 to 7 g per night. Sodium oxybate can also be used in association with antidepressant or stimulant therapy [204]. Sodium oxybate has been shown to reduce the frequency of hypnogogic hallucinations and sleep paralysis also [322,323]. On abrupt withdrawal of the drug, there is no rebound cataplexy as seen with use of tricyclic and SSRI antidepressants; effect can last for up to 2 weeks.

Treatment of Disrupted Nocturnal Sleep Associated With Narcolepsy

Sodium Oxybate

Several studies of sodium oxybate have shown a reduction in the number of nighttime awakenings with increased slow-wave sleep, making this drug a first-line treatment for narcoleptic patients with disturbed nighttime sleep [296]. Sodium oxybate helps consolidate sleep and increases the amount of delta sleep [105].

Hypnotic Medications

Benzodiazepines (clonazepam) and nonbenzodiazepine GABA agonists (zolpidem, zopiclone, and zaleplon) have also been used to improve nocturnal sleep; however, their use in narcolepsy has not been well established [307,324].

Future Directions

Despite major advances in our understanding of the neurobiological basis of narcolepsy, current treatment protocols all respond to specific symptoms but are not effective enough against the disease as a whole [204].

Based on the autoimmune hypothesis of narcolepsy, treatments such as intravenous immunoglobulins (IVIg) and plasmapheresis have shown promising results in a few cases, which need to be confirmed in larger series [129,130,325]. Steroid and immunosuppressive treatment in dogs with narcolepsy more than doubled the time to cataplexy onset, and the time spent in cataplexy was reduced by more than 90% [126]. A limitation of immunosuppressive treatments, however, will be the need to intervene at disease onset [204]. Treatment of 2 children with prednisone and 1 adult with azathioprine did not result in persistent improvement of symptoms [115–117]. In other studies, steroids, plasma exchange, and immunoglobulins have been given without clear benefit [127,130,325]. Immunoglobulins generated the most interest as some reported improvements in narcolepsy symptoms. Use of IVIg in 1 series resulted in improvement of cataplexy especially in the 3 patients who had the shortest time from onset of symptoms, but sleepiness persisted [129,131]. However, the improvement was more transient than sustained [130].

The replacement therapy for Hcrt deficiency remains the most logical approach for treating narcolepsy [306]. Such manipulations are effective when administered centrally in Hcrt-deficient mouse models [326]. In humans, part of the problem is getting Hcrt into the brain [306]. The peripheral administration has been disappointing because the peptides do not cross the blood-brain barrier [316,317]. An intranasal delivery method looks promising [77]. Hcrt-based therapies such as direct use of Hcrt agonists are currently under investigation in animal models [204]. Cell transplantation [327–329] and gene therapy [326] have also been examined in animal models too.

Thyrotrophin-releasing hormone (TRH) and TRH agonists have alerting properties [330,331]. TRH is excitatory on neurons and enhances dopamine and adrenergic transmission and may promote wakefulness by direct effect on thalamocortical pathways [330,332]. TRH has been shown to have anticataplectic activity in the narcoleptic canine [330]. Inhibition of the TRH-degrading enzyme inhibitor metallopeptidase may be a promising treatment in the future.

The histamine receptor has also been a target of different manipulations, as the drowsiness effects of antihistamine agents are well known [306]. Histamine 3 (H3) receptors regulate the release and synthesis of histamine. Stimulation of the H3 receptors causes sedation, whereas antagonism causes wakefulness [333]. H3 antagonists have been shown to be effective on sleepiness and cataplexy in canines and in mice with ablation of Hcrt neurons (orexin/ataxin-3) [334].

Conclusion

Despite significant advances in understanding the pathophysiology of narcolepsy, we do not have an ideal treatment to completely restore full and sustained alertness across the day. Early recognition and institution of effective therapy are keys to improving quality of life especially in the early formative years.

Currently, a number of different drug therapies are available for the treatment of the symptoms of narcolepsy. Modafinil and sodium oxybate have shown strong evidence of improvement in daytime alertness, and their combination appears to offer additional benefits. Sodium oxybate has demonstrated additional efficacy for the treatment of cataplexy. Other agents such as antidepressants of the TCA and SSRI classes are often effective but must be used in combination with hypnotic and stimulant medications if insomnia and/or EDS are coexistent symptoms.

Treatment approaches should be directed toward development of more effective and better tolerated therapies and primary prevention. Currently there are very few studies that involve special populations with hypersomnia such as children, older adults, and pregnant or breast-feeding women.

References

1. American Academy of Sleep Medicine. *The International Classification of Sleep Disorders Diagnostic and Coding Manual.* 2nd ed. Westchester, IL: American Academy of Sleep Medicine; 2005.
2. Guilleminault C, Pelayo R. Narcolepsy in children: a practical guide to its diagnosis, treatment and follow-up. *Paediatr Drugs*. 2000;2(1):1–9.
3. Nevsimalova S. Narcolepsy in childhood. *Sleep Med Rev*. 2009;13(2):169–180.
4. Gélineau J. [De la narcolepsie]. *Gaz Hôp Civil Milit*. 1880;53:626–628, 635–637.
5. Daniels L. Narcolepsy. *Medicine*. 1934;13(1):122.
6. Mignot E. A hundred years of narcolepsy research. *Arch Ital Biol*. 2001;139(3): 207–220.
7. Yoss RE, Daly DD. Criteria for the diagnosis of the narcoleptic syndrome. *Proc Staff Meet Mayo Clin*. 1957;32(12):320–328.
8. Vogel G. Studies in psychophysiology of dreams. III. The dream of narcolepsy. *Arch Gen Psychiatry*. 1960;3:421–428.
9. Ohayon MM, Priest RG, Zulley J, Smirne S, Paiva T. Prevalence of narcolepsy symptomatology and diagnosis in the European general population. *Neurology*. 2002;58(12):1826–1833.
10. Dement W, Zarcone W, Varner V, Hoddes E, Nassau S, Jacobs BL. The prevalence of narcolepsy. In: Sleep Research, Vol. 1, p. 148. Eds. M. H. Chase, W. C. Stern and P. L. Walter. Brain Information Service/Brain Research Institute, UCLA: Los Angeles, 1972.
11. Silber MH, Krahn LE, Olson EJ, Pankratz VS. The epidemiology of narcolepsy in Olmsted County, Minnesota: a population-based study. *Sleep*. 2002;25(2):197–202.
12. Longstreth WT Jr, Ton TG, Koepsell T, Gersuk VH, Hendrickson A, Velde S. Prevalence of narcolepsy in King County, Washington, USA. *Sleep Med*. 2009;10(4):422–426.
13. Longstreth WT Jr, Koepsell TD, Ton TG, Hendrickson AF, van Belle G. The epidemiology of narcolepsy. *Sleep*. 2007;30(1):13–26.
14. Franceschi M, Zamproni P, Crippa D, Smirne S. Excessive daytime sleepiness: a 1-year study in an unselected inpatient population. *Sleep*. 1982;5(3):239–247.
15. Hublin C, Kaprio J, Partinen M, et al. The prevalence of narcolepsy: an epidemiological study of the Finnish Twin Cohort. *Ann Neurol*. 1994;35(6):709–716.
16. Heier MS, Evsiukova T, Wilson J, Abdelnoor M, Hublin C, Ervik S. Prevalence of narcolepsy with cataplexy in Norway. *Acta Neurol Scand*. 2009;120(4):276–280.
17. Oksenberg J, Amar A, Cohen N, et al. HLA-D "BG" in Israel. A Japanese related allele population and family study. *Tissue Antigens*. 1983;21(4):271–280.
18. Lavie P, Peled R. Narcolepsy is a rare disease in Israel. *Sleep*. 1987;10(6):608–609.
19. Wilner A, Steinman L, Lavie P, Peled R, Friedmann A, Brautbar C. Narcolepsy-cataplexy in Israeli Jews is associated exclusively with the HLA DR2 haplotype. A study at the serological and genomic level. *Hum Immunol*. 1988;21(1):15–22.
20. Shin YK, Yoon IY, Han EK, et al. Prevalence of narcolepsy-cataplexy in Korean adolescents. *Acta Neurol Scand*. 2008;117(4):273–278.
21. al Rajeh S, Bademosi O, Ismail H, et al. A community survey of neurological disorders in Saudi Arabia: the Thugbah study. *Neuroepidemiology*. 1993;12(3):164–178.
22. Wing YK, Chiu HF, Ho CK, Chen CN. Narcolepsy in Hong Kong Chinese—a preliminary experience. *Aust N Z J Med*. 1994;24(3):304–306.
23. Wing YK, Li RH, Lam CW, Ho CK, Fong SY, Leung T. The prevalence of narcolepsy among Chinese in Hong Kong. *Ann Neurol*. 2002;51(5):578–584.
24. Honda K. Census of narcolepsy, cataplexy and sleep life among teenagers in Fujisawa City. *Sleep Res*. 1979;8: 191.
25. Tashiro T, Kanbayashi T, Iijima S, Hishikawa Y. An epidemiological prevalence of narcolepsy in Japanese. *J Sleep Res*. 1992;1(suppl):228.
26. Thorpy M. Therapeutic advances in narcolepsy. *Sleep Med*. 2007;8(4):427–440.
27. Vendrame M, Havaligi N, Matadeen-Ali C, Adams R, Kothare SV. Narcolepsy in children: a single-center clinical experience. *Pediatr Neurol*. 2008;38(5):314–320.
28. Ohayon MM, Ferini-Strambi L, Plazzi G, Smirne S, Castronovo V. How age influences the expression of narcolepsy. *J Psychosom Res*. 2005;59(6): 399–405.
29. Nevsimalova S, Buskova J, Kemlink D, Sonka K, Skibova J. Does age at the onset of narcolepsy influence the course and severity of the disease? *Sleep Med*. 2009;10(9):967–972.
30. Dauvilliers Y, Montplaisir J, Molinari N, et al. Age at onset of narcolepsy in two large populations of patients in France and Quebec. *Neurology*. 2001;57(11): 2029–2033.
31. Challamel MJ, Mazzola ME, Nevsimalova S, Cannard C, Louis J, Revol M. Narcolepsy in children. *Sleep*. 1994;17(8 suppl):S17–S20.
32. Thorpy M. Current concepts in the etiology, diagnosis and treatment of narcolepsy. *Sleep Med*. 2001;2(1):5–17.
33. Han F, Chen E, Wei H, et al. Childhood narcolepsy in North China. *Sleep*. 2001;24(3):321–324.
34. Guilleminault C, Mignot E, Grumet FC. Familial patterns of narcolepsy. *Lancet*. 1989;2(8676): 1376–1379.
35. Billiard M, Pasquie-Magnetto V, Heckman M, et al. Family studies in narcolepsy. *Sleep*. 1994;17 (8 suppl):S54–S59.
36. Krabbe E, Magnussen G. Familial narcolepsy. *Acta Psychiatr Neurol*. 1942;11:149–173.

37. Baraitser M, Parkes JD. Genetic study of narcoleptic syndrome. *J Med Genet*. 1978;15(4):254–259.
38. Hayduk R, Flodman P, Spence MA, Erman MK, Mitler MM. HLA haplotypes, polysomnography, and pedigrees in a case series of patients with narcolepsy. *Sleep*. 1997;20(10):850–857.
39. Nevsimalova S, Mignot E, Sonka K, Arrigoni JL. Familial aspects of narcolepsy-cataplexy in the Czech Republic. *Sleep*. 1997;20(11):1021–1026.
40. Maret S, Tafti M. Genetics of narcolepsy and other major sleep disorders. *Swiss Med Wkly*. 2005;135(45–46):662–665.
41. Mignot E. Genetics of narcolepsy and other sleep disorders. *Am J Hum Genet*. 1997;60(6): 1289–1302.
42. Honda M, Honda Y, Uchida S, Miyazaki S, Tokunaga K. Monozygotic twins incompletely concordant for narcolepsy. *Biol Psychiatry*. 2001;49(11):943–947.
43. Partinen M, Hublin C, Kaprio J, Koskenvuo M, Guilleminault C. Twin studies in narcolepsy. *Sleep*. 1994;17(8 suppl):S13–S16.
44. Pollmacher T, Schulz H, Geisler P, Kiss E, Albert ED, Schwarzfischer F. DR2-positive monozygotic twins discordant for narcolepsy. *Sleep*. 1990;13(4):336–343.
45. Neely S, Rosenberg R, Spire JP, Antel J, Arnason BG. HLA antigens in narcolepsy. *Neurology*. 1987;37(12):1858–1860.
46. Mignot E, Lin L, Rogers W, et al. Complex HLA-DR and -DQ interactions confer risk of narcolepsy-cataplexy in three ethnic groups. *Am J Hum Genet*. 2001;68(3):686–699.
47. Rogers AE, Meehan J, Guilleminault C, Grumet FC, Mignot E. HLA DR15 (DR2) and DQB1*0602 typing studies in 188 narcoleptic patients with cataplexy. *Neurology*. 1997;48(6):1550–1556.
48. Scammell TE. The neurobiology, diagnosis, and treatment of narcolepsy. *Ann Neurol*. 2003; 53(2):154–166.
49. Watson NF, Ton TG, Koepsell TD, Gersuk VH, Longstreth WT Jr. Does narcolepsy symptom severity vary according to HLA-DQB1*0602 allele status? *Sleep*. 2010;33(1):29–35.
50. Kales A, Cadieux RJ, Soldatos CR, et al. Narcolepsy-cataplexy. I. Clinical and electrophysiologic characteristics. *Arch Neurol*. 1982;39(3): 164–168.
51. Ohayon MM, Ferini-Strambi L, Plazzi G, Smirne S, Castronovo V. Frequency of narcolepsy symptoms and other sleep disorders in narcoleptic patients and their first-degree relatives. *J Sleep Res*. 2005;14(4):437–445.
52. Baust W, Holzbach E, Zechlin O. Phasic changes in heart rate and respiration correlated with PGO-spike activity during REM sleep. *Pflugers Arch*. 1972; 331(2):113–123.
53. Salin-Pascual R, Gerashchenko D, Greco M, Blanco-Centurion C, Shiromani PJ. Hypothalamic regulation of sleep. *Neuropsychopharmacology*. 2001;25(5 suppl):S21–S27.
54. John J, Wu MF, Boehmer LN, Siegel JM. Cataplexy-active neurons in the hypothalamus: implications for the role of histamine in sleep and waking behavior. *Neuron*. 2004;42(4): 619–634.
55. Chase M, Morales F. Control of motoneurons during sleep, *Principles and Practice of Sleep Medicine*. In: Kryger MH, Roth T, Dement W, eds. Philadelphia, PA: Elsevier Saunders; 2005:154–168.
56. Siegel JM. REM sleep, *Principles and Practice of Sleep Medicine*. In: Kryger MH, Roth T, Dement W, eds. Philadelphia, PA: Elsevier Saunders; 2005:120–135.
57. Taepavarapruk N, McErlane SA, Soja PJ. State-related inhibition by GABA and glycine of transmission in Clarke's column. *J Neurosci*. 2002;22(13):5777–5788.
58. Pace-Schott EF, Hobson JA. The neurobiology of sleep: genetics, cellular physiology and subcortical networks. *Nat Rev Neurosci*. 2002;3(8):591–605.
59. Strecker RE, Nalwalk J, Dauphin LJ, et al. Extracellular histamine levels in the feline preoptic/anterior hypothalamic area during natural sleep-wakefulness and prolonged wakefulness: an in vivo microdialysis study. *Neuroscience*. 2002;113(3):663–670.
60. Siegel JM. The neurobiology of sleep. *Semin Neurol*. 2009;29(4):277–296.
61. Siegel JM, Tomaszewski KS, Wheeler RL. Behavioral organization of reticular formation: studies in the unrestrained cat. II. Cells related to facial movements. *J Neurophysiol*. 1983;50(3): 717–723.
62. Siegel JM, Nienhuis R, Fahringer HM, et al. Neuronal activity in narcolepsy: identification of cataplexy-related cells in the medial medulla. *Science*. 1991;252(5010):1315–1318.
63. Lin, JS, Sakai K, Jouvet M. Evidence for histaminergic arousal mechanisms in the hypothalamus of cat. *Neuropharmacology*. 1988;27(2):111–122.
64. Steininger TL, Alam MN, Gong H, Szymusiak R, McGinty D. Sleep-waking discharge of neurons in the posterior lateral hypothalamus of the albino rat. *Brain Res*. 1999;840(1–2):138–147.
65. Vanni-Mercier G, Gigout S, Debilly G, Lin JS. Waking selective neurons in the posterior hypothalamus and their response to histamine H3-receptor ligands: an electrophysiological study in freely moving cats. *Behav Brain Res*. 2003; 144(1–2):227–241.
66. Watanabe T, Yanai K. Studies on functional roles of the histaminergic neuron system by using pharmacological agents, knockout mice and positron emission tomography. *Tohoku J Exp Med*. 2001;195(4):197–217.
67. Fenik VB, Davies RO, Kubin L. Noradrenergic, serotonergic and GABAergic antagonists injected together into the XII nucleus abolish the REM sleep-like depression of hypoglossal motoneuronal activity. *J Sleep Res*. 2005;14(4):419–429.
68. Jelev A, Sood S, Liu H, Nolan P, Horner RL. Microdialysis perfusion of 5-HT into hypoglossal motor nucleus differentially modulates genioglossus activity across natural sleep-wake states in rats. *J Physiol*. 2001;532(pt 2):467–481.

69. Sood S, Raddatz E, Liu X, Liu H, Horner RL. Inhibition of serotonergic medullary raphe obscurus neurons suppresses genioglossus and diaphragm activities in anesthetized but not conscious rats. *J Appl Physiol*. 2006;100(6):1807–1821.
70. Bourgin P, Huitron-Resendiz S, Spier AD, et al. Hypocretin-1 modulates rapid eye movement sleep through activation of locus coeruleus neurons. *J Neurosci*. 2000;20(20):7760–7765.
71. Saper CB, Scammell TE, Lu J. Hypothalamic regulation of sleep and circadian rhythms. *Nature*. 2005;437(7063):1257–1263.
72. Sakurai T, Amemiya A, Ishii M, et al. Orexins and orexin receptors: a family of hypothalamic neuropeptides and G protein-coupled receptors that regulate feeding behavior. *Cell*. 1998;92(4): 573–585.
73. de Lecea L, Kilduff TS, Peyron C, et al. The hypocretins: hypothalamus-specific peptides with neuroexcitatory activity. *Proc Natl Acad Sci U S A*. 1998;95(1):322–327.
74. Ebrahim IO, Howard RS, Kopelman MD, Sharief MK, Williams AJ. The hypocretin/orexin system. *J R Soc Med*. 2002;95(5):227–230.
75. Lin L, Faraco J, Li R, et al. The sleep disorder canine narcolepsy is caused by a mutation in the hypocretin (orexin) receptor 2 gene. *Cell*. 1999;98(3):365–376.
76. Chemelli RM, Willie JT, Sinton CM, et al. Narcolepsy in orexin knockout mice: molecular genetics of sleep regulation. *Cell*. 1999; 98(4):437–451.
77. John J, Wu MF, Siegel JM. Systemic administration of hypocretin-1 reduces cataplexy and normalizes sleep and waking durations in narcoleptic dogs. *Sleep Res Online*. 2000;3(1):23–28.
78. Deadwyler SA, Porrino L, Siegel JM, Hampson RE. Systemic and nasal delivery of orexin-A (Hypocretin-1) reduces the effects of sleep deprivation on cognitive performance in nonhuman primates. *J Neurosci*. 2007;27(52):14239–14247.
79. Tokita S, Chemelli RM, Willie JT, et al. Behavioral characterization of orexin-2 receptor (OX2R) knockout mice. *Sleep*. 2001;24:A20–A21.
80. Kisanuki Y, Chemelli RM, Tokita S, et al. Behavioral and polysomnographic characterization of orexin-1 receptor and orexin-2 receptor double knockout mice. *Sleep*. 2001;24:A22.
81. Peterson PC, Husain AM. Pediatric narcolepsy. *Brain Dev*. 2008;30(10):609–623.
82. Thannickal TC, Moore RY, Nienhuis R, et al. Reduced number of hypocretin neurons in human narcolepsy. *Neuron*. 2000;27(3):469–474.
83. Peyron C, Faraco J, Rogers W, et al. A mutation in a case of early onset narcolepsy and a generalized absence of hypocretin peptides in human narcoleptic brains. *Nat Med*. 2000;6(9):991–997.
84. Ripley B, Overeem S, Fujiki N, et al. CSF hypocretin/orexin levels in narcolepsy and other neurological conditions. *Neurology*. 2001;57(12):2253–2258.
85. Nishino S, Ripley B, Overeem S, GJ Lammers, Mignot E. Hypocretin (orexin) deficiency in human narcolepsy. *Lancet*. 2000;355(9197):39–40.
86. Kanbayashi T, Yano T, Ishiguro H, et al. Hypocretin-1 (orexin-A) levels in human lumbar CSF in different age groups: infants to elderly persons. *Sleep*. 2002;25(3):337–339.
87. Krahn LE, Pankratz VS, Oliver L, Boeve BF, Silber MH. Hypocretin (orexin) levels in cerebrospinal fluid of patients with narcolepsy: relationship to cataplexy and HLA DQB1*0602 status. *Sleep*. 2002;25(7): 733–736.
88. Nishino S, Ripley B, Overeem S, et al. Low cerebrospinal fluid hypocretin (Orexin) and altered energy homeostasis in human narcolepsy. *Ann Neurol*. 2001;50(3):381–388.
89. Mignot E, Lammers GJ, Ripley B, et al. The role of cerebrospinal fluid hypocretin measurement in the diagnosis of narcolepsy and other hypersomnias. *Arch Neurol*. 2002;59(10):1553–1562.
90. Dalal MA, Schuld A, Haack M, et al. Normal plasma levels of orexin A (hypocretin-1) in narcoleptic patients. *Neurology*. 2001;56(12): 1749–1751.
91. Knudsen S, Jennum PJ, Alving J, Sheikh SP, Gammeltoft S. Validation of the ICSD-2 criteria for CSF hypocretin-1 measurements in the diagnosis of narcolepsy in the Danish population. *Sleep*. 2010;33(2):169–176.
92. Tsukamoto H, Ishikawa T, Fujii Y, Fukumizu M, Sugai K, Kanbayashi T. Undetectable levels of CSF hypocretin-1 (orexin-A) in two prepubertal boys with narcolepsy. *Neuropediatrics*. 2002;33(1): 51–52.
93. Kubota H, Kanbayashi T, Tanabe Y, et al. Decreased cerebrospinal fluid hypocretin-1 levels near the onset of narcolepsy in 2 prepubertal children. *Sleep*. 2003;26(5):555–557.
94. Elias CF, Saper CB, Maratos-Flier E, et al. Chemically defined projections linking the mediobasal hypothalamus and the lateral hypothalamic area. *J Comp Neurol*. 1998; 402(4):442–459.
95. Peyron C, Tighe DK, van den Pol AN, et al. Neurons containing hypocretin (orexin) project to multiple neuronal systems. *J Neurosci*. 1998;18(23):9996–10015.
96. Hagan JJ, Leslie RA, Patel S, et al. Orexin A activates locus coeruleus cell firing and increases arousal in the rat. *Proc Natl Acad Sci U S A*. 1999;96(19):10911–10916.
97. Silber MH, Rye DB. Solving the mysteries of narcolepsy: the hypocretin story. *Neurology*. 2001;56(12):1616–1618.
98. Siegel JM. Hypocretin (orexin): role in normal behavior and neuropathology. *Annu Rev Psychol*. 2004;55:125–148.
99. Estabrooke IV, McCarthy MT, Ko E, et al. Fos expression in orexin neurons varies with behavioral state. *J Neurosci*. 2001;21(5):1656–1662.
100. Mileykovskiy BY, Kiyashchenko LI, Siegel JM. Behavioral correlates of activity in identified hypocretin/orexin neurons. *Neuron*. 2005;46(5): 787–798.
101. Lee MG, Hassani OK, Jones BE. Discharge of identified orexin/hypocretin neurons across the sleep-waking cycle. *J Neurosci*. 2005;25(28): 6716–6720.

102. Yoshida Y, Fujiki N, Nakajima T, Ripley B, et al. Fluctuation of extracellular hypocretin-1 (orexin A) levels in the rat in relation to the light-dark cycle and sleep-wake activities. *Eur J Neurosci.* 2001;14(7): 1075–1081.
103. Yoshimichi G, Yoshimatsu H, Masaki T, Sakata T. Orexin-A regulates body temperature in coordination with arousal status. *Exp Biol Med (Maywood).* 2001;226(5):468–476.
104. Matsumura K, Tsuchihashi T, Abe I. Central orexin-A augments sympathoadrenal outflow in conscious rabbits. *Hypertension.* 2001;37(6): 1382–1387.
105. Siegel JM, Boehmer LN. Narcolepsy and the hypocretin system—where motion meets emotion. *Nat Clin Pract Neurol.* 2006;2(10):548–556.
106. Gulyani S, Wu MF, Nienhuis R, John J, Siegel JM. Cataplexy-related neurons in the amygdala of the narcoleptic dog. *Neuroscience.* 2002;112(2): 355–365.
107. Kiyashchenko LI, Mileykovskiy BY, Maidment N, et al. Release of hypocretin (orexin) during waking and sleep states. *J Neurosci.* 2002;22(13): 5282–5286.
108. Erlich SS, Itabashi HH. Narcolepsy: a neuropathologic study. *Sleep.* 1986;9(1, pt 2):126–132.
109. Gerashchenko D, Murillo-Rodriguez E, Lin L, et al. Relationship between CSF hypocretin levels and hypocretin neuronal loss. *Exp Neurol.* 2003;184(2):1010–1016.
110. Thannickal TC, Lai YY, Siegel JM. Hypocretin (orexin) cell loss in Parkinson's disease. *Brain.* 2007;130(pt 6):1586–1595.
111. Fronczek R, Overeem S, Lee SY, et al. Hypocretin (orexin) loss and sleep disturbances in Parkinson's Disease. *Brain.* 2008;131(pt 1):e88.
112. Fronczek R, Overeem S, Lee SY, et al. Hypocretin (orexin) loss in Parkinson's disease. *Brain.* 2007;130(pt 6):1577–1585.
113. Overeem S, Dalmau J, Bataller L, et al. Hypocretin-1 CSF levels in anti-Ma2 associated encephalitis. *Neurology.* 2004;62(1):138–140.
114. Arii J, Kanbayashi T, Tanabe Y, et al. CSF hypocretin-1 (orexin-A) levels in childhood narcolepsy and neurologic disorders. *Neurology.* 2004; 63(12):2440–2442.
115. Kanbayashi T, Ishiguro H, Aizawa R, et al. Hypocretin-1 (orexin-A) concentrations in cerebrospinal fluid are low in patients with Guillain-Barre syndrome. *Psychiatry Clin Neurosci.* 2002; 56(3):273–274.
116. Rubin RL, Hajdukovich RM, Mitler MM. HLA-DR2 association with excessive somnolence in narcolepsy does not generalize to sleep apnea and is not accompanied by systemic autoimmune abnormalities. *Clin Immunol Immunopathol.* 1988;49(1):149–158.
117. Plazzi G, Montagna P, Provini F, Bizzi A, Cohen M, Lugaresi E. Pontine lesions in idiopathic narcolepsy. *Neurology.* 1996;46(5):1250–1254.
118. Fredrikson S, Carlander B, Billiard M, Link H. CSF immune variables in patients with narcolepsy. *Acta Neurol Scand.* 1990;81(3):253–254.
119. Tanaka S, Honda Y, Inoue Y, Honda M. Detection of autoantibodies against hypocretin, hcrtrl1, and hcrtr2 in narcolepsy: anti-Hcrt system antibody in narcolepsy. *Sleep.* 2006;29(5):633–638.
120. Black JL III, Silber MH, Krahn LE, et al. Studies of humoral immunity to preprohypocretin in human leukocyte antigen DQB1*0602-positive narcoleptic subjects with cataplexy. *Biol Psychiatry.* 2005; 58(6):504–9.
121. Black JL 3rd, Silber MH, Krahn LE, et al. Analysis of hypocretin (orexin) antibodies in patients with narcolepsy. *Sleep.* 2005;28(4): 427–431.
122. Overeem S, Black JL III, Lammers GJ. Narcolepsy: immunological aspects. *Sleep Med Rev.* 2008; 12(2):95–107.
123. Aran A, Lin L, Nevsimalova S, et al. Elevated anti-streptococcal antibodies in patients with recent narcolepsy onset. *Sleep.* 2009;32(8):979–983.
124. Dale RC. Post-streptococcal autoimmune disorders of the central nervous system. *Dev Med Child Neurol.* 2005;47(11):785–791.
125. Tanaka S, Honda M. IgG abnormality in narcolepsy and idiopathic hypersomnia. *PLoS One.* 5(3):e9555.
126. Boehmer LN, Wu MF, John J, Siegel JM. Treatment with immunosuppressive and anti-inflammatory agents delays onset of canine genetic narcolepsy and reduces symptom severity. *Exp Neurol.* 2004;188(2):292–299.
127. Hecht M, Lin L, Kushida CA, et al. Report of a case of immunosuppression with prednisone in an 8-year-old boy with an acute onset of hypocretin-deficiency narcolepsy. *Sleep.* 2003;26(7):809–810.
128. Dauvilliers Y, Abril B, Mas E, Michel F, Tafti M. Normalization of hypocretin-1 in narcolepsy after intravenous immunoglobulin treatment. *Neurology.* 2009;73(16):1333–1334.
129. Dauvilliers Y, Carlander B, Rivier F, Touchon J, Tafti M. Successful management of cataplexy with intravenous immunoglobulins at narcolepsy onset. *Ann Neurol.* 2004;56(6):905–908.
130. Lecendreux M, Maret S, Bassetti C, Mouren MC, Tafti M. Clinical efficacy of high-dose intravenous immunoglobulins near the onset of narcolepsy in a 10-year-old boy. *J Sleep Res.* 2003;12(4):347–348.
131. Plazzi G, Poli F, Franceschini C, et al. Intravenous high-dose immunoglobulin treatment in recent onset childhood narcolepsy with cataplexy. *J Neurol.* 2008;255(10):1549–1554.
132. Schatzberg SJ, Cutter-Schatzberg K, Nydam D, et al. The effect of hypocretin replacement therapy in a 3-year-old Weimaraner with narcolepsy. *J Vet Intern Med.* 2004;18(4):586–588.
133. Stores G. Recognition and management of narcolepsy. *Arch Dis Child.* 1999;81(6):519–524.
134. Wise MS, Lynch J. Narcolepsy in children. *Semin Pediatr Neurol.* 2001;8(4):198–206.
135. Okun ML, Lin L, Pelin Z, Hong S, Mignot E. Clinical aspects of narcolepsy-cataplexy across ethnic groups. *Sleep.* 2002;25(1): 27–35.
136. Benca RM. Narcolepsy and excessive daytime sleepiness: diagnostic considerations, epidemiology, and comorbidities. *J Clin Psychiatry.* 2007;68(suppl 13):5–8.

137. Wise MS. Narcolepsy and other disorders of excessive sleepiness. *Med Clin North Am.* 2004;88(3):597–610, vii–viii.
138. Kothare SV, Kaleyias J. Narcolepsy and other hypersomnias in children. *Curr Opin Pediatr.* 2008;20(6):666–675.
139. Stores G. The protean manifestations of childhood narcolepsy and their misinterpretation. *Dev Med Child Neurol.* 2006;48(4):307–310.
140. Harsh J, Peszka J, Hartwig G, Mitler M. Night-time sleep and daytime sleepiness in narcolepsy. *J Sleep Res.* 2000;9(3):309–316.
141. Vernet C, Arnulf I. Narcolepsy with long sleep time: a specific entity? *Sleep.* 2009;32(9):1229–1235.
142. Serra L, Montagna P, Mignot E, Lugaresi E, Plazzi G. Cataplexy features in childhood narcolepsy. *Mov Disord.* 2008;23(6):858–865.
143. Overeem S, Mignot E, van Dijk JG, Lammers GJ. Narcolepsy: clinical features, new pathophysiologic insights, and future perspectives. *J Clin Neurophysiol.* 2001;18(2):78–105.
144. Dahl RE, Holttum J, Trubnick L. A clinical picture of child and adolescent narcolepsy. *J Am Acad Child Adolesc Psychiatry.* 1994;33(6):834–841.
145. Thorpy MJ. Cataplexy associated with narcolepsy: epidemiology, pathophysiology and management. *CNS Drugs.* 2006;20(1):43–50.
146. Krahn LE, Lymp JF, Moore WR, Slocumb N, Silber MH. Characterizing the emotions that trigger cataplexy. *J Neuropsychiatry Clin Neurosci.* 2005;17(1):45–50.
147. Anic-LabatS,GuilleminaultC,KraemerHC,Meehan J, Arrigoni J, Mignot E. Validation of a cataplexy questionnaire in 983 sleep-disorders patients. *Sleep.* 1999;22(1):77–87.
148. Hayes D Jr. Narcolepsy with cataplexy in early childhood. *Clin Pediatr (Phila).* 2006;45(4): 361–363.
149. Stahl SM, Layzer RB, Aminoff MJ, Townsend JJ, Feldon S. Continuous cataplexy in a patient with a midbrain tumor: the limp man syndrome. *Neurology.* 1980;30(10):1115–1118.
150. Simon DK, Nishino S, Scammell TE. Mistaken diagnosis of psychogenic gait disorder in a man with status cataplecticus ("limp man syndrome"). *Mov Disord.* 2004;19(7):838–840.
151. Kandt RS, Emerson RG, Singer HS, Valle DL, Moser HW. Cataplexy in variant forms of Niemann-Pick disease.*Ann Neurol.* 1982;12(3):284–288.
152. Parkes JD. Genetic factors in human sleep disorders with special reference to Norrie disease, Prader-Willi syndrome and Moebius syndrome. *J Sleep Res.* 1999;8(suppl 1):14–22.
153. Martinez-Rodriguez JE, Lin L, Iranzo A, et al. Decreased hypocretin-1 (Orexin-A) levels in the cerebrospinal fluid of patients with myotonic dystrophy and excessive daytime sleepiness. *Sleep.* 2003;26(3):287–290.
154. Goode GB. Sleep paralysis. *Arch Neurol.* 1962; 6:228–234.
155. Girard TA, Cheyne JA. Timing of spontaneous sleep-paralysis episodes. *J Sleep Res.* 2006;15(2):222–229.
156. Guilleminault C, Pelayo R. Narcolepsy in prepubertal children. *Ann Neurol.* 1998;43(1):135–142.
157. Sturzenegger C, Bassetti CL. The clinical spectrum of narcolepsy with cataplexy: a reappraisal. *J Sleep Res.* 2004;13(4):395–406.
158. Dahmen N, Kasten M, Muller MJ, Mittag K. Frequency and dependence on body posture of hallucinations and sleep paralysis in a community sample. *J Sleep Res.* 2002;11(2):179–180.
159. Plazzi G, Serra L, Ferri R. Nocturnal aspects of narcolepsy with cataplexy. *Sleep Med Rev.* 2008;12(2):109–128.
160. Ohayon MM. Prevalence of hallucinations and their pathological associations in the general population. *Psychiatry Res.* 2000;97(2–3):153–164.
161. Ohayon MM, Priest RG, Caulet M, Guilleminault C. Hypnagogic and hypnopompic hallucinations: pathological phenomena? *Br J Psychiatry.* 1996;169(4):459–467.
162. Nobili L, Beelke M, Besset A, Billiard M, Ferrillo F. Nocturnal sleep features in narcolepsy: a model-based approach. *Rev Neurol (Paris).* 2001; 157(11, pt 2):S82–S86.
163. Dauvilliers Y, Rompre S, Gagnon JF, Vendette M, Petit D, Montplaisir J. REM sleep characteristics in narcolepsy and REM sleep behavior disorder. *Sleep.* 2007;30(7):844–849.
164. Schenck CH, Mahowald MW. Motor dyscontrol in narcolepsy: rapid-eye-movement (REM) sleep without atonia and REM sleep behavior disorder. *Ann Neurol.* 1992;32(1):3–10.
165. Ferri R, Franceschini C, Zucconi M, et al. Searching for a marker of REM sleep behavior disorder: submentalis muscle EMG amplitude analysis during sleep in patients with narcolepsy/cataplexy. *Sleep.* 2008;31(10):1409–1417.
166. Maski KP, Kothare SV. Searching for marker of REM sleep behavior disorder: submentalis muscle EMG amplitude analysis during sleep in patients with narcolepsy/cataplexy. *Sleep.* 2009;32(2):137.
167. Nightingale S, Orgill JC, Ebrahim IO, de Lacy SF, Agrawal S, Williams AJ. The association between narcolepsy and REM behavior disorder (RBD). *Sleep Med.* 2005;6(3):253–258.
168. Billiard M. REM sleep behavior disorder and narcolepsy. *CNS Neurol Disord Drug Targets.* 2009;8(4):264–270.
169. Bahammam A. Periodic leg movements in narcolepsy patients: impact on sleep architecture. *Acta Neurol Scand.* 2007;115(5):351–355.
170. Ferri R, Zucconi M, Manconi M, et al. Different periodicity and time structure of leg movements during sleep in narcolepsy/cataplexy and restless legs syndrome. *Sleep.* 2006;29(12):1587–1594.
171. Dahmen N, Kasten M, Wieczorek S, Gencik M, Epplen JT, Ullrich B. Increased frequency of migraine in narcoleptic patients: a confirmatory study. *Cephalalgia.* 2003;23(1):14–19.
172. Dahmen N, Querings K, Grun B, Bierbrauer J. Increased frequency of migraine in narcoleptic patients. *Neurology.* 1999;52(6):1291–1293.
173. Luc ME, Gupta A, Birnberg JM, Reddick D, Kohrman MH. Characterization of symptoms of

sleep disorders in children with headache. *Pediatr Neurol.* 2006;34(1):7–12.

174. Vandeputte M, de Weerd A. Sleep disorders and depressive feelings: a global survey with the Beck depression scale. *Sleep Med.* 2003;4(4): 343–345.
175. Chakravorty SS, Rye DB. Narcolepsy in the older adult: epidemiology, diagnosis and management. *Drugs Aging.* 2003;20(5):361–376.
176. Billiard M, Bassetti C, Dauvilliers Y, et al. EFNS guidelines on management of narcolepsy. *Eur J Neurol.* 2006;13(10):1035–1048.
177. Fortuyn HA, Swinkels S, Buitelaar J, et al. High prevalence of eating disorders in narcolepsy with cataplexy: a case-control study. *Sleep.* 2008;31(3):335–341.
178. Chabas D, Foulon C, Gonzalez J, et al. Eating disorder and metabolism in narcoleptic patients. *Sleep.* 2007;30(10):1267–1273.
179. Dahmen N, Becht J, Engel A, Thommes M, Tonn P. Prevalence of eating disorders and eating attacks in narcolepsy. *Neuropsychiatr Dis Treat.* 2008;4(1):257–261.
180. Bell I. Diet histories in narcolepsy. In: Guilleminault C, Dement W, Passouant P, eds. *Narcolepsy.* New York, NY: Spectrum Publications; 1976:221–227.
181. Kotagal S, Krahn LE, Slocumb N. A putative link between childhood narcolepsy and obesity. *Sleep Med.* 2004;5(2):147–150.
182. Baker TL, Guilleminault C, Nino-Murcia G, Dement WC. Comparative polysomnographic study of narcolepsy and idiopathic central nervous system hypersomnia. *Sleep.* 1986;9(1, pt 2):232–242.
183. Stores G, Montgomery P, Wiggs L. The psychosocial problems of children with narcolepsy and those with excessive daytime sleepiness of uncertain origin. *Pediatrics.* 2006;118(4):e1116–e1123.
184. Littner MR, Kushida C, Wise M, et al. Practice parameters for clinical use of the multiple sleep latency test and the maintenance of wakefulness test. *Sleep.* 2005;28(1):113–121.
185. Martin SK, Eastman CI. Sleep logs of young adults with self-selected sleep times predict the dim light melatonin onset. *Chronobiol Int.* 2002;19(4):695–707.
186. Bradshaw DA, Yanagi MA, Pak ES, Peery TS, Ruff GA. Nightly sleep duration in the 2-week period preceding multiple sleep latency testing. *J Clin Sleep Med.* 2007;3(6):613–619.
187. Hoddes E, Zarcone V, Smythe H, Phillips R, Dement WC. Quantification of sleepiness: a new approach. *Psychophysiology.* 1973;10(4):431–436.
188. Johns MW. A new method for measuring daytime sleepiness: the Epworth sleepiness scale. *Sleep.* 1991;14(6):540–545.
189. Drake C, Nickel C, Burduvali E, Roth T, Jefferson C, Pietro B. The pediatric daytime sleepiness scale (PDSS): sleep habits and school outcomes in middle-school children. *Sleep.* 2003;26(4):455–458.
190. Clinical practice guideline: diagnosis and management of childhood obstructive sleep apnea syndrome. *Pediatrics.* 2002; 109(4):704–712.
191. Nevsimalova S, Prihodova I, Kemlink D, Lin L, Mignot E. REM behavior disorder (RBD) can be one of the first symptoms of childhood narcolepsy. *Sleep Med.* 2007; 8(7–8):784–786.
192. Kothare SV, Kaleyias J. The clinical and laboratory assessment of the sleepy child. *Semin Pediatr Neurol.* 2008;15(2):61–69.
193. Carskadon MA, Dement WC, Mitler MM, Roth T, Westbrook PR, Keenan S. Guidelines for the multiple sleep latency test (MSLT): a standard measure of sleepiness. *Sleep.* 1986;9(4):519–524.
194. Arand D, Bonnet M, Hurwitz T, Mitler M, Rosa R, Sangal RB. The clinical use of the MSLT and MWT. *Sleep.* 2005;28(1):123–144.
195. Kotagal S, Hartse KM, Walsh JK. Characteristics of narcolepsy in preteenaged children. *Pediatrics.* 1990;85(2):205–209.
196. Aldrich MS, Chervin RD, Malow BA. Value of the multiple sleep latency test (MSLT) for the diagnosis of narcolepsy. *Sleep.* 1997;20(8):620–629.
197. Singh M, Drake CL, Roth T. The prevalence of multiple sleep-onset REM periods in a population-based sample. *Sleep.* 2006;29(7):890–895.
198. Wise MS. Childhood narcolepsy. *Neurology.* 1998;50(2)(suppl 1):S37–S42.
199. Gozal D, Wang M, Pope DW Jr. Objective sleepiness measures in pediatric obstructive sleep apnea. *Pediatrics.* 2001;108(3):693–697.
200. Palm L, Persson E, Elmqvist D, Blennow G. Sleep and wakefulness in normal preadolescent children. *Sleep.* 1989;12(4):299–308.
201. Fallone G, Owens JA, Deane J. Sleepiness in children and adolescents: clinical implications. *Sleep Med Rev.* 2002;6(4):287–306.
202. Mitler MM, Doghramji K, Shapiro C. The maintenance of wakefulness test: normative data by age. *J Psychosom Res.* 2000;49(5):363–365.
203. Mignot E, Young T, Lin L, Finn L. Nocturnal sleep and daytime sleepiness in normal subjects with HLA-DQB1*0602. *Sleep.* 1999;22(3):347–352.
204. Dauvilliers Y, Arnulf I, Mignot E. Narcolepsy with cataplexy. *Lancet.* 2007;369(9560):499–511.
205. Honda Y, Juji T, Matsuki K, et al. HLA-DR2 and Dw2 in narcolepsy and in other disorders of excessive somnolence without cataplexy. *Sleep.* 1986;9(1 pt 2): 133–142.
206. Mignot E, Hayduk R, Black J, Grumet FC, Guilleminault C. HLA DQB1*0602 is associated with cataplexy in 509 narcoleptic patients. *Sleep.* 1997; 20(11):1012–1020.
207. Gibson ES, Powles AC, Thabane L, et al. "Sleepiness" is serious in adolescence: two surveys of 3235 Canadian students. *BMC Public Health.* 2006;6(116):116.
208. Bassetti C, Aldrich MS. Idiopathic hypersomnia. A series of 42 patients. *Brain.* 1997;120(pt 8): 1423–1435.
209. Billiard M, Dauvilliers Y. Idiopathic Hypersomnia. *Sleep Med Rev.* 2001;5(5):349–358.
210. Sasai T, Inoue Y, Komada Y, Sugiura T, Matsushima E. Comparison of clinical characteristics among narcolepsy with and without cataplexy and idiopathic hypersomnia without long sleep time, focusing on HLA-DRB1(*)1501/DQB1(*)0602 finding. *Sleep Med.* 2009; 10(9):961–966.

211. Bruck D, Parkes JD. A comparison of idiopathic hypersomnia and narcolepsy-cataplexy using self report measures and sleep diary data. *J Neurol Neurosurg Psychiatry.* 1996;60(5):576–578.
212. Pizza F, Vandi S, Detto S, et al. Different sleep onset criteria at the multiple sleep latency test (MSLT): an additional marker to differentiate central nervous system (CNS) hypersomnias. *J Sleep Res.* 2010.
213. Arnulf I, Lin L, Gadoth N, et al. Kleine-Levin syndrome: a systematic study of 108 patients. *Ann Neurol.* 2008;63(4):482–493.
214. Critchley M, Hoffman HL. The syndrome of periodic somnolence and morbid hunger (Kleine-Levin syndrome). *Br Med J.* 1942;33:137–139.
215. Lamarche LJ, Driver HS, Wiebe S, Crawford L, DE.Koninck JM. Nocturnal sleep, daytime sleepiness, and napping among women with significant emotional/behavioral premenstrual symptoms. *J Sleep Res.* 2007;16(3):262–268.
216. Manber R, Bootzin RR. Sleep and the menstrual cycle. *Health Psychol.* 1997;16(3):209–214.
217. Regal AR, Amigo MC, Cebrian E. Sleep and women. *Rev Neurol.* 2009;49(7):376–382.
218. Guilleminault C, Stoohs R, Clerk A, Cetel M, Maistros P. A cause of excessive daytime sleepiness. The upper airway resistance syndrome. *Chest.* 1993;104(3):781–787.
219. Liu X, Buysse DJ, Gentzler AL, et al. Insomnia and hypersomnia associated with depressive phenomenology and comorbidity in childhood depression. *Sleep.* 2007;30(1):83–90.
220. Lim CG, Ooi YP, Fung DS, Mahendran R, Kaur A. Sleep disturbances in Singaporean children with attention deficit hyperactivity disorder. *Ann Acad Med Singapore.* 2008;37(8):655–661.
221. Krahn LE, Hansen MR, Shepard JW. Pseudocataplexy. *Psychosomatics.* 2001;42(4):356–358.
222. Krahn LE. Reevaluating spells initially identified as cataplexy. *Sleep Med.* 2005;6(6):537–542.
223. Nishino S, Kanbayashi T. Symptomatic narcolepsy, cataplexy and hypersomnia, and their implications in the hypothalamic hypocretin/orexin system. *Sleep Med Rev.* 2005;9(4):269–310.
224. Guilleminault C, Yuen KM, Gulevich MG, Karadeniz D, Leger D, Philip P. Hypersomnia after head-neck trauma: a medicolegal dilemma. *Neurology.* 2000;54(3):653–659.
225. Black JE, Brooks SN, Nishino S. Narcolepsy and syndromes of primary excessive daytime somnolence. *Semin Neurol.* 2004;24(3):271–282.
226. Manni R, Politini L, Nobili L, et al. Hypersomnia in the Prader-Willi syndrome: clinical-electrophysiological features and underlying factors. *Clin Neurophysiol.* 2001;112(5):800–805.
227. Vossler DG, Wyler AR, Wilkus RJ, Gardner-Walker G, Vlcek BW. Cataplexy and monoamine oxidase deficiency in Norrie disease. *Neurology.* 1996;46(5):1258–1261.
228. Zarowski M, Steinborn B, Gurda B, Dvorakova L, Vlaskova H, Kothare SV. Treatment of cataplexy in Niemann-Pick disease type C with the use of miglustat. *Eur J Paediatr Neurol.* 2010 Mar 5. [Epub ahead of print]
229. Schwartz WJ, Stakes JW, Hobson JA. Transient cataplexy after removal of a craniopharyngioma. *Neurology.* 1984;34(10):1372–1375.
230. Aldrich MS, Naylor MW. Narcolepsy associated with lesions of the diencephalon. *Neurology.* 1989;39(11):1505–1508.
231. Malik S, Boeve BF, Krahn LE, Silber MH. Narcolepsy associated with other central nervous system disorders. *Neurology.* 2001;57(3):539–541.
232. Arii J, Kanbayashi T, Tanabe Y, Ono J, Nishino S, Kohno Y. A hypersomnolent girl with decreased CSF hypocretin level after removal of a hypothalamic tumor. *Neurology.* 2001;56(12):1775–1776.
233. Scammell TE, Nishino S, Mignot E, Saper CB. Narcolepsy and low CSF orexin (hypocretin) concentration after a diencephalic stroke. *Neurology.* 2001;56(12):1751–1753.
234. Clavelou P, Tournilhac M, Vidal C, Georget AM, Picard L, Merienne L. Narcolepsy associated with arteriovenous malformation of the diencephalon. *Sleep.* 1995;18(3):202–205.
235. Mitler MM, Carskadon MA, Czeisler CA, Dement WC, Dinges DF, Graeber RC. Catastrophes, sleep, and public policy: consensus report. *Sleep.* 1988;11(1):100–109.
236. Findley LJ, Suratt PM, Dinges DF. Time-on-task decrements in "steer clear" performance of patients with sleep apnea and narcolepsy. *Sleep.* 1999;22(6):804–809.
237. Broughton R, Ghanem Q, Hishikawa Y, Sugita Y, Nevsimalova S, Roth B. Life effects of narcolepsy in 180 patients from North America, Asia and Europe compared to matched controls. *Can J Neurol Sci.* 1981;8(4):299–304.
238. Rogers AE, Aldrich MS, Lin X. A comparison of three different sleep schedules for reducing daytime sleepiness in narcolepsy. *Sleep.* 2001;24(4):385–391.
239. Mullington J, Broughton R. Scheduled naps in the management of daytime sleepiness in narcolepsy-cataplexy. *Sleep.* 1993;16(5):444–456.
240. Wise MS, Arand DL, Auger RR, Brooks SN, Watson NF. Treatment of narcolepsy and other hypersomnias of central origin. An American Academy of Sleep Medicine Review. *Sleep.* 2007;30(12):1712–1727.
241. Husain AM, Yancy WS Jr, Carwile ST, Miller PP, Westman EC. Diet therapy for narcolepsy. *Neurology.* 2004; 62(12):2300–2302.
242. Littner M, Johnson SF, McCall WV, et al. Practice parameters for the treatment of narcolepsy: an update for 2000. *Sleep.* 2001;24(4):451–466.
243. Pelayo R, Dubik M. Pediatric sleep pharmacology. *Semin Pediatr Neurol.* 2008;15(2):79–90.
244. Mitler MM, Aldrich MS, Koob GF, Zarcone VP. Narcolepsy and its treatment with stimulants. ASDA standards of practice. *Sleep.* 1994; 17(4):352–371.
245. Yoss RE, Daly DD. On the treatment of narcolepsy. *Med Clin North Am.* 1968;52(4):781–787.

246. Shindler J, Schachter M, Brincat S, Parkes JD. Amphetamine, mazindol, and fencamfamin in narcolepsy. *Br Med J (Clin Res Ed)*. 1985; 290(6476):1167–1170.
247. Mitler MM, Hajdukovic R, Erman M, Koziol JA. Narcolepsy. *J Clin Neurophysiol*. 1990;7(1): 93–118.
248. Mitler MM, Hajdukovic R, Erman MK. Treatment of narcolepsy with methamphetamine. *Sleep*. 1993;16(4):306–317.
249. Parkes JD, Dahlitz M. Amphetamine prescription. *Sleep*. 1993;16(3):201–203.
250. Guilleminault C. Amphetamines and narcolepsy: use of the Stanford database. *Sleep*. 1993; 16(3):199–201.
251. Aldrich MS. Narcolepsy. *N Engl J Med*. 1990;323(6):389–394.
252. Bassetti C, Aldrich MS. Narcolepsy. *Neurol Clin*. 1996;14(3):545–571.
253. Mitler MM, Shafor R, Hajdukovich R, Timms RM, Browman CP. Treatment of narcolepsy: objective studies on methylphenidate, pemoline, and protriptyline. *Sleep*. 1986;9(1 pt 2):260–264.
254. Greenhill LL, Biederman J, Boellner SW, et al. A randomized, double-blind, placebo-controlled study of modafinil film-coated tablets in children and adolescents with attention-deficit/hyperactivity disorder. *J Am Acad Child Adolesc Psychiatry*. 2006;45(5):503–511.
255. Honda Y, Hishikawa Y. A long-term treatment of narcolepsy and excessive daytime sleepiness with pemoline (Bentanamin). *Curr Ther Res*. 1980;27:429–441.
256. Knoll J. Deprenyl (selegiline): the history of its development and pharmacological action. *Acta Neurol Scand Suppl*. 1983;95:57–80.
257. Kuran W. Selegiline (Jumex) in the treatment of narcolepsy. *Neurol Neurochir Pol*. 1993; 27(1):131–133.
258. Mayer G, Ewert Meier K, Hephata K. Selegeline hydrochloride treatment in narcolepsy. A double-blind, placebo-controlled study. *Clin Neuropharmacol*. 1995;18(4):306–319.
259. Reinish LW, MacFarlane JG, Sandor P, Shapiro CM. REM changes in narcolepsy with selegiline. *Sleep*. 1995;18(5):362–367.
260. Hublin C, Partinen M, Heinonen EH, Puukka P, Salmi T. Selegiline in the treatment of narcolepsy. *Neurology*. 1994;44(11):2095–2101.
261. Schneider LS, Tariot PN, Goldstein B. Therapy with l-deprenyl (selegiline) and relation to abuse liability. *Clin Pharmacol Ther*. 1994;56(6 pt 2): 750–756.
262. Ferraro L, Antonelli T, O'Connor WT, Tanganelli S, Rambert FA, Fuxe K. Modafinil: an antinarcoleptic drug with a different neurochemical profile to d-amphetamine and dopamine uptake blockers. *Biol Psychiatry*. 1997;42(12):1181–1183.
263. Wyatt RJ, Fram DH, Buchbinder R, Snyder F. Treatment of intractable narcolepsy with a monoamine oxidase inhibitor. *N Engl J Med*. 1971;285(18):987–991.
264. Lin JS, Roussel B, Akaoka H, Fort P, Debilly G, Jouvet M. Role of catecholamines in the modafinil and amphetamine induced wakefulness, a comparative pharmacological study in the cat. *Brain Res*. 1992;591(2):319–326.
265. Mignot E, Nishino S, Guilleminault C, Dement WC. Modafinil binds to the dopamine uptake carrier site with low affinity. *Sleep*. 1994;17(5): 436–437.
266. Ferraro L, Tanganelli S, O'Connor WT, Antonelli T, Rambert F, Fuxe K. The vigilance promoting drug modafinil decreases GABA release in the medial preoptic area and in the posterior hypothalamus of the awake rat: possible involvement of the serotonergic 5-HT3 receptor. *Neurosci Lett*. 1996;220(1):5–8.
267. Randomized trial of modafinil for the treatment of pathological somnolence in narcolepsy. US Modafinil in Narcolepsy Multicenter Study Group. *Ann Neurol*. 1998;43(1):88–97.
268. Randomized trial of modafinil as a treatment for the excessive daytime somnolence of narcolepsy: US Modafinil in Narcolepsy Multicenter Study Group. *Neurology*. 2000;54(5):1166–1175.
269. Boivin DB, Montplaisir J, Petit D, Lambert C, Lubin S. Effects of modafinil on symptomatology of human narcolepsy. *Clin Neuropharmacol*. 1993;16(1):46–53.
270. Billiard M, Besset A, Montplaisir J, et al. Modafinil: a double-blind multicentric study. *Sleep*. 1994;17(suppl 8):S107–S112.
271. Biederman J, Swanson JM, Wigal SB, Boellner SW, Earl CQ, Lopez FA, *Modafinil ADHD Study Group*. A comparison of once-daily and divided doses of modafinil in children with attention-deficit/hyperactivity disorder: a randomized, double-blind, and placebo-controlled study. *J Clin Psychiatry*. 2006;67(5):727–735.
272. Biederman J, Swanson JM, Wigal SB, et al. Efficacy and safety of modafinil film-coated tablets in children and adolescents with attention-deficit/hyperactivity disorder: results of a randomized, double-blind, placebo-controlled, flexible-dose study. *Pediatrics*. 2005;116(6):e777–e784.
273. Swanson JM, Greenhill LL, Lopez FA, et al. Modafinil film-coated tablets in children and adolescents with attention-deficit/hyperactivity disorder: results of a randomized, double-blind, placebo-controlled, fixed-dose study followed by abrupt discontinuation. *J Clin Psychiatry*. 2006;67(1):137–147.
274. Gold LH, Balster RL. Evaluation of the cocaine-like discriminative stimulus effects and reinforcing effects of modafinil. *Psychopharmacology (Berl)*. 1996;126(4):286–292.
275. Jasinski DR. An evaluation of the abuse potential of modafinil using methylphenidate as a reference. *J Psychopharmacol*. 2000;14(1):53–60.
276. Mitler MM, Harsh J, Hirshkowitz M, Guilleminault C. Long-term efficacy and safety of modafinil (PROVIGIL((R))) for the treatment of excessive daytime sleepiness associated with narcolepsy. *Sleep Med*. 2000;1(3):231–243.
277. Dinges DF, Arora S, Darwish M, Niebler GE. Pharmacodynamic effects on alertness of single

doses of armodafinil in healthy subjects during a nocturnal period of acute sleep loss. *Curr Med Res Opin*. 2006;22(1):159–167.
278. Harsh JR, Hayduk R, Rosenberg R, et al. The efficacy and safety of armodafinil as treatment for adults with excessive sleepiness associated with narcolepsy. *Curr Med Res Opin*. 2006;22(4): 761–774.
279. Roth T, White D, Schmidt-Nowara W, et al. Effects of armodafinil in the treatment of residual excessive sleepiness associated with obstructive sleep apnea/hypopnea syndrome: a 12-week, multicenter, double-blind, randomized, placebo-controlled study in nCPAP-adherent adults. *Clin Ther.* 2006;28(5):689–706.
280. Laborit H. Sodium 4-Hydroxybutyrate. *Int J Neuropharmacol*. 1964;3:433–451.
281. Laborit H. Correlations between protein synthesis and serotonin in various activities of the central nervous system (slow and desynchronized sleep, learning and memory, sexual activity, morphine tolerance, aggressivity, Na gammahydroxybutyrate pharmacology). *Agressologie*. 1971;12(1):9–23.
282. Mamelak M, Escriu JM, Stokan O. Sleep-inducing effects of gammahydroxybutyrate. *Lancet*. 1973; 2(7824):328–329.
283. Mamelak M, Webster P. Treatment of narcolepsy and sleep apnea with gamma-hydroxybutyrate: a clinical and polysomnographic case study. *Sleep*. 1981;4(1):105–11.
284. Broughton R, Mamelak M. Effects of nocturnal gamma-hydroxybutyrate on sleep/waking patterns in narcolepsy-cataplexy. *Can J Neurol Sci*. 1980;7(1):23–31.
285. Scrima L, Hartman PG, Johnson FH Jr, Thomas EE, Hiller FC. The effects of gamma-hydroxybutyrate on the sleep of narcolepsy patients: a double-blind study. *Sleep*. 1990;13(6):479–490.
286. Lammers GJ, Arends J, Declerck AC, Ferrari MD, Schouwink G, Troost J. Gammahydroxybutyrate and narcolepsy: a double-blind placebo-controlled study. *Sleep*. 1993;16(3):216–220.
287. Brenneisen R, Elsohly MA, Murphy TP, et al. Pharmacokinetics and excretion of gamma-hydroxybutyrate (GHB) in healthy subjects. *J Anal Toxicol*. 2004;28(8): 625–630.
288. Borgen LA, Cook HN, Hornfeldt CS, Fuller DE. Sodium oxybate (GHB) for treatment of cataplexy. *Pharmacotherapy*. 2002;22(6):798–799, discussion 799.
289. Borgen LA, Okerholm R, Morrison D, Lai A. The influence of gender and food on the pharmacokinetics of sodium oxybate oral solution in healthy subjects. *J Clin Pharmacol*. 2003;43(1):59–65.
290. Borgen LA, Okerholm RA, Lai A, Scharf MB. The pharmacokinetics of sodium oxybate oral solution following acute and chronic administration to narcoleptic patients. *J Clin Pharmacol*. 2004;44(3): 253–257.
291. Abanades S, Farre M, Segura M, et al. Gamma-hydroxybutyrate (GHB) in humans: pharmacodynamics and pharmacokinetics. *Ann N Y Acad Sci*. 2006;1074:559–576.
292. Goodwin AK, Brown PR, Jansen EEW, Jakobs C, Gibson KM, Weerts EM. Behavioral effects and pharmacokinetics of gamma-hydroxybutyrate (GHB) precursors gamma-butyrolactone (GBL) and 1,4-butanediol (1,4-BD) in baboons. *Psychopharmacology (Berl)*. 2009;204(3):465–476.
293. A 12-month, open-label, multicenter extension trial of orally administered sodium oxybate for the treatment of narcolepsy. *Sleep*. 2003;26(1):31–35.
294. *U.S. Xyrem Multicenter Study Group*. Sodium oxybate demonstrates long-term efficacy for the treatment of cataplexy in patients with narcolepsy. *Sleep Med*. 2004;5(2):119–123.
295. *Xyrem International Study Group*. A double-blind, placebo-controlled study demonstrates sodium oxybate is effective for the treatment of excessive daytime sleepiness in narcolepsy. *J Clin Sleep Med*. 2005;1(4):391–397.
296. A randomized, double blind, placebo-controlled multicenter trial comparing the effects of three doses of orally administered sodium oxybate with placebo for the treatment of narcolepsy. *Sleep*. 2002;25(1):42–49.
297. Murali H, Kotagal S. Off-label treatment of severe childhood narcolepsy-cataplexy with sodium oxybate. *Sleep*. 2006;29(8):1025–1029.
298. Tarabar AF, Nelson LS. The gamma-hydroxybutyrate withdrawal syndrome. *Toxicol Rev*. 2004;23(1):45–49.
299. Hart CL, Haney M, Vosburg SK, Comer SD, Gunderson E, Foltin RW. Modafinil attenuates disruptions in cognitive performance during simulated night-shift work. *Neuropsychopharmacology.* 2006; 31(7):1526–1536.
300. Black J, Houghton WC. Sodium oxybate improves excessive daytime sleepiness in narcolepsy. *Sleep*. 2006;29(7):939–946.
301. Larrosa O, de la Llave Y, Bario S, Granizo JJ, Garcia-Borreguero D. Stimulant and anticataplectic effects of reboxetine in patients with narcolepsy: a pilot study. *Sleep*. 2001; 24(3):282–285.
302. Lammers GJ, Arends J, Declerck AC, Kamphuisen HA, Schouwink G, Troost J. Ritanserin, a 5-HT2 receptor blocker, as add-on treatment in narcolepsy. *Sleep*. 1991;14(2):130–132.
303. Mayer G. Ritanserin improves sleep quality in narcolepsy. *Pharmacopsychiatry*. 2003; 36(4):150–155.
304. Guilleminault C, Aftab FA, Karadeniz D, Philip P, Leger D. Problems associated with switch to modafinil—a novel alerting agent in narcolepsy. *Eur J Neurol*. 2000;7(4):381–384.
305. Akimoto H, Honda Y, Takahashi Y. Pharmacotherapy in narcolepsy. *Dis Nerv Syst*. 1960;21: 704–706.
306. Frenette E, Kushida CA. Primary hypersomnias of central origin. *Semin Neurol*. 2009;29(4):354–367.
307. Dauvilliers Y, Billiard M, Montplaisir J. Clinical aspects and pathophysiology of narcolepsy. *Clin Neurophysiol*. 2003;114(11):2000–2017.
308. Poryazova R, Siccoli M, Werth E, Bassetti CL. Unusually prolonged rebound cataplexy after withdrawal of fluoxetine. *Neurology*. 2005; 65(6):967–968.

309. Schmidt HS, Clark RW, Hyman PR. Protriptyline: an effective agent in the treatment of the narcolepsy-cataplexy syndrome and hypersomnia. *Am J Psychiatry*. 1977;134(2):183–185.
310. Schachter M, Parkes JD. Fluvoxamine and clomipramine in the treatment of cataplexy. *J Neurol Neurosurg Psychiatry*. 1980;43(2):171–174.
311. Guilleminault C, Raynal D, Takahashi S, Carskadon M, Dement W. Evaluation of short-term and long-term treatment of the narcolepsy syndrome with clomipramine hydrochloride. *Acta Neurol Scand*. 1976;54(1):71–87.
312. Shapiro WR. Treatment of Cataplexy with Clomipramine. *Arch Neurol*. 1975;32(10):653–656.
313. Langdon N, Shindler J, Parkes JD, Bandak S. Fluoxetine in the treatment of cataplexy. *Sleep*. 1986;9(2):371–373.
314. Frey J, Darbonne C. Fluoxetine suppresses human cataplexy: a pilot study. *Neurology*. 1994; 44(4):707–709.
315. Schrader H, Kayed K, Bendixen Markset AC, Treidene HE. The treatment of accessory symptoms in narcolepsy: a double-blind cross-over study of a selective serotonin re-uptake inhibitor (femoxetine) versus placebo. *Acta Neurol Scand*. 1986;74(4):297–303.
316. Abad VC, Guilleminault C. Emerging drugs for narcolepsy. *Expert Opin Emerg Drugs*. 2004;9(2):281–291.
317. Mignot E, Nishino S. Emerging therapies in narcolepsy-cataplexy. *Sleep*. 2005;28(6):754–763.
318. Roselaar SE, Langdon N, Lock CB, Jenner P, Parkes JD. Selegiline in narcolepsy. *Sleep*. 1987; 10(5):491–495.
319. Iijima S, Sugita Y, Teshima Y, Hishikawa Y. Therapeutic effects of mazindol on narcolepsy. *Sleep*. 1986;9(1 pt 2):265–268.
320. Vespignani H, Barroche G, Escaillas JP, Weber M. Importance of mazindol in the treatment of narcolepsy. *Sleep*. 1984;7(3):274–275.
321. *Xyrem International Study Group*. Further evidence supporting the use of sodium oxybate for the treatment of cataplexy: a double-blind, placebo-controlled study in 228 patients. *Sleep Med*. 2005;6(5):415–421.
322. Thorpy M. Orally administered sodium oxybate for the treatment of narcolepsy. *Curr Neurol Neurosci Rep*. 2004;4(2):155–156.
323. Thorpy MJ. Sodium oxybate for the treatment of narcolepsy. *Expert Opin Pharmacother*. 2005;6(2):329–335.
324. Thorpy MJ, Snyder M, Aloe FS, Ledereich PS, Starz KE. Short-term triazolam use improves nocturnal sleep of narcoleptics. *Sleep*. 1992;15(3):212–216.
325. Chen W, Black J, Call P, Mignot E. Late-onset narcolepsy presenting as rapidly progressing muscle weakness: response to plasmapheresis. *Ann Neurol*. 2005;58(3):489–490.
326. Mieda M, Willie JT, Hara J, Sinton CM, Sakurai T, Yanagisawa M. Orexin peptides prevent cataplexy and improve wakefulness in an orexin neuron-ablated model of narcolepsy in mice. *Proc Natl Acad Sci U S A*. 2004;101(13):4649–4654.
327. Arias-Carrion O, Murillo-Rodriguez E. Cell transplantation: a future therapy for narcolepsy? *CNS Neurol Disord Drug Targets*. 2009; 8(4):309–314.
328. Arias-Carrion O, Drucker-Colin R, Murillo-Rodriguez E. Survival rates through time of hypocretin grafted neurons within their projection site. *Neurosci Lett*. 2006;404 (1–2):93–97.
329. Arias-Carrion O, Murillo-Rodriguez E, Xu M, Blanco-Centurion C, Drucker-Colin R, Shiromani PJ. Transplantation of hypocretin neurons into the pontine reticular formation: preliminary results. *Sleep*. 2004;27(8): 1465–1470.
330. Riehl J, Honda K, Kwan M, Hong J, Mignot E, Nishino S. Chronic oral administration of CG-3703, a thyrotropin releasing hormone analog, increases wake and decreases cataplexy in canine narcolepsy. *Neuropsychopharmacology*. 2000;23(1):34–45.
331. Nishino S, Arrigoni J, Shelton J, Kanbayashi T, Dement WC, Mignot E. Effects of thyrotropin-releasing hormone and its analogs on daytime sleepiness and cataplexy in canine narcolepsy. *J Neurosci*. 1997;17(16):6401–6408.
332. Broberger C, McCormick DA. Excitatory effects of thyrotropin-releasing hormone in the thalamus. *J Neurosci*. 2005; 25(7):1664–1673.
333. Barbier AJ, Berridge C, Dugovic C, et al. Acute wake-promoting actions of JNJ-5207852, a novel, diamine-based H3 antagonist. *Br J Pharmacol*. 2004;143(5):649–661.
334. Tedford CE, Phillips JG, Gregory R, et al. Development of trans-2-[1H-imidazol-4-yl] cyclopropane derivatives as new high-affinity histamine H3 receptor ligands. *J Pharmacol Exp Ther*. 1999;289(2):1160–1168.

CHAPTER 13

Circadian Rhythm Disorders

Tifenn Raffray, Eliza Van Reen, Leila Tarokh, and Mary A. Carskadon

Introduction

Sleep changes dramatically across development. Among the many changes, perhaps the most readily observable is a decline in sleep duration with age. For example, one study, that followed 493 participants from birth to 16 years with maternal report found a decrease in average sleep duration per 24 hours from 14.2 hours at 6 months to 8.1 hours at 16 years [1] (see Figure 13.1). Furthermore, across the first year of life, sleep gradually becomes consolidated to the nighttime, but daytime napping is common. Iglowstein and colleagues, for example, reported that all participants less than 1 year of age napped, and napping showed a steady developmental decline such that there was essentially no napping at 7 years of age [1]. On the other hand, individual and racial differences in reported napping and nocturnal sleep exist. One study from the southern United States showed that at 8 years of age, more black children (39.1%) were reported to nap compared with non-Hispanic white children (4.9%) [2]. In addition, during the first year of life, it appears that circadian rhythms and the association of melatonin secretion with sleep-wake pattern become evident [3]. Moreover, a circadian rhythm in cortisol levels emerges between the third and sixth month after birth [4].

The transition to adolescence alters sleep-wake patterns: adolescents tend to go to bed later, get up later, and sleep less than prepubertal children. A common misperception is that adolescents need less sleep, but empirical data across a number of studies suggest that older adolescents need at least as much sleep as preadolescents, if not more [1,5].

Key Points

- Delayed sleep phase disorder (DSPD) is associated with excessive daytime sleepiness and excessive daytime sleepiness puts patients at increased risk for driving accidents.
- Comorbidity between DSPD and psychiatric disorders is high.
- Chronotherapy, timed light therapy, and timed exogenous melatonin are treatment options for circadian rhythm sleep disorder.
- Parental involvement in adolescents' sleep patterns is key.

A prevailing construct is that the adolescent delay in sleep is driven by biological processes that are exacerbated by factors such as increased assertion of autonomy and expanded opportunities for social interaction at nighttime [5,6]. Adolescents' increased striving toward independence translates into less parental influence on bedtime, taking on part-time jobs [5,7], and increased socialization with peers at night. The availability of media-related technology, such as computers, televisions, telephones, and music devices in the bedroom [8], offers an alluring alternative to sleep as well. Later bedtimes in adolescence are compounded by earlier school start times for older adolescents in the United States and elsewhere [5].

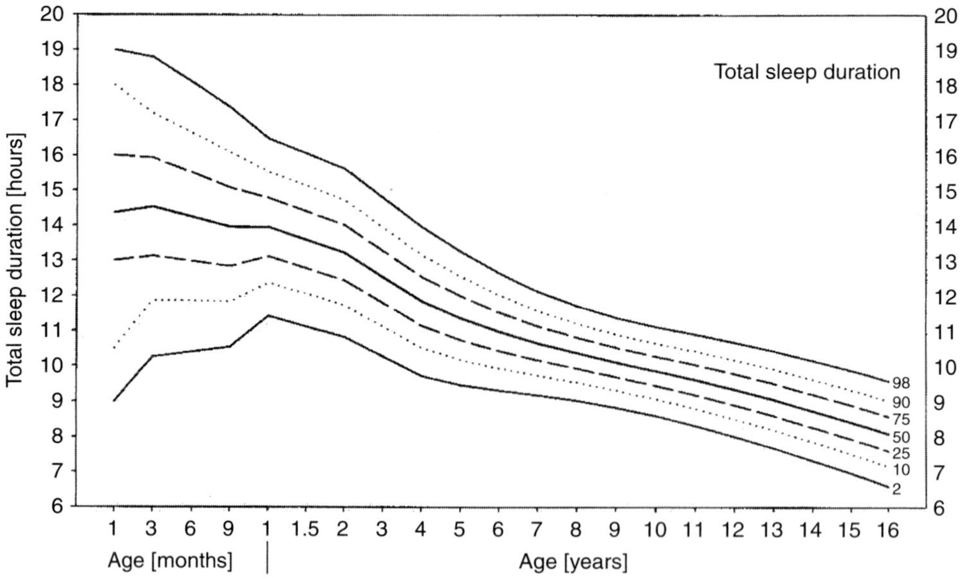

Figure 13.1 Percentiles for total sleep duration per 24 hours from infancy to adolescence. Reprinted with permission from Iglowstein and colleagues [1]. © 2003 *American Academy of Pediatrics.*

In a normally developing adolescent, all these factors contribute to the curtailment of sleep.

Distinguishing normal developmental phenomenon and circadian rhythm sleep disorders across childhood and adolescence can be challenging. This chapter first describes the biological processes that gate sleeping and waking, with an emphasis on circadian rhythms. Then, clinical assessment of circadian rhythm sleep disorder is detailed. Finally, circadian rhythm sleep disorders occurring in childhood and adolescence are reviewed with details on treatment options.

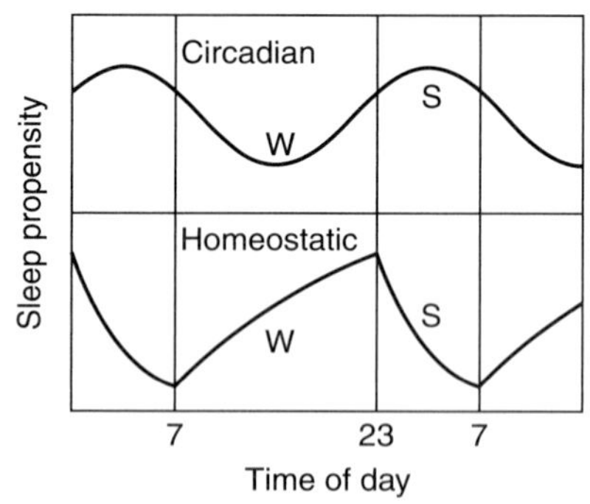

Figure 13.2 The 2-process model of sleep-wake regulation. Adapted from Refs. [40,85].

Sleep and Circadian Rhythms: An Overview

Intrinsic Processes

2-Process Model

The distribution of sleep-wake, as well as the distribution of stages within sleep are best understood using the 2-process model of sleep-wake regulation [9]. This model proposes 2 biological systems that regulate sleep-wake timing: a sleep-dependent homeostatic process (Process S) and a sleep-independent circadian process (Process C) [9]. The homeostatic process increases during waking and declines during sleep, whereas the circadian process is based on an internal daily biological rhythm or oscillation (see Figure 13.2).

Sleep Homeostatic System

The homeostatic process can be thought of as reflecting sleep "pressure." Physiological markers of the homeostatic process (Process S) include slow-wave sleep (SWS; non-rapid eye movement sleep stages 3 and 4) and sleep slow-wave activity (SWA; electroencephalogram [EEG] spectral power density in the 0.75- to 4.5-Hz range). Both features of sleep change predictably according to the length of prior waking and the progression of sleep across the night. For example, Webb and Agnew [10] demonstrated that longer bouts of prior waking were associated with increased stage 4 sleep in the subsequent sleep episode. Furthermore, Borbély and colleagues [11] showed that SWA during sleep after 40.5 hours of waking was greater than in sleep after roughly 16 hours of being awake. Shorter waking bouts examined in nap studies show more SWS and SWA during naps later in the day (following longer intervals of waking) compared with naps taken closer to waking [12]. In addition, SWA dissipates across the sleep episode with more SWA at the beginning of the sleep episode and less at the end of the sleep episode. In summary, Process S can be examined by looking at SWS and SWA: increases in these EEG phenomena are associated with increased pressure to sleep, and declines across sleep episodes are associated with recovery processes.

Circadian Timing System

A separate and independent process (Process C) gates the occurrence of sleep and wake and favors sleep or wake at different times relative to an internal daily oscillation. These oscillations have an intrinsic period of approximately 24 hours and are therefore referred to as circadian rhythms (circa = about, dies = day). The master mammalian circadian oscillator located in the suprachiasmatic nuclei (SCN) of the hypothalamus regulates the timing of sleep and wake and many other biological functions. Evidence for the role of the SCN in the timing of sleep comes from lesion studies showing that SCN destruction leads to arrhythmicity in sleeping and waking [13].

In addition to the gating of sleep and wakefulness, certain features of sleep and wake have strong circadian regulation. For example, rapid eye movement (REM) sleep is favored in the second half of a night's sleep because the second half of the night occurs at the trough of the core body temperature (CBT) rhythm—that is, the circadian phase when REM sleep is favored. A "wake-maintenance zone" linked to the circadian system occurs for a few hours in the evening before one's usual bedtime (see Figure 13.2).

Under typical circumstances, Process S and Process C interact to consolidate sleep at night and waking during the day (see Figure 13.2). Thus, as an individual's usual bedtime nears, high sleep pressure (Process S) supports falling asleep. Even though sleep pressure dissipates across the night, sleeping is sustained and consolidated in part by a strong circadian signal for sleep. The dissipation of Process S across the night meets the rising tide of the circadian wake promotion at the end of the night: the combination of the dissipation of Process S and the ramping up of Process C prepares us for wakefulness. Process S (sleep pressure) accumulates across the usual waking day and wakefulness is maintained into the evening; however, as the pressure to sleep encounters the crest of circadian wake promotion (wake-maintenance zone) wake is favored. The tendency for an afternoon slump in alertness appears to result when sleep pressure builds up earlier than the clock-dependent alerting strengthens.

Light and Measuring the Circadian Timing System

Ocular exposure to light is the most important stimulus involved in entraining circadian rhythms. Photic information from the eyes is transmitted to the SCN via the retinohypothalamic tract. In turn, the SCN sends information to the pineal gland, where the hormone melatonin is produced. The timing, intensity, and duration of light exposure are important factors for entraining circadian rhythms (see Figure 13.3). A phase response curve (PRC) describes how the timing of light affects circadian rhythms, because the effects of light are phase dependent. For example, light input occurring in the first half of the biological night leads to a delay of circadian rhythms, whereas, light input in the second half of the biological night produces an advance of circadian rhythms. Largest phase delays and phase advances occur toward the midpoint of the circadian night; smaller phase shifts to light result when light occurs near the fringes of night.

The intensity of light affects circadian phase shifts in a dose-dependent manner. For example, phase shifts are small or absent when

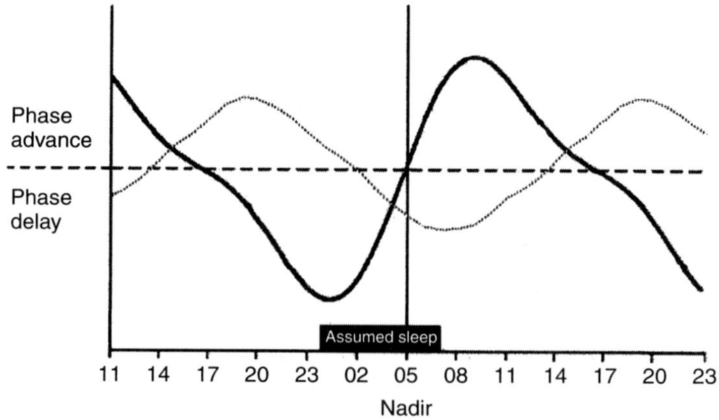

Figure 13.3 Schematic examples of phase response curves (PRCs) for light (solid line) and melatonin (dotted line) based on data from Khalsa and colleagues and Lewy and colleagues [59,85]. A PRC illustrates associations between the timing and the effects of a zeitgeber on circadian phase. Specific differences in effect between light and melatonin are not as shown in this figure; however, the general relationships are shown. Reprinted with permission from Bjorvatn and Pallesen [57]. © 2009 *Sleep Medicine Reviews*.

light exposure is dim (eg, less than 15 lux), but a saturating phase shift can be seen when using bright light (eg, greater than 500 lux) [14]. An important note, however, is that these studies indicate that room lighting can impact the circadian system, particularly for individuals who are not routinely exposed to bright light. Recently, studies have shown that the circadian system is sensitive to short-wavelength (blue) light. This sensitivity appears to arise from intrinsically photosensitive retinal ganglion cells (ipRGCs) that project directly to the SCN [15,16]. The photopigment melanopsin in these cells has peak sensitivity to light at approximately 482 to 484 nm [15].

How is the circadian system measured in humans? Early investigations used the CBT rhythm as a marker of circadian phase. This measure was difficult to obtain because the CBT rhythm is masked by sleep and activity. The CBT minimum was termed the "circadian trough," and the "circadian trough" is associated with changes in behavior (favors sleep), physiology (certain hormone production, eg, cortisol), and performance (decreased alertness and cognitive function).

A more common phase marker used currently is the hormone melatonin, which can be measured using serial samples of plasma, saliva, or urine for the urinary metabolite 6-sulfatoxymelatonin. Melatonin synthesis is suppressed by light; thus, melatonin collection (except from urine) needs to be performed in dim light conditions. Dim-light melatonin onset (DLMO) phase is the most common marker used to assess circadian phase. DLMO phase is estimated by collecting serial samples spaced about every 30 minutes in the subjective evening hours. Because melatonin is not produced in the circadian day, DLMO is captured at the clock time when melatonin levels are detectable. DLMO phase has been assessed using serial saliva samples in children and adolescents and has also been measured in infants and young children from urine collected in diapers, wherein estimates were made by curve fitting to the levels of 6-sulfatoxymelatonin in timed diaper collections [3,17].

The concept of phase angle is important in circadian biology and refers to the alignment of circadian phase markers and a reference marker such as clock time or sleep onset time. The importance of this concept in evaluating sleep behavior stems from the interaction of sleep patterns with circadian timing. The changes in phase angle that occur with jet travel, for example, lead to disrupted sleep and waking, as well as disruption in other activities such as eating and digestion. Children with abnormal phase angles on a consistent basis may suffer from chronic sleep problems.

Circadian period (also referred to as tau) can also be estimated in adolescents by taking serial saliva samples across a number of consecutive cycles during a protocol that creates an environmental day too long or too short for entrainment of the biological clock (typically 20-hour or 28-hour day lengths). This protocol is called "forced desynchrony" because of the free-running circadian rhythm that emerges on the background of the enforced sleep-wake schedule [18]. Intrinsic circadian period length may underlie sleep disruption in children and adolescents. Longer intrinsic period, for example, may be associated with delayed phase.

Assessing Circadian Rhythm Sleep Disorders in Clinical Practice

The *International Classification of Sleep Disorders* (ICSD) [19] defines circadian rhythm sleep disorders (CRSD) as:

> A persistent or recurrent pattern of sleep disturbance caused primarily by one of the following: alterations of the circadian timing system, misalignment between the endogenous circadian rhythm and exogenous factors that affect the timing or duration of sleep;
>
> The circadian-related sleep disruption leads to insomnia, excessive daytime sleepiness, or both;
>
> The sleep disturbance is associated with impairment of social, occupational, or other areas or functioning ([19], page 117).

As described in the previous section, DLMO is the gold standard measure of the phase of circadian rhythms. DLMO is mostly used in research; however, other tools such as actigraphy, and questionnaires assessing chronotype, sleep habits, and sleep pattern are available to the clinician for examining the behavioral outputs of the system.

An accurate assessment of sleep and wake always includes a thorough interview of the patient and his or her family and a physical examination. Clinical Pearl 1 describes key points about general assessment of sleep patterns in children and adolescents.

In most cases, a combination of questionnaires, sleep diaries, and actigraphy is used to address the diagnosis of CRSD, in which actigraphy and parental reports provide complimentary information about a child's sleep habits [20].

Polysomnography (PSG) is not indicated for the diagnosis of CRSD; however, PSG can be necessary to rule out another primary sleep disorder in patients whose symptoms suggest a primary sleep disorder in addition to CRSD.

Assessment of Chronotype

Morningness-eveningness preference, or chronotype, can be assessed using a Morningness-Eveningness Questionnaire (MEQ), such as the Horne and Ostberg questionnaire [21]. Insufficient evidence exists to recommend the routine use of the MEQ for the clinical evaluation of circadian rhythm sleep disorders [22,23]; however, a strong association is present for evening type with delayed sleep phase disorder (DSPD) and for morning type with advance sleep phase disorder (ASPD).

The MEQ has been validated in young adults, but not in children; however, 2 other scales have been developed for use to assess chronotype in children and adolescents: the morningness/eveningness scale for children, a self-report scale [24], and the children's chronotype questionnaire, a parental report [25]. Parents are often able to describe their children as night owls or morning larks, which may be as useful as questionnaires.

Sleep Diaries

Sleep diaries, or sleep logs, are daily records of estimated bedtime, sleep onset latency, awakenings (number, duration and time), wake-up time, rise time, and naps (number, duration, and time). Additional information, such as meal times, physical activity, or out of the ordinary events can also be useful. Parents are asked to fill in sleep diaries for children, and self-reports are common with adolescents. Sleep diaries recommended by the American Academy of Sleep Medicine are available online [26,27].

This inexpensive, simple tool is a valid source of information about sleeping patterns and most useful to provide information on the regularity of the timing and duration of sleep when collected for 2 weeks or longer. Use of sleep diaries is indicated in the assessment of patients with a suspected CRSD [22], and diaries are best used when sent to families before initial assessment if a CRSD is suspected. In this way, sleep patterns can be interpreted along with information obtained from other measures, interview, and physical examination. Sleep diaries are also useful during treatment in at least 2 ways: (1) they can help compliance with prescribed sleep-wake schedules (described in the next section of this chapter); (2) they provide information about efficacy of treatment (comparing sleep patterns pre- and postintervention).

Actigraphy

An actigraph is a small, wristwatchlike device containing an accelerometer for detecting and recording activity. The actigraph is a noninvasive, portable device worn on the nondominant wrist or on the ankle (only in very young children) that records and stores activity counts continuously for several weeks, thus providing information collected in habitual conditions over a long period of time. We note that actigraphy differs from actimetry or pedometry because the actigraph stores activity counts minute-by-minute rather than providing only a daily summary score. Estimates of sleep and wakefulness derived from the activity counts are produced using algorithms that have been validated against behavioral observation or PSG. Variables obtained include sleep start time, sleep endtime, wake after sleep onset, and sleep period. Actigraphy can overestimate sleep duration when an individual is awake and lying still (quiet wakefulness). At least 5 nights of usable recording are required to obtain reliable actigraph measures of sleep for children and adolescents [28]. Figure 13.4A provides examples of actigraphy recordings in adolescents. Actigraphy is used in combination with a sleep log (parental or adolescent's report) to help with interpretation of actigraphy data and to identify misperception of sleep.

Actigraphy results correlate well with other measurements of circadian rhythm such as melatonin and CBT. Observable sleep-wake rhythms are susceptible to masking effects, however, and do not always reflect the underlying endogenous rhythm [29].

The American Academy of Sleep Medicine recommends the use of actigraphy to delineate sleep pattern and to document treatment responses in infants, children, and adolescents [30].

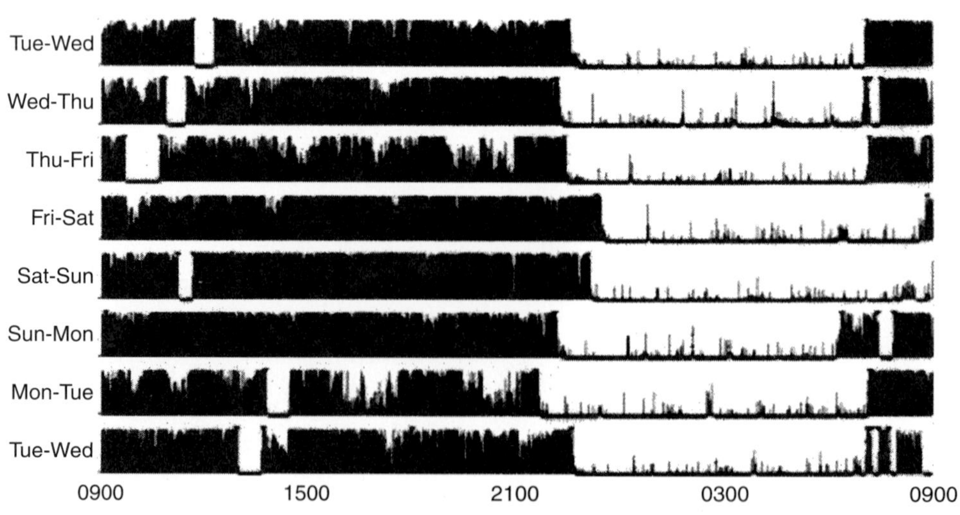

Figure 13.4A Eight days of actigraphy recording in adolescents sleeping on a self-selected schedule. A typically developing adolescent (15-year-old female). As is typical in adolescents, a delay in bedtime and rise time is observed on weekends (Friday and Saturday nights, Saturday and Sunday mornings), as well as a longer sleep period.

Circadian Rhythm Sleep Disorders Across Childhood and Adolescence

After describing normal developmental changes in the sleep regulatory processes, this section will review 4 (delayed sleep phase type, advanced sleep phase type, irregular sleep-wake type, free-running type) of the 9 types of CRSD described in the ICSD. The other types (jet lag disorder, shift work disorder, because of a medical condition, because of drug or substance, and other) are either covered in other chapters of this book or are not significant in childhood and adolescence.

Normal Changes in the Sleep Regulatory Process Across Adolescence

Developmental changes in the circadian (Process C) and homeostatic (Process S) processes in infancy and childhood are poorly understood. A number of studies have suggested that sleep homeostasis emerges in the second month of life and continues to manifest maturational changes well into adolescence [31–33]. Jenni and LeBourgeois [34] have proposed a model that postulates that sleep pressure accumulates more slowly with increasing age. According to this idea, young children accrue sleep pressure at a rapid rate necessitating a daytime nap; however, as they mature they are able to maintain wakefulness throughout the day. Experimental data supporting this conjecture in young children is lacking; however, experimental studies in older children and adolescents support a similar notion.

One such study examined the homeostatic regulatory process (Process S) cross-sectionally in prepubertal (Tanner 1) and postpubertal (Tanner 5) adolescents by fitting an exponential curve to SWA under conditions where prior sleep was held constant [35]. The decay time constant of SWA across the sleep episode did not differ between the younger and older participants (Tanner 1 average = 143.2 minutes, Tanner 5 average = 128.2 minutes). This finding suggests that the dissipation of sleep pressure is similar for adolescents across this developmental phase, supporting the notion that sleep need does not change. Conversely, a study modeling the accumulation of Process S examined in the context of extended wakefulness (36 hours) indicated that the buildup of homeostatic sleep pressure is slower in mature adolescents (12.1 hours) compared with prepubertal (Tanner 1) or early pubertal (Tanner 2) children (8.9 hours) [36]. The implication of these findings is that although the sleep recovery process is similar in early and late adolescence (as indicated by the dissipation of sleep pressure), more mature adolescents may find it easier to stay awake longer because of the slower accumulation rate of sleep pressure. No data are available in which these processes have been evaluated in children and adolescents with unusual or abnormal developmental trajectories or sleep disorders.

Circadian rhythms of CBT are present 1 month after birth and become more pronounced at 3 months [37]. Few studies have examined the circadian timing system across childhood, but data suggest that during adolescence, circadian timing tends toward a phase delay. A study of sixth-grade girls found that more mature sixth-grade girls also rated themselves as more evening types [38]. Intensive laboratory assessments indicated that DLMO phase under controlled conditions is positively correlated with Tanner stage [39]. Although the mechanism for the circadian delay has not been elucidated, one hypothesis is that postpubertal adolescents may have a longer circadian period compared with prepubertal adolescents. When compared with adults, circadian period is longer in adolescents [40]. The shift toward delayed sleep has also been reported in several nonhuman species such as the rhesus monkey and octodon degus [41].

Our working model is that the interaction of these 2 processes, set against the background of the behavioral and lifestyle changes that accompany adolescent development, can account for the observed adolescent sleep delay [6]. Thus, the lengthening of intrinsic period (Process C) may be the *driving* force behind the sleep delay, whereas the maturational decline in the accumulation of sleep pressure across the waking day may *permit* later bedtime. With these forces in place, the delay in bedtime may result in greater exposure to light in the evening, engaging the circadian system and further delaying sleep.

Delayed Sleep Phase Disorder

Delayed sleep phase disorder (DSPD) was initially described by Weitzman and colleagues in 1981 [42] who termed it "delayed sleep phase insomnia," as it occurred in patients younger than the general insomniac population who reported a chronic inability to fall asleep at a desired clock time, a normal sleep pattern, a restorative sleep when not on a strict schedule, and a history of unsuccessful attempts to treat the problem.

The defined characteristics of DSPD are delayed sleep onset and late awakening, expressed distress about the inability to fall asleep and wake-up at socially acceptable times, and unaltered sleep architecture and sleep quantity for age. The phase of entrainment to the 24-hour sleep-wake pattern is delayed but stable when a patient is allowed to choose his or her preferred schedule [19].

Onset of DSPD often occurs during adolescence [43], predominantly in males. Prevalence rates differ widely across studies, from less than 0.13% to 10% [19,44]. Most studies on DSPD have been performed in adolescents and young adults. The prevalence of DSPD in prepubertal children is unknown; however, behavioral sleep-onset insomnia of childhood could in some cases be a manifestation of an underlying DSPD.

As described above, a "normal" delay of sleep occurs in adolescence but without the distress or waking impairment of DSPD. In clinical practice, chief complaints can be sleep-onset insomnia, inability to wake up at a desired time, sleep deprivation, excessive daytime sleepiness in the morning, and impaired waking function. Clinical Pearl 2 provides details for clinical assessment of DSPD in children and adolescents. A thorough clinical interview with the patient and his or her family, along with a physical examination is required to screen for other etiologies or comorbid disorders. Indeed, one criterion for the diagnosis of DSPD is that the sleep disturbance is not better explained by another current sleep disorder (eg, restless legs syndrome, periodic limb movement, sleep-related breathing disorder, psychophysiological insomnia, inadequate sleep hygiene), medical or neurological disorder (eg, brain tumor), mental disorder (eg, mood disorder, anxiety disorder, schizophrenia), medication use (eg, theophylline, corticoids), or substance-use disorder (eg, caffeine, nicotine, other stimulants) [19].

A stable delay in the timing of the habitual sleep period is demonstrated by sleep diaries or actigraphy monitoring for at least 7 days to 2 weeks, including school days and nonschool days (see Figure 13.4B) [22,23,30]. Circadian phase markers, such as DLMO and CBT, are delayed in DSPD [45] but usually not available

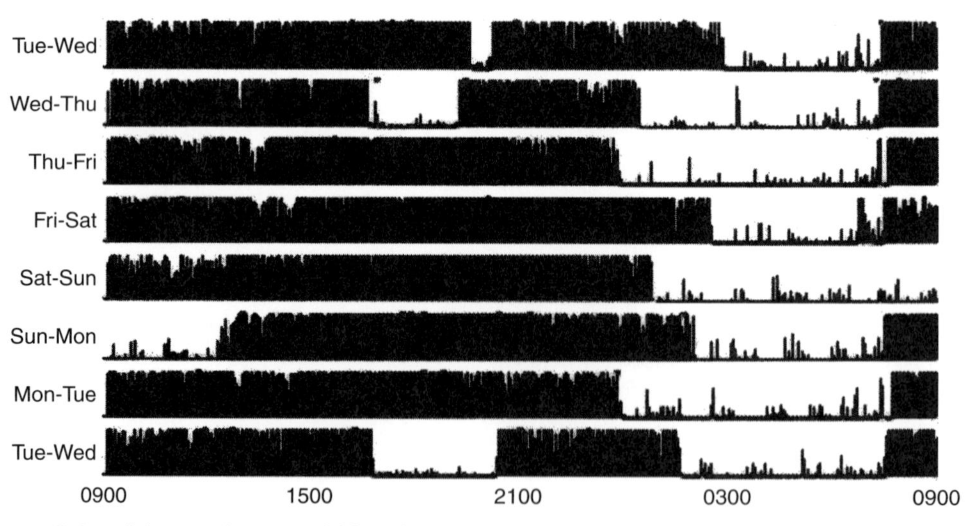

Figure 13.4B An adolescent (16-year-old female) with delayed sleep phase disorder (DSPD). As is typical in DSPD, a delay in bedtime is observed on school nights and nonschool nights (11:00 PM to 2:45 AM), and a delay in rise time on nonschool days (12:15 PM). Rise time is fixed on school days (7:15 AM). The combination of DSPD and early school start time resulting in a short sleep period on most school nights. [The two blank periods in the daytime on the second and the last day of recording correspond to period of working at a job that required removing the actigraph (restaurant's kitchen).]

in clinical practice [23]. Although PSG is not indicated in the routine assessment of DSPD [22], it may be useful to rule out other primary sleep disorders causing daytime sleepiness, such as periodic limb movement disorder or sleep-related breathing disorder.

The etiology of DSPD is unknown but predisposing and precipitating factors have been identified. As discussed previously, a natural shift toward delay occurs in the circadian timing system during adolescence because of a combination of environmental, behavioral, and biological changes [24,46]. Furthermore, modification in the homeostatic regulation of sleep during adolescence might play a role. Slower accumulation of sleep pressure after puberty allows later sleep onset and increased light exposure in the evening, thus delaying sleep onset and the circadian timing system.

A familial aggregation of DSPD has been reported [47], and several predisposing factors to DSPD have been identified: HLA DR1, arylalkylamine N-acetyltransferase gene, and PER3 gene polymorphism [48–52]. Life events, acute medical conditions, and psychiatric disorders appear to be precipitating factors for the onset of DSPD.

Secondary insomnia is a common complication of DSPD. Repeated attempts to fall asleep at an earlier time can lead to conditioned insomnia, with cognitions such as fear of inability to sleep and behaviors such as prolonged time in bed [53].

DSPD is associated with school absenteeism, academic failure, social isolation, family conflict, higher risk for driving accident, and psychiatric disorders. Depression, school phobia, substance abuse and dependence (alcohol, hypnotics, benzodiazepines, marijuana), schizoid and avoidant personalities, the posttraumatic stress disorder [43,54] are common comorbidities of DSPD; however, the direction of effects between these disorders is not clear.

Treatment consists of shifting the sleep phase to an earlier time, allowing the patient to sleep on socially acceptable schedules. Several therapeutic options are available: chronotherapy, timed light therapy, and timed exogenous melatonin. These 3 approaches can be combined or used as unique treatment options.

Chronotherapy, initially described by Weitzman and Czeisler in 1981 [42,55], consists of delaying bedtime and wake time by 3 hours every day until the desired bedtime is reached. The patient is then asked to keep a fixed sleep schedule 7 d/wk.

Morning *bright light exposure* (at the advance portion of the human PRC) over consecutive days phase advances the circadian timing system and is indicated in the treatment of DSPD [22]. Optimal timing, duration, and dosing have not been determined [22,23]; however, one light-pulse (2,500–10,000 lux) of 1- to 2-hour duration shortly after awakening is commonly prescribed [56], and 30 to 45 min of morning exposure to 10,000 lux also appears to be effective [57]. In addition to morning bright light exposure, dim light before bedtime is recommended to avoid delaying the sleep-wake cycle.

As previously mentioned, the circadian system is particularly sensitive to shortwave light; however, no studies have been published on the efficacy and safety of monochromatic light in adolescents. Indeed, effects of polychromatic and monochromatic light on a developing visual system are unknown.

Chronotherapy and phototherapy require the patient's high motivation, as they are very demanding. Close monitoring by regular follow-up appointments, daily sleep diaries, and parental involvement increase compliance.

Properly *timed exogenous melatonin* administration is also indicated as a therapy for DSPD [22,23], but there is no recommendation specific to children and adolescents. Physiologic (chronobiotic or phase shifting) doses of melatonin (0.1–0.5 mg) have shown efficacy in inducing phase advance shifting [58]. The melatonin PRC is nearly opposite to the light PRC: melatonin delays circadian rhythms when administered in the morning and advances them when administered in the afternoon or early evening [59] (see Figure 13.3). In DSPD, therefore, exogenous melatonin administration is recommended 5 to 6 hours before habitual sleep time [56]. Administration of exogenous melatonin in adults is safe for short-term use [60], and melatonin is now recommended in some neonatal care settings [61,62]. Chronic administration of exogenous melatonin (3.7 years of follow-up) in school-aged children with ADHD has exposed no safety concerns regarding serious adverse events [63,64]. Melatonin in children with treatment-resistant circadian rhythm sleep disorders shows positive long-term effectiveness (up to 3.8 years of follow-up) [65]. Potential toxicity of chronic administration of exogenous melatonin on a developing reproductive system is unknown. Melatonin has been shown to influence the secretion of several hormones such as luteinizing hormone, follicle stimulating hormone, and prolactin. Furthermore, melatonin can inhibit ovulation in women [66]. In the United States, melatonin is considered a dietary supplement and not regulated by the Food and Drug Administration. In the European Union, however, melatonin is considered a drug and is not recommended for children and adolescents under 18 years of age, as data are insufficient on safety and efficacy.

There is insufficient evidence supporting the use of hypnotic medications to promote sleep or the use of stimulant medications to promote alertness [22].

In addition to the 3 classical therapeutic approaches, advice on appropriate sleep hygiene, such as the avoidance of naps (to preserve sleep homeostasis), should be provided and parents and patients should be warned about consequences of daytime sleepiness, especially when driving.

Free-Running Disorder

In free-running disorder (FRD), also called non-24-hour sleep-wake syndrome or hypernycthemeral syndrome, the circadian clock is not entrained by external synchronizers. Isolating subjects from environmental synchronizers can experimentally model FRD.

The human intrinsic circadian period is on average longer than 24 hours, especially in adolescence when the period average is about 24.3 hours [67]. The period of the sleep-wake rhythm in FRD appears to correspond to the endogenous circadian period, resulting in a delay in sleep onset and wake times each 24-hour period (see Figure 13.5). When attempting to

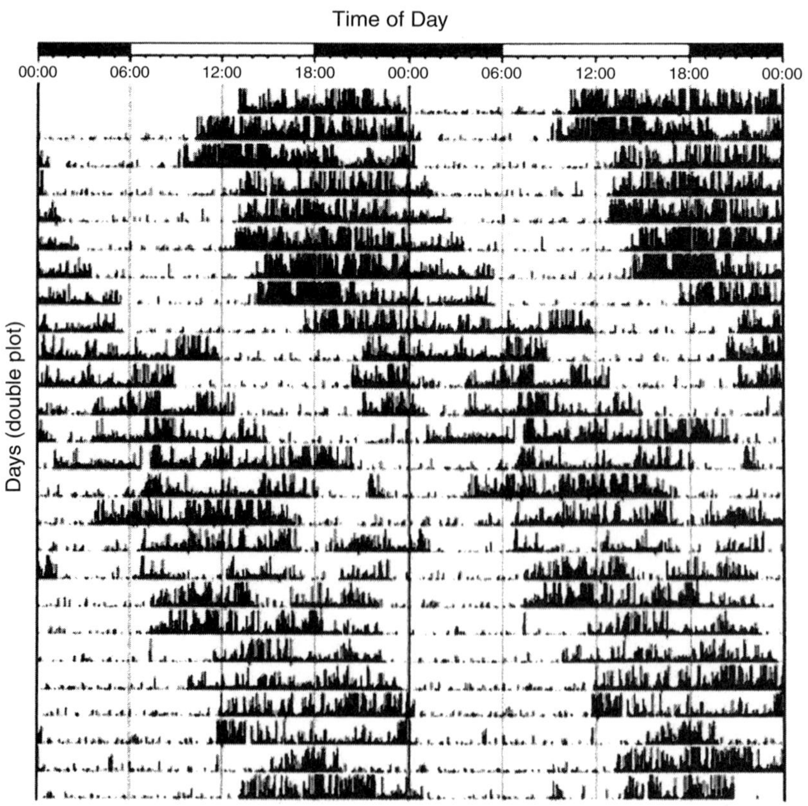

Figure 13.5 Actigraphy of an individual with free-running disorder (double plot). Reprinted with permission from Dagan and Ayalon [68]. © 2005 *Journal of the American Academy of Child and Adolescent Psychiatry.*

follow a 24-hour schedule, patients with FRD experience sleep-onset, sleep maintenance, and awakening difficulties that wax and wane as their endogenous rhythms cycle into and out of synchrony with the environment.

FRD is a rare condition in sighted people, although more common in psychiatric population. FRD can be a differential diagnosis of psychiatric disorders [68,69].

The most common cause of FRD is blindness. Yet, blind people with intact nonvisual light perception (eg, through intact ipRGCs) are entrained to the daily light and dark cycle. Thus, visual blindness is not always associated with "clock blindness." Circadian abnormalities in blind individuals have been well described over the past 50 years, with observed free-running circadian rhythms of CBT, cortisol, and melatonin secretion, as well as sleep [70–74]. Nonsighted individuals often report sleep complaints [75] and impaired wakefulness [76], resulting in a higher risk for accidents [77]. Blindness is often associated with mental retardation, as part of an overall syndrome. In these patients, FRD is more frequent as they are lacking not only the photic entrainment of light but also the nonphotic entrainment of social activities.

Sleep logs and actigraphy are useful for assessment of FRD, showing a systematic delay of the sleep-wake cycle (see Figure 13.3). Circadian phase markers (CBT, DLMO) are recommended to determine the circadian phase and confirm the diagnosis of FRD in sighted and unsighted patients [22,23,30].

The therapeutic approach to FRD consists of entraining the circadian pacemaker.

Timed light exposure has shown to entrain sighted patients with FRD [23] and may also be useful in blind individuals with intact ipRGCs and retinohypothalamic pathway. Nonphotic synchronizers can help entrain the human circadian pacemaker and permit blind individuals to have a 24-hour day [78]. Therefore, *fixed sleep-wake schedules* are recommended in patients with FRD [22,23]. *Daily timed administration of exogenous melatonin* can entrain the circadian timing system in FRD patients [79] and thereby improve sleep and reduce daytime sleepiness. Exogenous melatonin is entraining at 0.1 to 0.5 mg, and such low physiological doses may be more effective than at pharmacological levels [22,23,80,81]. Administration is started when the patient's free-running period approaches the desired phase. Exogenous melatonin is given 2 hours before bedtime or near the expected time of DLMO [56].

Irregular Sleep-Wake Rhythm

Irregular sleep-wake rhythm (ISWR) is characterized by an absence of a predictable, regular sleep-wake circadian rhythm [19]. The total sleep duration over 24 hours is normal, but sleep is fragmented into bouts of variable duration and with unpredictable schedules. Patients complain of excessive daytime sleepiness and insomnia.

The etiology of ISWR is unknown, but lesion of the circadian pacemaker in the SCN is a theoretical etiological factor, because animal models after SCN ablation show arrhythmicity of activity patterns [82]. Poor sleep hygiene and absence of exposure to external synchronizers such as light or social activities also predispose, precipitate, and perpetuate ISWR. Children with severe neurological disorders and children with mental retardation are at a higher risk of ISWR, likely because of lesions of the retinohypothalamic tract and/or the SCN, alteration of melatonin secretion, and inadequate exposure to environmental synchronizers. The greatest incidence of ISWR, however, is in adults with dementia.

Sleep logs and actigraphy are indicated to identify ISWR and monitor treatment outcomes [22,30].

Timed exogenous melatonin, timed bright light exposure, physical activity, and other behavioral elements are therapeutic options available for children with ISWR associated with psychomotor and/or mental retardation [22].

Advance Sleep Phase Disorder

Characterized by early sleep onset and early awakening, expressed distress of inability to sleep at conventional schedule, and no alteration of sleep architecture and sleep quantity, advanced sleep phase disorder (ASPD) is a rare condition, more common in middle-aged and older adults and unusual in children and teenagers.

Genetic causes should be suspected in younger patients. A familial advance sleep phase disorder (FASPD) has been described, with 2 causative mutations identified: a Per2 mutation with autosomal dominant transmission and high

Clinical Pearl 1 Key Points for Assessing Sleep Patterns in Children and Adolescents

- Intraindividual differences: assessment of several nights.
- School year (weekdays and weekends) and vacation sleep patterns.
- Sleep logs for diagnosis and compliance.
- Goodness of fit of sleep pattern and sleep duration with age and family habits.
- Seasonal variations of sleep duration, pattern, and daytime functioning.

Clinical Pearl 2 Clinical Evaluation of Delayed Sleep Phase Disorder

History of presenting problem**:** onset, precipitating factor.

Bedtime
Chief complaint: difficulty initiating sleep.
Sleep hygiene: bedtime routine, evening/bedtime activities, evening/bedtime light exposure, snacks after dinner (composition and time).
Substance use (type, quantity, and time): stimulants, caffeine in the evening, sleeping pills, other drugs or illicit substance to fall asleep (eg, benzodiazepines, marijuana, alcohol).
Bedtime on school, nonschool, and vacation nights.
Sleep onset latency on school, nonschool, and vacation nights. Shorter sleep onset latency at a later time?
Rule out other etiologies of prolonged sleep onset latency: restless legs syndrome, insomnia (psychophysiological or secondary to delayed sleep phase disorder [DSPD]), and anxiety.

Main sleep period
Chief complaint: short sleep duration or no complaint.
Total sleep duration on school, nonschool, and vacation nights. Is total sleep duration appropriate for age?
Rule out: OSA and PLMS.

Awakening
Chief complaint: difficulty waking up.
Wake-up time and rise time on school, nonschool, and vacation nights. Spontaneous or provoked awakening? Spontaneous at a later time? Late in class or missed school days because of inability to wake up (frequency).
Refreshing sleep on school, nonschool, and vacation nights?
Light exposure on awakening, breakfast time.
Rule out etiologies of difficulty on awakening: OSA, PLMS, narcolepsy, Kleine-Levin syndrome, school phobia, and depression.

Daytime
Chief complaint: excessive daytime sleepiness.
Daytime sleepiness: severity (fell asleep in class? while driving?), time of the day (morning, afternoon, evening), frequency.
Naps: planned or unplanned, duration, time, refreshing or unrefreshing.
Daytime functioning: academic performance, social and familial interaction, mood (depression, anxiety, irritability), concentration.
Synchronizers: light exposure, meals regularity, duration and time of physical activity.
Substance and drugs to stay awake: type, quantity, and time of intake (eg, stimulants, caffeine).
Rule out etiologies of impaired daytime functioning: psychiatric disorder (eg, depression, school phobia), narcolepsy with or without cataplexy, Kleine-Levin syndrome, medical causes of hypersomnia, and medications.
Family history of DSPD, other sleep disorders, psychiatric disorder.
Physical examination: oriented by the findings and conclusion from the interview with patient and family, and review of sleep diaries and/or actigraphy. Within normal limits in DSPD.

Directions for Future Research

- Clinical trials on efficacy, modality, and safety of exogenous melatonin in children and adolescents with DSPD and FRD.
- Clinical trials on efficacy, modality, and safety of melatonin receptor agonists in children and adolescents with CRSD.
- Clinical trials on modality, safety, and efficacy of chronotherapy in DSPD.
- Establishment of PRCs to light for children and adolescents.

penetrance or a misense mutation that impairs hCKIδ [83,84].

Sleep logs and actigraphy monitoring for at least a week showing stable earlier timing of the habitual sleep period confirm the diagnosis [19,23,30]. Early awakenings of ASPD should be distinguished from depressive symptom and sleep maintenance insomnia.

Prescribed sleep-wake scheduling, bright light exposure in the evening, and timed melatonin administration are recommended treatment options [22]; however, efficacy of these treatments in FASPD is unknown. Further research is required to assess efficacy of chronotherapy, modality of bright light therapy, and safety and efficacy of exogenous melatonin administration in patients with ASPD.

References

1. Iglowstein I, Jenni OG, Molinari L, Largo RH. Sleep duration from infancy to adolescence: reference values and generational trends. *Pediatrics.* 2003;111(2):302–307.
2. Crosby B, LeBourgeois MK, Harsh J. Racial differences in reported napping and nocturnal sleep in 2- to 8-year-old children. *Pediatrics.* 2005; 115(suppl 1):225–232.
3. Sadeh A. Sleep and melatonin in infants: a preliminary study. *Sleep.* 1997;20(3):185–191.
4. Rivkees SA, Mirmiran M, Ariagno RL. Circadian rhythms in infants. *NeoReviews.* 2003;4:298–304.
5. Carskadon M. Patterns of sleep and sleepiness in adolescents. *Pediatrician.* 1990;17:5–12.
6. Carskadon M. Maturation of processes regulating sleep in adolescents. In: Marcus C, Carroll JL, Donnelly D, Loughlin GM, eds. *Sleep in Children: Developmental Changes in Sleep Patterns.* New York, NY: Informa Healthcare; 2008:95–114.
7. Carskadon MA, Mancuso J, Rosekind MR. Impact of part-time employment on adolescent sleep patterns. *Sleep Res.* 1989;18:114.
8. Calamaro CJ, Mason TB, Ratcliffe SJ. Adolescents living the 24/7 lifestyle: effects of caffeine and technology on sleep duration and daytime functioning. *Pediatrics.* 2009;123(6):1005–1010.
9. Borbély AA. A two process model of sleep regulation. *Hum Neurobiol.* 1982;1(3):195–204.
10. Webb WB, Agnew HW Jr. Stage 4 sleep: influence of time course variables. *Science.* 1971;174(16): 1354–1356.
11. Borbély AA, Baumann F, Brandeis D, Strauch I, Lehmann D. Sleep deprivation: effect on sleep stages and EEG power density in man. *Electroencephalogr Clin Neurophysiol.* 1981; 51(5):483–495.
12. Feinberg I, Maloney T, March JD. Precise conservation of NREM period 1 (NREMP1) delta across naps and nocturnal sleep: implications for REM latency and NREM/REM alternation. *Sleep.* 1992;15(5):400–403.
13. Edgar DM, Dement WC, Fuller CA. Effect of SCN lesions on sleep in squirrel monkeys: evidence for opponent processes in sleep-wake regulation. *J Neurosci.* 1993;13(3):1065–1079.
14. Zeitzer JM, Dijk DJ, Kronauer R, Brown E, Czeisler C. Sensitivity of the human circadian pacemaker to nocturnal light: melatonin phase resetting and suppression. *J Physiol.* 2000;526(3):695–702.
15. Berson DM, Dunn FA, Takao M. Phototransduction by retinal ganglion cells that set the circadian clock. *Science.* 2002;295(5557):1070–1073.
16. Gooley JJ, Lu J, Chou TC, Scammell TE, Saper CB. Melanopsin in cells of origin of the retinohypothalamic tract. *Nat Neurosci.* 2001;4(12):1165.
17. Thomas KA. 6-Sulfatoxymelatonin collected from infant diapers: feasibility and implications for urinary biochemical markers. *Biol Res Nurs.* 2010;11(3):288–292.
18. Czeisler CA, Kronauer RE. A method for assaying the effects of therapeutic agents on the period of the endogenous circadian pacemaker in man. In: Montplaisir J, Godbout R, eds. *Sleep and Biological Rhythms: Basic Mechanisms and Applications to Psychiatry.* USA: Oxford University Press; 1990:87–98.
19. American Academy of Sleep Medicine. *International Classification of Sleep Disorders, 2nd ed.: Diagnostic and Coding Manual.* Westchester, IL: American Academy of Sleep Medicine; 2005.
20. Holley S, Hill C, Stevenson J. A comparison of actigraphy and parental report of sleep Habits in typically developing children aged 6 to 11 Years. *Behav Sleep Med.* 2010;8(1):16–27.
21. Horne JA, Ostberg O. A self-assessment questionnaire to determine morningness-eveningness in human circadian rhythms. *Int J Chronobiol.* 1976;4(2):97–110.
22. Morgenthaler TI, Lee-Chiong T, Alessi C, et al. Practice parameters for the clinical evaluation and treatment of circadian rhythm sleep disorders. An American Academy of Sleep Medicine report. *Sleep.* 2007;30(11):1445–1459.
23. Sack RL, Auckley D, Auger RR, et al., American of Sleep Medicine. Circadian rhythm sleep disorders: part II, advanced sleep phase disorder, delayed sleep phase disorder, free-running disorder, and irregular sleep-wake rhythm. An American Academy of Sleep Medicine review. *Sleep.* 2007;30(11):1484–1501.
24. Carskadon MA, Vieira C, Acebo C. Association between puberty and delayed phase preference. *Sleep.* 1993;16(3):258–4262.
25. Werner H, Lebourgeois MK, Geiger A, Jenni OG. Assessment of chronotype in four- to eleven-year-old children: reliability and validity of the Children's Chronotype Questionnaire (CCTQ). *Chronobiol Int.* 2009;26(5):992–1014.
26. Learn About Your Sleep. Sleep for kids—teaching kids the importance of sleep. Also available at http://www.sleepforkids.org/html/learn.html. Accessed March 16, 2010.

27. SleepEducation.com. Also available at http://www.sleepeducation.com/EvaluateSleep.aspx. Accessed March 16, 2010.
28. Acebo C, Sadeh A, Seifer R, et al. Estimating sleep patterns with activity monitoring in children and adolescents: how many nights are necessary for reliable measures? *Sleep*. 1999;22(1):95–103.
29. Ancoli-Israel S, Cole R, Alessi C, Chambers M, Moorcroft W, Pollak CP. The role of actigraphy in the study of sleep and circadian rhythms. *Sleep*. 2003;26:342–392.
30. Morgenthaler T, Alessi C, Friedman L, et al. Practice parameters for the use of actigraphy in the assessment of sleep and sleep disorders: an update for 2007. *Sleep*. 2007;30(4):519–529.
31. Jenni OG, Borbély AA, Achermann P. Development' of the nocturnal sleep electroencephalogram in human infants. *Am J Physiol Regul Integr Comp Physiol*. 2004;286(3):528–538.
32. Peirano P, Algarín C, Uauy R. Sleep-wake states and their regulatory mechanisms throughout early human development. *J Pediatr*. 2003;143 (suppl 4):S70–S79.
33. Salzarulo P, Fagioli I. Post-natal development of sleep organization in man: speculations on the emergence of the 'S process'. *Neurophysiol Clin*. 1992;22(2):107–115.
34. Jenni OG, LeBourgeois MK. Understanding sleep-wake behavior and sleep disorders in children: the value of a model. *Curr Opin Psychiatry*. 2006;19(3):282–287.
35. Jenni OG, Carskadon MA. Spectral analysis of the sleep electroencephalogram during adolescence. *Sleep*. 2004;27(4):774–783.
36. Jenni OG, Achermann P, Carskadon MA. Homeostatic sleep regulation in adolescents. *Sleep*. 2005;28:1446–1454.
37. Glotzbach SF, Edgar DM, Boeddiker M, Ariagno RL. Biological rhythmicity in normal infants during the first 3 months of life. *Pediatrics*. 1994;94(4):482–488.
38. Carskadon M, Vieira C, Acebo C. Association between puberty and delayed phase preference. *Sleep*. 1993;16:258–262.
39. Carskadon MA, Acebo C, Richardson GS, Tate BA, Seifer R. An approach to studying circadian rhythms of adolescent humans. *J Biol Rhythms*. 1997;12(3):278–289.
40. Carskadon MA, Acebo C, Jenni OG. Regulation of adolescent sleep: implications for behavior. *Ann N Y Acad Sci*. 2004;1021:276–291.
41. Hagenauer MH, Perryman JI, Lee TM, Carskadon MA. Adolescent changes in the homeostatic and circadian regulation of sleep. *Dev Neurosci*. 2009;31(4):276–284.
42. Weitzman ED, Czeisler CA, Coleman RM, et al. Delayed sleep phase syndrome. A chronobiological disorder with sleep-onset insomnia. *Arch Gen Psychiatry*. 1981;38(7):737–746.
43. Thorpy MJ, Korman E, Spielman AJ, Glovinsky PB. Delayed sleep phase syndrome in adolescents. *J Adolesc Health Care*. 1988;9:22–27.
44. Ohayon MM, Roberts RE, Zulley J, Smirne S, Priest RG. Prevalence and patterns of problematic sleep among older adolescents. *J Am Acad Child Adolesc Psychiatry*. 2000;39(12):1549–1556.
45. Wyatt JK, Stepanski EJ, Kirkby J. Circadian phase in delayed sleep phase syndrome: predictors and temporal stability across multiple assessments. *Sleep*. 2006;29(8):1075–1080.
46. Crowley SJ, Acebo C, Carskadon MA. Sleep, circadian rhythms, and delayed phase in adolescence. *Sleep Med*. 2007;8(6):602–612.
47. Ancoli-Israel S, Schnierow B, Kelsoe J, Fink R. A pedigree of one family with delayed sleep phase syndrome. *Chronobiol Int*. 2001;18(5):831–840.
48. Ebisawa T, Uchiyama M, Kajimura N, et al. Association of structural polymorphisms in the human period3 gene with delayed sleep phase syndrome. *EMBO Rep*. 2001;2:342–346.
49. Hohjoh H, Takahashi Y, Hatta Y, et al. Possible association of human leucocyte antigen DR1 with delayed sleep phase syndrome. *Psychiatry Clin Neurosci*. 1999;53(4):527–529.
50. Hohjoh H, Takasu M, Shishikura K, et al. Significant association of the arylalkylamine N-acetyltransferase (AA-NAT) gene with delayed sleep phase syndrome. *Neurogenetics*. 2003;4(3):151–153.
51. Iwase T, Kajimura N, Uchiyama M, et al. Mutation screening of the human Clock gene in circadian rhythm sleep disorders. *Psychiatry Res*. 2002;109:121–128.
52. Takahashi Y, Hohjoh H, Matsuura K. Predisposing factors in delayed sleep phase syndrome. *Psychiatry Clin Neurosci*. 2000;54:356–358.
53. Ferber R. Sleep schedule-dependent causes of insomnia and sleepiness in middle childhood and adolescence. *Pediatrician*. 1990;17(1):13–20.
54. Dagan Y, Stein D, Steinbock M, Yovel I, Hallis D. Frequency of delayed sleep phase syndrome among hospitalized adolescent psychiatric patients. *J Psychosom Res*. 1998;45:15–20.
55. Czeisler CA, Richardson GS, Coleman RM, et al. Chronotherapy: resetting the circadian clocks of patients with delayed sleep phase insomnia. *Sleep*. 1981;4(1):1–21.
56. Reid KJ, Zee PC. Circadian disorders of the sleep-wake cycle. In: Kryger M, Roth T, Dement WC, eds. *Principles and Practice of Sleep Medicine*. 4th ed. Philadelphia, PA: Elsevier Saunders; 2005:691–701.
57. Bjorvatn B, Pallesen S. A practical approach to circadian rhythm sleep disorders. *Sleep Med Rev*. 2009;13(1):47–60.
58. Lewy AJ, Ahmed S, Sack RL. Phase shifting the human circadian clock using melatonin. *Behav Brain Res*. 1996;73(1–2):131–134.
59. Lewy AJ, Ahmed S, Jackson JM, Sack RL. Melatonin shifts human circadian rhythms according to a phase-response curve. *Chronobiol Int*. 1992;9(5):380–392.
60. Buscemi N, Vandermeer B, Hooton N, et al. Efficacy and safety of exogenous melatonin for secondary sleep disorders and sleep disorders

accompanying sleep restriction: meta-analysis. *BMJ*. 2006;332(7538):385–393.
61. Gitto E, Pellegrino S, Gitto P, et al. Oxidative stress of the newborn in the pre- and postnatal period and the clinical utility of melatonin. *J Pineal Res*. 2009;46(2):128–139.
62. Jan JE, Wasdell MB, Freeman RD, Bax M. Evidence supporting the use of melatonin in short gestation infants. *J Pineal Res*. 2007;42(1):22–27.
63. Bendz LM, Scates AC. Melatonin treatment for insomnia in pediatric patients with attention-deficit/hyperactivity disorder. *Ann Pharmacother*. 2010;44(1):185–191.
64. Hoebert M, van der Heijden KB, van Geijlswijk IM, Smits MG. Long-term follow-up of melatonin treatment in children with ADHD and chronic sleep onset insomnia. *J Pineal Res*. 2009;47(1):1–7.
65. Carr R, Wasdell MB, Hamilton D, et al. Long-term effectiveness outcome of melatonin therapy in children with treatment-resistant circadian rhythm sleep disorders. *J Pineal Res*. 2007;43(4):351–359.
66. Voordouw BC, Euser R, Verdonk RE, et al. Melatonin and melatonin-progestin combinations alter pituitary-ovarian function in women and can inhibit ovulation. *J Clin Endocrinol Metab*. 1992;74(1):108–117.
67. Carskadon MA, Labyak SE, Acebo C, Seifer R. Intrinsic circadian period of adolescent humans measured in conditions of forced desynchrony. *Neurosci Lett*. 1999;260(2):129–132.
68. Dagan Y, Ayalon L. Case study: psychiatric misdiagnosis of non-24-hours sleep-wake schedule disorder resolved by melatonin. *J Am Acad Child Adolesc Psychiatry*. 2005;44(12):1271–1275.
69. Hayakawa T, Uchiyama M, Kamei Y, et al. Clinical analyses of sighted patients with non-24-hour sleep-wake syndrome: a study of 57 consecutively diagnosed cases. *Sleep*. 2005;28(8):945–952.
70. Leger D, Prevot E, Philip P, et al. Sleep disorders in children with blindness. *Ann Neurol*. 1999;46(4):648–651.
71. Migeon CJ, Tyler FH, Mahoney JP, et al. The diurnal variation of plasma levels and urinary excretion on 17-hydroxycorticosteroids in normal subjects, night workers and blind subjects. *J Clin Endocrinol Metab*. 1956;16(5):622–633.
72. Miles LE, Raynal DM, Wilson MA. Blind man living in normal society has circadian rhythms of 24.9 hours. *Science*. 1977;198(4315):421–423.
73. Okawa M, Nanami T, Wada S, et al. Four congenitally blind children with circadian sleep-wake rhythm disorder. *Sleep*. 1987;10(2):101–110.
74. Sadeh A, Klitzke M, Anders TF, Acebo C. Case study: sleep and aggressive behavior in a blind, retarded adolescent. A concomitant schedule disorder? *J Am Acad Child Adolesc Psychiatry*. 1995;34(6):820–824.
75. Leger D, Guilleminault C, Defrance R, Domont A, Paillard M. Prevalence of sleep/wake disorders in persons with blindness. *Clin Sci*. 1999;97(2):193–199.
76. Lockley SW, Dijk D, Kosti O, Skene DJ, Arendt J. Alertness, mood and performance rhythm disturbances associated with circadian sleep disorders in the blind. *J Sleep Res*. 2008;17(2):207–216.
77. Leger D, Guilleminault C, Santos C, Paillard M. Sleep/wake cycles in the dark: sleep recorded by polysomnography in 26 totally blind subjects compared to controls. *Clin Neurophysiol*. 2002;113(10):1607–1614.
78. Klerman EB, Rimmer DW, Dijk DJ, Kronauer RE, Rizzo JF 3rd, Czeisler CA. Nonphotic entrainment of the human circadian pacemaker. *Am J Physiol*. 1998;274(4):991–996.
79. Lockley SW, Skene DJ, James K, Thapan K, Wright J, Arendt J. Melatonin administration can entrain the free-running circadian system of blind subjects. *J Endocrinol*. 2000;164(1):1–6.
80. Hack LM, Lockley SW, Arendt J. The effects of low-dose 0.5-mg melatonin on the free-running circadian rhythms of blind subjects. *J Biol Rhythms*. 2003;18(5):420–429.
81. Lewy AJ, Bauer VK, Hasler BP, Kendall AR, Pires ML, Sack RL. Capturing the circadian rhythms of free-running blind people with 0.5 mg melatonin. *Brain Res*. 2001;918(1–2):96–100.
82. Eastman CI, Mistlberger RE, Rechtschaffen A. Suprachiasmatic nuclei lesions eliminate circadian temperature and sleep rhythms in the rat. *Physiol Behav*. 1984;32(3):357–368.
83. Toh KL, Jones CR, He Y, et al. An hPer2 phosphorylation site mutation in familial advanced sleep phase syndrome. *Science*. 2001;291(5506):1040–1043.
84. Xu Y, Padiath QS, Shapiro RE, et al. Functional consequences of a CKIdelta mutation causing familial advanced sleep phase syndrome. *Nature*. 2005;434(7033):640–644.
85. Khalsa SB, Jewett ME, Cajochen C, Czeisler CA. A phase response curve to single bright light pulses in human subjects. *J Physiol*. 2003;549(3):945–952.
86. Achermann P, Borbély AA. Mathematical models of sleep regulation. *Frontiers in Bioscience*. 2003;8:683–693.

CHAPTER 14

Sleep and Circadian Dysfunction in Children With Mental Retardation or Cerebral Palsy

Jonathan Lipton

Introduction

Sleep comprises dynamic and developmentally regulated neurophysiological states that have important influences on waking behavior. Sleep affects neurocognitive function including learning and memory, attention, emotion and mood, and behavior. Despite its ubiquity in the animal kingdom, the biological function of sleep remains a matter of debate. In humans, sleep undergoes remarkable changes during the first year of human life, suggesting an important role in neural development; however, direct evidence for this assumption is lacking [1–5]. Sleep disruption has been associated with increased behavioral problems, attentional deficits, and metabolic problems in children; conversely, children with neurocognitive disorders have an increased risk of sleep problems [6,7]. Sleep dysfunction is more common in children with developmental disorders than in normal children and contributes to morbidity in both children and their families. It is important to recognize that terms such as "intellectual disability" (ID) and "mental retardation" are not equivalent. "Intellectual disability" is a *legal* term defined in the American with Disabilities Act as: "...with respect to an individual as (A) a physical or mental impairment [8] that substantially limits one or more of the major life activities of such individual; (B) a record of such an impairment; or (C) being regarded as having such an impairment" [8]. In contrast, mental retardation (MR) is defined by an intelligence quotient less than 70 or 75. In this review, I have combined available data on patients with ID and MR and use the terms interchangeably because the reported sleep dysfunction in cohorts using either term is similar: bedtime resistance, sleep-onset insomnia, nocturnal arousals, and/or early morning terminal waking. These symptoms are nonspecific and may be the manifestation of sleep disorders as disparate as psychophysiological insomnia and delayed sleep phase disorder.

Clinical Approach to Sleep in the Mentally or Physically Disabled Child

The clinical approach to sleep in the developmentally disabled child should initially be the same as that in the normal child. Because pediatric sleep disorders are dependent on both chronological age and developmental stage, both must be carefully considered, especially in the developmentally challenged child. A detailed birth history, family history, and physical examination should be performed with an eye toward understanding as much as possible about the underlying pathophysiological mechanisms that may underlie the child's developmental milieu. A detailed medication history along with precise timing of administration is crucial. Comorbid medical and neurological conditions should be reviewed in detail. Particularly pertinent conditions include epilepsy, gastroesophageal reflux, and asthma, all of which can have major impact on sleep.

Physical examination must include assessment of the oropharynx for tonsillar size, palate, and the relative position of the maxilla and mandible. Because sleep is a complex behavior and is influenced by many potential environmental factors, close attention should be paid to the sleeping environment, including bedtime ritual, sleeping quarters, nocturnal gastrostomy tube feeding, seizures, difficulty clearing oropharyngeal secretions, and light exposure in, and around, the sleeping berth. The presence of co-sleeping should be investigated as it may contribute to behavioral attachments at sleep onset and foment nocturnal arousals; alternatively, co-sleeping is accepted in certain cultures and may be an important coping mechanism for some parents. An understanding of family dynamics and knowledge of primary and secondary care providers are absolutely critical elements for delineating potential factors that disrupt sleep.

A parental sleep log or, if possible, a child's sleep diary can be useful to determine sleep timings and patterns of arousal. This can be particularly useful to clarify circadian rhythm disorders that otherwise cannot be gleaned from review of a single night's sleep. A careful history should address sleep timings over several days to weeks. The presence of regular snoring (more than 3 times weekly), gasping arousals, witnessed apneas, mouth breathing, leg movements, and parasomniac activity should be assessed.

There are no established guidelines that specify when polysomnography is indicated for normally developing children. Polysomnography is prudent, however, when there is clear evidence of sleep-disordered breathing (SDB) (eg, chronic snoring, witnessed apneas, gasping arousals, snorting), report of rhythmic movements in sleep, or if reported nocturnal events are concerning for seizures. Stereotyped movements during sleep or those regularly associated with arousals from sleep should be investigated by 24-hour electroencephalogram (EEG) or by polysomnography with full "10–20–20" electrode placement. Liberal use of a 16-channel EEG montage should be made during polysomnography when there is a history of nocturnal spells, whether related to epileptic or non-epileptic in nature.

Sleep Dysfunction in MR

Sleep problems have been reported in 13% to 86% of individuals with intellectual disabilities, depending on the study however [9,10]. The high prevalence and persistence of such problems in children with severe learning difficulties is particularly worrying because sleep problems are associated with child and maternal stress and add further morbidity to families already challenged by the stress of a developmentally disabled child [11–13]. Sleep problems are commonly reported in cohorts with MR; however, there is little direct evidence that MR *itself* predisposes an individual to sleep dysfunction. Cognitive dysfunction is poorly understood on a pathophysiological level and it is unknown to what extent the processes that contribute to, or cause MR, contribute to sleep dysfunction. Because MR frequently occurs in the context of other comorbidities that can significantly impact sleep including epilepsy, blindness, motor disabilities, and/or in the context of neurodevelopmental syndromes, it is a challenge for the clinician to investigate sleep complaints in the context of the comorbidities and their treatments.

Most assessments of sleep in cohorts with ID or MR have relied on parental report with the use of questionnaire-based methodologies, and there are few, if any, formal longitudinal studies that use objective measures of sleep quality, sleep maintenance, or circadian function. The most commonly reported problems are difficulty settling to sleep, nocturnal arousals, and bedtime resistance. Thus, sleep problems reported in disabled children are similar to those in normal school-aged children but occur with greater frequency [14]. This exemplifies the importance of careful determination and consideration of the *developmental* age of the child that may be a greater contributor to the nature of the sleep disorder than the *chronological* age. Importantly, 2 longitudinal studies have demonstrated persistence of sleep dysfunction during development, suggesting either stagnation sleep patterns with developmental age or difficulty adequately addressing sleep dysfunction during intervals examined [11,15].

The relationship between sleep and optimal cognitive and physical function is bidirectional and can be mutually beneficial or detrimental. Consistently, sleep problems in developmentally disabled children are associated with a number of associated clinical outcomes: poor communication skills, poor academic skills, poor self-help skills, incontinence, daytime behavior problems, and epilepsy [10,11,16] (Table 14.1). Reports of an increase in daytime behavior problems have been reported in intellectually disabled children with reported sleep dysfunction [6,10].

Several studies have demonstrated that both the number and degree of comorbid disability individually predict sleep-wake disturbances [17]. Sleep disorders such as early morning waking, daytime sleepiness, abnormal sleep latency, and insomnia are more commonly reported in otherwise healthy children with blindness with impaired light perception when compared with children with proper eyesight [18]. Circadian disruption may manifest as variable patterns of nocturnal awakenings, daytime somnolence, sleep-onset insomnia, and altered circadian phase in these individuals. Indeed, light is a major *zeitgeber* (timegiver) that entrains the endogenous circadian timekeeping mechanism to the ambient light-dark cycle [19,20]. Visual impairments associated with total or partial loss of light perception can render unresponsiveness to the entraining effect of light on the endogenous circadian timekeeper in the suprachiasmatic nucleus [21–24] (Figure 14.1). Food and social cues may also be effective *zeitgebers*; indeed, a true "free-running" (nonentrained) rest-activity rhythm is found in only 32% to 50% of totally blind individuals, suggesting that other mechanisms may compensate for ineffective light entrainment [25–27]. Supplemental melatonin has been used with success as a chronotherapeutic *zeitgeber* in blind patients, including those with MR [9,28].

Table 14.1 Clinical factors that correlate with an increased risk of sleep dysfunction in developmentally disabled children

- severity of intellectual disability (15, 17)
- poor communication skills (10)
- poor academic skills (10)
- poor self-help skills (10)
- incontinence (10)
- daytime behavior problems (10)
- epilepsy (10, 15, 17)
- medication (15)
- younger chronological age (15)
- cerebral palsy (15, 18)

Comorbid Epilepsy

Epilepsy has been repeatedly described as a significant risk factor for sleep disorders perhaps as a result of nocturnal arousals associated with seizure or epileptiform discharges; the pathophysiological basis for this association has not been described [29–33]. Depending on the degree of cognitive impairment, a sleep history may be difficult in the MR population and the clinician may require the participation of caregivers; this may be especially true for institutionalized individuals. Sleep diaries, detailed sleep hygiene, and actigraphy may be useful. Knowledge of the presence and luminosity of ambient light in the environment, medication timings, social cues, and meal schedules are important in discriminating factors that might significantly alter circadian phase and contribute to sleep disruption. Such a detailed approach may enable interventions such as scheduling, chronotherapy, or adjustments in daytime activity without the use of medications [34].

Cerebral Palsy

Cerebral palsy (CP) is a static neurodevelopmental disorder characterized by motor dysfunction with or without associated encephalopathy affecting 2 to 2.5 of 1000 of live births worldwide. CP is the clinical manifestation of perinatally acquired brain injury, most commonly the result of perinatal asphyxia and hypoxic-ischemic encephalopathy or intraventricular hemorrhage. Subsequent periventricular white matter damage may culminate in periventricular leukomalacia. The location of injury may predict the type of motor symptom: involvement of the periventricular white matter results in spasticity, involvement of the basal ganglia results in extrapyramidal symptoms such as athetosis and/or dystonia, and involvement of the cerebellum results in hypotonia or ataxia and mixed involvement. Spastic plegia or paresis accounts for about 75% of cases and is classified according to the topography of the motor deficit. The main risk factor for CP is prematurity even though the overall incidence is higher in full-term infants.

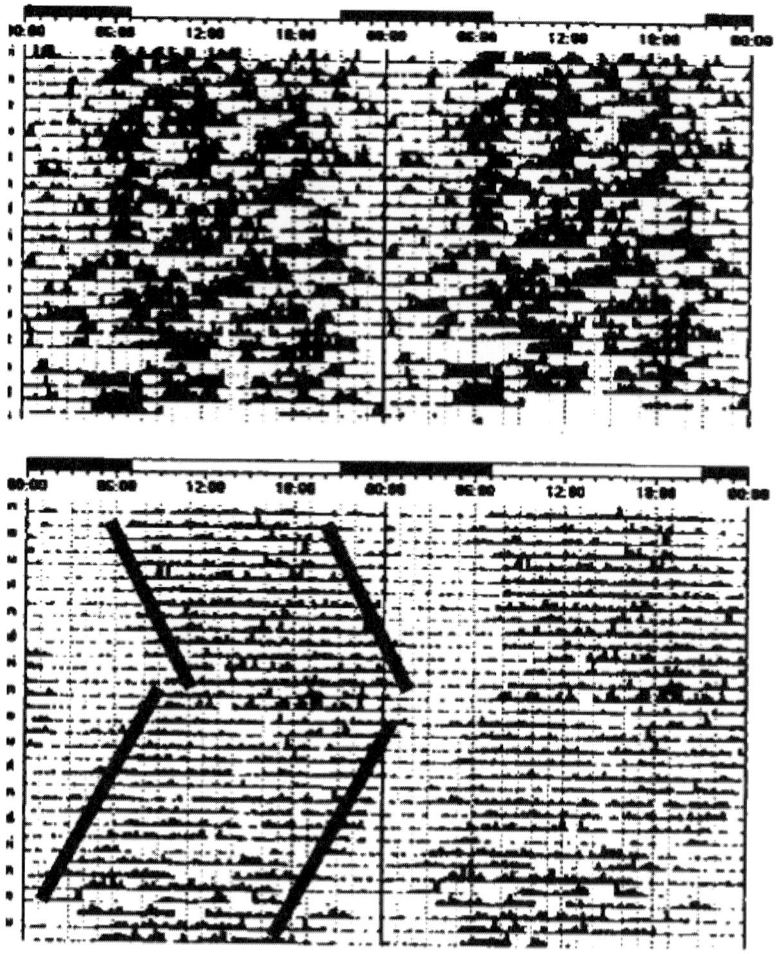

Figure 14.1 Actograms bi-plotted over 48 hours per line demonstrating disrupted circadian entrainment to the light-dark cycle and fragmented circadian rhythmicity in a child with septo-optic dysplasia (top) and free-running rhythm in a child with optic nerve glioma (bottom). Adapted from Rivkees, 2003 (ref 94).

Sleep dysfunction is frequent in patients in CP; however, there are few studies formally assessing sleep dysfunction and its risk factors in these children. Not surprisingly, patients with more severe CP (and by implication, a greater area of affected brain) have a greater likelihood of sleep dysfunction. Thus, functional impairment seems to correlate with both the number and severity of reported sleep disorders [10,35,36]. Risk factors for sleep dysfunction in individuals with CP include comorbid epilepsy, MR, visual impairment, and degree of functional motor impairment. There is some evidence that children with spastic quadriparesis and psychomotor impairment demonstrate poorly organized sleep likely complicated by an intermittent slow and epileptiform EEG, making sleep scoring highly challenging [36]. Visual impairment associated with abnormal light perception (eg, from associated retinopathy or other cause) may affect the retinohypothalamic tract and subsequently, the ability to adequately respond to the entraining circadian influence of the light-dark cycle, as discussed above. Exogenous melatonin supplementation may be particularly useful in these individuals [35,37–40].

Spasticity, contractures, limitation of movement, and associated pain can adversely contribute to positioning during sleep. Severe CP can be associated with scoliosis and restricted lung volumes thus placing affected patients at risk for sleep-related hypoventilation. Involvement of the bulbar musculature may contribute to crowding of the oropharynx and arching of the palate further increasing the risk of SDB. The results of 1 study suggested that sleep problems in children with severe CP may be exacerbated by nighttime oxygen desaturation (associated with apnea) caused by the inability to compensate for it by changes in body position [36]. The prevalence of sleep apnea has not been formally assessed in the CP population.

Sleep, CP, and Assessment of the Quality of Life

The Pediatric Quality of Life Inventory (PedsQL) developed by Varni et al has been validated in various languages and cultures and has been refined over time [96]. It uses a modular approach that varies by age of the subject and integrates both parental and child self-reports on QOL. A questionnaire has also been developed for specific use in children with CP. Ideally, the Generic scale should be combined with the disease-specific scale. The PedsQL 4.0 Generic Core Scale contains a parent report form that is applicable from infancy to age 18 years. The parent report form has 23 items, each organized on a 5-point Likert scale (0 = never, 1 = almost never, 2 = sometimes, 3 = often, and 4 = almost always). The items address 4 domains—physical, emotional, social, and school function. Each questionnaire takes about 5 minutes to complete and 5 minutes to score. The *higher* the score, the *better* is the quality of life. The PedsQL is reliable (*r* value of total child self-report scale = 0.88, parent proxy form = 0.9), valid in the sense that it distinguishes between healthy children and those with acute/chronic health conditions, and sensitive to change [96]. There is a need for longitudinal studies to determine whether improvement in sleep quality of children with CP leads to a commensurate improvement in the quality of life.

Specific Disorders

Fragile X Syndrome

Fragile X syndrome (FXS) is the most common inherited cause of MR. The incidence is about 1 in 4000 live male births and 0.6 in 1000 in females. FXS manifests physically with an elongated face, large ears, macroorchidism, and MR. Males with FXS manifest behavioral abnormalities that can include language deficits, social avoidance, anxiety, and stereotypes such as hand-flapping, hyperactivity, deficits in executive function, and deficits in visual-spatial recognition [41,42]. About 30% of children meet criteria for diagnosis of autism [43]. Cytogenitically, chromosome spreads demonstrate the eponymic gap or break on the X chromosome at Xq27.3. FXS results from replication of CGG repeats in the 5' untranslated region of the Fragile X Mental Retardation 1 (*FMR1*) gene which encodes the Fragile X Mental Retardation Protein (FMRP) [44,45]. Hypermethylation of the expanded CGG repeats and upstream CpG island leads to transcriptional silencing of *FMR1* [46]. Fifty-four or fewer repeats renders a normal phenotype, 55 to 200 repeats are referred to as "pre-mutated" and can contribute to expansion of the repeats. FMRP is a messenger RNA (mRNA)–binding polysome-associated protein that acts as a negative regulator of protein translation, facilitates mRNA trafficking, and influences mRNA stability [47–50]. Activity-dependent alterations in local protein synthesis at synapses may underlie the neurobehavioral manifestation of FXS [51,52]. Interestingly, orthologs of *FMR1* have been implicated in the regulation of sleep homeostasis in flies and circadian rhythms in both mice and fruit flies [53–56].

The full scope of sleep problems in children with FXS is unknown. In 1 study, 77% of parents of children with FXS reported a significant sleep disorder and these include primarily sleep-onset insomnia and sleep maintenance difficulties [14,57]. Abnormal melatonin profiles have been reported, suggesting circadian dysfunction [58]. There have been reports of some benefit to supplemental melatonin in FXS.

There have been a few physiological studies of children with FXS. Increased stage N3 sleep, decreased REM, increased first REM latency, and decreased total sleep have been reported in FXS boys compared with typically developing boys [58]. Compared with normally developing children, subtle changes in sleep macroarchitecture such as shorter total sleep time, longer REM latency, and decreased REM have been described in children with FXS that are more similar to changes seen in children with autism compared with those of normally developing children. There are correlations between sleep dysfunction and poorer nonverbal communication, social relatedness, and perceptual measures; these are consistent with previous associations seen in children with MR (Table 14.1) [11]. Interictal epileptiform activity with features similar to centrotemporal spikes of Rolandic epilepsy has been described in FXS children; however, the generalizability of these findings to all individuals with FXS is less clear [59–62]. Sleep apnea has been reported; however, follow-up studies demonstrated normal breathing in a cohort of FXS patients; thus, the risk of SDB in individuals with FXS remains unknown relative to the normal population [63,64].

Trisomy 21 (Down Syndrome)

Trisomy 21 is the most common known chromosomal cause of MR with an incidence of 1 per 660 live births [65]. The resulting clinical syndrome is characterized by obesity, growth retardation, congenital atrioventricular canal defects, hypotonia, atlanto-axial instability, and stereotyped craniofacial features. Sleep dysfunction is common in trisomy 21 and may contribute to cognitive dysfunction [66,67]. Sleep abnormalities include prolonged sleep latency, increased sleep fragmentation, a reduction in REM sleep, and SDB, particularly SDB in the form of the obstructive sleep apnea syndrome (OSAS) [67–70].

OSAS affects 30% to 55% of children with trisomy 21 compared with about 2% of normal children [71–74]. In 1e large study, hypoventilation ($P_{ET}CO_2$>45 mmHg) was present in 81% of patients with trisomy 21 suspected of obstructive sleep apnea (OSA) [73]. Untreated hypoventilation may contribute to pulmonary hypertension and congestive heart failure. Obstructive hypoventilation and cor pulmonale have been reported in infants with trisomy 21 [75]. The etiology of SDB in trisomy 21 is likely multifactorial. Several factors contribute to crowding of the airway including an oropharynx that is relatively wide in the lateral dimension and narrow in the anterior-posterior dimension, glossoptosis, macroglossia, and hypotonia of the upper airway muscles [76]. One study of snoring in nonobese children with trisomy 21 found OSA in 97%. Thus, although there are no agreed upon published guidelines, the threshold for polysomnography in individuals with trisomy 21 should be low. The risk of OSAS in trisomy continues into adulthood [67,77].

The waking EEG in trisomy 21 demonstrates a relative decrease in waking alpha frequency with an increased theta frequency. The degree of slowing seems to correlate with the level of cognitive dysfunction [78,79]. To what extent this relative slowing of the waking EEG represents a dysfunction of the arousal system is unknown.

Tuberous Sclerosis Complex

Tuberous sclerosis complex (TSC) is a neurogenetic disorder characterized by a variable degree of MR, developmental delay, epilepsy, autism, and multiorgan tumors [80]. TSC is caused by heterozygous mutation in either the Tsc1 or Tsc2 genes, whose products indirectly suppress the mechanistic target of rapamycin (mTOR), a key integrator of cell growth in response to nutritional status [81]. Thus, a result of TSC dysfunction is activation of mTOR [82]. How mTOR overactivation results in the neurological phenotype of TSC remains unclear, but abnormal neuronal plasticity, stress-response and apoptotic pathways, and aberrant connectivity have been described [83–86]. Sleep problems are frequently reported in studies of neurobehavioral aspects of TSC, affecting 50% to 80% of affected individuals. The sleep problems reported in TSC do not constitute a single phenotypic class and include insomnia, frequent arousals, premature awakening, and abnormal REM sleep [87–90]. The presence of sleep dysfunction seems to correlate with comorbid epilepsy and/or autism [87,89]. Treatment of sleep dysfunction with melatonin has been attempted with equivocal efficacy [90–92]. No systematic study of circadian function has been reported in individuals with TSC.

Septooptic Dysplasia

Septooptic dysplasia (SOD) is a clinically heterogeneous disorder defined by a combination of optic nerve hypoplasia, pituitary gland hypoplasia, and midline abnormalities of the brain, including absence of the corpus callosum and septum pellucidum. Visual impairment and/or blindness are frequent in patients with SOD placing them at risk for inability to entrain to the light-dark cycle and circadian disruption. Irregular or even nonentrained (ie, "free-running") rest-activity patterns have been described in individuals with SOD and in patients with other disorders affecting the midline subcortical structures [93–95]. Exogenous melatonin supplementation prescribed at the same time nightly is a reasonable therapy. Comorbid hypopituitarism can result in obesity and other hypothalamic dysfunction, predisposing to sleep apnea.

Conclusion

Sleep disorders are common in children with cognitive and/or physical disabilities yet remain poorly understood and understudied. Sleep is critical to daytime functioning in all children and may be of particular importance in children with cognitive and/or developmental disorders given the frequency of comorbid epilepsy, gastrointestinal, and musculoskeletal dysfunction—all of which may be detrimental interactions in contributing to sleep dysfunction. Improvement of sleep disorders in children with disability benefits daytime functioning and quality of life, making sleep a key interface for clinical intervention. A working of knowledge of sleep and circadian mechanisms stand to significantly benefit the lives of patients with disabilities and potentially spare them unnecessary pharmacological intervention. More research is needed to longitudinally examine sleep disorders in children with MR, CP, and other neurodevelopmental disorders. The biology underlying cognitive and physical disability may make important contributions to understanding the basic mechanisms by which sleep contributes to development and vice versa.

References

1. Marks GA, Shaffery JP, Oksenberg A, Speciale SG, Roffwarg HP. A functional role for REM sleep in brain maturation. *Behav Brain Res.* 1995; 69(1–2):1.
2. Anders TF, Roffwarg HP. The effects of selective interruption and deprivation of sleep in the human newborn. *Dev Psychobiol.* 1973;6(1):77.
3. Finkelstein JW, Anders TF, Sacher EJ, Roffwarg HP, Hellman LD. Behavioral state, sleep stage and growth hormone levels in human infants. *J Clin Endocrinol Metab.* 1971; 32(3):368.
4. Anders TF, Sachar EJ, Kream J, Roffwarg HP, Hellman L. Behavioral state and plasma cortisol response in the human newborn. *Pediatrics.* 1970;46(4):532.
5. Roffwarg HP, Muzio JN, Dement WC. Ontogenetic development of the human sleep-dream cycle. *Science.* 1966;152(3722):604.
6. Dorris L, Scott N, Zuberi S, Gibson N, Espie C. Sleep problems in children with neurological disorders. *Dev Neurorehabil.* 2008;11(2):95.
7. Tirosh E, Tal Y, Jaffe M. CPAP treatment of obstructive sleep apnoea and neurodevelopmental deficits. *Acta Paediatr.* 1995;84(7):791.
8. U.S.C., in *110–325* U. S. Congress, Ed. (2008).
9. Braam W, Smits MG, Didden R, Korzilius H, Van Geijlswijk IM, Curfs LM. Exogenous melatonin for sleep problems in individuals with intellectual disability: a meta-analysis. *Dev Med Child Neurol.* 2009;51(5):340.
10. Didden R, Korzilius H, van Aperlo B, van Overloop C, de Vries M. Sleep problems and daytime problem behaviours in children with intellectual disability. *J Intellect Disabil Res.* 2002; 46(pt 7):537.
11. Quine L. Sleep problems in children with mental handicap. *J Ment Defic Res.* 1991;35(pt 4):269.
12. Chu J, Richdale AL. Sleep quality and psychological wellbeing in mothers of children with developmental disabilities. *Res Dev Disabil.* 2009;30(6):1512.
13. Robinson AM, Richdale AL. Sleep problems in children with an intellectual disability: parental perceptions of sleep problems, and views of treatment effectiveness. *Child Care Health Dev.* 2004;30(2):139.
14. Lipton J, Becker RE, Kothare SV. Insomnia of childhood. *Curr Opin Pediatr.* 2008;20(6):641.
15. Wiggs L, Stores G. Severe sleep disturbance and daytime challenging behaviour in children with severe learning disabilities. *J Intellect Disabil Res.* 1996;40(pt 6):518.
16. Touchette E, Petit D, Séguin JR, Boivin M, Tremblay RE, Montplaisir JY. Associations between sleep duration patterns and behavioral/cognitive functioning at school entry. *Sleep.* 2007;30(9):1213.
17. Lindblom N, Heiskala H, Kaski M, et al. Neurological impairments and sleep-wake behaviour among the mentally retarded. *J Sleep Res.* 2001;10(4):309.
18. Leger D, Prevot E, Philip P, et al. Sleep disorders in children with blindness. *Ann Neurol.* 1999;46(4):648.
19. Duffy JF, Czeisler CA. Effect of light on human circadian physiology. *Sleep Med Clin.* 2009;4(2):165.
20. Czeisler CA, Gooley JJ. Sleep and circadian rhythms in humans. *Cold Spring Harb Symp Quant Biol.* 2007;72:579.
21. Bjorvatn B, Pallesen S. A practical approach to circadian rhythm sleep disorders. *Sleep Med Rev.* 2009;13(1):47.
22. Hofstra WA, de Weerd AW. How to assess circadian rhythm in humans: a review of literature. *Epilepsy Behav.* 2008;13(3):438.
23. Lack LC, Wright HR. Chronobiology of sleep in humans. *Cell Mol Life Sci.* 2007;64(10):1205.

24. Saper CB, Lu J, Chou TC, Gooley J. The hypothalamic integrator for circadian rhythms. *Trends Neurosci.* 2005;28(3):152.
25. Leger D, Guilleminault C, Defrance R, Domont A, Paillard M. Prevalence of sleep/wake disorders in persons with blindness. *Clin Sci (Lond).* 1999;97(2):193.
26. Leger D, Guilleminault C, Defrance R, Domont A, Paillard M. Blindness and sleep patterns. *Lancet.* 1996;348(9030):830.
27. Sack RL, Lewy AJ, Blood ML, Keith LD, Nakagawa H. Circadian rhythm abnormalities in totally blind people: incidence and clinical significance. *J Clin Endocrinol Metab.* 1992;75(1):127.
28. Wirojanan J, Jacquemont S, Diaz R, et al. The efficacy of melatonin for sleep problems in children with autism, fragile X syndrome, or autism and fragile X syndrome. *J Clin Sleep Med.* 2009;5(2):145.
29. Hofstra WA, de Weerd AW. The circadian rhythm and its interaction with human epilepsy: a review of literature. *Sleep Med Rev.* 2009;13(6):413.
30. Malow BA. The interaction between sleep and epilepsy. *Epilepsia.* 2007;48(suppl 9):36.
31. Malow BA. Sleep and epilepsy. *Neurol Clin.* 2005;23(4):1127.
32. Stores G, Wiggs L, Campling G. Sleep disorders and their relationship to psychological disturbance in children with epilepsy. *Child Care Health Dev.* 1998;24(1):5.
33. Shouse MN, da Silva AM, Sammaritano M. Circadian rhythm, sleep, and epilepsy. *J Clin Neurophysiol,* 1996;13(1):32.
34. Hylkema T, Vlaskamp C. Significant improvement in sleep in people with intellectual disabilities living in residential settings by non-pharmaceutical interventions. *J Intellect Disabil Res.* 2009;53(8):695.
35. Zucconi M, Bruni O. Sleep disorders in children with neurologic diseases. *Semin Pediatr Neurol.* 2001;8(4):258.
36. Kotagal S, Gibbons VP, Stith JA. Sleep abnormalities in patients with severe cerebral palsy. *Dev Med Child Neurol.* 1994;36(4):304.
37. Lockley SW, Dijk DJ, Kosti O, Skene DJ, Arendt J. Alertness, mood and performance rhythm disturbances associated with circadian sleep disorders in the blind. *J Sleep Res.* 2008;17(2):207.
38. Palm L, Blennow G, Wetterberg L. Long-term melatonin treatment in blind children and young adults with circadian sleep-wake disturbances. *Dev Med Child Neurol.* 1997;39(5):319.
39. Lapierre O, Dumont M. Melatonin treatment of a non-24-hour sleep-wake cycle in a blind retarded child. *Biol Psychiatry.* 1995;38(2):119.
40. Tzischinsky O, Skene D, Epstein R, Lavie P. Circadian rhythms in 6-sulphatoxymelatonin and nocturnal sleep in blind children. *Chronobiol Int.* 1991;8(3):168.
41. Crawford DC, Acuna JM, Sherman SL. FMR1 and the fragile X syndrome: human genome epidemiology review. *Genet Med.* 2001;3(5):359.
42. Mazzocco MM. Advances in research on the fragile X syndrome. *Ment Retard Dev Disabil Res Rev.* 2000;6(2):96.
43. Rogers SJ, Wehner DE, Hagerman R. The behavioral phenotype in fragile X: symptoms of autism in very young children with fragile X syndrome, idiopathic autism, and other developmental disorders. *J Dev Behav Pediatr.* 2001;22(6):409.
44. Fu YH, Kuhl DP, Pizzuti A, et al. Variation of the CGG repeat at the fragile X site results in genetic instability: resolution of the Sherman paradox. *Cell.* 1991;67(6):1047.
45. Verkerk AJ, Pieretti M, Sutcliffe JS, et al. Identification of a gene (FMR-1) containing a CGG repeat coincident with a breakpoint cluster region exhibiting length variation in fragile X syndrome. *Cell.* 1991;65(5):905.
46. Garber K, Smith KT, Reines D, Warren ST. Transcription, translation and fragile X syndrome. *Curr Opin Genet Dev.* 2006;16(3):270.
47. Laggerbauer B, Ostareck D, Keidel EM, Ostareck-Lederer A, Fischer U. Evidence that fragile X mental retardation protein is a negative regulator of translation. *Hum Mol Genet.* 2001;10(4):329.
48. Zalfa F, Giorgi M, Primerano B, Moro A, Di Penta A, Reis S, Oostra B, Bagni C. The fragile X syndrome protein FMRP associates with BC1 RNA and regulates the translation of specific mRNAs at synapses. *Cell.* 2003;112(3):317.
49. Sung YJ, Dolzhanskaya N, Nolin SL, Brown T, Currie JR, Denman RB. The fragile X mental retardation protein FMRP binds elongation factor 1A mRNA and negatively regulates its translation in vivo. *J Biol Chem.* 2003;278(18):15669.
50. Siomi H, Siomi MC, Nussbaum RL, Dreyfuss G. The protein product of the fragile X gene, FMR1, has characteristics of an RNA-binding protein. *Cell.* 1993;74(2):291.
51. Bassell GJ, Warren ST. Fragile X syndrome: loss of local mRNA regulation alters synaptic development and function. *Neuron.* 2008;60(2):201.
52. Ramocki MB, Zoghbi HY. Failure of neuronal homeostasis results in common neuropsychiatric phenotypes. *Nature.* 2008;455(7215):912.
53. Gatto CL, Broadie K. The fragile X mental retardation protein in circadian rhythmicity and memory consolidation. *Mol Neurobiol.* 2009;39(2):107.
54. Sofola O, Sundram V, Ng F, et al. The Drosophila FMRP and LARK RNA-binding proteins function together to regulate eye development and circadian behavior. *J Neurosci.* 2008;28(41):10200.
55. Zhang J, Fang Z, Jud C, et al. Fragile X-related proteins regulate mammalian circadian behavioral rhythms. *Am J Hum Genet.* 2008;83(1):43.
56. Bushey D, Tononi G, Cirelli C. The Drosophila fragile X mental retardation gene regulates sleep need. *J Neurosci.* 2009;29(7):1948.
57. Gould EL, Loesch DZ, Martin MJ, Hagerman RJ, Armstrong SM, Huggins RM. Melatonin profiles and sleep characteristics in boys with fragile X syndrome: a preliminary study. *Am J Med Genet.* 2000;95(4):307.

58. Musumeci SA, Ferri R, Elia M, et al. Sleep neurophysiology in fragile X syndrome patients. *Dev Brain Dysfunct.* 1995;8:218.
59. Musumeci SA, Colognola RM, Ferri R, et al. Fragile-X syndrome: a particular epileptogenic EEG pattern. *Epilepsia.* 1988;29(1):41.
60. Musumeci SA, Ferri R, Scuderi C, Bosco P, Elia M. Seizures and epileptiform EEG abnormalities in FRAXE syndrome. *Clin Neurophysiol.* 2001;112(10):1954.
61. Elia M, Ferri R, Musumeci SA, et al. Sleep in subjects with autistic disorder: a neurophysiological and psychological study. *Brain Dev.* 2000;22(2):88.
62. Ferri R, Bergonzi P, Elia M, Ferri P, Musumeci SA. Modulation of the interictal epileptiform EEG activity during sleep: from oscillations to complex dynamics. *Neurophysiol Clin.* 1991;21(1):1.
63. Musumeci SA, Ferri R, Elia M, Del Gracco S, Scuderi C, Stefanini MC. Normal respiratory pattern during sleep in young fragile X-syndrome patients. *J Sleep Res.* 1996;5(4):272.
64. Tirosh E, Borochowitz Z. Sleep apnea in fragile X syndrome. *Am J Med Genet.* 1992;43(1–2):124.
65. Smith DW. *Recognizable Patterns of Human Malformation.* Philadelphia, PA: WB Saunders; 1982:10–13.
66. Harvey MT, Kennedy CH Polysomnographic phenotypes in developmental disabilities. *Int J Dev Neurosci.* 2002;20(3–5):443.
67. Andreou G, Galanopoulou C, Gourgoulianis K, Karapetsas A, Molyvdas P. Cognitive status in Down syndrome individuals with sleep disordered breathing deficits (SDB). *Brain Cogn.* 2002;50(1):145.
68. Levanon A, Tarasiuk A, Tal A. Sleep characteristics in children with Down syndrome. *J Pediatr.* 1999;134(6):755.
69. Hamaguchi H, Hashimoto T, Mori K, Tayama M. Sleep in the Down syndrome. *Brain Dev.* 1989;11(6):399.
70. Grubar JC, Gigli GL, Colognola RM, Ferri R, Musumeci SA, Bergonzi P. Sleep patterns of Down's syndrome children: effects of butoctamide hydrogen succinate (BAHS) administration. *Psychopharmacology (Berl).* 1986;90(1):119.
71. de Miguel-Diez J, Villa-Asensi JR, Alvarez-Sala JL. Prevalence of sleep-disordered breathing in children with Down syndrome: polygraphic findings in 108 children. *Sleep.* 2003;26(8):1006.
72. Ferri R, Curzi-Dascalova L, Del Gracco S, Elia M, Musumeci SA, Stefanini MC. Respiratory patterns during sleep in Down's syndrome: importance of central apnoeas. *J Sleep Res.* 1997;6(2):134.
73. Marcus CL, Keens TG, Bautista DB, von Pechmann WS, Ward SL. Obstructive sleep apnea in children with down syndrome. *Pediatrics.* 1991;88(1):132.
74. Stebbens VA, Dennis J, Samuels MP, Croft CB, Southall DP. Sleep related upper airway obstruction in a cohort with down's syndrome. *Arch Dis Child.* 1991;66(11):1333.
75. Levine OR, Simpser M. Alveolar hypoventilation and cor pulmonale associated with chronic airway obstruction in infants with down syndrome. *Clin Pediatr (Phila).* 1982;21(1):25.
76. Fink GB, Madaus WK, Walker GF. A quantitative study of the face in down's syndrome. *Am J Orthod.* 1975;67(5):540.
77. Trois MS, Capone GT, Lutz JA, et al. Obstructive sleep apnea in adults with down syndrome. *J Clin Sleep Med.* 2009;5(4):317.
78. Politoff AL, Stadter RP, Monson N, Hass P. Cognition-related EEG abnormalities in nondemented down syndrome subjects. *Dementia.* 1996;7(2):69.
79. Katada A, Hasegawa S, Ohira D, et al. On chronological changes in the basic EEG rhythm in persons with down syndrome—with special reference to slowing of alpha waves. *Brain Dev.* 2000;22(4):224.
80. Crino PB, Nathanson KL, Henske EP. The tuberous sclerosis complex. *N Engl J Med.* 2006;355(13):1345.
81. Laplante M, Sabatini DM. mTOR signaling at a glance. *J Cell Sci.* 2009;122(pt 20):3589.
82. Wullschleger S, Loewith R, Hall MN. TOR signaling in growth and metabolism. *Cell.* 2006;124(3):471.
83. Di Nardo A, Kramvis I, Cho N, Sadowski A, Meikle L, Kwiatkowski DJ, Sahin M. Tuberous sclerosis complex activity is required to control neuronal stress responses in an mTOR-dependent manner. *J Neurosci.* 2009;29(18):5926.
84. Choi YJ, Di Nardo A, Kramvis I, et al. Tuberous sclerosis complex proteins control axon formation. *Genes Dev.* 2008;22(18):2485.
85. Meikle L, Pollizzi K, Egnor A, et al. Response of a neuronal model of tuberous sclerosis to mammalian target of rapamycin (mTOR) inhibitors: effects on mTORC1 and Akt signaling lead to improved survival and function. *J Neurosci.* 2008;28(21):5422.
86. Nie D, Di Nardo A, Han JM, et al. Tsc2-Rheb signaling regulates EphA-mediated axon guidance. *Nat Neurosci.* 2010;13:163.
87. Asato MR, Hardan AY. Neuropsychiatric problems in tuberous sclerosis complex. *J Child Neurol.* 2004;19(4):241.
88. Bruni O, Cortesi F, Giannotti F, Curatolo P. Sleep disorders in tuberous sclerosis: a polysomnographic study. *Brain Dev.* 1995;17(1):52.
89. Hunt A, Stores G. Sleep disorder and epilepsy in children with tuberous sclerosis: a questionnaire-based study. *Dev Med Child Neurol.* 1994;36(2):108.
90. Hunt A. Development, behaviour and seizures in 300 cases of tuberous sclerosis. *J Intellect Disabil Res.* 1993;37(pt 1):41.
91. Hancock E, O'Callaghan F, Osborne JP. Effect of melatonin dosage on sleep disorder in tuberous sclerosis complex. *J Child Neurol.* 2005;20(1):78.
92. Hancock E, O'Callaghan F, English J, Osborne JP. Melatonin excretion in normal children and

in tuberous sclerosis complex with sleep disorder responsive to melatonin. *J Child Neurol.* 2005;20(1):21.

93. Rivkees SA. Arrhythmicity in a child with septo-optic dysplasia and establishment of sleep-wake cyclicity with melatonin. *J Pediatr.* 2001;139(3):463.
94. Rivkees SA. Rest-activity patterns in children with hypopituitarism. *Pediatrics.* 2003;111(6, pt 1): e720.
95. Lipton J, Megerian JT, Kothare SV, et al. Melatonin deficiency and disrupted circadian rhythms in pediatric survivors of craniopharyngioma. *Neurology.* 2009;73(4):323.
96. Varni JW, Limbers CA. The pediatric quality of life inventory: measuring pediatric health-related quality of life from the perspective of children and their parents. *Pediatr Clin North Am.* 2009;56(4):843.

CHAPTER 15

Sleep-Related Breathing Disorders in Children With Miscellaneous Neurological Disorders

Madeleine Grigg-Damberger and Jeffrey J. Stanley

Introduction

Sleep disorders in children with certain neurological disorders are often more common, frequent, severe, and persistent, further impairing quality of life (QOL) (and sleep) for both the child and the caregivers. Their problems are associated with greater cognitive impairment, impaired learning, and more problematic behaviors [1,2]. Children with particular neurological disorders are at increased risk for sleep-disordered breathing (SDB) including sleep apnea syndromes, nocturnal hypoxemia, and/or sleep-related hypoventilation. Often unrecognized and untreated, SDB may further compromise their intellectual capacity, ability to learn, provoke problematic behaviors, and lead some to sudden death. Awareness of the nature, prevalence, and treatments of SDB in children with neurological disorders can greatly improve QOL for these children (and the caregivers).

Neurodevelopmental Disorders

Down Syndrome

Down syndrome (DS) is the most common genetic cause of mental retardation with an incidence ranging from 1 per 1000 births in mothers younger than 40 years to 1 in 50 births for mothers 40 years or older [3]. DS accounts for approximately 30% of all cases of moderate-to-severe intellectual disability (ID) [4]. Contrary to common expectation, the prevalence of DS is increasing (now 10.3 per 10,000 children in the United States) the effects of childbearing later in life and increasing longevity of individuals with DS [5].

DS is most often caused by an extra chromosome 21 (Trisomy 21) in the distal long arm of chromosome 21 (21q22.3). The phenotypic expression of the Trisomy 21 genotype shows great interindividual variability, seemingly modified by allelic variation, genomic imbalances, epigenetic, and/or environmental factors [6]. Early intervention programs and parental nurturing may contribute to better cognitive outcomes for children with DS. Children with DS compared to the general pediatric population have significantly greater bedtime resistance, sleep anxiety, night waking, parasomnias, SDB, and daytime sleepiness [7].

Two to 3% of children between ages 2 to 7 years in the general pediatric population have obstructive sleep apnea-hypopnea-hypoventilation syndrome (OSA with $\geq$ 1.5 obstructive apneas and hypopneas per hour of sleep after excluding central events); whereas, the prevalence of OSA in children with DS ranges from 30% to 60% [8]. A prospective cohort study reported that 57% of DS children ages 2 to 4 years had OSA [9]. The craniofacial features common in DS that predispose to OSA include maxillary hypoplasia, a relatively large and/or posteriorly positioned tongue in relatively smaller oral cavities, glossoptosis, a small nose with a low nasal bridge, absent frontal and sphenoid sinuses, maxillary sinus hypoplasia, and increased salivary secretions [10]. Uong et al (2001) found that children with DS (mean age 3.2 ± 1.4 years) have smaller airway volume, a smaller mid- and lower-face skeleton, shorter hard palate length, and mandible volume compared to age-matched controls [11]. The volume of their adenoids, tonsils, or tongue was not larger than control subjects, but these soft tissues were crowded with their smaller mid- and lower-face skeletons.

Many young children with DS have pharyngeal hypotonia, oral aversion, dysphagia, laryngomalacia, tracheomalacia, and/or tracheal abnormalities. Because of impaired cellular immunity, children with DS have a 12-fold greater risk for infections, especially pneumonia. Obesity, pulmonary arterial hypertension, and hypothyroidism may further predispose to SDB [10]. Children with DS are thought to be at increased risk for pulmonary arterial hypertension because of reduced number of alveoli, thinner media of pulmonary arterioles, and impaired endothelial function [12,13]. Reduced hypoxic drive in some may lead to sleep-related hypoventilation, central apneas, and rarely respiratory failure [14]. Mitchell et al (2003) found upper airway obstruction was most often related to laryngomalacia in DS infants younger than 1 month and due to OSA in those 2 years or older (further complicated by gastroesophageal reflux disease in nearly two-thirds) [15].

Several recent prospective studies have found OSA is much more common in children with DS compared to the general pediatric population. Schott et al (2006) found OSA on overnight polysomnography (PSG) in 57% of 65 DS children (mean age 42 months), increasing to 80% if cases of upper airway resistance (with snoring and increased work of breathing, triggering frequent arousals) were included [9]. Ng et al (2006) found OSA (AHI >1.5/h) in 59% of 22 DS children compared with 32% of children without DS who snored [16]. Dyken et al (2003) found OSA in 79% of 19 unselected children with DS with a mean AHI of 6/h [17]. Parents of DS often under- or overestimated the likelihood their child would have OSA on a PSG [9,18]. One study found 62% of the DS children with PSG-confirmed OSA did not habitually snore [19]. OSA when present in children with DS is often much more severe than that in children without DS: a mean AHI of 12.9/h consistent with severe OSA for age was found on overnight PSG in 33 *nonobese* DS children (mean age 4.9 years) who snored [8]. OSA is so common in DS children that some argue a PSG should be done for *all* between ages 3 to 4 years [9]. The diagnosis of OSA in DS should be confirmed by overnight PSG because afternoon nap studies often underestimate the severity of the disorder [18].

If a DS child with OSA has relatively enlarged tonsils and/or adenoids, the first treatment strategy is adenotonsillectomy (AT). Before surgery, cervical x-rays in extension and lateral flexion are recommended to screen for atlantoaxial subluxation or instability, which is present in 10% to 20% of infants and children with DS [20]. AT under endoscopic guidance may be useful to ensure maximal removal of their adenoidal tissue [21]. Children with DS have smaller airways, and intubation in a child with DS should be performed initially using an endotracheal tube that is at least two times smaller than would be used in a child of the same age without DS [22]. Children with DS, particularly those with SDB, are at increased risk for postoperative respiratory complications and should be hospitalized for close observation following upper airway surgeries. A retrospective survey by Goldstein et al (1998) found respiratory complications occurred in 25% of 87 children with DS following AT compared to 5% in age-matched "uncomplicated" control subjects [23]. DS have longer length of stay following AT (mean 1.6 days vs. 0.8 days), and 25% of the children with DS required airway management or observation in the pediatric intensive care unit compared to none of the controls [23].

A PSG should be repeated 2 to 3 months after AT in children with DS because significant residual OSA was found on postoperative PSG despite parental report of subjective "cure" [24]. AT usually lessens OSA severity but does not normalize SDB in children with DS [25,26]. AHI decreased significantly following AT in children with DS (mean age 101 months) but not as much as the children without DS [26]. No significant improvement in REM–AHI or SpO_2 nadir occurred in the DS group, and 73% required further treatment (CPAP, BPAP, or oxygen) for significant residual OSA following AT [26].

Residual (or recurrence) of OSA following AT in a child with DS warrants evaluation for the presence of lingual tonsils or regrowth of adenoidal tissue. Donnelly et al (2004) used cine magnetic resonance imaging (MRI) under sedation in 27 children with DS (mean age 9.9 years) who had recurrence or persistence of OSA following AT [27]. They found multiple causes for OSA: 74% had macroglossia, 63% glossoptosis, 63% recurrence of adenoids, and 30% enlarged lingual tonsils. Lingual tonsils were present in 35% to 50% of DS children who had persistent OSA following palatine tonsillectomy [28,29]. Enlarged lingual tonsils can be visualized on flexible nasopharyngoscopy or identified using cine MRI. Lingual tonsils on MRI are defined as >10 mm abutting both the dorsal posterior border of the tongue and the posterior pharyngeal wall [28,29].

Persistent OSA in a child with DS following removal of all adenoidal and tonsillar tissues warrants consideration of continuous positive airway pressure (CPAP), or bilevel postivie airway pressure (BPAP) if needed for tolerance or hypoventilation. Nasal or oronasal CPAP is an effective treatment for OSA in those who tolerate it. Unfortunately, too many DS children dislike placement of anything on their face (even a nasal cannula), so extensive mask desensitization play therapy is often required to improve PAP compliance [30,31]. Oral appliances should be considered for older children with DS who will not tolerate or use PAP [32]. Weight management, good orodental care and medical treatment of rhinitis and allergies may also help when indicated [33–35]. For infants and young children with severe persistent OSA who will not tolerate PAP and who have severe retrognathia, mid-face hypoplasia, and/or macroglossia consideration of mandibular distraction osteogenesis, tongue base reduction, and/or maxillary/midface advancement is recommended as an alternative to the frequently refused tracheostomy [10,36–38].

Prader-Willi Syndrome

Prader-Willi syndrome (PWS) is the most common genetic form of obesity in children, occurring in about 1 of 15,000 births [39,40]. PWS arises from the lack of expression of paternally inherited imprinted genes on chromosome 15q11-q13. These genes are imprinted and silenced on the maternally inherited chromosome (which is normally nonfunctional). Seventy to 75% acquire PWS as a result of a deletion of the paternally acquired portion of the gene, 20% to 25% inherit both copies of this region of chromosome 15 from their mother (maternal uniparental disomy), and 2% to 5% have a sporadic or inherited microdeletion in a genetic element termed the imprinting center, and 1% have translocations [39,41]. The likelihood of a paternal deletion recurring with another pregnancy is less than 1%. Maternal uniparental disomy is more common in older (than younger) mothers. Molecular genetic testing confirms the particular genetic defect in more than 99% of individuals with PWS and is especially useful in those with atypical features or too young to make the diagnosis based on clinical features. Dysfunction of the hypothalamic-pituitary axis is thought to lead to the clinical and behavioral symptoms and signs of PWS. The clinical features of PWS are summarized in Table 15.1 [39,42–44].

SDB is often observed in PWS even in those without sleep-wake complaints. Moreover, SDB in PWS is often associated with behavior problems including skin picking, food foraging, self-injury, mood lability, impulsiveness, and repetitive speech [45,46]. Sleep problems are the strongest predictor for maladaptive behavior. Behavioral problems in PWS are highly associated with excessive daytime sleepiness (EDS) [47,48]. Treating SDB in PWS can lessen these behavioral problems.

Sleep-related hypoventilation, either primarily or during REM sleep only, is the most common pattern of SDB in PWS. Risks for sleep hypoventilation in PWS are increased by obesity and hypotonia [48–56]. Figure 15.1 shows sleep-related central hypoventilation during REM sleep in a morbidly obese adolescent boy with PWS. Profound tachypnea was observed during NREM 3 sleep in the same boy (Figure 15.2).

Hypoventilation in PWS is thought to reflect a primary disorder of ventilatory control [57]. Absent or depressed peripheral chemoreceptor function responses to acute hypoxic and hypercapnic challenges have been found in children with PWS whether obese or not [58]. PWS subjects compared to controls rarely aroused

Table 15.1 Clinical features of Prader-Willi syndrome

- Severe central hypotonia at birth with a poor suck, weak cry, lethargy, and decreased movement during infancy;
- Hyperphagia and insatiable appetite develop between ages 1 and 6 years which leads to morbid obesity usually by age 4;
- Short stature (50% at or below the third percentile for age);
- Characteristic facies (almond-shaped eyes, strabismus, narrow bifrontal diameter, a thin upper lip, and downturned mouth);
- Fat storage in the abdomen, buttocks, and thighs even nonobese;
- Small hands and feet;
- Hypothalamic hypogonadism (genital hypoplasia, incomplete pubertal development and, in most, infertility);
- Delayed language development;
- Delayed motor milestones (usually first sit at 12 months of age, and walk by 24 months);
- Prone to stubbornness, temper tantrums, self-injury, skin-picking, food foraging, impulsiveness, mood lability, and repetitive speech;
- Learning difficulties, poor academic performance and mean IQs in the 60s to 70s;
- Impaired social cognition, literal mindness, and cognitive inflexibility;
- Sleep-disordered breathing (especially sleep-related hypoventilation, often mild obstructive sleep apnea);
- Central hypersomnia attributed to hypothalamic dysfunction;
- Impaired GH secretion and low serum insulin-like growth factor-I (IGF-I) levels;
- Increased body fat mass, decreased lean body mass, and low bone mineral content.

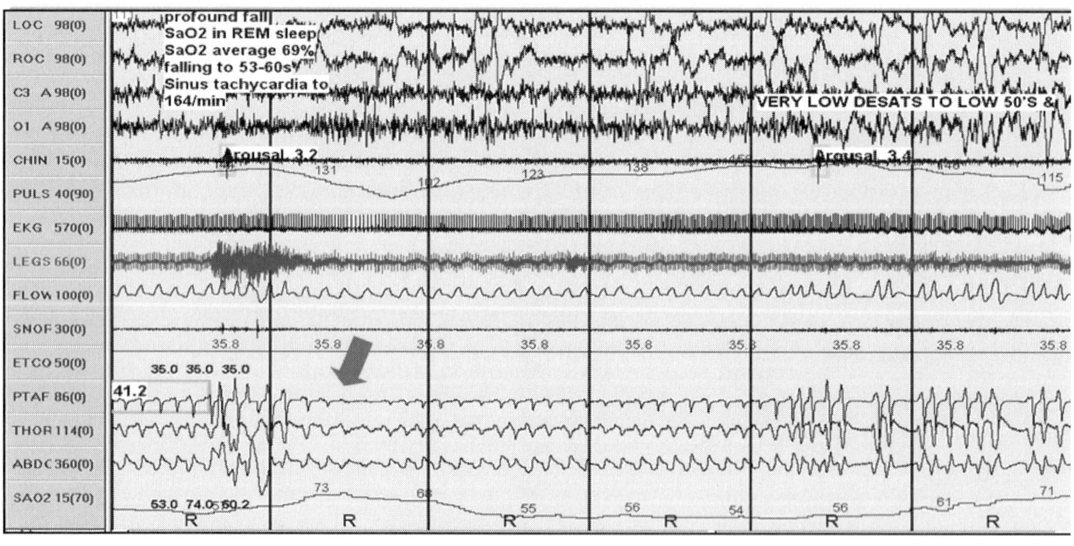

Figure 15.1 Sleep-related central hypoventilation during REM sleep in a morbidly obese adolescent boy with Prader-Willi syndrome.

from NREM sleep in response to hypoxia and failed to demonstrate the appropriate tachycardia response to it [59]. The level of pCO_2 needed to provoke an arousal from sleep has been shown to be much higher in subjects with PWS compared to controls [60].

Apneas observed in overnight PSG of PWS patients are more often central in type [61]. Several studies have found only 10% to 20% of PWS patients will have OSA on overnight PSG [56,62,63]. Obstructive apnea when present in PWS is often mild with an AHI of 5 to less than 10/h of sleep [56,63,64]. Lin et al (2007) in their study of overnight PSG of 30 PWS children (mean age 7 ± 4 years) found their AHI averaged only 6 ± 4/h of sleep, desaturations

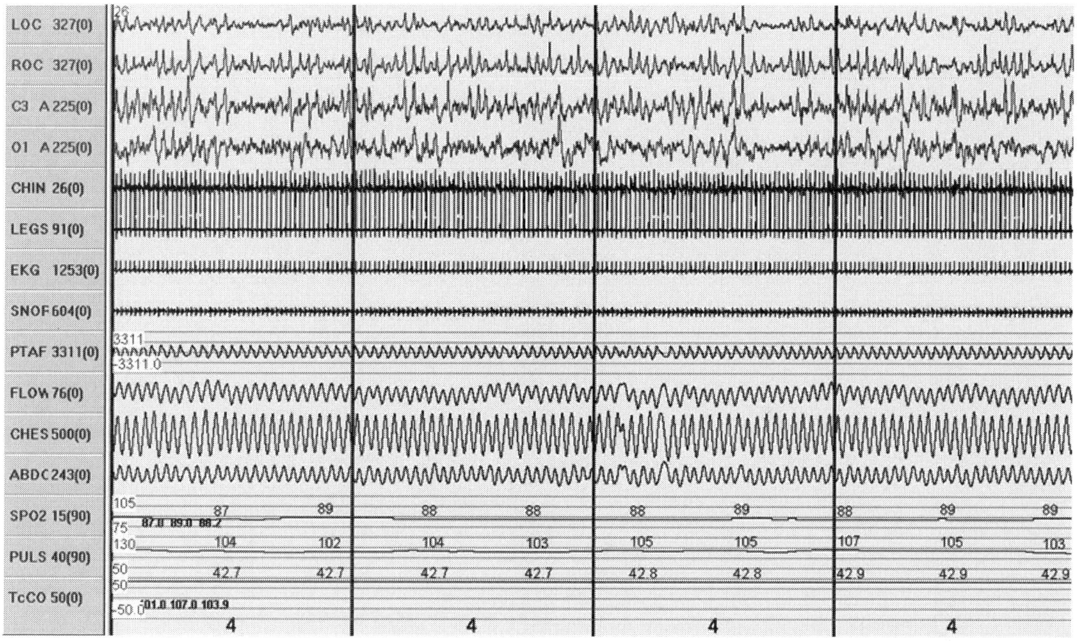

Figure 15.2 Profound tachypnea observed during NREM 3 sleep in the same boy with Prader-Willi syndrome.

8 ± 7/h, but nadir SpO_2 was 77 ± 10% [63]. The severity or type(s) of SDB could not be predicted by BMI Z-score, particular PWS gene mutation, or Epworth sleepiness scale score [55]. However, Hertz et al (1995) found higher BMI correlated with higher AHI and lower arterial oxygen desaturations on the PSG of 43 children and adults with PWS [65].

Yee et al (2007) evaluated 19 adolescents and adults with PWS: 95% had an AHI >5/h, 21% had severe OSA (AHI ≥ 30/h), and 47% were diagnosed with obesity-hypoventilation syndrome [66]. Patients with PWS, as compared with a control group, had significantly greater amounts of nocturnal hypoxemia, lower nadir SpO_2, and higher percentages of sleep time with oxyhemoglobin saturation <80%. Sleep-related hypoventilation with hypercapnia is often present and will go undetected without reliable carbon dioxide (CO_2) monitoring (simultaneously recording end-tidal and transcutaneous CO_2 recommended).

Infants with PWS who are not overweight but have hypotonia can have sleep-related central hypoventilation and central apneas, especially during REM sleep (Figure 15.3). Hypotonia in PWS improves with age, but PWS adults remain mildly hypotonic and are often prone to develop scoliosis. Scoliosis in an adult with PWS may add a pulmonary restrictive component to the person's SDB.

Treating Sleep-Disordered Breathing in Prader-Willi Syndrome

Reducing the likelihood and severity of sleep-related hypoventilation in PWS begins with avoiding or reducing obesity. Stringent caloric intake and restricting access to food are needed for a child or adolescent with PWS to avoid or lose excessive weight gain [67,68]. This often makes them unhappy [69]. A strict 10 kcal/cm height fat-reduced and carbohydrate-modified diet is effective in controlling excessive weight gain in children with PWS if started before age 2 [70]. The same diet started at a mean age of 16 years led to gradual weight reductions in adolescents with PWS from an initial mean BMI of 41.3 kg/m^2 to 30.5 kg/m^2 6 years later [71]. Some debate whether preventing patients with PWS from "eating themselves to death" is unethical, interfering with their autonomy [69,72]. Early recognition of the diagnosis by genetic testing in a floppy infant, early introduction of exogenous growth hormone (GH) therapy, and strict caloric restriction has reduced, but not eliminated, obesity or excessive weight among children with PWS.

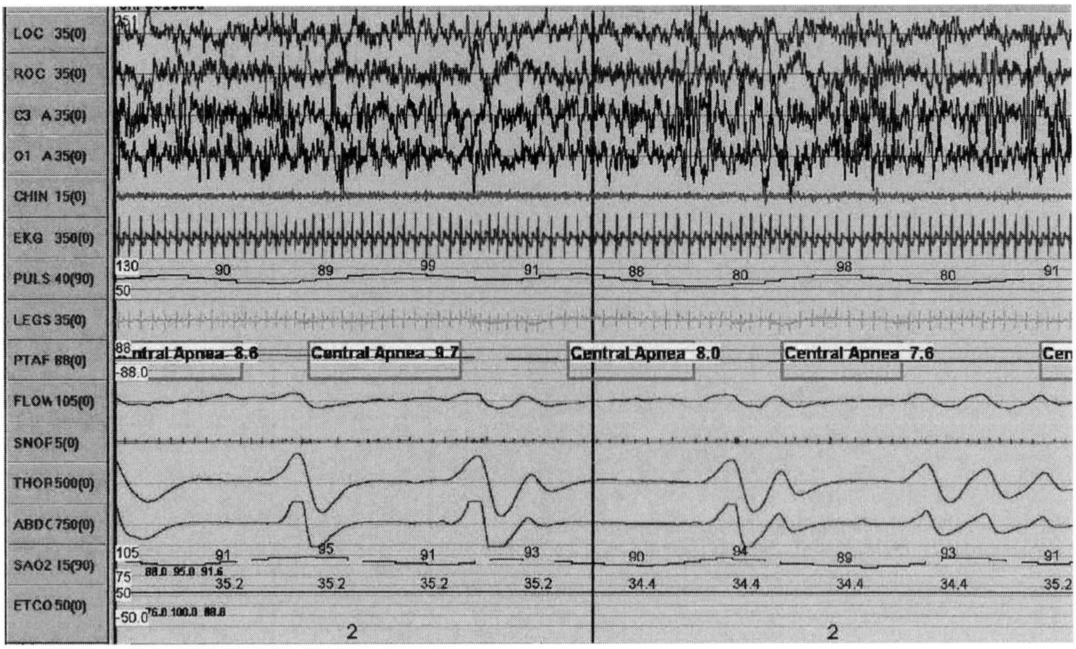

Figure 15.3 Central apneas, especially during REM sleep in Prader-Willi syndrome.

OSA without sleep-related central hypoventilation in patients with PWS may respond to CPAP [62,73]. Sleep-related central hypoventilation in PWS (with or without a component of OSA) is usually best treated by bilevel PAP, sometimes requiring a timed or backup rate. Treating SDB in children with PWS improved their cognitive function, improved daytime performance and sleep quality [51]. If significant adenotonsillar hypertrophy and OSA on the PSG are present, AT can be considered. However, PWS patients are at increased risk for postoperative complications [54,74], and residual SDB is likely to remain following surgery, requiring PAP [74].

Risks and Benefits of Exogenous Growth Hormone in Children With Prader-Willi Syndrome

Exogenous GH treatment for children with PWS is now recommended to increase height and the ratio of lean muscle-to-fat body composition in PWS [75–77]. A randomized, placebo-controlled trial found that PWS chidren (ages 4–16) treated with GH showed significant increased height velocity, decreased mean body fat, increased mean lean body mass, physical strength, respiratory muscle function, and sleep quality [78,79], prompting a recommendation for its use in PWS [76], preferably started before age 3 years [77].

Another randomized controlled trial in 91 prepubertal PWS children (42 infants, 49 children ages 3–14 years) showed that GH (1 mg/m^2/d) significantly improved height, BMI, body proportions, body fat percentage, and normalized head circumference [80]. A recently published longitudinal study found 21 children with PWS treated with GH for 6 years (beginning at age 13 ± 6 months) had lower body fat (mean 36% vs. 45%), greater height (131 vs. 114 cm), greater motor strength, and better lipid profiles compared to 27 children of a similar age (ages 5–9 years) before GH treatment was available [75]. These and other studies support the efficacy of GH use in PWS [80–85], preferably started before age 3 years [77]. Improvements in subtle NREM sleep microarchitecture (cyclic alternating patterns [CAP]) were found in PWS following GH treatment [86].

Increased Risk for Sudden Death in Prader-Willi Syndrome

Individuals with PWS have an annual death rate of 3% and are at increased risk for sudden or premature death. A large case series found respiratory failure or infections were the most common cause of death in PWS, present in 61% of 64 PWS children [61]. Childhood sudden death in PWS is often associated with respiratory infection and high temperature [87,88]. Impaired central (hypothalamic) body temperature regulation may contribute to sudden death in PWS infants and children when sick. Sudden death in infants with PWS is more often secondary to milk aspiration; viral infections in older children and adolescents; and respiratory failure, pulmonary embolism, cellulites, or other complications of morbid obesity in adults [88].

Initial reports raised great concern that exogenous GH therapy contributed to or caused sudden death in PWS. More studies that are recent refute this. Festen et al (2006) found a mean AHI in 53 prepubertal PWS children (mean age 5.4 years) before receiving GH (1 mg/m^2) of 5.1/h; 4.8/h after 6 months of treatment [89]. More than half of the respiratory events (2.8/h) in the pretreatment PSG were central apneas (mean duration 15 sec); the rest were hypopneas. Central apneas did not correlate with BMI, but did decrease with age. One child died unexpectedly during a mild upper respiratory tract infection (although he had a nearly normal PSG). Miller et al (2009) found *no* significant effect on SDB in 20 infants with PWS (ages 2 to 21 months) before and 6 weeks after starting GH therapy [90]. However, 12 had an increase in the frequency of obstructive events associated with either GER or an URI at the time of the second sleep study, which normalized on repeat PSG studies.

Recent studies found that 60% of patients with PWS exhibit central adrenal insufficiency during stress [91,92]. Researchers from the Netherlands hypothesized that PWS patients might suffer from central adrenal insufficiency during stressful conditions [91]. They showed that 60% of 25 randomly selected patients with PWS (mean age 9.7 years) had central adrenal insufficiency [91]. Patients were considered as having central adrenal insufficiency when their ACTH levels remained below 33 pmol/l at 07:30 hours after receiving metyrapone (30 mg/kg) at 23:30 hours the night before. The authors suggested that the high percentage of central adrenal insufficiency in PWS might explain the high rate of sudden death in these patients, particularly during infection-related stress. Based on their data, they recommended treating PWS patients during acute illnesses with stress doses of hydrocortisone unless central adrenal insufficiency has recently been ruled out with a metyrapone test [91].

The same investigators found SDB was worse in 10 healthy PWS children (median age 8.4 years) who had diagnostic testing consistent with central adrenal insufficiency (ACTH levels during the metyrapone test were below 33 pmol/l at 07:30 hours) [92]. They also found the median central apnea index increased from 2.2 to 5.2/h after metyrapone administration (a pharmacological stressor), and the increase was significantly higher among the children with central adrenal insufficiency [2.8 vs. 1.0/h). PSG performed before the metyrapone stress test showed that PWS children with central adrenal insufficiency (compared to those without it) had significantly higher central apnea index and lower nadir SpO_2.

Central Hypersomnia Common in Prader-Willi Syndrome

EDS in 29 patients with PWS was unrelated to body mass index or weight, a distinctive characteristic of PWS, and it is thought to be related to "hypothalamic dysfunction" (hence the term "central hypersomnia") [93,94]. Hypersomnia in PWS often persists after successful treatment of SDB *and* weight loss [95,96]. Manni et al (2001) recorded overnight PSG in 14 subjects with PWS (mean age 17 years) unselected for sleep-wake complaints followed by a multiple sleep latency test (MSLT) in 10 [97]. Short mean sleep latencies confirming hypersomnia were present on an MSLT in 8 of 10 PWS subjects unselected for sleep-wake complaints [97]. Five had 2 or more sleep onset REM periods (SOREMPs) [97]. Others have found that some patients with PWS have SOREMPs in MSLT [65,97,98]. Abnormalities in REM sleep architecture (marked fragmentation of REM sleep resulting in multiple brief REM periods across a night) have been observed in PSG of patients with PWS [86].

Central hypersomnia in PWS is not due to a deficiency of hypocretin-1 (as seen in narcolepsy with cataplexy). Fronczek et al (2005) found no loss of hypocretin-secreting hypothalamic neurons in PWS subjects compared to controls [99]. Cerebrospinal fluid levels of hypocretin-1 were mildly reduced (but not low) in PWS subjects compared with healthy controls [100]. Studies of NREM sleep microarchitecture using CAP scoring have shown increased NREM instability in children and adults with PWS compared to healthy controls [86,101]. Adults with PWS who had less instability of NREM sleep had less severe GH deficiency. Verrillo et al (2009) evaluated CAP in 30 PWS children (13 treated with GH) and found the severity of the NREM instability was less in the PWS children treated with GH compared to those who were not. Modafinil and other CNS stimulants are prescribed for hypersomnia in PWS patients who continue to have EDS after treating SDB and weight loss, even though supportive medical literature for this is lacking.

Mucopolysaccharidoses Including Hurler and Hunter Syndromes

Mucopolysaccharidoses (MPSs) are a group of inherited lysosomal storage disorders caused by various single-gene defects, which lead to progressive cellular accumulation of glycosaminoglycans within various organ systems including the central nervous, musculoskeletal, and cardiorespiratory systems [102]. MPS occur in as many as 1 in 10,000 live births. So far, 7 distinct MPS types and 11 different enzyme deficiencies have been described [103]. Phenotypic expression varies between different MPS syndromes depending upon which glycosaminoglycan accumulates in which cells, tissues, and organs. Even among a particular MPS type, severe and attenuated phenotypes are observed [104].

Three MPS syndromes that often present to pediatric sleep specialists are Hurler (MPS I), Hunter (MPS II), and Sanfilippo (MPS III): the first 2 for OSA, the last for severe pediatric insomnia. Hunter syndrome (MPS II) is an X-linked recessive disorder due to genetic defect in the X chromosome at Xq27–q28. MPS II leads to accumulation of chondroitin sulfate B and heparan sulfate in various body tissues. Hurler syndrome (MPS I) has an autosomal recessive pattern of inheritance, is due a deficiency of α-L-uronidase, and the genetic defect maps to chromosome 4p16.3.

MPS II (Hunter) syndrome has early and late onset forms. Boys with early onset Hunter syndrome (MPS IIa) tend to have much more severe and rapidly progressive disease than those with the late-onset form of the disease. Boys with early onset Hunter syndrome are normal at birth and then have a decline in their development, which usually begins between 2 to 4 years, followed by a progressive loss of skills, eventually leading to a profound ID. Boys with Hunter syndrome have coarse facial features (with thickening of the lips, nostrils, and tongue), a large head set on a short neck, and a short stocky build. They have progressive loss of hearing and vision, hepatosplenomegaly, early cardiovascular disease, and aggressive behavior. Their life expectancy is reduced to 12 years with death most often due to airway obstruction or cardiac failure.

In contrast, the symptoms of late-onset Hunter syndrome (MPS IIb) are milder, usually diagnosed after age 10, and may go undetected until adulthood. Intellectual and social development in MPS IIb is usually nearly normal (although verbal and reading skills may be impaired). Abnormal bone size, stunted growth, poor peripheral vision, hearing loss, diarrhea, joint stiffness, and sleep apnea are often present. Patients with MPS IIb can live into their 50s.

The symptoms and signs of Hurler syndrome (MPS I) are very similar to early-onset Hunter syndrome, but their symptoms often progress even much more rapidly. Affected children may be large at birth and appear normal. Their growth in height initially may be faster than normal, but begins to slow before the end of the first year, and often ends around age 3. Developmental delay often appears by the end of their first year. By age 2, the distinctive coarse facies, short body trunk with widened oar-shaped ribs, cardiomyopathy, and hepatosplenomegaly are usually present. Development usually ceases between ages 2 to 4 years, followed by progressive, cognitive decline and loss of physical skills. Language is limited by intellectual decline, macroglossia, and deafness. They often die before age 10 from obstructive airway disease, respiratory infections, or cardiovascular complications.

Children with Hurler or Hunter syndromes often present to pediatric otolaryngologists between ages 4 to 5 years with chronic middle ear effusions, recurrent otitis, hearing loss, OSA, and progressive upper airway obstruction [105–107] sufficiently severe to require tracheotomy in 11% [107]. Vocal cord abnormalities in children with MPS tend to present later (mean age 9.2 years) [108]. Progressive upper airway narrowing and OSA in these children is often severe and progressive, and untreated can lead to chronic respiratory failure and premature death [109,110]. Hypertrophy of the tongue, adenoids, tonsils, laryngeal, and tracheobronchial mucosa due in part to depositions of glycosaminoglycans coupled with thoracic kyphoscoliosis predispose them to OSA [106,110]. Nashed et al (2009) retrospectively reviewed PSG data on 11 children (median age 5.2 years, BMI 19.9) with different MPSs referred to their teaching hospital [111]. Sixty-four percent had OSA with a median OAHI of 6.6/h, and severe in 3 (OAHI >10). OSA was treated in some, with variable success.

Leighton et al (2001) found OSA on cardiopulmonary studies in 92% of 26 children with ng MPS, most severe in those with Hurler or Hunter syndromes [109]. The clinical history underestimated the severity of OSA in one-third. Santamaria et al (2007) found severe OSA on overnight PSG in all 5 children with various types of MPS (AI 10.4/h, AHI 14.7/h), whereas mild OSA was present in only one of 6 MPS adults (AI 2.3/h, AHI 7.4/h) [112]. All 5 of the children had marked adenoidal hypertrophy (and adenoid regrowth had recurred in 4 who had undergone previous adenotonsillectomy).

In contrast, children with Sanfilippo syndrome (MPS III) are particularly susceptible to pediatric behavioral insomnia. There are 4 types of MPS-III, each due to a different enzyme deficiency affecting the degradation of the glycosaminoglycan heparin sulfate, leading to its accumulation in various brain and body tissues. MPS III affects 1 in 20 000 live births [113].

The 4 types of MPS III are clinically indistinguishable, the brain being the primary organ system affected. Following normal birth, children with MPS III begin to exhibit delay in language and motor skills, followed in the second stage by severe behavioral and sleep disturbances when the child is 3 or 4 years old [114]. Behavioral problems include hyperactivity, temper tantrums, pica, and aggressive–destructive behaviors. Their strength and mobility is initially unaffected, making the management of their behaviors even more challenging. The final stage of the disease is characterized by seizures, dysphagia, increasing immobility, and unresponsiveness, which leads to an early death most often due to inanition.

Fraser et al (2005) found that often, severe pediatric behavioral insomnia was reported by the parents of 141 children with MPS III [115]. Children with MPS III had significantly more difficulty falling asleep, nighttime waking, and daytime napping than their unaffected siblings [115]. A small case-control study recorded 48 hours of ambulatory EEG, PSG, and sleep diaries in 6 patients with MPS III [116]. Extremely chaotic sleep patterns with several sleep periods of inconstant duration irregularly distributed across 24 hours were observed in the 4 oldest MPS III subjects. Sleep maintenance insomnia with several nocturnal awakenings was observed in the younger two. Treatment strategies for insomnia in children with MPS III include behavioral modification, often coupled with medication (particularly oral melatonin, less often benzodiazepines) and co-sleeping with the parents [117].

Management of Obstructive Sleep Apnea in Children With Mucopolysaccharidoses

OSA identified on PSG in a child with MPS warrants a repeat sleep study titrating CPAP, and if needed bilevel PAP titration, often preceded by a mask desensitization trial. Consideration of adenotonsillectomy for OSA in MPS requires thoughtful reflection because OSA often persists postoperatively, adenoids frequently recur, and these patients are at increased risk for postoperative complications [118,119]. PAP may initially relieve their OSA but secondarily fail due to continued deposition of glycosaminoglycans at multiple levels in their airways. When this occurs, repeat PSG with PAP titration is indicated. If PAP is ineffective (or not tolerated) and the OSA is severe, tracheotomy should be considered.

However, tracheotomy can be an ineffective treatment in MPS children with tracheal stenosis and/or tracheomalacia (which was present in one-fifth of MPS children in one case series) [119]. Adachi effectively treated mucopolysaccharide tracheal obstruction in 2 children with Hurler syndrome using CO_2 laser [119]. Jeong et al (2006) found 86% of 7 children with Hunter syndrome had infrastomal tracheal stenosis and 71% stomal narrowing [120].

Recent identification of which lysosomal enzyme(s) are deficient in different types of MPS has led to the development and use of specific enzyme replacement therapy (ERT) for MPS I, II and VI [103,121,122]. ERT seems to reduce the peripheral (including upper airway obstruction and hypertrophy) but not central manifestations of these diseases [121]. ERT significantly reduced upper airway obstruction in 13 of 14 MPS children, avoiding tracheotomy [107]. Decreased AHI attributed to reduced glycoaminoglycan storages in upper airway tissues have been demonstrated after α-L-iduronidase administration in MPS I [121,123].

ERT is beneficial to some patients with MPS 1, II, or VI but does not improve neurocognitive function because of its inability to cross the blood brain barrier [121]. Bone marrow, allogenic hematopoietic stem cell (HSCT) from a donor, and most recently unrelated donor umbilical cord blood (UCBT) transplants are being used to treat young children with MPS [102]. When started early in the course of the disease, transplant-derived enzyme-producing cells can cross the blood-brain barrier and to other organs replacing the missing enzymes, improve neurocognitive and organ system function, prolong survival, and improve QOL in some MPSs [102,124].

Tonsillar biopsy before bone marrow transplant in a 3-year-old boy with Hurler syndrome and severe OSA showed more than half the tissue volume was due to abnormal lysosomal inclusions in macrophages. Six months following the transplant, upper airway patency markedly improved, and repeat tonsillar biopsy showed complete absence of lysosomal inclusions. ERT started sufficiently at early stage (perhaps even before significant upper airway obstruction and hypertrophy has developed) may reduce or reverse upper airway obstruction in MPS.

Coman et al (2008) queried 249 caregiver(s) of children with MPS as to whether they wanted their child to receive ERT [122]. Ninety-two percent favored ERT when the particular MPS caused severe physical problems but did not affect intellect, 69% when physical limitations were mild and intellect spared, but only 47% when severe intellectual and physical disease was already present [122]. ERT and transplant for MPS demonstrates how identifying the genetic and molecular basis of a disease process can lead to innovative therapies, and perhaps one day provide a cure for these patients.

Children with Intellectual Disabilities and/or Cerebral Palsy

Sleep problems are very common in children with ID and/or cerebral palsy (CP). Newman et al (2006) found 44% of 173 CP children (mean age 8.8 years) had at least one sleep problem compared with 5% of the general pediatric population [125]. EDS was present in 19%, SDB 15%, and NREM arousal disorders 8% [125]. The risk for a sleep disorder was 21-fold higher if the child had dyskinetic CP, 17 times greater with active epilepsy, and 13 times greater with either spastic quadriplegia or visual impairment [125]. Didden et al (2002) reported 16% of children with mild to profound ID had at least one type of sleep problem: 4% had severe settling problems, 11% night waking, and 4% early morning awakening [2]. They found that the children with severe sleep problems tended to have more severe ID, CP, and/or epilepsy, daytime sleepiness, and problem behaviors (aggression, hyperactivity, and opposition) compared to those children without a severe sleep problem [2].

Particularly debilitating for caregivers, sleep problems in children with severe ID tend to be persistent [126]. Teaching cognitive–behavioral insomnia therapy to caregivers of sleepless ID children improved sleep, increased sense of control, and reduced stress of the sleep-deprived caregivers [127]. PSG studies in children with CP have shown they are more likely to have altered sleep architecture, increased arousals, delayed REM sleep latency, decreased numbers of gross body movements, fewer body position shifts, and decreased duration of REM sleep compared to healthy controls [128,129].

Sleep-related Breathing Disorders in Children With Cerebral Palsy or Intellectual Disability

SDB in children with CP often consists of varying combinations of obstructive and central events, and central or obstructive hypoventilation with hypoxemia during REM sleep. SDB in children with severe CP is often more severe compared to children with suspected sleep apnea without chronic medical conditions [129]. Repeated pulmonary aspiration, airway colonization with pathogenic bacteria, bronchiectasis, *and* SDB are major contributors to mortality and morbidity in individuals with CP [130]. Kotagal et al

(1994) found children with severe CP and spastic quadriparesis have far fewer body position changes compared with controls (0.3/h vs. 6.6/h, respectively), often failing to change their body position when arterial oxyhemoglobin saturations fell as low as 70% [129].

Adenotonsillectomy is often the first treatment strategy for CP children with OSA and adenotonsillar hypertrophy. Margardino et al (1999) found OSA remitted in 84% of 27 children with CP following adenotonsillectomy in 19, and adenoidectomy in 6. However, 4 children later required tracheotomy to control their OSA [131]. Other studies have shown that children with moderate-to-severe CP (especially those with spastic quadriparesis and/or epilepsy) are more likely to suffer postoperative respiratory complications, and residual OSA on their postoperative PSGs with lower "cure rates" following AT [132–134].

Since residual postoperative OSA is likely to remain, a PSG should be performed 2 to 3 months following surgery [133]. If significant SDB persists, consider the following: (1) a repeat sleep study titrating CPAP for OSA, or BPAP if needed for tolerance or concomitant hypoventilation, best preceded by a PAP desensitization trial; (2) for pediatric ENT reevaluation consider whether other upper airway surgeries (including mandibular distraction, tongue base reduction, and/or skeletal advancement or expansion) would be useful (especially if PAP is not well-tolerated) [131,135–137]; and (3) aggressive treatment of comorbidities including excessive oral secretions, swallowing problems, epilepsy, and reflux to possibly improve overall sleep quality [138].

Treating OSA with either adenotonsillectomy or positive airway pressure in 51 children with CP significantly improved their QOL (especially for sleep disturbances, caregiver concerns, and daytime functioning) compared to the children in whom treatment was refused [139]. Other treatment strategies for SDB in children with CP, with or without ID or spastic quadriparesis are as follows: (1) nocturnal postural devices as long as they do not worsen the SDB [140]; (2) oral appliances [141]; and (3) botulinum toxin injections of submandibular salivary glands to reduce hypersalivation [142].

The prognosis and QOL for individuals with CP has changed, particularly in those with mild to moderate impairment [143–145]. A cross-sectional telephone survey found the majority of patients with CP report a *high* level of life satisfaction, 79% had completed ≥ 12 years of schooling, 25% had served in the military, and 23% work in competitive environments, and have a driver's license [145]. An even larger cross-sectional survey found severity of CP predicted QOL, and QOL was rated very good or excellent by 57% of the youth and 46% of the adults with CP [143]. Addressing and treating chronic pain in patients with CP can improve their QOL [146]. Children with CP and multiple developmental disabilities should be encouraged to enroll in therapy programs, which use treadmills or walkers with microswitches and contingent stimulation. Studies show these therapies improve their ability to walk [147].

Sleep-Disordered Breathing in Children with Epilepsy

Epilepsy affects 4% to 10% of children before age 16, and 5% to 10% have seizures, which occur primarily or only during sleep. Children with epilepsy have significantly more sleep problems than their siblings or healthy controls [148]. Compared to the general pediatric population, children with idiopathic epilepsy had more bedtime difficulties, sleep fragmentation, daytime drowsiness, and parasomnias, particularly if their seizures were poorly controlled [148]. Poor sleep has been shown to correlate with daytime inattention in children with epilepsy [149]. Children with epilepsy compared with control subjects had more daytime sleepiness, less on-task behavior, and more inattention [150]. Unfortunately, sleep complaints in children with epilepsy are rarely brought up at a pediatric visit and are often misdiagnosed [151].

Undiagnosed OSA is common in children with epilepsy who have "sleep problems" [148,149,152,153]. One case-control study found 43% of 40 children with epilepsy referred for various sleep complaints had OSA on overnight PSG. Children with epilepsy who had OSA on overnight PSG had a lower mean AHI (3.4/h) but longer sleep latency (51 vs. 16 minutes), higher arousal index (49 vs. 21/h of sleep), lower nadir SpO_2 (86% vs. 90%), and higher BMI

(29 vs. 21.5) and more often had a BMI >95th percentile (62% vs. 18%) compared to children with moderate OSA without comorbidities (AHI 6.9/h) [153]. Identifying and treating OSA in patients with epilepsy can improve their daytime functioning and epilepsy [154–157].

Vagal nerve stimulation (VNS), a treatment for medically refractory epilepsy, can worsen or unmask OSA. Decreases in airflow and respiratory effort and frank obstructive events during the 30-second period the vagal nerve stimulator activates (typically every 5 minutes) have been observed in children and adults [158–161]. OSA was present in 15%, and subsequently developed in another 15% of 26 children in whom a VNS stimulator was implanted [158]. OSA when identified in children or adults with epilepsy treated with VNS responded to adenotonsillectomy or CPAP [158]. Reducing the pulse width of the VNS can sometimes lessen the effect upon breathing during sleep.

Craniocervical Junction Disorders

The craniocervical junction (CCJ) is an intricate pathway of interlocking muscles, ligaments and skeletal components, which act in concert to preserve neurological function. Infants and children with CCJ disorders are at increased risk for sleep apnea, prolonged breath holding, and sudden death. Children or adolescents at risk for CCJ dysfunction include those with Chiari 1 malformations (CM1) but also craniofacial syndromes such as Conradi, Goldenhar, Klippel-Feil, Larsen, Morquio, Weaver, and Pierre-Robin [162]. Early diagnosis and prevention of neurological compromise is critical. Inspiratory stridor and central sleep apnea (CSA) with/without obstructive sleep apnea in varying combinations are often present in patients with CCJ disorders, and may be the *sole* manifestation of potentially life-threatening cervicomedullary junction compression. Early diagnosis and prevention of neurological compromise are crucial.

The clinical symptoms of craniocervical junction disorders causing medullary and/or high cervical spinal compression are summarized in Table 15.2. The diagnostic approach for evaluating for cervicomedullary compression begins with history and physical examination searching for its symptoms and signs (Table 15.2). Plain x-rays with patients in cervical lateral flexion and extension are the best first neuroimaging technique, avoiding additional radiation exposure in young children. A computed tomography (CT) scan of the craniocervical junction and cervical spine evaluates the bony structures and is sometimes easier to obtain in young children, avoiding the need for sedation. Relationships between the soft tissue structures, ligaments, and brain regarding compression can be further evaluated by static or dynamic MRI of the craniovertebral junction with the patient first in cervical flexion and then repeated in extension. MRI often requires conscious sedation in infants and young children, and

Table 15.2 Clinical symptoms of craniocervical junction dysfunction in children with medullary compression

Neck or occipital pain (85%)

- Myelopathy (either mono-, hemi-, para- or quadriparesis) that may develop acutely following a seemingly mild head or neck injury;
- Sleep apnea (central, obstructive, mixed, and/or pulmonary restrictive disease);
- Apneic episodes awake;
- Severe breath holding spells, syncope, and/or sudden death when sleeping;
- Abnormal sensation in hands or feet (manifested in an infant or young child by constant rubbing of the affected limbs);
- Transient visual field deficits, vertigo, altered consciousness, and/or confusional states (sometimes provoked or reproduced by neck extension or rotation of the head or neck);
- Unilateral or bilateral paralysis or dysfunction of soft palate or pharynx;
- Vertical downbeat nystagmus;
- Hearing loss;
- Basilar migraine (25%).

sedation may unmask their SDB; anticipation of this can be useful. Comprehensive pediatric PSG with endtidal and transcutaneous CO_2 monitoring should be done to evaluate for varying combinations of central or mixed sleep apneas, bradypnea, nocturnal hypoxemia, and OSA. Some neurosurgeons assess for impaired central conduction in primary somatosensory pathways across the cervicomedullary junction using upper extremity somatosensory evoked potentials.

Achondroplasia

Achondroplasia (AC) is the most common cause of short-limbed dwarfism (more than 250,000 individuals worldwide) and occurs in 1 of 10,000 to 40,000 live births [163]. AC is due to a heterozygous mutation in the FGFR3 gene on chromosome 4p16.3, which codes for production of the FGFR3 (Fibroblast growth receptor-3) protein [164]. FGFR3 protein is a *negative* regulator of linear bone growth, which inhibits proliferation of chondrocytes. The mutant gene in AC increases FGFR3 protein activity, which severely inhibits bone and cartilage growth [165,166].

AC has an autosomal dominant pattern of inheritance. Phenotypic expression of the mutant gene in AC is 100%; all who have the mutant gene will have AC. Eighty percent of cases of AC are a result of a spontaneous mutation. Almost all AC patients have mutation of FGFR3 gene and more than 95% have the same point mutation [164]. The FGFR3 protein is a negative regulator of linear bone growth inhibiting chondrocyte proliferation. The FGFR3 mutant AC gene causes gain of function by increasing FGFR3 protein activity, which then severely inhibits bone and cartilage growth.

The AC mutant gene decreases the rate of endochondral bone formation, which limits linear bone growth. This leads to the characteristic skeletal manifestation of AC: short stature (average adult height 4 feet), large heads with frontal bossing set on a small short cranial base, short squat long bones, shorter proximal limbs, and hyperextensible joints (especially at the knees) [166]. Normal intelligence is typical in AC. Infants with AC exhibit poor head control, which improves by 3 to 4 months of age. These infants are particularly vulnerable to craniocervical injury at this age with their large heads sitting on a small skull base.

Infants with AC have varying degrees of thoracolumbar kyphosis (gibbus) attributed to a combination of a large head, cervical ligamentous laxity and delayed motor milestones. Most AC children begin to walk by 24 to 36 months. Once they begin to walk, their lumbar kyphosis resolves only to be replaced by exaggerated lumbar lordosis. However, thoracolumbar kyphosis in AC resolves in 90% of AC children once they start walking. If the kyphosis does not resolve, bracing from ages 4 to 7 or 8 years until the curvature is ≤ 10 degrees is recommended. Four percent will need spinal surgery or spinal fusion by age 15 years. Pulmonary restrictive disease occurs in less than 5% of children with AC younger than 3 years of age. Severe kyphosis or lordosis can add pulmonary restrictive component to SDB.

Sudden death occurs in 7.5% of young AC children during the first year of life; 2.5% between ages 1 to 4 years. Foramen magnum stenosis in infants and children with AC predisposes them to brainstem kinking, compression, and/or ischemia, which may also involve the cervical spinal cord. This can lead to myelopathy, hypotonia, central, and/or obstructive SDB, severe breath holding spells, severe bradypnea during sleep, apneic episodes with impaired arousal awake or asleep, and sudden death [167–170]. Pauli et al (1984) reviewed the records of 13 AC infants with sudden unexpected death (some associated with sudden unexplained apnea) [171]. The cause of death in many was acute or chronic compression of the lower brainstem or cervical spinal cord. The risk of sudden death was greatest between ages 1 month to 1 year. Pauli et al (1995) found that 5 of 53 prospectively followed AC infants subsequently developed compression and required craniocervical junction decompression [172]. The following are best predictors of need for decompression: lower-limb hyperreflexia or clonus on physican exam *and* central hypopneas on PSG.

King et al (2009) found 2 peak ages for symptomatic foramen magnum compression in AC, less than 2 years (mean 23 mo) and 9 years. Eleven percent require reoperation for secondary compression (mean age 5.5 years) [170]. Possible mechanisms for sudden death in AC include compression of the pontomedullary junction, obstruction of the Sylvian aqueduct, ischemic injury to vital brainstem nuclei, and/or cranio-cervical dislocations from minor trauma with poor neck support.

Minor head or cervical injuries can lead to acute or subacute cervicomedullary compression. Good neck support in hypotonic AC infants is crucial. Symptoms of cervicomedullary compression in an AC include cervical or occipital pain, cranial nerve dysfunction, paresis, ankle clonus, hyperreflexia, hypotonia, and/or abnormal central apneas on PSG [173]. More subtle reasons to consider decompression are poor feeding, transient visual deficits, syncope, and/or "basilar" migraine.

Varying Combinations of Sleep-Disordered Breathing in Achondroplasia

SDB is present in 38% to 42% of children or adults with AC and characterized by *varying* combinations of pulmonary restrictive disease, OSA, CSA, and/or abnormal EMG activity of accessory muscles [174–179]. Factors that predispose infants and children with AC to SDB appear in summary in Table 15.3. AC children who have symptomatic cervicomedullary compression with or without obstructive hydrocephalus are more likely to have CSA on their PSGs; whereas, AC children who only have adenotonsillar hypertrophy tend to have OSA.

Onodera et al (2006) found the craniofacial/airway morphology, which was most often present in AC children *with* OSA, was upper airway stenosis, mandibular retrognathia, an increased mandibular plane angle due to partial early ossification of cranial bones, and an increased lower facial height due to an increased mandibular angle [175]. Tasker et al (1998) found OSA was mild in 17 AC infants who only had adenotonsillar hypertrophy, more severe in those who also had a small foramen magnum and obstructive hydrocephalus, and led to sudden death in 3 of the 5 with cor pulmonale [180].

Table 15.3 Factors which predispose infants or children with achondroplasia to sleep-disordered breathing (SDB)

- Propensity for recurrent infections (especially the first 5–6 years probably due to abnormal Eustachian tube drainage and faulty bone development);
- Small caliber upper airway with relative adenotonsillar hypertrophy;
- Airway muscle hypotonia;
- Narrow trunk and small thoracic cage;
- Foramen magnum stenosis;
- Dental crowding and malocclusion;
- Obesity.

One study of 88 AC children (1 month to 12.6 years) found 44% had nocturnal hypoxemia (attributed to pulmonary restrictive disease); only 4% had OSA, but it was severe enough to require treatment with CPAP in two, and tracheotomy in 3 patients [177]. The authors argued that SDB in AC was most often nocturnal hypoxemia due to pulmonary restrictive disease. Sisk et al (1999) found OSA in 38% of 95 AC children (mean age 3.7 years) [181]. Symptoms that best predicted OSA on their PSG were snoring, observed apnea, glottal stops, and apneic episodes during wakefulness. Neither severe (4+) tonsillar hypertrophy, a small oropharyngeal size, nor redundant oropharyngeal tissue predicted OSA.

Ednick et al (2009) found 67% of 12 AC infants (mean age 1.5 ± 0.5 months) had a RDI > 5 (mean 14 ± 11/h) vs. 2 ± 1/h in controls [182]. These young infants with AC had fewer spontaneous or respiratory-related arousals (12/h) compared to 19/h in the control subjects. The investigators further found no correlation between foramen magnum size and SDB or arousal frequency. Zucconi et al (1996) argued that the most common SDB in AC children (mean age 4.7 years) was OSA, present in overnight PSG in 75% of 16 AC children [178]. The mean AHI was not higher in the children with foramen magnum stenosis. However, King et al (2009) found CSA on PSG was a common and distinctive pattern of SDB in AC infants and children with symptomatic cervicomedullary compression (which presented before age 2 in 14 of their 18 cases) [170]. CSA was present in preoperative PSG in 12 of 18 children who had pre- and postoperative PSGs. CSA improved or resolved following surgery in all but one child. Persistence of CSA following surgery prompted at least in part early reoperation. With further decompression, the CSA resolved. Eleven percent of the AC children needed their decompressive surgeries repeated years later (mean age 5.5 years). The need for repeat decompressive surgery in older children with AC was often heralded by return of the central apnea.

Treatment Strategies for Achondroplasia

Patients with AC often have OSA that more often responds best to CPAP (or BPAP if concomitant pulmonary restrictive disease is present). OSA in 17 AC patients (median age 6.6 years) was treated by CPAP in 13, adenotonsillectomy in 3, and weight loss in one [183]. CSA on a PSG in a child with AC (especially those younger than 2 years of age or who have had decompressive surgery when younger) should have craniocervical junction MRI to evaluate for cervicomedullary compression and obstructive hydrocephalus.

SDB in AC with significant symptomatic cervicomedullary compression (even with concomitant adenotonsillar hypertrophy) is first best treated by surgical decompression. A repeat sleep study should be done 2 to 3 months following decompressive surgery to assess whether further intervention is needed (PAP, adenotonsillectomy, and/or further decompressive surgery). A craniocervical MRI should be done *before* adenotonsillectomy: a retrospective review of 22 AC children referred to a tertiary pediatric otolaryngology clinic found 50% had sufficient foramen magnum stenosis to warrant decompressive surgery before adenotonsillectomy [184].

AC children are at increased risk for perioperative complications during upper airway surgeries [185]. They have difficulty in visualizing small caliber airways, and some also have pulmonary restrictive disease [181]. Neck extension or uncontrolled head movement during intubation and surgery should be avoided. Endotracheal tube placement requires direct visualization and the tube size should be based on age rather than weight. Ain et al (2008) found 61% of 98 AC adolescents or young adults who underwent lumbar decompressive surgery had at least one perioperative complication, including neurological complications in 23% [186].

The indication for cervicomedullary decompressive surgery in 18 children with AC was the following: (1) a T2-weighted signal change in the cervical spinal cord (56%), (2) documented CSA on a PSG (39%), (3) a history of cyanotic or apneic episodes (28%), (4) focal neurological deficits or myelopathy (17%), and (5) impairment of consciousness in two. The authors favor a suboccipital craniectomy with C1 laminectomy and division of fibrous extradural bands without formal dural opening for cervicomedullary decompression in infants and children with AC [170]. They find preserving the muscle attachment at C2 may reduce postoperative pain and/or instability. Of 18 patients, one failed to improve and required early reoperation to relieve the residual stenosis, and another patient who presented in comatose state never recovered, suffered a respiratory arrest, and died. CSA in these patients often improved over weeks following surgery, requiring PAP, or BPAP support in some.

King et al recommend MRI imaging and a PSG for all children with AC in the first 6 months of life [170]. Symptomatic patients with notable cervicomedullary compression should be treated. Close clinical follow-up searching of symptoms of CCJ dysfunction and yearly MRI imaging should be done for at least the first 2 years of life in those with "asymptomatic" cervicomedullary compression, as symptoms usually manifest in the first 2 years of life.

AC children who have dental malocclusion or crowding should be referred for orthodontic evaluation. We refer AC who are overweight to a pediatric weight management clinic and screen them for hyperlipidemia, insulin resistance, fatty liver, hypothyroidism, and hypertension. AC children between ages 5 to 6 years have frequent middle ear infections, which should be treated aggressively to avoid permanent conductive hearing loss [187]. Families and caregivers of people with AC should be encouraged to join patient- and family support groups, including Little People of America (www.lpaonline.org) and the Magic Foundation for Children's Growth (www.magicfoundation.org).

Chiari Malformations, Spina Bifida, and Meningomyelocele

Clinical presentations of Chiari malformation (CM) vary with CM type. CM1 is defined as a caudal herniation of the cerebellar tonsils more than 5 mm below the foramen magnum as measured by a line from the inner margins of the foramen magnum to the most inferior part of the cerebellar tonsils. Syringomyelia (a central cavitation or tubular fluid-filled cavity in several spinal cord segments) is present in 40% to 75% of cases of CM1. Syringomyelia is thought to arise from abnormal cerebrospinal fluid flow dynamics through the central spinal canal. Syringomyelia can occur as early as 12 months of age in CM1. Ninety percent of patients with syringomyelia have CMs.

Chiari 2 (CM2) is a caudal herniation of the brain stem, caudal cerebellar vermis, and 4th ventricle through the foramen magnum into the cervical spinal canal. Individuals with Chiari 3 (CM3) malformations have some of the CM2 defects accompanied by an occipital encephalocele. CM is often associated with varying combinations of spina bifida, meningomyelocele (MM), bilateral abductor vocal cord paralysis (BAVP), SDB, and sudden unexplained death [188–195].

Symptoms and Signs of Cervicomedullary Compression in Children With Chiari 1 Malformations

Symptoms of cervicomedullary compression in CM1 usually present in the second or third decade of life (younger in those with syringomyelia). Symptomatic cervicomedullary compression was diagnosed in 38% of 130 symptomatic CM1 patients (mean age 11 years), 58% of whom also had syringomyelia [196]. Twenty-two presented with headache or neck pain, 22% migraine-like headaches, 18% progressive scoliosis, 15% dysphagia, 9% ataxia, 8% apnea or bradypnea, 5% hoarseness, and 2% drop attacks [196].

Physical signs of symptomatic cervicomedullary compression in the same cohort are as follows: (1) a short or bull-like neck (25%); (2) levoscoliosis in those with syringomyelia; (3) motor neuron signs (initially generalized hyperreflexia, spasticity involving particularly the legs with bilateral plantar extensor responses; later atrophy, weakness and fasciculations, and areflexia particularly of the arms); (4) lower cranial nerve dysfunction in 15% to 25% (including BAVP, soft palate weakness, lingual atrophy, circopharyngeal achalasia, facial numbness, and absent gag reflexes); (5) central spinal cord syndrome in those with syringomyelia; (6) cerebellar symptoms (ataxia, nystagmus and/or dysmetria); and (7) syringomyelia.

A recently published case series reviewed the clinical presentation of cervicomedullary compression in 39 CM1 children younger than 6 years [197]. They found that children up to 2 years of age commonly presented with oropharyngeal dysfunction (78%); whereas, those aged 3 to 5 years presented with syringomyelia (86%), scoliosis (38%), and/or headache (57). The headache in some children would increase in severity with coughing, sneezing, or bowel movement. Neck pain was often worse with the Valsalva maneuver and head movements could provoke vertigo and/or tinnitus.

Sleep-Disordered Breathing in Chiari Malformation, Spina Bifida, Syringomyelia, and/or Meningomyelocele

Brainstem compression in children with CM1 may present with SDB only [190, 199]. Murray et al (2006) ordered craniocervical junction MRI when they observed central apneas (lasting longer than 15 seconds) and severe bradypnea when sleeping (4–7 breaths/min) in 3 children referred for intermittent snoring, witnessed apnea, and/or paroxysmal nocturnal headaches [190]. Their symptoms and SDB improved or resolved following surgical decompression. Brown et al (2010) ordered a PSG in a morbidly obese 12-year-old girl with a 2-year history of nocturnal enuresis [198]. Long runs of central apneas lasting 15 seconds during NREM 1 sleep that caused oxygen desaturations to 87% on her PSG prompted the authors to order a craniocervical MRI. They found she had CM1. Her CSA and the nocturnal enuresis resolved following decompression.

A study of 46 children and adults with CM found SDB in 70% with CM1 and 50% CM2 [189]. Sixty percent of the 20 children with CM had SDB: primarily obstructive in type in 35% obstructive and central in 25%. Seventy-three percent of the adults with CM had SDB, but it was primarily obstructive in type in 58%, central in only 17%. The authors found that young age, more severe CM2, and/or vocal cord paralysis best predicted the central apnea index (mean number of central apneas per hour of sleep) [189].

Risk factors for SDB and cervicomedullary compression in children with CM2 include the following: (1) mechanical compression of the medulla at the level of the upper cervical cord (the atlas); (2) caudal displacement of the brainstem into the spinal canal by a small posterior fossa; (3) obstructive hydrocephalus; (4) BAVP; and (5) spastic paraparesis. Children with CM2 who undergo closure of their MM may acutely develop severe CSA (at times with an obstructive component) due to postoperative obstructive hydrocephalus and brainstem compression (as the brain tries to adjust to alternative pathways for cerebrospinal fluid drainage).

MM is a small, moist cystic sac which protrudes through the spinal defect which contains a portion of the spinal cord, meninges, nerve roots, and CSF fluid. It can leak CSF when the infant cries. Spina bifida or MM occurs in 3% to 7.8% of 10,000 live births and develops 28 days before conception. SB/MM results from incomplete closure of posterior spine. It is most common in lumbar region. Periconceptional folic acid supplementation may reduce but has not eliminated posterior neural tube defects.

Children with CM2 may also present with apneic episodes or severe breath holding spells awake or suffer sudden death often when sleeping. BAVP manifests as inspiratory stridor at rest, worse with agitation, progressive airway obstruction but near-normal phonation, and CSA [199]. MM when surgically closed can cause acute obstructive hydrocephalus with sudden onset or increase in the severity of SDB, at times life-threatening, requiring urgent intubation and mechanical ventilation.

Wealthall et al (1974) reported that 26 infants with spina bifida had life-threatening apnea and/or stridor accompanied by profound bradycardia particularly during phasic periods of REM sleep, and showed a delay or failure to self-resuscitate [195]. Waters et al (1998) found mild OSA in 42% and moderate to severe OSA in 20% of 83 unselected children attending an MM clinic [191]. The risk for SDB in a child or adolescent with MM increased 11.6 times if the child had abnormal pulmonary function tests, 9.2 times with thoracic spinal cord lesions, 3.5 times with a history of a previous posterior fossa decompression, and threefold for those with CM2 (as opposed to CM1) [191]. Another study of 73 children with MM by Kirk et al (2000) found SDB was most often obstructive in type (41%, mean OAHI 17/h) although 34% had predominantly CSA (CAHI 17/h), 16% central sleep-related hypoventilation (peak $etCO_2$ 67 ± 11 mm Hg), and 8% sleep-exacerbated restrictive lung disease, which caused nocturnal hypoxemia (nadir SpO_2 67 ± 14%) with apnea and/or hypercapnia [193].

Diagnostic Approach to Evaluating Sleep Breathing Disorders in Children With Chiari Malformations, Meningomyelocele, Syringomyelia, and/or Bilateral Abductor Vocal Cord Paralysis

A diagnostic approach to evaluating sleep breathing disorders in CM begins (as usually recommended) with a thorough neurological and sleep history and examination, followed by combinations of neuroimaging beginning with cervical x-rays in flexion and extension (which avoids additional radiation exposure in young children). CT imaging of the CCJ is useful for evaluating the skeletal structures. However, optimal neuroimaging is static or dynamic MRI of CCJ in cervical extension and flexion. Comprehensive overnight PSG with CO_2 monitoring is done to evaluate for OSA, CSA, stridor, central, or obstructive sleep-related hypoventilation and/or pulmonary restrictive disease. Somatosensory evoked potentials may assess for impaired central conduction through the CCJ.

Potentially *reversible* causes for SDB in children with CM2 include the following: (1) obstructive hydrocephalus; (2) BAVP; (3) caudal displacement of brainstem into spinal canal because of obstructive hydrocephalus and small posterior fossa; and (4) mechanical compression of medulla by vermian peg in cervical spinal cord, most often at level of atlas. Potentially *irreversible* causes for SDB in children with CM are as follows: (1) developmental immaturity of brainstem networks and respiratory centers; (2) lower brainstem cranial nerve nuclei aplasia or hypoplasia; (3) ischemic or hemorrhagic changes in brainstem; and/or (4) chronic chemical meningitis and arachnoiditis due to CSF contamination by amniotic fluid squames and lanugo hairs.

BAVP can be observed in children with CM with or without MM. The vocal cords in BAVP are flaccid and lie stationary in the midline. This can lead to obstruction, inspiratory stridor at rest (often worse with agitation), various forms of apnea, but normal or near-normal vocalization [200]. SDB in children with BAVP can include combinations of inspiratory stridor, central, and/or obstructive apnea [188]. Central apneas in children with BAVP can be cyanotic expiratory apnea of long duration [188].

Choi et al (1999) found BAVP in 12.5% of 6 patients with CM2 and none of 18 with CM1

[201]. CSA was present in overnight PSG in 83% of the 6 patients with CM2, none of the 18 with CM1. Central apnea and BAVP often improved following posterior fossa decompression (or less often, it would worsen). There are isolated case reports of BVAP occurring in patients with CM1. Central apnea in children with BAVP, CM2, and cervicomedullary compression with or without obstructive hydrocephalus may persist following cervicomedullary compression and ventriculoperitoneal shunting, leading to sudden death in some despite full resuscitative efforts [194,200].

Treating Sleep-Disordered Breathing in Chiari Malformations and Meningomyelocele

Posterior fossa decompression in 130 patients with symptomatic CM1 resulted in improvement or stabilization of symptoms: (1) the sleep apnea resolved in 100%, headache in 90%; (2) scoliosis improved in 43%; (3) the syrinx in those with syringomyelia would often "stabilize" (and sometimes decrease in size); (4) motor or sensory deficits present before surgery were likely to persist; and (5) scoliosis was less likely with decompression if the angle before surgery was more than 40 degrees [196]. Sometimes, acute hydrocephalus developed in the immediate postoperative period heralded by worsening of the SDB. Outcomes for decompression were better if the symptoms had been present for less than 2 years.

Posterior fossa decompression in symptomatic CM2 may reverse obstructive hydrocephalus, vocal cord paralysis and CSA. Potentially irreversible causes of SDB in infants or children with CM2 include the following: (1) developmentally immature brainstem networks and respiratory centers; (2) lower brainstem cranial nerve nuclei aplasia or hypoplasia; (3) ischemic or hemorrhagic changes in the brainstem; and/or (4) chronic chemical meningitis and arachnoiditis due to cerebrospinal fluid contamination by amniotic fluid squames and lanugo hairs.

OSA in a child with CM (with/without MM) and adenotonsillar hypertrophy often persists following upper airway surgery. Evaluation for symptomatic posterior fossa compression is crucial before proceeding with surgery. Persistent OSA following adenotonsillectomy is effectively treated with CPAP in those who tolerate it. CSA may respond to supplemental oxygen: if ineffective, NIPPV may be needed. If the SDB is central hypoventilation, bilevel PAP (with or without a timed or backup rate) may suffice.

Clinicians when unexpectedly finding frequent central apneas and/or severe sleep bradypnea in a PSG of an infant, child or adult should consider whether the patient has a symptomatic craniocervical junction disorder. We request the patient return to the sleep center, reexamine the patient, seek for symptoms and signs of compression, and perform neuroimaging. Appreciate the variety of SDB that can occur in these patients and how treating them can reduce their risk for sudden unexpected death.

Neuromuscular Disorders

Sleep-related breathing disorders are common in children with neuromuscular disease (NMD), often misdiagnosed or unrecognized, but usually treatable. The prevalence of SDB in children with NMD is greater than 40%, 10-fold higher than in the general pediatric population [202]. The diaphragm is the major muscle for inspiration during wakefulness and sleep. Diaphragmatic weakness predisposes NMD patients to hypercapnic hypoventilation, which first appears during REM sleep. NMD patients with diaphragmatic weakness depend upon their intercostal and accessory respiratory muscles to breathe; when these become hypotonic during REM sleep, they are prone to hypoventilation. Weak cough reflexes, kyphoscoliosis, obesity, impaired central respiratory control, restrictive pulmonary disease, medication effects, malnutrition, and/or obesity when present further predispose NMD patients to SDB.

Nocturnal or sleep-related hypoventilation is defined in the second edition of the *International Classification of Sleep Disorders* (ICSD-2) as a rise in arterial carbon dioxide above 45 mm Hg (torr) or disproportionately increased relative to wake levels [203]. Sleep-induced hypoxemia is defined as a SpO_2 <90% for ≥ 5 minutes with a nadir of <85% or >30% of the total sleep time with a SpO_2 <90%. In 2007, the American Academy of Sleep Medicine published sleep scoring guidelines, and sleep-related hypoventilation in children was defined as above 25% of the total sleep time with a CO_2 >50 mm Hg, and a ≥10 torr rise in CO_2 in sleep compared to wakefulness in adults [204].

The most common symptoms of sleep-related hypoventilation in slowly progressive NMD are the new or recent onset of the following: morning headache, nocturnal arousals, need to be repositioned more frequently, restless sleep, daytime fatigue, difficulty awakening from sleep, impaired concentration, orthopnea (difficulty breathing supine), or a decline in academic or work performance [205]. However, symptoms are poorly predictive of which children with NMD will have SDB even when using a structured sleep questionnaire [206–208], made more difficult by low intellectual functioning present in some patients.

Many NMD patients who have moderate to severe sleep-related hypoventilation look "normal" when awake with little to tax their respiratory systems when they are wheelchair-bound. NM patients should be routinely examined for paradoxical breathing when lying supine. The abdomen normally moves outward during inspiration. In paradoxical breathing, the abdomen inappropriately flattens or moves inward during inspiration. Paradoxical breathing in a child with NMD is a sign of diaphragmatic weakness and usually is not obvious until the diaphragmatic strength is <25% of normal.

Sleep-related central hypoventilation is the primary pattern of SDB in children with DMD, spinal muscular atrophies [209], congential myotonic dystrophy[210], limb girdle muscular dystrophies[211], and childhood-onset acid maltase deficiency [212]. Sleep-related hypoventilation could be predicted with a high sensitivity and specificity in 27 children with congenital and limb girdle muscular dystrophies (present in 42%) by a vital capacity less than 40% [211]. Superimposed OSA can be observed in patients with NMD, especially those in those with kyphoscoliosis, bulbar muscle weakness, adenotonsillar hypertrophy, and/or obesity.

Predicting Which Children With Neuromuscular Disease Will Have Sleep-Disordered Breathing

Serial monitoring of lung function is mandated for all children with NMD once they are able to participate in testing (usually after age 5 years) [35,214]. Pulmonary function test abnormalities may help predict which NMD patients are more likely to have sleep-related hypoventilation and appear more reliable than symptoms [23]. Sleep-related central hypoventilation is likely to be present in a child with NMD once their inspiratory vital capacity (IVC) falls below 40% of predicted [207,213] or they have a daytime $paCO_2$ >40 mm Hg [207]. Mellies et al (2003) found that a daytime $paCO_2$ level >40 mm Hg had a 92% sensitivity and 72% specificity and an IVC of <40% had a 96% sensitivity and 88% specificity for predicting sleep-related hypoventilation in children or adolescents with NMD [207]. However, children with NMD may develop sleep-related hypoventilation with IVC of only less than 60% predicted when they are obese, have concomitant lung disease, or during an acute respiratory infection. Given all this, overnight PSG should be considered in children with NMD from the time the child becomes a wheelchair user, when their FVC is less than 40% (less than 60% if they are obese, have concomitant pulmonary disease, or symptoms), their maximal inspiratory pressure is less than 60%, and/or their daytime $paCO_2$ > 40 mm Hg. Monitoring CO_2 during PSG is critical in patients with NMD: one in-laboratory PSG study found 12% of 609 children with low apnea-hypopnea indexes had hypercapnia; their SDB would go undetected without CO_2 monitoring [214].

Common Polysomnographic Findings in Children With Neuromuscular Diseases

Ragette et al (2002) described patterns of SDB in 42 patients with primary myopathies [215]. They found that patients with IVC less than 60% only had hypopneas during REM sleep, REM sleep hypoventilation developed when their IVC was less than 40%, hypoventilation during both NREM and REM sleep with an IVC of <30%, and respiratory failure when the IVC was less than 25% predicted [215]. The common PSG findings in NMD are shown in summary in Table 15.4.

Cardiorespiratory Management in Patients With Duchenne Muscular Dystrophy

One of the most common muscular dystrophies that present in childhood is Duchenne muscle dystrophy (DMD). DMD is due to mutation in the short arm of the X chromosome (Xp21), which results in the absence of dystrophin

Table 15.4 Common polysomnographic findings in children with neuromuscular disease

- Sleep-related fall in baseline $SpO_2$and rise in the $etCO_2$, $tcCO_2$or $paCO_2$ especially during REM sleep;
- At first elevated mean $etCO_2$ and low mean SpO_2 present only during REM sleep, later in all sleep stages;
- Some have no apneas or hypopneas;
- Others have apneas or short hypopneas only during REM sleep, most are central, or combinations of central, mixed and obstructive.
- Periods of nonapneic oxygen desaturation;
- ntermittent periodic or shallow breathing;
- Tachycardia and tachypnea;
- Reduced or absent REM sleep often abbreviated by arousals when their SpO_2 drops and/or $etCO_2$ rises in transition to REM sleep;
- Progressive fall in the baseline SaO_2 and rise in $etCO_2$ as the period of REM sleep proceeds;
- In severe REM sleep, hypoventilation may observe prolonged hypopneas, which last more than 30–70 seconds causing arterial oxygen desaturations less than 70% and are finally terminated by an arousal.

(a muscle protein). DMD occurs almost exclusively in males with an incidence of 1 of 3500 [216]. SDB in patients with DMD have a bimodal presentation of SDB: OSA in the first decade of life and sleep-related hypoventilation later when they become wheelchair-bound [208].

SDB in young boys with DMD is often "uncomplicated" OSA. Suresh et al (2005) found SDB in children with DMD had a bimodal presentation with OSA found at a median age of 8 years with sleep-related hypoventilation most often developing at the beginning of the second decade (median age 14 years) [208]. Sleep-related hypoventilation in DMD most often develops after the child becomes wheelchair-bound. Boys with DMD often become wheelchair-dependent around 12 years of age [208,217–221]. Once ambulation is lost, kyphoscoliosis accelerates. Forced vital capacity (FVC) falls approximately 4% for each 10° increase in the thoracic spine curvature.

The American Thoracic Society in 2004 recommended that DMD patients should visit a physician with expertise in pediatric or pulmonary disease every 6 months once wheelchair-dependent, 12 years or older, and their IVC falls <80% predicted [222]. Quality of sleep and symptoms of SDB should be discussed at every patient encounter. Overnight PSG with CO_2 monitoring should be done at least annually once boys with DMD become wheelchair-bound.

The DMD Care Considerations Group in 2010 recently published detailed recommendations for diagnosing and managing DMD [223–225]. They recommend boys with DMD once nonambulatory should have peak cough flow, MIP, MEP, sitting FVC, and SpO_2 oximetry measured every 6 months [224,225]. CO_2 levels awake should be assessed at least annually if the FVC is less than 50% predicted, patient is already using assisted ventilation, and/or hypoventilation is suspected [224]. Overnight PSG with CO_2 monitoring should be done if the FVC is below 1.25 L, baseline FVC less than 40% predicted, baseline or blood $etCO_2$ awake less than 45 mm Hg, and/or awake baseline SpO_2 less than 95%.

Cardiac disease in DMD most often presents with cardiomyopathy and/or cardiac arrhythmia. Clinical signs of heart failure in DMD (fatigue, weight loss, abdominal pain, inability to tolerate daily activities, and sleep disturbances) often go unrecognized until late because of musculoskeletal limitations. Table 15.5 summarizes their recommendations for respiratory interventions in DMD. These recommendations are often useful when managing children and adolescents with other NMDs, which affect breathing during sleep.

Over the past decade, Iannaccone et al have developed and validated the Pediatric Quality of Life Inventory (PedQL) Neuromuscular Module for use as a secondary outcome measure in phase III clinical trials. Recently, they tested the

Table 15.5 Recommendations by the DMD considerations working group for managing respiratory complications in patients with Duchenne muscular dystrophy

- Use volume recruitment/deep lung inflation techniques when FVC less than 40% predicted.
- Manual and mechanically assisted cough techniques should be employed when:
  - Respiratory infection is present and the baseline peak cough flow is below 270 L/min;
  - Baseline peak cough flow is below 160 L/min or maximum expiratory pressure less than 40 cm water;
  - Baseline FVC less than 40% predicted or below 1.25 L in an older teen or adult.
- Nocturnal ventilation indicated for either:
  - Signs or symptoms of hypoventilation;
  - Baseline SpO_2 less than 95% and/or blood or end-tidal CO_2 more than 45 mm Hg awake;
  - Apnea-hypopnea index above 10/h on overnight PSG;
  - $\geq$ 4 episodes of SpO_2 less than 92% or at least 4% per hour of sleep.
- Daytime ventilation recommended when:
  - Dyspnea when swallowing relieved by ventilator assistance;
  - Symptoms and signs of hypoventilation when awake;
  - Unable to speak a full sentence without breathlessness;
  - Patient feels more comfortable breathing with it when awake.
- Tracheostomy:
  - Patient and/or clinician preference;
  - Unable to use needed noninvasive ventilation;
  - Three failures to achieve extubation during critical illness despite optimal use of noninvasive ventilation and mechanically assisted cough;
  - Failure of noninvasive ventilation to prevent aspiration of secretions and drops in SpO_2 less than 95% or the patient's baseline requiring frequent tracheal suctioning via tracheostomy.

feasibility, reliability, and validity of the PedsQL NMM in 54 children with DMD and their caregivers. They found it a reliable measure of disease-specific health-related QOL in the DMD population, which can be used as outcome measure in future clinical trials [225].

Rationale for Home Noninvasive Nocturnal Ventilation in Patients With Neuromuscular Disease

As reviewed above, sleep-related hypoventilation in NMD is most often central in type, and best treated by either bilevel positive airway pressure (BPAP) or nocturnal intermittent positive pressure ventilation (NIPPV) [206,208,209,212,226–230]. Home noninvasive nocturnal ventilation (NIV) has contributed to longer survival times in NMD patients with hypercapnic hypoventilation: the mean age of survival for DMD has increased from 19 to 25 years [231] and spinal muscular atrophy type 1 (SMA-1, Werdnig-Hoffman disease) from 10 ± 4 months to 65 ± 46 months [232].

The benefits of nocturnal nasal intermittent positive pressure ventilation (NIPPV) in patients with severe kyphoscoliosis and chronic alveolar hypoventilation due to NMD, spinal cord injury, or skeletal deformity include the following: (1) improved daytime and nighttime arterial blood gases. [233]; (2) fewer hospitalizations [233] (3) fewer nocturnal oxyhemoglobin desaturations [233, 234]; and (4) improved exercise capacity [234].

A longitudinal study of 14 children with NMD treated with BPAP (13) or CPAP (1) followed a mean of 30 (6–84) months found symptoms of daytime sleepiness and morning headache lessened, hospitalization rates and health care costs decreased, and QOL remained stable despite disease progression [206]. Another study found the use of NIPPV in children with various NMDs: (1) reduced their mean nocturnal $tcCO_2$ from 54 to 42 torr and diurnal $paCO_2$ from 48 to 41 torr; (2) decreased arousals from sleep, reduced nocturnal heart rates, and improved respiratory disturbance index and sleep architecture; (3) effects persisted over 25 ± 13 months; and (4) 3 nights withdrawal of NIV in 10 previously stable patients resulted in prompt deterioration of SDB and gas exchange back to baseline, which was reversed by resumption of NIV [228].

A case-control study found NIPPV via a nasal or oronasal mask improved QOL and longevity, and avoided or delayed the need for tracheostomy among 48 patients with DMD [226]. Treating SDB in 10 of 15 patients with different types of spinal muscular atrophy with NIPPV increased their NREM 3 sleep, reduced their mean nocturnal heart rate by 12 beats/min, and "normalized" their sleep architecture, and led to improved concentration, appetite, and lessening of morning headaches [209]. Ninety percent of the DMD patients in the untreated control group developed diurnal hypercapnia or respiratory complications within a mean of 8 months.

Patients With Sleep-related Hypoventilation Require Serial Adjustments of Their Nocturnal Ventilation Treatment

Patients with progressive NMD need close follow-up, reassessing and retitrating their nocturnal ventilation treatments. A retrospective review of 61 sleep studies recorded over a 12-month period in 45 children with NMD (median age 8.3 years, 27 boys) found changes in sleep-related respiratory support were needed in 66% of the studies [230]. No clinical parameters predicted that children would require a change in respiratory support settings.

Another longitudinal study of 20 patients with NMD initially treated their sleep-related hypoventilation with BPAP using a spontaneous mode in 18 [229]. One patient required his BPAP set to a timed rate 1 year later. The mean inspiratory positive airway pressure (IPAP) in these adolescents and young adults was 11.5 (9–14) and expiratory positive airway pressure (EPAP) was 4.5 (ranging from 4 to 5) cm H_2O. Over the 3.5-year follow-up period, supplemental oxygen (0.5–1.0 L/min) was added to PPV in 3 patients and 3 others switched to nasal volume controlled NIPPV. Patients with myotonic dystrophy can have central hypersomnia (unrelated to their SDB) and 3 who remained excessively sleep despite PAP therapy, requiring the addition of CNS stimulants.

In Closing

Compared to the general pediatric population, various forms of SDB are more common in children with neurodevelopmental, cervicomedullary compressive, and neuromuscular disorders. Many infants, children or adolescents with CP, epilepsy, and/or ID also have varying forms of SDB. Treatment strategies are available and often effective for most. Awareness of treatments for them is crucial toward improving health-related QOL, longevity, and well-being for them.

References

1. Dorris L, Scott N, Zuberi S, Gibson N, Espie C. Sleep problems in children with neurological disorders. *Dev Neurorehabil.* 2008;11(2):95–114.
2. Didden R, Korzilius H, van Aperlo B, van Overloop C, de Vries M. Sleep problems and daytime problem behaviours in children with intellectual disability. *J Intellect Disabil Res.* 2002;46 (pt 7):537–547.
3. Habayeb O, Goodburn S, Chudleigh T, et al. The NTplus method of screening for Down syndrome: achieving the 2010 targets? *Prenat Diagn.* 2010;30(5):434–437.
4. Rachidi M, Lopes C. Molecular and cellular mechanisms elucidating neurocognitive basis of functional impairments associated with intellectual disability in Down syndrome. *Am J Intellect Dev Disabil.* 2010;115(2):83–112.
5. Shin M, Besser LM, Kucik JE, Lu C, Siffel C, Correa A; Congenital Anomaly Multistate Prevalence and Survival Collaborative. Prevalence of Down syndrome among children and adolescents in 10 regions of the United States. *Pediatrics.* 2009;124(6):1565–1571.
6. Lott IT, Dierssen M. Cognitive deficits and associated neurological complications in individuals with Down's syndrome. *Lancet Neurol.* 2010;9(6): 623–633.
7. Carter M, McCaughey E, Annaz D, Hill CM. Sleep problems in a Down syndrome population. *Arch Dis Child.* 2009;94(4):308–310.
8. Fitzgerald DA, Paul A, Richmond C. Severity of obstructive apnoea in children with Down syndrome who snore. *Arch Dis Child.* 2007;92(5): 423–425.
9. Shott SR, Amin R, Chini B, Heubi C, Hotze S, Akers R. Obstructive sleep apnea: Should all children with Down syndrome be tested? *Arch Otolaryngol Head Neck Surg.* 2006;132(4):432–436.
10. Guimaraes CV, Donnelly LF, Shott SR, Amin RS, Kalra M. Relative rather than absolute macroglossia in patients with Down syndrome: implications for treatment of obstructive sleep apnea. *Pediatr Radiol.* 2008;38(10):1062–1067.
11. Uong EC, McDonough JM, Tayag-Kier CE. Magnetic resonance imaging of the upper airway in children with Down syndrome. *Am J Respir Crit Care Med.* 2001;163(3, pt 1):731–736.
12. Cua CL, Blankenship A, North AL, Hayes J, Nelin LD. Increased incidence of idiopathic persistent pulmonary hypertension in Down syndrome neonates. *Pediatr Cardiol.* 2007;28(4):250–254.

13. Shah PS, Hellmann J, Adatia I. Clinical characteristics and follow up of Down syndrome infants without congenital heart disease who presented with persistent pulmonary hypertension of newborn. *J Perinat Med.* 2004;32(2):168–170.
14. Levine OR, Simpser M. Alveolar hypoventilation and cor pulmonale associated with chronic airway obstruction in infants with Down syndrome. *Clin Pediatr (Phila).* 1982;21(1):25–29.
15. Mitchell RB, Call E, Kelly J. Diagnosis and therapy for airway obstruction in children with Down syndrome. *Arch Otolaryngol Head Neck Surg.* 2003;129(6):642–645.
16. Ng DK, Hui HN, Chan CH. Obstructive sleep apnoea in children with Down syndrome. *Singapore Med J.* 2006;47(9):774–779.
17. Dyken ME, Lin-Dyken DC, Poulton S, Zimmerman MB, Sedars E. Prospective polysomnographic analysis of obstructive sleep apnea in down syndrome. *Arch Pediatr Adolesc Med.* 2003;157(7): 655–660.
18. Marcus CL, Keens TG, Bautista DB, von Pechmann WS, Ward SL. Obstructive sleep apnea in children with Down syndrome. *Pediatrics.* 1991;88(1):132–139.
19. Ng DK, Chan CH, Cheung JM. Children with Down syndrome and OSA do not necessarily snore. *Arch Dis Child.* 2007;92(11):1047–1048.
20. Harley EH, Collins MD. Neurologic sequelae secondary to atlantoaxial instability in Down syndrome. Implications in otolaryngologic surgery. *Arch Otolaryngol Head Neck Surg.* 1994;120(2): 159–165.
21. Schaffer SR, Wong GH. Endoscopic visualization facilitates adenoidectomy. *Otolaryngol Head Neck Surg.* 2007;136(3):510.
22. Shott SR. Down syndrome: analysis of airway size and a guide for appropriate intubation. *Laryngoscope.* 2000;110(4):585–592.
23. Goldstein NA, Armfield DR, Kingsley LA, Borland LM, Allen GC, Post JC. Postoperative complications after tonsillectomy and adenoidectomy in children with Down syndrome. *Arch Otolaryngol Head Neck Surg.* 1998;124(2):171–176.
24. Kavanagh KT, Kahane JC, Kordan B. Risks and benefits of adenotonsillectomy for children with Down syndrome. *Am J Ment Defic.* 1986;91(1):22–29.
25. Tauman R, Gulliver TE, Krishna J, et al. Persistence of obstructive sleep apnea syndrome in children after adenotonsillectomy. *J Pediatr.* 2006;149(6):803–808.
26. Shete MM, Stocks RM, Sebelik ME, Schoumacher RA. Effects of adeno-tonsillectomy on polysomnography patterns in Down syndrome children with obstructive sleep apnea: a comparative study with children without Down syndrome. *Int J Pediatr Otorhinolaryngol.* 2010;74(3): 241–244.
27. Donnelly LF, Shott SR, LaRose CR, Chini BA, Amin RS. Causes of persistent obstructive sleep apnea despite previous tonsillectomy and adenoidectomy in children with down syndrome as depicted on static and dynamic cine MRI. *AJR Am J Roentgenol.* 2004;183(1):175–181.
28. Fricke BL, Donnelly LF, Shott SR, et al. Comparison of lingual tonsil size as depicted on MR imaging between children with obstructive sleep apnea despite previous tonsillectomy and adenoidectomy and normal controls. *Pediatr Radiol.* 2006;36(6):518–523.
29. Guimaraes CV, Kalra M, Donnelly LF, et al. The frequency of lingual tonsil enlargement in obese children. *AJR Am J Roentgenol.* 2008;190(4): 973–975.
30. Kirk VG, O'Donnell AR. Continuous positive airway pressure for children: a discussion on how to maximize compliance. *Sleep Med Rev.* 2006;10(2):119–127.
31. Rains JC. Treatment of obstructive sleep apnea in pediatric patients. Behavioral intervention for compliance with nasal continuous positive airway pressure. *Clin Pediatr (Phila).* 1995;34(10): 535–541.
32. Waldman HB, Hasan FM, Perlman S. Down syndrome and sleep-disordered breathing: the dentist's role. *J Am Dent Assoc.* 2009;140(3):307–312.
33. Trois MS, Capone GT, Lutz JA. Obstructive sleep apnea in adults with Down syndrome. *J Clin Sleep Med.* 2009;5(4):317–323.
34. Sato K, Shirakawa T, Niikuni N, Sakata H, Asanuma S. Effects of oral care in Down syndrome children with obstructive sleep apnea. *J Oral Sci.* 2010;52(1):145–147.
35. Mannan SE, Yousef E, Hossain J. Prevalence of positive skin prick test results in children with Down syndrome: a case-control study. *Ann Allergy Asthma Immunol.* 2009;102(3):205–209.
36. Bell RB, Turvey TA. Skeletal advancement for the treatment of obstructive sleep apnea in children. *Cleft Palate Craniofac J.* 2001;38(2):147–154.
37. Miloro M. Mandibular distraction osteogenesis for pediatric airway management. *J Oral Maxillofac Surg.* 2010;68(7):1512–1523.
38. Brooker GE, Cooper MG. Airway management for infants with severe micrognathia having mandibular distraction osteogenesis. *Anaesth Intensive Care.* 2010;38(1):43–49.
39. Cassidy SB, S.S., S.-. I Seattle (WA): University of Washington, and O.u.S. 03]. *Prader-Willi Syndrome.* In: Pagon RA, Bird TC, Dolan CR, Stephens K, eds. *Gene Reviews [Internet].* Seattle, WA: University of Washington; 2009.
40. Kousta E, Hadjiathanasiou CG, Tolis G, Papathanasiou A. Pleiotropic genetic syndromes with developmental abnormalities associated with obesity. *J Pediatr Endocrinol Metab.* 2009;22(7): 581–592.
41. Goldstone, AP. Prader-Willi syndrome: advances in genetics, pathophysiology and treatment. *Trends Endocrinol Metab.* 2004;15(1):12–20.
42. Whittington J, Holland A, Webb T, Butler J, Clarke D, Boer H. Cognitive abilities and genotype in a population-based sample of people with Prader-Willi syndrome. *J Intellect Disabil Res.* 2004; 48(pt 2):172–187.

43. Holm VA, Cassidy SB, Butler MG, et al. Prader-Willi syndrome: consensus diagnostic criteria. *Pediatrics*. 1993;91(2):398–402.
44. Whittington J, Holland A, Webb T, Butler J, Clarke D, Boer H. Academic underachievement by people with Prader-Willi syndrome. *J Intellect Disabil Res*. 2004;48(pt 2): 188–200.
45. Morgan JR, Storch EA, Woods DW, Bodzin D, Lewin AB, Murphy TK. A preliminary analysis of the phenomenology of skin-picking in Prader-Willi syndrome. *Child Psychiatry Hum Dev*. 2010;41(4):448–463.
46. Schepis C, Failla P, Siragusa M, Romano C. Skin-picking: the best cutaneous feature in the recognization of Prader-Willi syndrome. *Int J Dermatol*. 1994;33(12):866–867.
47. Clarke DJ, Waters J, Corbett JA. Adults with Prader-Willi syndrome: abnormalities of sleep and behaviour. *J R Soc Med*. 1989;82(1):21–24.
48. O'Donoghue FJ, Camfferman D, Kennedy JD, et al. Sleep-disordered breathing in Prader-Willi syndrome and its association with neurobehavioral abnormalities. *J Pediatr*. 2005;147(6):823–829.
49. Festen DA, de Weerd AW, van den Bossche RA, Joosten K, Hoeve H, Hokken-Koelega AC. Sleep-related breathing disorders in prepubertal children with Prader-Willi syndrome and effects of growth hormone treatment. *J Clin Endocrinol Metab*. 2006;91(12):4911–4915.
50. Festen DA, Wevers M, de Weerd AW, van den Bossche RA, Duivenvoorden HJ, Hokken-Koelega AC. Cognition and behavior in pre-pubertal children with Prader-Willi syndrome and associations with sleep-related breathing disorders. *Am J Med Genet A*. 2008;146A(23):3018–3025.
51. Festen DA, Wevers M, de Weerd AW, et al. Psychomotor development in Infants with Prader-Willi syndrome and associations with sleep-related breathing disorders. *Pediatr Res*. 2007;62(2): 221–224.
52. Lin HY, Lin SP, Lin CC. Polysomnographic characteristics in patients with Prader-Willi syndrome. *Pediatr Pulmonol*. 2007;42(10):881–887.
53. Miller J, Silverstein J, Shuster J, Driscoll DJ, Wagner M. Short-term effects of growth hormone on sleep abnormalities in Prader-Willi syndrome. *J Clin Endocrinol Metab*. 2006;91(2):413–417.
54. Pavone M, Paglietti MG, Petrone A, Crinò A, De Vincentiis GC, Cutrera R. Adenotonsillectomy for obstructive sleep apnea in children with Prader-Willi syndrome. *Pediatr Pulmonol*. 2006;41(1): 74–79.
55. Williams K, Scheimann A, Sutton V, Hayslett E, Glaze DG. Sleepiness and sleep disordered breathing in Prader-Willi syndrome: relationship to genotype, growth hormone therapy, and body composition. *J Clin Sleep Med*. 2008;4(2): 111–118.
56. Hertz G, Cataletto M, Feinsilver SH, Angulo M. Sleep and breathing patterns in patients with Prader-Willi syndrome (PWS): effects of age and gender. *Sleep*. 1993;16(4):366–371.
57. Arens R, Gozal D, Omlin KJ, et al. Hypoxic and hypercapnic ventilatory responses in Prader-Willi syndrome. *J Appl Physiol*. 1994;77(5):2224–2230.
58. Gozal D, Arens R, Omlin KJ, Ward SL, Keens TG. Absent peripheral chemosensitivity in Prader-Willi syndrome. *J Appl Physiol*. 1994;77(5): 2231–2236.
59. Arens R, Gozal D, Burrell BC, et al. Arousal and cardiorespiratory responses to hypoxia in Prader-Willi syndrome. *Am J Respir Crit Care Med*. 1996;153(1):283–287.
60. Livingston FR, Arens R, Bailey SL, Keens TG, Ward SL. Hypercapnic arousal responses in Prader-Willi syndrome. *Chest*. 1995;108(6):1627–1631.
61. Tauber M, Diene G, Molinas C, Hébert M. Review of 64 cases of death in children with Prader-Willi syndrome (PWS). *Am J Med Genet A*. 2008;146(7):881–887.
62. Clift S, Dahlitz M, Parkes JD. Sleep apnoea in the Prader-Willi syndrome. *J Sleep Res*. 1994;3(2):121–126.
63. Lin HY, Lin SP, Lin CC, et al. Polysomnographic characteristics in patients with Prader-Willi syndrome. *Pediatr Pulmonol*. 2007;42(10):881–887.
64. Kaplan J, Fredrickson PA, Richardson JW. Sleep and breathing in patients with the Prader-Willi syndrome. *Mayo Clin Proc*. 1991;66(11):1124–1126.
65. Hertz G, Cataletto M, Feinsilver SH, Angulo M. Developmental trends of sleep-disordered breathing in Prader-Willi syndrome: the role of obesity. *Am J Med Genet*. 1995;56(2):188–190.
66. Yee BJ, Buchanan PR, Mahadev S, et al. Assessment of sleep and breathing in adults with Prader-Willi syndrome: a case control series. *J Clin Sleep Med*. 2007;3(7):713–718.
67. van Mil EA, Westerterp KR, Gerver WJ, et al. Energy expenditure at rest and during sleep in children with Prader-Willi syndrome is explained by body composition. *Am J Clin Nutr*. 2000;71(3): 752–756.
68. Holland AJ, Treasure J, Coskeran P, Dallow J. Characteristics of the eating disorder in Prader-Willi syndrome: implications for treatment. *J Intellect Disabil Res*. 1995;39(pt 5):373–381.
69. Dykens EM, Goff BJ, Hodapp RM, et al. Eating themselves to death: have "personal rights" gone too far in treating people with Prader-Willi syndrome? *Ment Retard*. 1997;35(4):312–314.
70. Schmidt H, Pozza SB, Bonfig W, Schwarz HP, Dokoupil K. Successful early dietary intervention avoids obesity in patients with Prader-Willi syndrome: a ten-year follow-up. *J Pediatr Endocrinol Metab*. 2008;21(7):651–655.
71. Bonfig W, Dokoupil K, Schmidt H. A special, strict, fat-reduced, and carbohydrate-modified diet leads to marked weight reduction even in overweight adolescents with Prader-Willi syndrome (PWS). *ScientificWorldJournal*. 2009;9:934–939.
72. Hooren RH, Widdershoven GA, Borne HW, Curfs LM. Autonomy and intellectual disability: the case of prevention of obesity in Prader-Willi syndrome. *J Intellect Disabil Res*. 2002;46(pt 7):560–568.

73. Sforza E, Krieger J, Geisert J, Kurtz D. Sleep and breathing abnormalities in a case of Prader-Willi syndrome. The effects of acute continuous positive airway pressure treatment. *Acta Paediatr Scand.* 1991;80(1): 80–85.
74. Tanna N, Choi SS. Efficacy and safety of adenotonsillectomy for pediatric obstructive sleep apnea in Prader-Willi syndrome. *Ann Otol Rhinol Laryngol.* 2009;118(4):267–269.
75. Carrel AL, Myers SE, Whitman BY, Eickhoff J, Allen DB. Long-term growth hormone therapy changes the natural history of body composition and motor function in children with prader-willi syndrome. *J Clin Endocrinol Metab.* 2010; 95(3):1131–1136.
76. Eggermann T, Schönherr N, Spengler S, et al. Identification of a 21q22 duplication in a Silver-Russell syndrome patient further narrows down the Down syndrome critical region. *Am J Med Genet A.* 2010;152A(2):356–359.
77. Myrelid A, Bergman S, Elfvik Strömberg M, et al. Late effects of early growth hormone treatment in Down syndrome. *Acta Paediatr.* 2010;99(5):763–769.
78. Contestabile A, Benfenati F, Gasparini L. Communication breaks-Down: from neurodevelopment defects to cognitive disabilities in Down syndrome. *Prog Neurobiol.* 2010;91(1):1–22.
79. Ruby NF, Fernandez F, Zhang P, Klima J, Heller HC, Garner CC. Circadian locomotor rhythms are normal in Ts65Dn "Down syndrome" mice and unaffected by pentylenetetrazole. *J Biol Rhythms.* 2010;25(1):63–66.
80. Cho CK, Smith CR, Diamandis EP. Amniotic fluid proteome analysis from Down syndrome pregnancies for biomarker discovery. *J Proteome Res.* 2010;9(7):3574–3582.
81. Shaw SW, Lin SY, Lin CH, et al. Second-trimester maternal serum quadruple test for Down syndrome screening: a Taiwanese population-based study. *Taiwan J Obstet Gynecol.* 2010;49(1):30–34.
82. Koster MP, Heetkamp KM, Pennings JL, de Vries A, Visser GH, Schielen PC. Down syndrome screening: imagining the screening test of the future. *Expert Rev Mol Diagn.* 2010;10(4):445–457.
83. Andriolo RB, El Dib RP, Ramos L, Atallah AN, da Silva EM. Aerobic exercise training programmes for improving physical and psychosocial health in adults with Down syndrome. *Cochrane Database Syst Rev.* 2010;5: CD005176.
84. Esbensen AJ, Bishop S, Seltzer MM, Greenberg JS, Taylor JL. Comparisons between individuals with autism spectrum disorders and individuals with Down syndrome in adulthood. *Am J Intellect Dev Disabil.* 2010;115(4):277–290.
85. Mendonca GV, Pereira FD, Fernhall B. Oxygen uptake kinetics during exercise in adults with Down syndrome. *Eur J Appl Physiol.* 2010;110(3):575–583.
86. Verrillo E, Bruni O, Franco P, et al. Analysis of NREM sleep in children with Prader-Willi syndrome and the effect of growth hormone treatment. *Sleep Med.* 2009;10(6):646–650.
87. Vogels A, Van Den Ende J, Keymolen K, et al. Minimum prevalence, birth incidence and cause of death for Prader-Willi syndrome in Flanders. *Eur J Hum Genet.* 2004;12(3):238–240.
88. Nagai T, Obata K, Tonoki H, et al. Cause of sudden, unexpected death of Prader-Willi syndrome patients with or without growth hormone treatment. *Am J Med Genet A.* 2005;136(1):45–48.
89. Reuland-Bosma W, Reuland MC, Bronkhorst E, Phoa KH. Patterns of tooth agenesis in patients with Down syndrome in relation to hypothyroidism and congenital heart disease: an aid for treatment planning. *Am J Orthod Dentofacial Orthop.* 2010;137(5):584 e1-9.
90. Miller JL, Shuster J, Theriaque D, Driscoll DJ, Wagner M. Sleep disordered breathing in infants with Prader-Willi syndrome during the first 6 weeks of growth hormone therapy: a pilot study. *J Clin Sleep Med.* 2009;5(5):448–453.
91. de Lind van Wijngaarden RF, Otten BJ, Festen DA. High prevalence of central adrenal insufficiency in patients with Prader-Willi syndrome. *J Clin Endocrinol Metab.* 2008;93(5):1649–1654.
92. de Lind van Wijngaarden RF, Joosten KF, van den Berg S, et al. The relationship between central adrenal insufficiency and sleep-related breathing disorders in children with Prader-Willi syndrome. *J Clin Endocrinol Metab.* 2009;94(7): 2387–2393.
93. Maas AP, Didden R, Bouts L, Smits MG, Curfs LM. Scatter plot analysis of excessive daytime sleepiness and severe disruptive behavior in adults with Prader-Willi syndrome: a pilot study. *Res Dev Disabil.* 2009;30(3):529–537.
94. Richdale AL, Cotton S, Hibbit K. Sleep and behaviour disturbance in Prader-Willi syndrome: a questionnaire study. *J Intellect Disabil Res.* 1999; 43(pt 5):380–392.
95. Harris JC, Allen RP. Is excessive daytime sleepiness characteristic of Prader-Willi syndrome? The effects of weight change. *Arch Pediatr Adolesc Med.* 1996;150(12):288–293.
96. Hiroe Y, Inoue Y, Higami S, Suto Y, Kawahara R. Relationship between hypersomnia and respiratory disorder during sleep in Prader-Willi syndrome. *Psychiatry Clin Neurosci.* 2000;54(3):323–325.
97. Manni R, Politini L, Nobili L, et al. Hypersomnia in the Prader Willi syndrome: clinical-electrophysiological features and underlying factors. *Clin Neurophysiol.* 2001;112(5):800–805.
98. Vela-Bueno A, Kales A, Soldatos CR, et al. Sleep in the Prader-Willi syndrome. Clinical and polygraphic findings. *Arch Neurol.* 1984;41(3): 294–296.
99. Fronczek R, Lammers GJ, Balesar R, Unmehopa UA, Swaab DF. The number of hypothalamic hypocretin (orexin) neurons is not affected in Prader-Willi syndrome. *J Clin Endocrinol Metab.* 2005;90(9):5466–5470.
100. Nevsimalova S, Vankova J, Stepanova I, Seemanova E, Mignot E, Nishino S. Hypocretin deficiency in Prader-Willi syndrome. *Eur J Neurol.* 2005;12(1):70–72.

101. Priano L, Grugni G, Miscio G, et al. Sleep cycling alternating pattern (CAP) expression is associated with hypersomnia and GH secretory pattern in Prader-Willi syndrome. *Sleep Med.* 2006;7(8):627–633.
102. Prasad VK, Kurtzberg J. Transplant outcomes in mucopolysaccharidoses. *Semin Hematol.* 2010; 47(1):59–69.
103. Clarke LA. The mucopolysaccharidoses: a success of molecular medicine. *Expert Rev Mol Med.* 2008;10:e1.
104. Muenzer J. The mucopolysaccharidoses: a heterogeneous group of disorders with variable pediatric presentations. *J Pediatr.* 2004;144(5 suppl): S27–S34.
105. Wold SM, Derkay CS, Darrow DH, Proud V. Role of the pediatric otolaryngologist in diagnosis and management of children with mucopolysaccharidoses. *Int J Pediatr Otorhinolaryngol.* 2010;74(1):27–31.
106. Simmons MA, Bruce IA, Penney S, Wraith E, Rothera MP. Otorhinolaryngological manifestations of the mucopolysaccharidoses. *Int J Pediatr Otorhinolaryngol.* 2005;69(5):589–595.
107. Yeung AH, Cowan MJ, Horn B, Rosbe KW. Airway management in children with mucopolysaccharidoses. *Arch Otolaryngol Head Neck Surg.* 2009;135(1):73–79.
108. Shih SL, Lee YJ, Lin SP, Sheu CY, Blickman JG. Airway changes in children with mucopolysaccharidoses. *Acta Radiol.* 2002;43(1):40–43.
109. Leighton SE, Papsin B, Vellodi A, Dinwiddie R, Lane R. Disordered breathing during sleep in patients with mucopolysaccharidoses. *Int J Pediatr Otorhinolaryngol.* 2001;58(2):127–138.
110. Semenza GL, Pyeritz RE. Respiratory complications of mucopolysaccharide storage disorders. *Medicine (Baltimore).* 1988;67(4):209–219.
111. Nashed A, Al-Saleh S, Gibbons J, et al. Sleep-related breathing in children with mucopolysaccharidosis. *J Inherit Metab Dis.* 2009;32(4):544–550.
112. Santamaria F, Andreucci MV, Parenti G, et al. Upper airway obstructive disease in mucopolysaccharidoses: polysomnography, computed tomography and nasal endoscopy findings. *J Inherit Metab Dis.* 2007;30(5):743–749.
113. Cleary MA, Wraith JE. Management of mucopolysaccharidosis type III. *Arch Dis Child.* 1993;69(3):403–406.
114. Malm G, Mansson JE. Mucopolysaccharidosis type III (Sanfilippo disease) in Sweden: clinical presentation of 22 children diagnosed during a 30-year period. *Acta Paediatr.* 2010;99(8):1253–1257.
115. Fraser J, Gason AA, Wraith JE, Delatycki MB. Sleep disturbance in Sanfilippo syndrome: a parental questionnaire study. Arch Dis Child. 2005;90(12):1239–1242.
116. Mariotti P, Della Marca G, Iuvone L, et al. Sleep disorders in Sanfilippo syndrome: a polygraphic study. *Clin Electroencephalogr.* 2003;34(1):18–22.
117. Fraser J, Wraith JE, Delatycki MB. Sleep disturbance in mucopolysaccharidosis type III (Sanfilippo syndrome): a survey of managing clinicians. *Clin Genet.* 2002;62(5):418–421.
118. Belani KG, Krivit W, Carpenter BL, et al. Children with mucopolysaccharidosis: perioperative care, morbidity, mortality, and new findings. *J Pediatr Surg.* 1993;28(3):403–408, discussion 408–410.
119. Adachi K, Chole RA. Management of tracheal lesions in Hurler syndrome. *Arch Otolaryngol Head Neck Surg.* 1990;116(10):1205–1207.
120. Jeong HS, Cho DY, Ahn KM, Jin DK. Complications of tracheotomy in patients with mucopolysaccharidoses type II (Hunter syndrome). *Int J Pediatr Otorhinolaryngol.* 2006;70(10):1765–1769.
121. Wraith JE. Enzyme replacement therapy for the management of the mucopolysaccharidoses. *Int J Clin Pharmacol Ther.* 2009;47(suppl 1):S63–S65.
122. Coman DJ, Hayes IM, Collins V, Sahhar M, Wraith JE, Delatycki MB. Enzyme replacement therapy for mucopolysaccharidoses: opinions of patients and families. *J Pediatr.* 2008;152(5):723–727.
123. Kakkis ED, Muenzer J, Tiller GE. Enzyme-replacement therapy in mucopolysaccharidosis I. *N Engl J Med.* 2001;344(3):182–188.
124. Whitley CB, Belani KG, Chang PN, et al. Long-term outcome of Hurler syndrome following bone marrow transplantation. *Am J Med Genet.* 1993;46(2):209–218.
125. Newman CJ, O'Regan M, Hensey O. Sleep disorders in children with cerebral palsy. *Dev Med Child Neurol.* 2006; 48(7):564–568.
126. Wiggs L, Stores G. Severe sleep disturbance and daytime challenging behaviour in children with severe learning disabilities. *J Intellect Disabil Res.* 1996;40(pt 6): 518–528.
127. Wiggs L, Stores G. Behavioural treatment for sleep problems in children with severe intellectual disabilities and daytime challenging behaviour: effect on mothers and fathers. *Br J Health Psychol.* 2001;6(pt 3):257–269.
128. Hayashi M, Inoue Y, Iwakawa Y, Sasaki H. REM sleep abnormalities in severe athetoid cerebral palsy. *Brain Dev.* 1990;12(5):494–497.
129. Kotagal S, Gibbons VP, Stith JA. Sleep abnormalities in patients with severe cerebral palsy. *Dev Med Child Neurol.* 1994;36(4):304–311.
130. Fitzgerald DA, Follett J, Van Asperen PP. Assessing and managing lung disease and sleep disordered breathing in children with cerebral palsy. *Paediatr Respir Rev.* 2009;10(1):18–24.
131. Magardino TM, Tom LW. Surgical management of obstructive sleep apnea in children with cerebral palsy. *Laryngoscope.* 1999;109(10):1611–1615.
132. Biavati MJ, Manning SC, Phillips DL. Predictive factors for respiratory complications after tonsillectomy and adenoidectomy in children. *Arch Otolaryngol Head Neck Surg.* 1997;123(5):517–521.
133. Wiet GJ, Bower C, Seibert R, Griebel M. Surgical correction of obstructive sleep apnea in the complicated pediatric patient documented by polysomnography. *Int J Pediatr Otorhinolaryngol.* 1997;41(2):133–43.

134. Kerschner JE, Lynch JB, Kleiner H, Flanary VA, Rice TB. Uvulopalatopharyngoplasty with tonsillectomy and adenoidectomy as a treatment for obstructive sleep apnea in neurologically impaired children. *Int J Pediatr Otorhinolaryngol.* 2002;62(3):229–235.
135. Preciado DA, Sidman JD, Sampson DE, Rimell FL. Mandibular distraction to relieve airway obstruction in children with cerebral palsy. *Arch Otolaryngol Head Neck Surg.* 2004;130(6): 741–745.
136. Cohen SR, Holmes RE, Machado L, Magit A. Surgical strategies in the treatment of complex obstructive sleep apnoea in children. *Paediatr Respir Rev.* 2002;3(1):25–35.
137. Cohen SR, Simms C, Burstein FD, Thomsen J. Alternatives to tracheostomy in infants and children with obstructive sleep apnea. *J Pediatr Surg.* 1999;34(1):182–6, discussion 87.
138. Cohen SR, Lefaivre JF, Burstein FD, et al. Surgical treatment of obstructive sleep apnea in neurologically compromised patients. *Plast Reconstr Surg.* 1997;99(3):638–646.
139. Hsiao KH, Nixon GM. The effect of treatment of obstructive sleep apnea on quality of life in children with cerebral palsy. *Res Dev Disabil.* 2008;29(2):133–140.
140. Hill CM, Parker RC, Allen P, Paul A, Padoa KA. Sleep quality and respiratory function in children with severe cerebral palsy using night-time postural equipment: a pilot study. *Acta Paediatr.* 2009;98(11):1809–1814.
141. Yoshida K. Elastic retracted oral appliance to treat sleep apnea in mentally impaired patients and patients with neuromuscular disabilities. *J Prosthet Dent.* 1999;81(2):196–201.
142. Sriskandan N, Moody A, Howlett DC. Ultrasound-guided submandibular gland injection of botulinum toxin for hypersalivation in cerebral palsy. *Br J Oral Maxillofac Surg.* 2010;48(1):58–60.
143. Young NL, Rochon TG, McCormick A, Law M, Wedge JH, Fehlings D. The health and quality of life outcomes among youth and young adults with cerebral palsy. *Arch Phys Med Rehabil.* 2010;91(1):143–148.
144. Tarsuslu T, Livanelioglu A. Relationship between quality of life and functional status of young adults and adults with cerebral palsy. *Disabil Rehabil.* 2010;32(20):1658–1665.
145. Mesterman R, Leitner Y, Yifat R. Cerebral palsy—long-term medical, functional, educational, and psychosocial outcomes. *J Child Neurol.* 2010; 25(1):36–42.
146. Doralp S, Bartlett DJ. The prevalence, distribution, and effect of pain among adolescents with cerebral palsy. *Pediatr Phys Ther.* 2010;22(1): 26–33.
147. Lancioni GE, Singh NN, O'Reilly MF, et al. Fostering locomotor behavior of children with developmental disabilities: an overview of studies using treadmills and walkers with microswitches. *Res Dev Disabil.* 2009; 30(2):308–322.
148. Cortesi F, Giannotti F, Ottaviano S. Sleep problems and daytime behavior in childhood idiopathic epilepsy. *Epilepsia.* 1999;40(11):1557–1565.
149. Stores G, Wiggs L, Campling G. Sleep disorders and their relationship to psychological disturbance in children with epilepsy. *Child Care Health Dev.* 1998;24(1):5–19.
150. Didden R, de Moor JM, Korzilius H. Sleepiness, on-task behavior and attention in children with epilepsy who visited a school for special education: a comparative study. *Res Dev Disabil.* 2009; 30(6):1428–1434.
151. Nunes ML. Sleep disorders. *J Pediatr (Rio J).* 2002;78(suppl 1):S63–S72.
152. Maganti R, Hausman N, Koehn M, Sandok E, Glurich I, Mukesh BN. Excessive daytime sleepiness and sleep complaints among children with epilepsy. *Epilepsy Behav.* 2006;8(1):272–277.
153. Kaleyias J, Cruz M, Goraya JS, et al. Spectrum of polysomnographic abnormalities in children with epilepsy. *Pediatr Neurol.* 2008;39(3):170–176.
154. Miano S, Pelliccia A, Evangelisti M, Pagani J, Villa MP. Role of continuous positive airway pressure therapy on the pathogenesis of sleep-related frontal lobe epilepsy in a child with obstructive sleep apnea syndrome. *J Child Neurol.* 2008;23(1):124–128.
155. Malow BA, Foldvary-Schaefer N, Vaughn BV, et al. Treating obstructive sleep apnea in adults with epilepsy: a randomized pilot trial. *Neurology.* 2008;71(8):572–577.
156. Chihorek AM, Abou-Khalil B, Malow BA. Obstructive sleep apnea is associated with seizure occurrence in older adults with epilepsy. *Neurology.* 2007;69(19):1823–1827.
157. Malow BA, Weatherwax KJ, Chervin RD, et al. Identification and treatment of obstructive sleep apnea in adults and children with epilepsy: a prospective pilot study. *Sleep Med.* 2003;4(6): 509–515.
158. Khurana DS, Reumann M, Hobdell EF, et al. Vagus nerve stimulation in children with refractory epilepsy: unusual complications and relationship to sleep-disordered breathing. *Childs Nerv Syst.* 2007;23(11):1309–1312.
159. Malow BA, Edwards J, Marzec M, Sagher O, Fromes G. Effects of vagus nerve stimulation on respiration during sleep: a pilot study. *Neurology.* 2000;55(10):1450–1454.
160. Marzec M, Edwards J, Sagher O, Fromes G, Malow BA. Effects of vagus nerve stimulation on sleep-related breathing in epilepsy patients. *Epilepsia.* 2003;44(7):930–935.
161. Nagarajan L, Walsh P, Gregory P, Stick S, Maul J, Ghosh S. Respiratory pattern changes in sleep in children on vagal nerve stimulation for refractory epilepsy. *Can J Neurol Sci.* 2003;30(3):224–227.
162. Menezes AH, Vogel TW. Specific entities affecting the craniocervical region: syndromes affecting the craniocervical junction. *Childs Nerv Syst.* 2008;24(10):1155–1163.

163. Bellus GA, Hefferon TW, Ortiz de Luna RI, et al. Achondroplasia is defined by recurrent G380R mutations of FGFR3. *Am J Hum Genet.* 1995;56(2):368–373.
164. Nahar R, Saxena R, Kohli S, Puri R, Verma IC. Molecular studies of achondroplasia. *Indian J Orthop*. 2009;43(2):194–196.
165. Martinez-Frias ML, de Frutos CA, Bermejo E, Nieto MA; ECEMC Working Group. Review of the recently defined molecular mechanisms underlying thanatophoric dysplasia and their potential therapeutic implications for achondroplasia. *Am J Med Genet A*. 2010;152A(1):245–255.
166. Shirley ED, Ain MC. Achondroplasia: manifestations and treatment. *J Am Acad Orthop Surg.* 2009;17(4):231–241.
167. Majdalany DS, Burkhart HM, Connolly HM, et al. Adults with Down syndrome: safety and long-term outcome of cardiac operation. *Congenit Heart Dis*. 2010; 5(1):38–43.
168. Rupela V, Manjula R, Velleman SL. Phonological processes in Kannada-speaking adolescents with Down syndrome. *Clin Linguist Phon*. 2010;24(6): 431–450.
169. Looper J, Ulrich DA. Effect of treadmill training and supramalleolar orthosis use on motor skill development in infants with Down syndrome: a randomized clinical trial. *Phys Ther.* 2010;90(3):382–390.
170. King JA, Vachhrajani S, Drake JM, Rutka JT. Neurosurgical implications of achondroplasia. *J Neurosurg Pediatr*. 2009;4(4):297–306.
171. Pauli RM, Scott CI, Wassman ER Jr, et al. Apnea and sudden unexpected death in infants with achondroplasia. *J Pediatr*. 1984;104(3):342–348.
172. Pauli RM, Horton VK, Glinski LP, Reiser CA. Prospective assessment of risks for cervicomedullary-junction compression in infants with achondroplasia. *Am J Hum Genet*. 1995;56(3):732–744.
173. Danielpour M, Wilcox WR, Alanay Y, Pressman BD, Rimoin DL. Dynamic cervicomedullary cord compression and alterations in cerebrospinal fluid dynamics in children with achondroplasia. Report of four cases. *J Neurosurg*. 2007;107(6 suppl): 504–507.
174. Nelson FW, Hecht JT, Horton WA, Butler IJ, Goldie WD, Miner M. Neurological basis of respiratory complications in achondroplasia. *Ann Neurol*. 1988;24(1):89–93.
175. Onodera K, Niikuni N, Chigono T, Nakajima I, Sakata H, Motizuki H. Sleep disordered breathing in children with achondroplasia. Part 2. Relationship with craniofacial and airway morphology. *Int J Pediatr Otorhinolaryngol*. 2006;70(3):453–461.
176. Hankinson TC, Anderson RC. Craniovertebral junction abnormalities in Down syndrome. *Neurosurgery*. 2010;66(3 suppl): 32–38.
177. Mogayzel PJ Jr, Carroll JL, Loughlin GM, Hurko O, Francomano CA, Marcus CL. Sleep-disordered breathing in children with achondroplasia. *J Pediatr*. 1998; 132(4):667–671.
178. Zucconi M, Weber G, Castronovo V, et al. Sleep and upper airway obstruction in children with achondroplasia. *J Pediatr*. 1996;129(5):743–749.
179. Lloyd M, Burghardt A, Ulrich DA, Angulo-Barroso R. Physical activity and walking onset in infants with Down syndrome. *Adapt Phys Activ Q*. 2010;27(1):1–16.
180. Tasker RC, Dundas I, Laverty A, Fletcher M, Lane R, Stocks J. Distinct patterns of respiratory difficulty in young children with achondroplasia: a clinical, sleep, and lung function study. *Arch Dis Child*. 1998;79(2):99–108.
181. Sisk EA, Heatley DG, Borowski BJ, Leverson GE, Pauli RM. Obstructive sleep apnea in children with achondroplasia: surgical and anesthetic considerations. *Otolaryngol Head Neck Surg*. 1999;120(2):248–254.
182. Ednick M, Tinkle BT, Phromchairak J, Egelhoff J, Amin R, Simakajornboon N. Sleep-related respiratory abnormalities and arousal pattern in achondroplasia during early infancy. *J Pediatr*. 2009;155(4):510–515.
183. Dabrowska A, Pisula E. Parenting stress and coping styles in mothers and fathers of pre-school children with autism and Down syndrome. *J Intellect Disabil Res*. 2010;54(3):266–280.
184. Collins WO, Choi SS. Otolaryngologic manifestations of achondroplasia. *Arch Otolaryngol Head Neck Surg*. 2007;133(3):237–244.
185. Vaglio A, Milunsky A, Quadrelli A, et al. Clinical, cytogenetic, and molecular characterization of a girl with some clinical features of Down syndrome resulting from a pure partial trisomy 21q22.11-qter due to a de novo intrachromosomal duplication. *Genet Test Mol Biomarkers*. 2010;14(1):57–65.
186. Sangani M, Shahid A, Amina S, Koubeissi M. Improvement of myoclonic epilepsy in Down syndrome treated with levetiracetam. *Epileptic Disord*. 2010;12(2):151–154.
187. Moncaster JA, Pineda R, Moir RD, et al. Alzheimer's disease amyloid-beta links lens and brain pathology in Down syndrome. *PLoS ONE*. 2010;5(5):e10659.
188. Cochrane DD, Adderley R, White CP, Norman M, Steinbok P. Apnea in patients with myelomeningocele. *Pediatr Neurosurg*. 1990;16(4-5):232–239.
189. Dauvilliers Y, Stal V, Abril B, et al. Chiari malformation and sleep related breathing disorders. *J Neurol Neurosurg Psychiatry*. 2007;78(12):1344–1348.
190. Murray C, Seton C, Prelog K, Fitzgerald DA. Arnold Chiari type 1 malformation presenting with sleep disordered breathing in well children. *Arch Dis Child*. 2006;91(4):342–343.
191. Waters KA, Forbes P, Morielli A, et al. Sleep-disordered breathing in children with myelomeningocele. *J Pediatr*. 1998;132(4):672–681.
192. Kirk VG, Morielli A, Brouillette RT. Sleep-disordered breathing in patients with myelomeningocele: the missed diagnosis. *Dev Med Child Neurol*. 1999;41(1):40–43.
193. Kirk VG, Morielli A, Gozal D, et al. Treatment of sleep-disordered breathing in children with

myelomeningocele. *Pediatr Pulmonol*. 2000;30(6): 445–452.
194. Holinger PC, Holinger LD, Reichert TJ, Holinger PH. Respiratory obstruction and apnea in infants with bilateral abductor vocal cord paralysis, meningomyelocele, hydrocephalus, and Arnold-Chiari malformation. *J Pediatr*. 1978;92(3):368–373.
195. Wealthall SR, Whittaker GE, Greenwood N. The relationship of apnoea and stridor in spina bifida to other unexplained infant deaths. *Dev Med Child Neurol*. 1974;16(6 suppl 32):107–116.
196. Di Filippo M, Tozzi A, Ghiglieri V, et al. Impaired plasticity at specific subset of striatal synapses in the Ts65Dn mouse model of Down syndrome. *Biol Psychiatry*. 2010;67(7):666–671.
197. Albert GW, Menezes AH, Hansen DR, Greenlee JD, Weinstein SL. Chiari malformation Type I in children younger than age 6 years: presentation and surgical outcome. *J Neurosurg Pediatr*. 2010;5(6):554–561.
198. Brown BJ, Habelt S, Koral K, Sacco D, Herman JH, Baker LA. Secondary nocturnal enuresis caused by central sleep apnea from Chiari malformation type 1. *J Pediatr Urol*. 2010;6(3): 265–269.
199. Luke A, Sutton M, Schoeller DA, Roizen NJ. Nutrient intake and obesity in prepubescent children with Down syndrome. *J Am Diet Assoc*. 1996;96(12):1262–1267.
200. Holinger LD, Holinger PC, Holinger PH. Etiology of bilateral abductor vocal cord paralysis: a review of 389 cases. *Ann Otol Rhinol Laryngol*. 1976;85(4 pt 1):428–436.
201. Choi SS, Tran LP, Zalzal GH. Airway abnormalities in patients with Arnold-Chiari malformation. *Otolaryngol Head Neck Surg*. 1999;121(6):720–724.
202. Goldstein H. Utilisation of health services over a one-year period by an adolescent population with Down syndrome. *Dan Med Bull*. 1988;35(6):585–588.
203. *The International Classification of Sleep Disorders: Diagnostic & Coding Manual*. 2nd ed. Westchester, IL: American Academy of Sleep Medicine; 2005.
204. Iber C, Ancoli-Israel S, Chesson A Jr, Quan S. *The AASM Manual for the Scoring of Sleep and Associated Events: Rules, Terminology and Technical Specifications*. 1st ed. Westchester, IL: American Academy of Sleep Medicine; 2007.
205. Bach JR, Alba AS. Management of chronic alveolar hypoventilation by nasal ventilation. *Chest*. 1990;97(1):52–57.
206. Young HK, Lowe A, Fitzgerald DA, et al. Outcome of noninvasive ventilation in children with neuromuscular disease. *Neurology*. 2007;68(3):198–201.
207. Mellies U, Ragette R, Schwake C, Boehm H, Voit T, Teschler H. Daytime predictors of sleep disordered breathing in children and adolescents with neuromuscular disorders. *Neuromuscul Disord*. 2003;13(2):123–128.
208. Suresh S, Wales P, Dakin C, Harris MA, Cooper DG. Sleep-related breathing disorder in Duchenne muscular dystrophy: disease spectrum in the paediatric population. *J Paediatr Child Health*. 2005;41(9–10):500–503.
209. Mellies U, Dohna-Schwake C, Stehling F, Voit T. Sleep disordered breathing in spinal muscular atrophy. *Neuromuscul Disord*. 2004;14(12):797–803.
210. Quera Salva MA, Blumen M, Jacquette A, et al. Sleep disorders in childhood-onset myotonic dystrophy type 1. *Neuromuscul Disord*. 2006; 16(9–10):564–570.
211. Dohna-Schwake C, Ragette R, Mellies U, Straub V, Teschler H, Voit T. Respiratory function in congenital muscular dystrophy and limb girdle muscular dystrophy 2I. *Neurology*. 2004;62(3):513–514.
212. Nabatame S, Taniike M, Sakai N, et al. Sleep disordered breathing in childhood-onset acid maltase deficiency. *Brain Dev*. 2009;31(3):234–239.
213. Ejskjaer K, Uldbjerg N, Goldstein H. Menstrual profile and early menopause in women with Down syndrome aged 26–40 years. *J Intellect Dev Disabil*. 2006;31(3):166–171.
214. Kirk VG, Batuyong ED, Bohn SG. Transcutaneous carbon dioxide monitoring and capnography during pediatric polysomnography. *Sleep*. 2006;29(12):1601–1608.
215. Ragette R, Mellies U, Schwake C, Voit T, Teschler H. Patterns and predictors of sleep disordered breathing in primary myopathies. *Thorax*. 2002;57(8):724–728.
216. Velazquez-Wong AC, Hernández-Huerta C, Márquez-Calixto A. Identification of duchenne muscular dystrophy female carriers by fluorescence in situ hybridization and RT-PCR. *Genet Test*. 2008;12(2):221–223.
217. Brooke MH, Fenichel GM, Griggs RC, et al. Duchenne muscular dystrophy: patterns of clinical progression and effects of supportive therapy. *Neurology*. 1989;39(4):475–481.
218. Manni R, Ottolini A, Cerveri I, et al. Breathing patterns and HbSaO2 changes during nocturnal sleep in patients with Duchenne muscular dystrophy. *J Neurol*. 1989;236(7):391–394.
219. Khan Y, Heckmatt JZ. Obstructive apnoeas in Duchenne muscular dystrophy. *Thorax*. 1994;49(2):157–161.
220. Smith PE, Calverley PM, Edwards RH. Hypoxemia during sleep in Duchenne muscular dystrophy. *Am Rev Respir Dis*. 1988;137(4):884–888.
221. Barbe F, Quera-Salva MA, McCann C, et al. Sleep-related respiratory disturbances in patients with Duchenne muscular dystrophy. *Eur Respir J*. 1994;7(8):1403–1408.
222. Finder JD, Birnkrant D, Carl J, et al; American Thoracic Society. Respiratory care of the patient with Duchenne muscular dystrophy: ATS consensus statement. *Am J Respir Crit Care Med*. 2004;170(4):456–465.
223. Bushby K, Finkel R, Birnkrant DJ, et al; DMD Care Considerations Working Group. Diagnosis and management of Duchenne muscular dystrophy,

part 1: diagnosis, and pharmacological and psychosocial management. *Lancet Neurol.* 2010;9(1): 77–93.
224. Bushby K, Finkel R, Birnkrant DJ, et al; DMD Care Considerations Working Group. Diagnosis and management of Duchenne muscular dystrophy, part 2: implementation of multidisciplinary care. *Lancet Neurol.* 2010;9(2):177–189.
225. Davis SE, Hynan LS, Limbers CA, et al. The PedsQL™ in pediatric patients with Duchenne muscular dystrophy: feasibility, reliability, and validity of the pediatric quality of life inventory neurmuscular module and generic core scales. *J Clin Neuromusc Dis.* 2010;11:97–109.
226. Ward S, Chatwin M, Heather S, Simonds AK. Randomised controlled trial of non-invasive ventilation (NIV) for nocturnal hypoventilation in neuromuscular and chest wall disease patients with daytime normocapnia. *Thorax.* 2005;60(12): 1019–1824.
227. Edwards EA, Hsiao K, Nixon GM. Paediatric home ventilatory support: the Auckland experience. *J Paediatr Child Health.* 2005;41(12):652–658.
228. Mellies U, Ragette R, Dohna Schwake C, Boehm H, Voit T, Teschler H. Long-term noninvasive ventilation in children and adolescents with neuromuscular disorders. *Eur Respir J.* 2003;22(4):631–636.
229. Guilleminault C, Philip P, Robinson A. Sleep and neuromuscular disease: bilevel positive airway pressure by nasal mask as a treatment for sleep disordered breathing in patients with neuromuscular disease. *J Neurol Neurosurg Psychiatry.* 1998;65(2):225–232.
230. Tan E, Nixon GM, Edwards EA. Sleep studies frequently lead to changes in respiratory support in children. *J Paediatr Child Health.* 2007;43(7–8):560–563.
231. Eagle M, Baudouin SV, Chandler C, Giddings DR, Bullock R, Bushby K. Survival in Duchenne muscular dystrophy: improvements in life expectancy since 1967 and the impact of home nocturnal ventilation. *Neuromuscul Disord.* 2002;12(10):926–929.
232. Bach JR. Medical considerations of long-term survival of Werdnig-Hoffmann disease. *Am J Phys Med Rehabil.* 2007;86(5):349–355.
233. Bach JR, Robert D, Leger P, Langevin B. Sleep fragmentation in kyphoscoliotic individuals with alveolar hypoventilation treated by NIPPV. *Chest.* 1995; 107(6):1552–1558.
234. Fuschillo S, De Felice A, Gaudiosi C, Balzano G. Nocturnal mechanical ventilation improves exercise capacity in kyphoscoliotic patients with respiratory impairment. *Monaldi Arch Chest Dis.* 2003;59(4):281–286.

CHAPTER 16

Management of Sleep-Disordered Breathing in Children With Neuromuscular Disease

Eliot S. Katz and Carolyn M. D'Ambrosio

Overview

Children with neuromuscular disease (NMD) and chest wall deformities (CWD) frequently develop sleep-disordered breathing, including obstructive sleep apnea (OSA), central sleep apnea, and nocturnal hypoventilation. The pathophysiology includes respiratory muscle weakness, altered brainstem control of breathing, craniofacial abnormalities, impaired upper airway motor control, and decreased chest wall compliance (obesity or scoliosis). The resultant intermittent hypoxemia, hypercapnia, and sleep fragmentation may produce considerable cardiovascular and neurocognitive morbidity. The pattern of sleep-disordered breathing is predicated on the type of impairment present. Diaphragmatic and intercostal muscle weakness may lead to profound hypoventilation, whereas upper airway weakness may produce OSA.

Children with NMD/CWD tend to breathe with fast respiratory rates and low tidal volumes during wakefulness. During sleep, upper airway resistance increases and central chemoreceptor sensitivity decreases, resulting in impaired respiratory load compensation. Thus, minute ventilation declines an estimated 10% to 15% with sleep onset, which may result in respiratory insufficiency in NMD/CWD. Also, children with NMD/CWD frequently have low baseline oxygen saturation and therefore operate on the steeper portion of their oxygen dissociation curve, leading to rapid oxygen desaturation with ventilatory disturbances. Children with CWD have a mechanical disadvantage leading to an increased work of breathing and can develop hypoventilation during sleep, particularly during rapid eye movement (REM) sleep.

This chapter will review the available treatment options for sleep-disordered breathing in children with NMD/CWD, and the outcome data in special populations.

Key Points

Sleep-disordered breathing is common in children with NMD, resulting in metabolic, cardiovascular, and neurocognitive morbidity. There appear to be important individual differences in genetic susceptibility that influence the expression of OSA sequelae. In some children, even mild OSA can result in adverse neurocognitive and cardiovascular sequelae.

Diagnostic and Treatment Paradigm

The optimal methodology and criteria for the diagnosis of sleep-disordered breathing in children with NMD/CWD have not been established. Previous efforts to define OSA severity with threshold levels of the apnea-hypopnea index (AHI, mild 1–5 per hour, moderate 5–10 per hour, severe > 10 per hour), gas exchange abnormalities, or sleep fragmentation have proven unsatisfactory, because they fail to account for the individual trait susceptibility to the neurocognitive, cardiovascular, and metabolic sequelae of OSA. Similarly, the consequences of hypercapnia are highly variable, with some children remaining remarkably asymptomatic in the setting of respiratory insufficiency. Thus, the threshold amount of hypoxemia, hypercapnia, and sleep disruption associated with adverse consequences varies widely among children. Therefore, a hybrid approach to the diagnosis and treatment of sleep-disordered breathing in NMD/CWD in children is necessary, considering polysomnographic indices, symptoms, the natural history of the condition, and the risk-benefit ratio of the available therapies.

Regarding OSA, most clinicians consider adenotonsillectomy the first-line treatment in the setting of adenotonsillar hypertrophy. However, with a compatible clinical history and physical examination suggestive of allergy, the threshold level of OSA necessary for treatment with intranasal steroids and leukotriene antagonists is quite low. By contrast, it is recognized that the initiation of *continuous positive airway pressure* (CPAP) is fraught with difficulties in tolerance and may itself be disruptive of sleep. Thus, initiating CPAP therapy requires more polysomnographic evidence of obstruction (usually AHI >5 events per hour), more profound gas exchange abnormalities (SpO_2 <90%), increased sleep fragmentation (arousal index >15 per hour), and/or neurobehavioral symptoms. Finally, children with severe OSA polysomnographically, and severe manifestations including failure to thrive, pulmonary hypertension, marked aberrations in daytime functioning, would mandate consideration of all available therapies, including medically supervised weight loss, and, if life-threatening, tracheotomy.

For respiratory insufficiency, in most cases there is no specific therapy available for the underlying neuromuscular weakness. Similarly, the surgical correction of CWD may at best stabilize the mechanical disadvantage observed. Thus, the therapeutic approach is predicated on considering the severity of the sleep-associated gas exchange abnormalities, sleep fragmentation, and symptoms, along with the morbidities associated with noninvasive and invasive mechanical ventilation. Bilevel ventilation using a nasal or oro-nasal interface is beneficial in most patients, though tolerance is often poor. Invasive ventilation through a tracheostomy is highly effective in reversing the respiratory insufficiency, but it interferes with speech and predisposes toward infections. General measures for patients with OSA or respiratory insufficiency include the avoidance of sedating medications, weight reduction if appropriate, and proper sleep hygiene measures.

Obstructive Sleep Apnea

There is little evidence-based data on the treatment of OSA specifically in children with NMD. The etiology of OSA in this population is often multifactorial, and successful therapy may require combination therapy tailored to the individual child. The available therapeutic approaches that are useful in the general population, and routinely used in children with neuromuscular disorders, are described below.

Pharmacologic Therapy

Leukotrienes and their receptors are increased in adenotonsillar tissue [1] and exhaled condensate [2] of children with OSA. Topical intranasal steroids have been shown to decrease adenoidal hypertrophy and improve symptom scores of obstructed breathing [3]. Aqueous beclomethasone decreased the adenoid-choanae ratio from 91% at baseline, to 77% at 1 month, and to 62% after 6 months [3]. Several studies have documented reduction in the AHI following a course of nasal steroids; (1) 5 weeks of intranasal fluticasone decreased the AHI from 11 to 6 per hour [4]; (2) 6 weeks of intranasal budesonide decreased the AHI from 3.7 to 1.3 per hour [5]; and (3) 4 weeks of intranasal budesonide reduced the AHI from 5.2 to 3.2 per hour [6]. The improvement in OSA severity after discontinuing intranasal steroid therapy appears to be stable at least 2 months polysomnographically [5], and after at least 9 months symptomatically [6]. Children whose symptoms improve with nasal steroids are less likely to have an adenotonsillectomy within 2 years, compared with nonresponders

(54% vs 83%) [7]. The combination of budesonide and montelukast in children with mild residual OSA following adenotonsillectomy resulted in a reduction in the AHI from 3.9 to 0.3 per hour, after 3 months of therapy [8]. The long-term success of anti-inflammatory therapy has not been established.

Positive Pressure/Oxygen Therapy

CPAP delivered noninvasively through nasal or oro-nasal interface is a highly efficacious therapy for pediatric OSA, though long-term compliance is often problematic [9–11]. CPAP is typically reserved for moderate-severe OSA and not amenable to surgical or pharmacologic treatment. A properly fitted mask and adequate age-appropriate behavioral training is crucial to the success of CPAP therapy [12,13]. The minimum daily duration of CPAP therapy required to mitigate the adverse effects of OSA is unknown. In a prospective study of children with severe OSA, CPAP compliance monitored electronically after approximately 1 month of therapy revealed that CPAP usage greater than 4 hours per night, greater than 5 hours per night greater than 6 hours per night were observed in only 54%, 48%, and 31% of patients, respectively [14]. Most new CPAP machines digitally record compliance data, which should be reviewed at 1- to 3-month intervals to identify barriers to usage. The reported side effects of CPAP in children include skin erythema, eye irritation, congestion, and rhinorrhea [15]. CPAP was reported to be equally efficacious compared with bilevel ventilation for the treatment of OSA in children [15]. However, children with hypoventilation during sleep despite successful treatment of OSA, should be considered for bilevel ventilation (see below).

Oxygen therapy has a limited role in the treatment of children with OSA. Two studies have evaluated the effect of supplemental oxygen in children with OSA, with disappointing results. Improvements in oxygen saturation are evident, but there is no significant decrease in OSA severity [16,17]. In addition, 2 children with OSA developed a marked increase in PCO_2 on supplemental oxygen (>75 torr) [16]. Thus, oxygen therapy will not alleviate the sleep fragmentation or hypoventilation associated with OSA, which may have significant adverse consequences.

Surgical Therapy

Successful treatment of children with OSA is predicated upon identifying the origin of the increased upper airway resistance. In most children with documented OSA and adenotonsillar hypertrophy, an adenotonsillectomy is the recommended first-line therapy. Following adenotonsillectomy, children with OSA have reported improvements in quality of life [18], behavior [19], attention [20], growth [21], cognitive scores [22,23], and school performance [24]. However, residual OSA may be present polysomnographically in more than 40% of cases postoperatively [25,26]. Moreover, there is no consensus on whether the adenoids, tonsils, or both, need to be removed. A retrospective study in children undergoing adenoidectomy for obstructive symptoms reported that 27% subsequently had a tonsillectomy [27]. Selected patients may benefit from treatment of additional sites of obstruction such as turbinectomy, deviated septum repair, maxillary expansion, mandibular distraction, maxillary distraction, tongue reduction/advancement, or lingual tonsillar removal [28].

Parental reports of OSA symptomotology post-adenotonsillectomy are usually favorable, though objective testing often reveals considerable residual obstruction. Complete normalization of OSA (AHI < 1) following adenotonsillectomy was observed in only 25% of patients, with 46% having persistent mild OSA ($1 < \text{AHI} < 5$) and 29% having at least moderate OSA (AHI >5) [25]. Children with residual OSA following adenotonsillectomy are most likely to have obesity, severe OSA, enlarged turbinates, deviated septum, neurological disorders, and/or craniofacial malformations [25,26]. Together, these studies indicate that adenotonsillar hypertrophy is only one of several important determinants of OSA in children. A recent meta-analysis of the cure rate of adenotonsillectomy for OSA (defined as an AHI <1) was only 60%, though there was a marked improvement in OSA in the majority of children [29].

Adenotonsillectomy for OSA is associated with postoperative bleeding (3% of cases), pain, and respiratory decompensation (20% of cases), including pulmonary edema, upper airway obstruction and, rarely, death [30–32]. The first postoperative night may be associated with significant OSA, resulting in profound desaturation [33]. However, the majority of children with mild OSA will improve on the first postoperative night [34]. Patients at high risk for postoperative complications include children less than 3 years of age or those with prematurity, craniofacial abnormalities, obesity, neuromuscular weakness, cerebral palsy (CP), cor pulmonale, or severe OSA [35,36]. Careful postoperative monitoring of high-risk patients in a pediatric intensive care unit is recommended. Children experiencing respiratory distress postoperatively have been reported to benefit from positive airway pressure [35]. Adenoidectomy alone has a lower risk of postoperative bleeding (<0.5%) and other complications.

Dental Therapy

Craniofacial growth in children is determined by both genetic and environmental factors. Chronic mouth breathing results in aberrant facial development, including maxillary constriction. Rapid maxillary expansion, using an orthodontic appliance to deliver a lateral force to the upper posterior molars, opens the midpalatal suture transversely and therefore widens the nasal cavity. Over a period of about 3 weeks, the intermolar distance increases approximately 3.9 mm, and the nasal pyriform opening increases 1.3 mm [37]. After 4 months of therapy, rapid maxillary expansion decreases nasal resistance [37] and improves OSA in children with maxillary constriction [37–39]. Children with OSA caused by both maxillary constriction and adenotonsillar hypertrophy may require both rapid maxillary expansion and adenotonsillectomy to resolve the OSA.

Children with OSA and dysgnathia (87% deep/retrusive bite, 13% cross-bite) were randomized into a 6-month trial of a custom mandibular advancement device versus an untreated control group [40]. Twenty-six percent of the children in the treatment group discontinued therapy for unknown reasons. As a group, follow-up polysomnography revealed a decrease in the AHI from 7.1 to 2.6 events per hour, but 20% of the patients had a residual AHI above 5 events per hour [40]. Another pediatric study similarly demonstrated that mandibular advancement devices reduced the AHI from 8 to 4 events per hour [41]. Nevertheless, there are insufficient long-term efficacy data using mandibular advancement devices to treat OSA in children with dysgnathia.

Weight Loss

The prevalence of childhood obesity has tripled in the last 25 years and is presently estimated to be 17% to 18% of the general population. Moreover, the incidence of obesity is increased in children with developmental disabilities and therefore merits special attention in these children [42]. Obese children are more likely to snore than lean children [43]. The incidence of OSA in obese children is high at 36% [44] and may exceed 60% if habitual snoring is present [45]. Both OSA and obesity are considered chronic, low-grade systemic inflammatory states and may contribute to the cardiovascular, metabolic, and neurocognitive morbidities.

Most obese children with OSA will also have adenotonsillar hypertrophy [45]. However, when obese and lean children with OSA are matched for disease severity, the obese children have less adenotonsillar hypertrophy, but significantly higher Mallampati scores (indicating more crowding of the oropharynx) [46]. This finding supports the concept that a central distribution of adiposity poses the greatest risk for OSA. Obese children with OSA have more obstructive events in the supine position, whereas nonobese children with OSA are more severe in the prone or side positions [47]. Preferential sleep positioning may be helpful in reducing the severity of OSA in obese children.

Adenotonsillectomy in obese children with OSA results in a marked reduction in AHI, but 76% have residual OSA [25,26]. One series reported that 56% of obese children with OSA required CPAP following adenotonsillectomy [48]. Weight loss in obese children of 18.7 kg over 20 weeks resulted in a reduction in the AHI from 14.1 to 1.6 per hour [49]. However, another study reported that 38% of obese children had an AHI greater than 2 per hour after a 24-kg weight loss over 5 months [50]. Bariatric surgery in adolescents resulting in an average 58-kg weight loss over 5 months resulted in a reduction in the AHI from a median of 9.1 to 0.7 per hour, with only 1 child with residual OSA [51]. Postoperative respiratory complications are higher in obese children with suspected OSA.

Respiratory Insufficiency During Sleep

Noninvasive Positive Pressure Ventilation: Overview

Respiratory failure occurs when the alveolar ventilation is insufficient to meet the needs of cellular metabolism, resulting in hypercapnia and possibly hypoxemia (see Figure 16.1). Patients with NMD/CWD frequently develop hypoventilation initially during sleep. The risk factors for hypercapnia include neuromuscular weakness, thoracic cage abnormalities, obesity, upper airway obstruction, and/or impaired central respiratory drive. By contrast, hypoxemia with normal P_aCO_2 is most commonly observed in parenchymal lung disease, which also frequently occurs in neuromuscularly impaired children following aspiration or recurrent pneumonia. Polysomnography is essential to distinguish the components of sleep-disordered breathing including central hypoventilation, central apnea, and/or obstructive apnea.

Noninvasive positive pressure ventilation (NIPPV) is indicated in symptomatic patients with nocturnal hypoventilation, even before the development of daytime hypoventilation. Symptoms include morning headaches, fatigue, and dyspnea arising from the hypercapnia, as well as hypersomnolence secondary to sleep fragmentation. Also, patients with significant daytime hypoventilation (P_aCO_2 >50 torr) should be considered for nocturnal NIPPV, even if they are not aware of daytime symptomotology. However, there are no data to support the prophylactic use of NIPPV to mitigate the deterioration of respiratory muscle strength [52]. Long-term positive pressure ventilation may be delivered by noninvasive (nasal or oro-nasal mask) or invasive techniques (tracheostomy). Complications from the use of a tracheostomy tube are common, including infection, tracheomalacia, bleeding, accidental decannulation, and mucous plugging.

NIPPV is the preferred choice in most patients with hypoventilation during sleep, but may be contraindicated in children with dysphagia or laryngeal dysfunction associated with aspiration. Also, continuous NIPPV may also be a poor choice for most patients requiring long-term daytime ventilatory assistance, as it interferes with feeding and speech. Contraindications for NIPPV are few, but

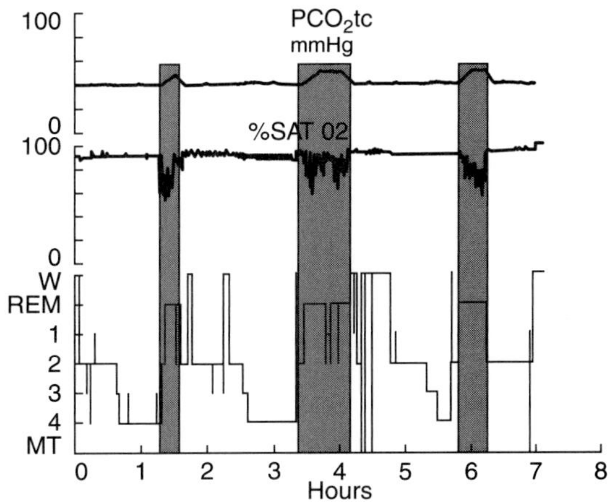

Figure 16.1 Overnight hypnogram from a patient with restrictive lung disease because of obesity. Rapid eye movement–related oxygen desaturation and hypercapnia are evident. This pattern is also seen in chest wall disorders and neuromuscular weakness. Reprinted with permission from Ref. [55].

technical difficulties often arise with uncooperative patients. Patients likely to succeed with NIPPV include cooperative, motivated patients, with adequate caregiver support. A careful mask fitting is important to ensure that there are no pressure sores or air leaks. Nasal masks are preferred, except in mouth-breathing children who require an oro-nasal mask. Oro-nasal masks are less desirable because they may interfere with coughing and could need to be removed urgently in patients with excessive upper airway secretions or vomiting. Mouthpieces may also be configured to provide NIPPV during wakefulness and/or sleep. Positive pressure ventilation can also be delivered via a tracheostomy tube using a continuous-flow ventilator.

NIPPV: Technical Aspects and Outcomes

NIPPV typically consists of a pressure-limited ventilator that is delivered through a nasal or oro-nasal interface. In the *spontaneous* mode, the patient receives a baseline *expiratory positive airway pressure* (EPAP), which is increased to the *inspiratory positive airway pressure* (IPAP) during patient breaths that are detected. Typically, the *spontaneous* mode results in an increase in the tidal volume, but a slowing of respiratory rate tends to limit overall increases in minute ventilation. The *spontaneous/timed* mode also synchronizes the IPAP to the patient's spontaneous breaths, but in addition, provides machine-initiated breaths if the patient's respiratory rate drops below a user-adjustable level. Generally, the EPAP is set to eliminate apneas, hypopneas, and respiratory effort–related arousals. The typical EPAP settings are 4 to 10 cm H_2O (10–14 cm H_2O in obesity) in children. To facilitate ventilation, a minimum IPAP to EPAP difference of 6 cm H_2O is recommended. IPAP settings are generally 10 to 20 cm H_2O (20–30 cm H_2O in obesity). The back-up respiratory rate is empirically set slightly below the patient's spontaneous respiratory rate (10–20 breaths per minute). Some ventilators facilitate patient comfort by allowing adjustment of the inspiratory time, rise time, and triggering sensitivity.

Bilevel titration in the sleep laboratory requires empirically determining the EPAP, IPAP, rate, and the level of oxygen supplementation. Monitoring end-tidal CO_2 while on NIPPV is often inaccurate because of the air leak in the mask. Transcutaneous CO_2 measurements should be validated with blood gases and can be useful to monitor ventilation changes during sleep. In addition to a properly fitting mask, the principal determinant of NIV tolerance is patient-ventilator synchrony. Asynchrony between the patient and ventilator may arise from a mask leak or inability to trigger the machine and lead to gas exchange abnormalities, increased work of breathing, and sleep disruption. Air leaks through the mouth are common during nasal NIPPV and may be disruptive of sleep [53]. The adaptation process to NIPPV may take several weeks of practice during wakefulness, with gradual usage during sleep at lower than optimal pressures, and trials of different interfaces (mask, headgear, and chin strap). Follow-up of patients with NMD/CWD includes ensuring symptom resolution and documenting adequate gas exchange.

The treatment objective for NIPPV in NMD/CWD is to improve gas exchange parameters, and therefore symptomatology. Documentation of NIPPV efficacy with blood gases is essential because noninvasive CO_2 monitoring may be quite inaccurate in the setting of positive pressure ventilation and oxygen supplementation [54]. NIPPV improves sleep quality, hypersomnolence, and headache in many NMD/CWD patients, including increased sleep efficiency and slow-wave sleep [55–57]. However, the symptoms of nocturnal respiratory insufficiency recur immediately following the withdrawal of NIPPV [58]. Nocturnal ventilation may also improve daytime ventilation by resetting the central chemoreceptors [57]. There are many case series reporting the effectiveness of noninvasive ventilation in the treatment of nocturnal respiratory insufficiency [57,59,60]. The common side effects of NIPPV are listed in Table 16.1.

Table 16.1 Side effects of noninvasive positive pressure ventilation

Skin breakdown
Areophagia/gastric distention
Aspiration
Eye irritation
Mouth leaks/dry mouth
Nasal congestion
Claustrophobia
Epistaxis
Pneumothorax
Decreased cardiac output

NIPPV is often initiated in the inpatient setting for patients being treated for acute respiratory failure. Children with NMD/CWD with chronic respiratory failure are most often started on NIPPV at home or in the sleep laboratory, along with a titration study to optimize ventilator settings. Monitors are an important part of the therapeutic regimen, especially in patients with limited mobility or communication skills. A low-pressure alarm within the ventilator circuit is mandatory to alert caregivers of a disconnection. An oximeter with alarm is helpful to readily adjust the levels of oxygen supplementation in the setting of intercurrent viral illnesses. Patients with congenital central hypoventilation syndrome should also be monitored continuously with a capnometer during sleep.

Treatment of Sleep-Disordered Breathing in Special Populations

Congenital Central Hypoventilation Syndrome

Congenital central hypoventilation syndrome (CCHS) is a rare disorder characterized by alveolar hypoventilation that is particularly pronounced during non-rapid eye movement (NREM) sleep. CCHS patients have a diminished integration of CO_2 tension by the medullary chemoreceptors in the absence of any structural brainstem lesion, parenchymal lung disease, cardiac disease, or neuromuscular weakness. Patients with CCHS present with life-threatening hypercapnia and hypoxemia. Lifelong ventilatory support is necessary, and the sleep laboratory is an important resource for ensuring optimal ventilator settings. A comprehensive consensus statement on the diagnosis and health care needs of CCHS patients was published in 2010 [61].

The spectrum of hypoventilation is related to the underlying genotype, with the longer polyalanine repetitions associated with more severe disease. Late-onset CCHS in childhood [62] and adults is most often reported with the 20/24 [62] and 20/25 [63–65] genotype. Approximately 10% of CCHS cases have a 20/20 genotype, with a missense, nonsense, or frameshift mutation in the PHOX2B gene (*non-polyalanine repeat expansion mutations*). Most of these are de novo mutations and tend to have a very severe phenotype, with neural crest tumors, Hirschsprung disease, and a 24-h/d ventilator requirement.

Respiratory Abnormalities in CCHS

Children with CCHS who can maintain a CO_2 below 45 torr during wakefulness generally do not need daytime ventilatory support. CCHS genotypes are highly predictive of the requirement for nocturnal versus continuous mechanical ventilation. Individuals with the 20/24 genotype often present as late-onset cases and typically need nocturnal ventilation alone. The 20/25 genotype not only usually presents at birth but also generally requires only nocturnal ventilation. The 20/26 genotype frequently requires additional daytime ventilatory assistance in the setting of exercise or viral illness. Finally, the 20/27 to 20/33 genotypes mostly require 24-h/d mechanical ventilation. Most CCHS patients with the non-polyalanine repeat expansion mutations also need uninterrupted 24-hour ventilatory assistance. Overall, approximately 1/3 of children with CCHS need 24-hour a day ventilatory support. Though exercise does stimulate breathing to some extent in CCHS patients, hypoventilation may become apparent during moderate exercise [66].

To ensure optimal neurocognitive development, it is essential to maintain proper gas exchange during resting wakefulness, exercise, and sleep. Comprehensive monitoring is indicated in each of these states using respiratory inductance plethysmography, oximetry, end-tidal CO_2, and electrocardiogram. Overnight polysomnography with continuous end-tidal CO_2 monitoring is recommended at least twice per year. Importantly, though supplemental oxygen alone will correct the oxygenation deficit, it does not reverse the underlying hypoventilation, which will eventually contribute to pulmonary hypertension. The target end-tidal CO_2 during sleep ranges between 35 and 40 torr, with normal oxygenation. Some authors recommend maintaining the sleeping CO_2 at or below 35 torr, to facilitate daytime ventilation [67]. Careful attention to monitoring alarms during sleep, emergency plans, and availability of an electrical back-up source for the ventilator are essential. The recent American Thoracic Society clinical policy statement on care for CCHS patients recommends continuous monitoring during sleep by a trained nurse with knowledge of ventilator management [61]. It is important that a monitor be placed *before* sleep onset, as hypoventilation can occur fulminantly immediately after sleep onset. Patients with CCHS should sleep with a documenting oximeter (alarm set at 85%) and end-tidal CO_2 monitor (alarm set at 55 torr) at all times.

The mainstay of therapy for young children with CCHS is positive pressure ventilation through a tracheostomy. Pressure-cycled ventilation using a portable, battery-powered, continuous-flow ventilator using a small tracheostomy tube is typically sufficient during the first 6 to 8 years of life. Patients with CCHS should have an extra tracheostomy tube and ventilation bag with them at all times, including visits to the sleep laboratory. Noninvasive ventilation is an option in older children with CCHS (after 6–8 years of age) who require ventilatory support only during sleep. Typically, a nasal mask with a fixed leak is used in combination with a bilevel ventilator with a back-up rate. Strict adherence to the aforementioned monitoring regimen is also essential with noninvasive ventilation. Some children requiring daytime ventilation may consider diaphragmatic pacing to free themselves from a more cumbersome ventilator

[67]. Diaphragmatic pacing involves bilateral thoracoscopic placement of phrenic nerve electrodes that activate the diaphragm, and thus provide ventilatory support. The external device is small and easily portable. Diaphragmatic pacing should be limited to 12 to 15 h/d because of concerns regarding diaphragmatic fatigue. Thus, an alternative form of respiratory support will be necessary for those patients requiring continuous ventilation. Though large data sets are not available, it is believed that at least 50% of children using diaphragmatic pacers exclusively at night will tolerate decannulation [67]. Some children with diaphragmatic pacer develop obstructive apnea during sleep. Insertion and care of diaphragmatic pacers should be limited to institutions with particular experience in the technique. In the event of a pacing malfunction, noninvasive or tracheostomy ventilation will be necessary emergently. Patients with a diaphragmatic pacer cannot obtain magnetic resonance imaging (MRI).

Children with CCHS are vulnerable to acute respiratory failure during anesthesia, intercurrent viral illnesses, and with the use of respiratory depressants. Viral upper respiratory illnesses pose a considerable risk to CCHS patients as they are unable to perceive elevations of CO_2 that may accompany parenchymal lung disease or soft tissue swelling of the upper airway. Similarly, great caution should be taken during swimming because patients with CCHS lack the perception of asphyxia and are at risk of drowning. Alcohol and illicit drugs are known to be respiratory depressants, and death or coma has been reported in adolescents with CCHS after ingesting alcohol [68]. Patients with CCHS should be counseled regarding the risks of substance abuse. A recent report in 2 female CCHS patients documented a restoration of CO_2 chemosensitivity in response to a progestin contraceptive, desogestrel [69]. Progestins are known to augment ventilatory drive and chemosensitivity. This is a potentially important proof of concept that requires further evaluation.

Rett Syndrome

Rett syndrome (RS) is a heterogeneous disorder affecting females and is caused by a mutation of the MECP2 gene on the X chromosome. Breathing abnormalities, including hyperventilation, central apnea, valsalva breathing (expiring against a closed glottis), and apneusis (prolonged inspiration) usually begin after 2 years of age and are often confined to wakefulness [70], but may also occur during sleep [71]. The apneustic breathing pattern predominates in the first 10 years of life. Older individuals also frequently demonstrate valsalva breathing, central apnea, and shallow breathing [70]. The sleep abnormalities are frequently observed at sleep onset transitions, but prolonged central apneas have been reported in all stages of sleep. Typically, RS patients have normal sleep architecture and NREM breathing, with an occasional prolonged central apnea during REM sleep [72]. Parenchymal lung disease on the basis of gastroesophageal reflux and oropharyngeal dysfunction may contribute to the hypoxemia observed during respiratory pauses. Supplemental oxygen via nasal cannula will mitigate the severity of hypoxemia during the central apneas, though the respiratory pauses persist.

Hyperventilation is associated with hypocarbia, whereas apnea produces hypercarbia and hypoxemia. Hypocapnic alkalosis may result in vasoconstriction, reduction in cerebral/coronary artery perfusion, and even sudden death [70]. During hyperventilation episodes, there is widespread activation of the ventrolateral medulla, including autonomic excitation. Autonomic symptoms often include flushing, pupillary dilatation, and cold extremities. Breath-holding spells are often interspersed with hyperventilation. Brief, nonepileptic staring episodes, termed "vacant spells," may be associated with respiratory dysrhythmias. During valsalva maneuvers, forced expiration against a closed glottis increases intrapleural pressure, which impairs systemic venous return and leads to arterial hypotension. Dystonic posturing or repetitive movements are frequently seen during breathing dysrhythmias, although epileptiform discharges are rare. Impairment in parasympathetic circuitry gives rise to exaggerated sympathetic responses and an increased risk of cardiac arrhythmias. Aerophagia has been reported to occur during hyperventilation and breath-holding episodes, resulting in gastric distension that may interfere with respiratory gas exchange. Successful treatment of the gastric distension may require gastrostomy tube placement [73]. The termination of inspiration is serotonin dependent, and agonists to serotonin 1A receptors have been used to treat apneustic breathing in RS [74].

Prader-Willi Syndrome

Prader-Willi syndrome (PWS) is characterized by dysfunction of the hypothalamus, peripheral chemoreceptors, and autonomic nervous system. Symptoms include pain insensitivity, temperature instability, diminished salivation, poor satiety, excessive daytime sleepiness (EDS), and an altered sleep-wake cycle.

EDS in PWS

Children with PWS have a central abnormality of sleep-state cycling including REM sleep fragmentation, sleep-onset REM cycles, and increased cyclic alternating patterns [75]. Over half of children with PWS report EDS, that is, more severe than in other developmental disabilities [76]. Children with PWS are both objectively [77] and subjectively [76] sleepy. EDS in PWS may arise from OSA, obesity, or as a primary feature of PWS. Some PWS patients have objective EDS based on multiple sleep latency testing, even in the absence of obesity or OSA [75,78,79]. Thus, sleepiness in PWS may be a feature of primary hypothalamic dysfunction. Low cerebrospinal fluid hypocretin levels were reported in 2 PWS patients with objective sleepiness, but minimal OSA [80]. The wakefulness promoting agent, Modafinil, may be helpful to reduce the level of sleepiness in PWS.

Sleep-Disordered Breathing in PWS

Children with PWS have multiple risk factors for sleep-related breathing including respiratory muscle weakness, obesity, midfacial hypoplasia, micrognathia, pharyngeal muscle weakness, impaired peripheral chemoreceptors, and scoliosis. Longstanding OSA in PWS may lead to pulmonary hypertension, behavioral disturbances [81], and cognitive impairment [82]. Most studies in PWS children have demonstrated little or no OSA in the absence of obesity [78]. However, even lean PWS patients frequently demonstrate oxygen desaturation associated with normal, brief respiratory pauses and during REM sleep [83]. Children with PWS may be particularly vulnerable to OSA during intercurrent viral respiratory infections [84–86].

PWS patients with severe sleep-disordered breathing and daytime respiratory failure have been successfully treated with nocturnal NIPPV, resulting in normalization of daytime gas exchange [87]. The hypercapnic ventilatory drive has been documented to increase after tracheotomy in an obese PWS patient. Weight reduction has also been documented to improve both alveolar ventilation and OSA in PWS, but not EDS [79,88]. Treating the OSA in PWS patients with adenotonsillectomy or CPAP reduces the EDS in some patients [89].

Influence of Growth Hormone on Sleep Apnea in PWS

Growth hormone (GH) therapy in PWS may improve behavior, physical activity, hypersomnolence, respiratory muscle strength, hypercapnic ventilatory responsiveness, and basal ventilation [90,91]. Safety concerns were raised by a series of case reports of sudden death after starting GH in PWS [92]. These deaths occurred mostly during sleep, within 4 months of starting therapy, and OSA was suspected as a contributor. Also, there are several reports of OSA worsening in PWS patients during an intercurrent viral illness [84,86]. Children with PWS may be particularly vulnerable to the effects of increased upper airway resistance, given their peripheral chemoreceptor dysfunction. Nevertheless, 3 prospective trials of GH in children with PWS have not demonstrated a consistent worsening of OSA on therapy [84,86,93].

There is no clear consensus on the optimal serial screening protocol for OSA in PWS children treated with GH, but practice guidelines from an expert panel are available [94]. Before starting GH therapy, a detailed clinical sleep history, physical examination, and overnight polysomnography are recommended. If OSA is present, treatment is initiated before beginning GH. PWS children treated with GH should have repeat polysomnography after 2 months initially, and every 6 months thereafter. A routine clinical history and airway examination should be performed every 3 months. GH therapy is started in low doses and gradually increased over several months. Symptoms of OSA should prompt an immediate reevaluation, including polysomnography, airway physical examination, weight, and serum insulin-like growth factor-1 levels. GH therapy should be discontinued in the setting of worsening OSA. PWS patients started on GH should be placed on a strict dietary regimen to ensure that weight gain does not accompany GH usage. Following the OSA screening, there should be a low threshold for adenotonsillectomy in suitable patients. PWS children with OSA that is adequately treated with positive pressure may continue GH. The first 3 to 4 months of GH therapy appear to be the greatest risk of sudden death and heightened vigilance is recommended.

Chiari Malformations

Chiari malformations (CM) are characterized by congenital or acquired herniations of the cerebellum or brainstem through the foramen magnum, potentially causing symptoms of brainstem compression. Symptomatic CM are usually accompanied by headache, neck pain, ataxia, or oculomotor disturbances. Occasionally, asymptomatic children with CM may present with sudden death because of an unrecognized CM [95]. Because the brainstem regulates central respiratory drive, upper airway motor control, and arousal from sleep, a combination of central apnea, obstructive apnea, and hypoventilation may be observed. In 1 series, 25% of the children with CM had central apnea and 35% obstructive apnea [96]. The incidence of central apnea increases to 57% if the CM is associated with myelomeningocele [97]. Children with CM/ myelomeningocele may also demonstrate prolonged expiratory apnea with cyanosis [97–99] and have parenchymal lung disease. Individual events may resolve spontaneously or require resuscitation; occasionally death will ensue [99]. Expiratory apnea events do not resolve with surgical decompression, and may be fatal even after tracheotomy and mechanical ventilation.

From a surgical perspective, older children with a new onset of brainstem dysfunction often respond to craniocervical decompression, though the response of infants is more variable. Some case series of early decompression surgery reported improvement in brainstem dysfunction, whereas others have not [100–104]. In our experience, infants are most often not symptomatic at birth, but rather develop symptoms of brainstem dysfunction over time and may respond favorably to decompression, though some residual central apnea often remains. The early recognition and treatment of symptoms of brainstem compression is critical in preserving function. Patients with CM undergoing repair are at high risk of worsening respiratory failure in the postoperative period, likely related to swelling of the brainstem [96]. Even following successful decompression surgery, a relapse of brainstem compression symptoms are common, often in the first 2 to 3 years, and central apnea may be an early sign [105]. Thus, close follow-up is essential. Shunt malfunction in myelomeningocele may lead to sudden brainstem compression and respiratory arrest [106]. Infants who are symptomatic at birth or those with bilateral vocal cord paralysis have a poor prognosis with irreversible damage to the brainstem and often require tracheotomy.

The choice of medical therapies depends in part on the consequences of the central apnea observed, including hypoxemia, hypercapnia, and electroencephalography arousal. Patients with hypercapnia will likely need positive pressure ventilation with a back-up rate. Patients with isolated episodes of hypoxemia may benefit from supplemental oxygen alone. Oxygen may also regularize cyclic breathing patterns in some cases. Patients who are unresponsive to supplemental oxygen, or who are experiencing frequent sleep fragmentation, will also need positive pressure ventilation. The optimal settings should be established by performing a titration study during overnight polysomnography. In the majority of cases, there will be coexisting OSA that may respond to CPAP. An adenotonsillectomy is frequently unsuccessful in resolving OSA in children with CM, suggesting impairment in pharyngeal motor control.

Cerebral Palsy

CP is a nonprogressive abnormality of the developing brain resulting in disorders of movement, posture, and sometimes, cognitive function. CP is a heterogeneous condition frequently characterized by muscle weakness (pharyngeal and thoracic), decreased chest wall compliance, scoliosis, and impairments of motor control. Children with CP have a high incidence of disorders of arousal, disorders initiating or maintaining sleep, movement disorders, and sleep-disordered breathing [107]. Polysomnographically, children with CP have a high incidence of OSA and hypoxemia [108]. Many children with CP will have oral-motor dysfunction and gastroesophageal reflux producing aspiration, and therefore parenchymal lung disease. The gas exchange abnormalities are generally most pronounced during REM sleep.

Irregular sleep-wake cycles and insomnia are commonly observed in CP and can be problematic for both the children and their caregivers. Some children with CP may have diminished light perception resulting in a free-running circadian rhythm or chronic pain disrupting sleep [109]. Treatment of circadian rhythm disturbances usually consists of strict adherence to a schedule of feeding, activity, and sleep. Poor sleep quality may adversely affect daytime functioning. Seizures may result in sleep fragmentation and anti-epileptic medications may also cause sleepiness.

Children with CP have an increased incidence of OSA because of pharyngeal hypotonia, adenotonsillar hypertrophy, glossoptosis, and craniofacial abnormalities. The hypoxemia and sleep disruption induced by complete or partial obstruction may further impair neurocognitive development. Treatment of OSA with either adenotonsillectomy or CPAP has been reported to improve OSA and quality of life in CP [110]. If central respiratory drive is diminished, NIPPV may be indicated. However, an adenotonsillectomy is frequently only partially effective in reducing the severity of OSA in children with CP. Uvulopalatopharyngoplasty has been reported to successful in some children with CP and OSA [56,63]. In our experience, children with CP often do not tolerate dental appliances, CPAP, or nasal pharyngeal airways. Successful surgical management of OSA in individuals with CP has been reported by treating other sites of airway obstruction, including an enlarged and retropositioned tongue, nasal septal deviation, enlarged inferior turbinates, retrognathia, or maxillary hypoplasia [63]. If surgical and medical management of severe OSA fails in individuals with CP, a tracheostomy may be indicated.

Down Syndrome

Children with Down syndrome (DS) frequently demonstrate sleep-disordered breathing, including OSA and REM-predominant hypoxemia. The prevalence of OSA in children and adults with DS is 31% to 60% [111,112] and 94% [113], respectively. In DS children with snoring, 97% had documented OSA [114]. Interestingly, 1 study reported that 38% of DS children with OSA did not habitually snore [115]. Thus, some authors have recommended polysomnographic screening for OSA in all children with DS. Obesity is an important risk factor for OSA in DS and weight loss may be helpful [113,116]. The etiology of sleep-disordered breathing is related to increased upper airway resistance, parenchymal lung disease, and respiratory muscle weakness. Upper airway obstruction is particularly common throughout life in DS as the result of micrognathia, maxillary hypoplasia, relative macroglossia, nasopharyngeal narrowing, and hypotonia. In addition, congenital heart disease may result in right-to-left shunts, baseline hypoxemia, and pulmonary hypertension.

Polysomnographically, OSA may be very severe in DS, with marked oxygen desaturation and hypercapnia. Although an adenotonsillectomy is usually effective in patients with mild OSA, it is often insufficient to reverse the upper airway obstruction in severe OSA [117,118]. Approximately one half to three quarters of children with DS will have residual OSA following adenotonsillectomy requiring additional therapy, including CPAP, bilevel positive airway pressure, and supplemental oxygen [117–119]. CPAP is effective therapy for most patients with DS, even with hypercapnia, resulting in a reduction in daytime sleepiness [113,116]; however, compliance may be poor. In some series, 5% of DS children with OSA require tracheostomy [117]. Both endoscopy and cine-MRI may be useful to identify the multiple sites of obstruction in severe cases, permitting a personalized approach to surgery [120,121] (see Figure 16.2). Following an adenotonsillectomy, children with DS have a high incidence of postoperative respiratory distress including upper airway obstruction, oxygen desaturation, and hypoventilation [122]. Rapid maxillary expansion has been reported to improve subjective symptoms of OSA in DS [123]. Successful treatment of OSA in DS children often requires auxillary therapy for comorbidities including gastroesophageal reflux, laryngomalacia, parenchymal lung disease, and congenital heart disease [124].

Duchenne Muscular Dystrophy

Duchenne muscular dystrophy (DMD) is characterized by progressive muscular weakness resulting

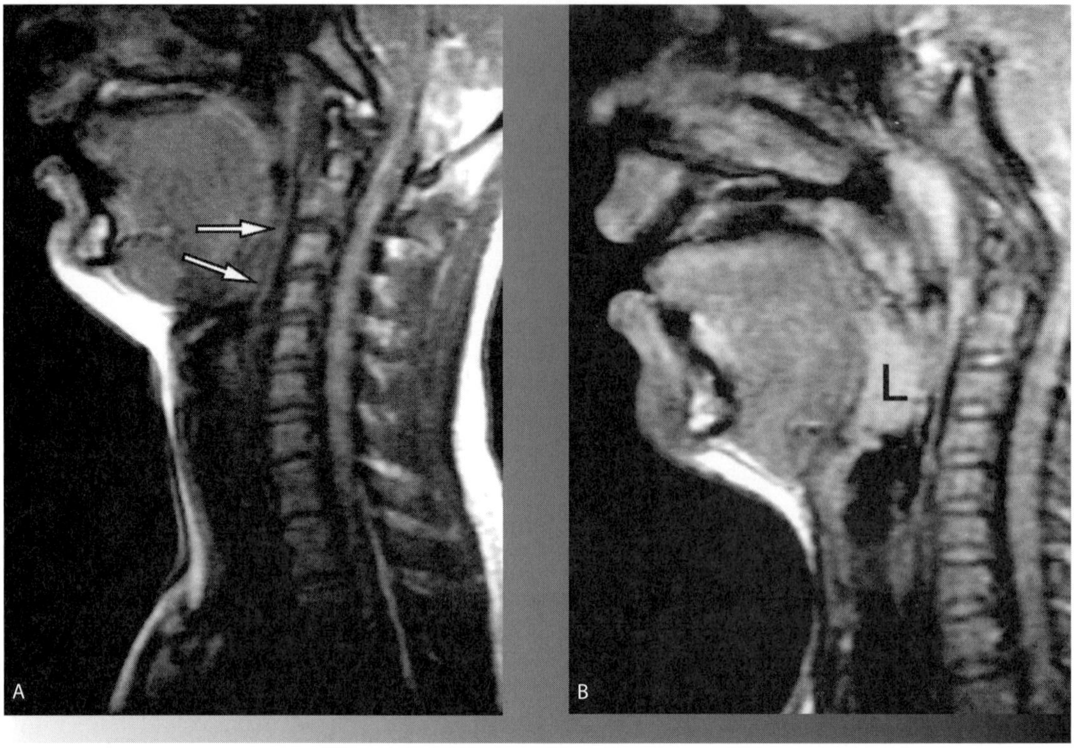

Figure 16.2 Causes of persistent obstructive sleep apnea in Down syndrome (DS) patients following adenotonsillectomy. (A) 18-Year-old female with DS. Relative macroglossia resulting in glossoptosis and hypopharyngeal collapse. (B) 10-Year-old male with DS. Cine-magnetic resonance imaging abnormalities include a recurrence of adenoidal tissue and an enlarged lingual tonsil obstructing the hypopharynx. Adapted with permission from Ref. [120].

in the development of OSA (5–12 years of age), nocturnal hypoventilation (15–17 years of age), progression to daytime hypercapnia (16–18 years of age), and death (20–25 years of age). Respiratory failure is the cause of death in 80% to 90% of cases, with the remainder succumbing to cardiac disease. Respiratory failure in DMD patients results from a combination of respiratory muscle weakness, scoliosis, decreased compliance of the chest wall, and parenchymal lung disease (recurrent aspiration). Hypercapnia is rare in DMD until very late in the course because there is a relative sparing of diaphragm function and a normal central respiratory drive. Thus, daytime hypercapnia is seen late in the course of DMD. However, nocturnal gas exchange abnormalities are frequently observed during adolescence when the vital capacity is less than 1.1 to 1.2 L.

Patients with DMD have a high incidence of OSA during the first decade of life [125]. Many of these children have adenotonsillar hypertrophy. Obesity appears to be an important risk factor for OSA in DMD patients. In consecutive DMD patients with a mean age of 18 years, 4 of 6 were observed to have symptoms of respiratory insufficiency and moderate-to-severe OSA [126]. During wakefulness, DMD patients rely on a higher respiratory rate to maintain their minute ventilation. During sleep, there is a greater reduction in the respiratory rate in DMD, resulting in a proportionately larger decline in minute ventilation, particularly during REM sleep. REM sleep is particularly problematic because of a reduction in the activity of intercostal muscles and pharyngeal airway dilator muscles, resulting in a decrease in alveolar ventilation and an increase in airway resistance. The earliest sign of respiratory insufficiency in DMD is REM-related hypoxemia [127,128].

There is a slight improvement in OSA following adenotonsillectomy, but most patients will have residual OSA [125]. Treatment of nocturnal hypoxemia with oxygen is effective at reversing the desaturation, but may worsen the OSA and/or hypoventilation [129]. In view of the progressive nature of the disease, early institution of nocturnal ventilatory support should be considered when nocturnal hypoxemia develops. Noninvasive ventilation has been evaluated in patients with DMD as an *imperative* measure in treating respiratory failure and as a *preventative* therapy in nonfailure patients. A randomized trial of *preventative* NIPPV in patients with DMD patients before respiratory failure revealed no benefits in terms of the decline in pulmonary function and survival was worse in the treated patients [52]. By contrast, *imperative* NIPPV has been demonstrated to be effective in improving symptoms of respiratory failure and increase survival, although the natural history of pulmonary function decline is unchanged [57,130–132].

Spinal Muscular Atrophy

Children with spinal muscular atrophy (SMA) have a spectrum of clinical severity in ventilatory deficits, ranging from complete paralysis necessitating mechanical ventilation support at birth, to mild muscle weakness that may not require ventilatory support. SMA patients have a high incidence of OSA, nocturnal hypoventilation, and sleep fragmentation [133]. Sleep-disordered breathing most often precedes daytime respiratory insufficiency. NIPPV is an effective long-term therapy in children with SMA to improve sleep quality, normalize $PaCO_2$ (during wakefulness and sleep), and alleviate the symptoms of hypercapnia [133,134].

Craniofacial Anomalies

Craniofacial dysmorphology is a common comorbidity in NMD. Craniofacial anomalies may predispose to upper airway obstruction on the basis of abnormal airway size, collapsibility, or neuromuscular control [3]. Despite the apparent increased incidence of OSA in children with micrognathia and mid-facial hypoplasia, little longitudinal data have been presented documenting its natural history and response to therapy.

Micrognathia

During early fetal development, a hypoplastic mandible results in displacement of the tongue posteriorly toward the pharyngeal wall and superiorly between the palatal shelves. The constellation of micrognathia, glossoptosis, and U-shaped cleft palate is termed the Robin sequence. Crowding of the oral and pharyngeal space in this condition has been associated with OSA [135]. In most instances, Robin sequence will occur in association with other anomalies such as Stickler syndrome, velocardiofacial syndrome, and fetal alcohol syndrome [136]. A retrospective series of 50 micrognathic infants revealed that 72% required an intervention for airway obstruction [137]. The site of airway collapse is variable and not syndrome specific [138,139]. Thus, treatment options must be based on the underlying pathophysiology. The natural history of OSA in children with micrognathia, and optimal therapy, has not been established.

OSA often improves during the first year of life, particularly in nonsyndromic Robin sequence [137]. However, worsening of OSA during the first few weeks of life has also been observed [135,137]. In addition, follow-up studies of micrognathic patients reveal that 65% have a history of chronic snoring or OSA [140]. Polysomnography has been used to demonstrate the acute resolution of OSA in 4 infants with the Pierre Robin sequence after tongue-lip adhesion [141]. Prone positioning [142], CPAP [10,143,144], nasopharyngeal stenting [142,145], adenotonsillectomy [137], and mandibular distraction [146,147] have also been successfully used to treat OSA in patients with micrognathia [135]. Late resolution of OSA associated with micrognathia has also been observed in a case report after mandibular growth occurring between 12 and 15 years of age [148].

Midface Hypoplasia

Syndromic craniosynostosis is characterized by abnormalities of the cranium, orbit, and midface. Airway anomalies are frequently present including choanal atresia, septal deviation, and pharyngeal narrowing. The prevalence of OSA in these children ranges from 24% to 88% of patients [149,150]. In 1 large series, 48% of patients with syndromic craniosynostosis required tracheotomy for airway obstruction [151]. The midface grows poorly in patients with syndromic craniosynostosis and OSA develops with increasing size of the tonsils and adenoids during childhood. As the lymphoid tissue decreases in size during late adolescence, there are reports of OSA resolution [152]. CPAP has been reported to successfully treat OSA in young children with Crouzon syndrome [152]. However, the external maxillary pressure posed by nasal CPAP may retard the growth of the midfacial bones [153]. Midfacial advancement has been reported to improve OSA in some patients, but not others [154–156].

Directions for Future Research

Though children with NMD have a high incidence of sleep-disordered breathing, there are little data available regarding diagnosis, consequences, and efficacy of treatment in this population. The threshold levels of OSA, hypercapnia, or hypoxemia that necessitate therapy have not been established using evidence-based criteria. In neurologically impaired children, it may be difficult to clearly distinguish the consequences of sleep-disordered breathing from the underlying disease, and therefore, proper treatment may be delayed. Better outcome measures for sleep-disordered breathing need to be developed including neurocognitive testing and serum markers for inflammation, oxidation, and autonomic dysfunction. Many neurologically impaired children also have craniofacial dysmorphology that precludes the use of commercially available masks.

The choice of therapy is predicated on the etiology, severity, natural history, and therapeutic options available for the OSA or hypoventilation. For OSA, most clinicians consider adenotonsillectomy the first-line treatment in the setting adenotonsillar hypertrophy. However, anti-inflammatory therapy with intranasal steroids and leukotriene antagonists is helpful in many cases. CPAP is generally reserved for children without surgically correctable obstruction, or significant residual OSA following other treatments. For hypoventilation, noninvasive positive pressure ventilation through a nasal or oro-nasal mask is recommended for symptomatic patients or those with daytime hypercapnia. Preliminary data suggest that the consequences of sleep-disordered breathing are at least partially reversible with appropriate therapy. However, there is concern that exposure to hypoxemia and hypercapnia during critical developmental intervals may result in lasting neurocognitive deficits.

Clinical Pearls

- Sleep-disordered breathing, including central apnea, hypoventilation, and obstructive sleep apnea, is common in children with NMD.
- Sleep-disordered breathing is associated with neurocognitive, cardiovascular, and metabolic impairment.
- Polysomnography is the gold standard for diagnosing sleep-disordered breathing.
- Treatment of respiratory insufficiency with noninvasive positive pressure ventilation improves sleep quality, gas exchange abnormalities, and daytime symptoms.
- The success of noninvasive ventilation is highly dependent on a well-fitting nasal or oro-nasal interface and proper titration of ventilator settings.

References

1. Goldbart AD, Goldman JL, Li RC, et al. Differential expression of cysteinyl leukotriene receptors 1 and 2 in tonsils of children with obstructive sleep apnea syndrome or recurrent infection. *Chest.* 2004;126:13–18.
2. Goldbart AD, Krishna J, Li RC, et al. Inflammatory mediators in exhaled condensate of children with obstructive sleep apnea syndrome. *Chest.* 2006;130:143–148.
3. Demain JG, Goetz DW. Pediatric adeniodal hypertrophy and nasal airway obstruction: reduction with aqueous nasal beclomethasone. *Pediatrics.* 1995;95:355–364.

4. Brouillette RT, Manoukian JJ, Ducharme FM, et al. Efficacy of fluticasone nasal spray for pediatric obstructive sleep apnea. *J Pediatr*. 2001;138: 838–844.
5. Kheirandish-Gozal L, Gozal D. Intranasal budesonide treatment for children with mild obstructive sleep apnea syndrome. *Pediatrics*. 2008;122:e149–e155.
6. Alexopoulos EI, Kaditis AG, Kalampouka E, et al. Nasal corticosteroids for children with snoring. *Pediatr Pulmonol*. 2004;38:161–167.
7. Criscuoli G, D'Amora S, Ripa G, et al. Frequency of surgery among children who have adenotonsillar hypertrophy and improve after treatment with nasal beclomethasone. *Pediatrics*. 2003;111(3): e236–e238.
8. Kheirandish L, Goldbart AD, Gozal D. Intranasal steroids and oral leukotriene modifier therapy in residual sleep-disordered breathing after tonsillectomy and adenoidectomy in children. *Pediatrics*. 2006;117:e61–e66.
9. Waters KA, Everett FM, Bruderer JW, Sullivan CE. Obstructive sleep apnea: the use of nasal CPAP in 80 children. *Am J Respir Crit Care Med*. 1995;152:780–785.
10. Marcus C, Ward SL, Mallory GM, et al. Use of nasal continuous positive airway pressure as treatment of childhood obstructive sleep apnea. *J Pediatr*. 2002;127:88–94.
11. Downey R III, Perkin RM, MacQuarrie J. Nasal continuous positive airway pressure use in children with obstructive sleep apnea younger than 2 years of age. *Chest*. 2000;117(6):1608–1612.
12. Rains J. Treatment of obstructive sleep apnea in pediatric patients. Behavioral intervention for compliance with nasal continuous positive airway pressure. *Clin Pediatr*. 1995;34:535–541.
13. Koontz KL, Slifer KJ, Cataldo MD, Marcus CL. Improving pediatric compliance with positive airway pressure therapy: the impact of behavioral intervention. *Sleep*. 2003;26(8):1010–1015.
14. Castorena-Maldonado A, Torre-Bouscoulet L, Meza-Vargas S, et al. Preoperative continuous positive airway pressure compliance in children with obstructive sleep apnea syndrome: assessed by a simplified approach. *Int J Pediatr Otorhinolaryngol*. 2008;72:1795–1800.
15. Marcus CL, Rosen G, Davidson-Ward SL, et al. Adherence to and effectiveness of positive airway pressure in children with obstructive sleep apnea. *Pediatrics*. 2006;117:e442–e451.
16. Marcus CL, Carroll JL, Bamford O, et al. Supplemental oxygen during sleep in children with sleep-disordered breathing. *Am J Respir Crit Care Med*. 1995;152:1297–1301.
17. Aljadeff G, Gozal D, Bailey-Wahl SL, et al. Effects of overnight supplemental oxygen in obstructive sleep apnea in children. *Am J Respir Crit Care Med*. 1996;153:51–55.
18. Colen TY, Seidman C, Weedon J, Goldstein NA. Effect of intracapsular tonsillectomy on quality of life for children with obstructive sleep-disordered breathing. *Arch Otolaryngol Head Neck Surg*. 2008;134:124–127.
19. Wei JL, Bond J, Mayo MS, et al. Improved behavior and sleep after adenoidectomy in children with sleep-disordered breathing: long-term follow-up. *Arch Otolaryngol Head Neck Surg*. 2009;135:642–646.
20. Dillon JE, Blunden S, Ruzicka DL, et al. DSM-IV diagnoses and obstructive sleep apnea in children before and 1 year after adenotonsillectomy. *J Am Acad Child Adolesc Psychiatry*. 2007;46: 1425–1436.
21. Nieminen P, Lopponen T, Tolonen U, et al. Growth and biochemical markers of growth in children with snoring and obstructive sleep apnea. *Pediatrics*. 2002;109:e55–e61.
22. Montgomery-Downs HE, Crabtree VM, Gozal D. Cognition, sleep and respiration in at-risk children treated for obstructive sleep apnea. *Eur Respir J*. 2005;25:216–217.
23. Friedman BC, Hendeles-Amitai A, Kozminsky E, et al. Adenotonsillectomy improves neurocognitive function in children with obstructive sleep apnea syndrome. *Sleep*. 2003;15:999–1005.
24. Gozal D. Sleep-disordered breathing and school performance in children. *Pediatrics*. 1998;102: 616–620.
25. Tauman R, Gulliver TE, Krishna J, et al. Persistence of obstructive sleep apnea syndrome in children after adenotonsillectomy. *J Pediatr*. 2006;149:803–808.
26. Guilleminault C, Huang Y, Glamann C, et al. Adenotonsillectomy and obstructive sleep apnea in children: a prospective survey. *Otolaryngol Head Neck Surg*. 2007;136:169–175.
27. Brietzke S, Kenna M, Katz ES, et al. Pediatric adenotonsillectomy: what is the effect of obstructive symptoms on the likelihood of future surgery? *Int J Pediatr Otorhinolaryngol*. 2006;70:1467–1472.
28. Cohen S, Simms C, Burstein F, Thomsen J. Alternatives to tracheostomy in infantsand children with obstructive sleep apnea. *J Pediatr Surg*. 1999;34(1):182–187.
29. Friedman M, Wilson M, Lin HC, Chang HW. Updated systemic review of tonsillectomy and adenoidectomy for treatment of pediatric obstructive sleep apnea/hypopnea syndrome. *Otolaryngol Head Neck Surg*. 2009;140:800–808.
30. Tami TA, Parker GS, Taylor RE. Post-tonsillectomy bleeding: an evaluation of risk factors. *Laryngoscope*. 1987;97:1307–1311.
31. Wilkinson AR, McCormick MS, Freeland AP, Pickering D. Electrocardiographic signs of pulmonary hypertension in children who snore. *Br Med J*. 1981;282:1579–1581.
32. Yates DW. Adenotonsillar hypertrophy and cor pulmonale. *Br J Anaesth*. 1988;61:355–359.
33. Nixon GM, Kermack AS, McGreagor CD, et al. Sleep and breathing on the first night after adenotonsillectomy for obstructive sleep apnea. *Pediatr Pulmonol*. 2005;39:332–338.
34. Helfaer MA, McColley SA, Pyzik PL, et al. Polysomnography after adenotonsillectomy in

mild pediatric obstructive sleep apnea. *Crit Care Med*. 1996;24:1323–1327.
35. Rosen GM, Muckle RP, Mahowald MW, Goding GS, Ullevig C. Post-operative respiratory compromise in children with obstructive sleep apnea syndrome: can it be anticipated? *Pediatrics*. 1994;93:784–788.
36. Ruboyianes JM, Cruz RM. Pediatric adenotonsillectomy for obstructive sleep apnea. *Ear Nose Throat J*. 1996;75:430–433.
37. Pirelli P, Saponara M, Guilleminault C. Rapid maxillary expansion in children with obstructive sleep apnea syndrome. *Sleep*. 2004;27:761–766.
38. Pirelli P, Saponara M, Attanasio G. Obstructive sleep apnoea syndrome (OSAS) and rhino-tubaric disfunction in children: therapeutic effects of RME therapy. *Prog Ortho*. 2005;6:48–61.
39. Villa MP, Malagola C, Pagani J, et al. Rapid maxillary expansion in children withobstructive sleep apnea syndrome: 12-month follow-up. *Sleep Med*. 2007;8:128–134.
40. Villa MP, Bernkopf E, Pagani J, et al. Randomized controlled study of an oral jaw-positioning appliance for the treatment of obstructive sleep apnea in children with malocclusion. *Am J Respir Crit Care Med*. 2002;165:123–127.
41. Cozza P, Gatto R, Ballanti F, Prete L. Management of obstructive sleep apnoea in children with modified monobloc appliances. *Eur J Pediatr Dent*. 2004;5:24–29.
42. Emerson E. Overweight and obesity in 3- and 5-year-old children with and without developmental delay. *Public Health*. 2009;123:130–133.
43. Urschitz MS, Guenther A, Eitner S, et al. Risk factors and natural history of habitual snoring. *Chest*. 2004;126:790–800.
44. Marcus CL, Curtis S, Koerner CB, et al. Evaluation of pulmonary function and polysomnography in obese children and adolescents. *Pediatr Pulmonol*. 1996;21:176–183.
45. Silvestri JM, Weese-Meyer DE, Bass MT, et al. Polysomnography in obese children with a history of sleep-associated breathing disorders. *Pediatr Pulmonol*. 1993;16:124–129.
46. Dayyat E, Kheirandish-Gozal L, Capdevila OS, et al. Obstructive sleep apnea in children. Relative contributions of body mass index and adenotonsillar hypertrophy. *Chest*. 2009;136:137–144.
47. Dayyat E, Maarafeya MMA, Capdevila OS, et al. Nocturnal body position in sleeping children with and without obstructive sleep apnea. *Pediatr Pulmonol*. 2007;42:374–379.
48. Shine NP, Lannigan FJ, Coates HL, Wilson A. Adenotonsillectomy for obstructive sleep apnea in obese children: effects on respiratory parameters and clinical outcome. *Arch Otolaryngol Head Neck Surg*. 2006;132:1123–1127.
49. Willi SM, Oexmann MJ, Wright NM, et al. The effects of a high protein, low-fat, ketogenic diet on adolescents with morbid obesity: body compensation, blood chemistries, and sleep abnormalities. *Pediatrics*. 1998;101:61–67.
50. Verhulst SL, Franckx H, Van Gaal L, et al. The effect of weight loss on sleep-disordered breathing in obese teenagers. *Obesity*. 2009;17:1178–1183.
51. Kalra M, Inge T, Garcia V, et al. Obstructive sleep apnea in extremely overweight adolescents undergoing bariatric surgery. *Obes Res*. 2005;13:1175–1179.
52. Raphael JC, Chevret S, Chastang C, Bouvet F. Randomised trial of preventive nasal ventilation in Duchenne muscular dystrophy. *Lancet*. 1994;343:1600–1604.
53. Meyer TJ, Pressman MR, Benditt J, et al. Air leaking through the mouth during nocturnal nasal ventilation: effect on sleep quality. *Sleep*. 1997;20:561–569.
54. Sanders MH, Kern NB, Costantino JP, et al. Accuracy of end-tidal and transcutaneous PCO2 monitoring during sleep. *Chest*. 1994;106(2):472–483.
55. Masa JF, Celli BR, Riesco JA, d et al. Noninvasive positive pressure ventilation and not oxygen may prevent overt ventilatory failure in patients with chest wall diseases. *Chest*. 1997;112(1):207–213.
56. Windisch W, Dreher M, Storre JH, Sorichter S. Nocturnal non-invasive positive pressure ventilation: physiological effects on spontaneous breathing. *Respir Physiol Neurobiol*. 2006;150(2–3):251–260.
57. Barbe F, Quera-Salva MA, de Lattre J, et al. Long-term effects of nasal intermittent positive-pressure ventilation on pulmonary function and sleep architecture in patients with neuromuscular diseases. *Chest*. 1996;110:1179–1183.
58. Hill NS, Eveloff SE, Carlisle CC, Goff SG. Efficacy of nocturnal nasal ventilation in patients with restrictive thoracic disease. *Am Rev Respir Dis*. 1992;145:365–371.
59. Laserna E, Barrot E, Beiztegui A, et al. Non-invasive ventilation in kyphoscoliosis. A comparison of a volumetric ventilator and a BIPAP support pressure device. *Arch Bronconeumol*. 2003;39:13–18.
60. Ellis ER, Bye PTP, Bruderer JW, Sullivan CE. Treatment of respiratory failure during sleep in patients with neuromuscular disease. Positive-pressure ventilation through a nose mask. *Am Rev Respir Dis*. 1987;135:148–152.
61. Weese-Mayer DE, Berry-Kravis EM, Ceccherini I, et al. An official ATS clinical policy statement: congenital central hypoventilation syndrome: genetic basis, diagnosis, and management. *Am J Respir Crit Care Med*. 2010;181(6):626–644.
62. Repetto GM, Corrales RJ, Abara SG, et al. Later-onset congenital central hypoventilation syndrome due to a heterozygous 24-polyalanine repeat expansion mutation in the PHOX2B gene. *Acta Paediatr*. 2009;98:190–198.
63. Fine-Goulden MR, Manna S, Durward A. Cor pulmonale due to congenital central hypoventilation syndrome presenting in adolescence. *Pediatr Crit Care Med*. 2009;10:e41–e42.

64. Weese-Mayer DE, Berry-Kravis EM, Zhou L. Adult identified with congenital central hypoventilation syndrome-mutation in PHOX2B gene and late-onset CHS. *Am J Respir Crit Care Med.* 2005;171:88.
65. Antic NA, Malow BA, Lange N, et al. PHOX2B mutation-confirmed congenital central hypoventilation syndrome: presentation in adulthood. *Am J Respir Crit Care Med.* 2006;174(8):923–927.
66. Silvestri JM, Weese-Mayer DE, Flanagan EA. Congenital central hypoventilation syndrome: cardiorespiratory responses to moderate exercise, simulating daily activity. *Pediatr Pulmonol.* 1995;20(2):89–93.
67. Chen ML, Tablizo MA, Kun S, Keens TG. Diaphram pacers as a treatment for congenital central hypoventilation syndrome. *Expert Rev Med Devices.* 2005;2:577–585.
68. Chen ML, Turkel SB, Jacobson JR, Keens TG. Alcohol use in congenital central hypoventilation syndrome. *Pediatr Pulmonol.* 2006;41:283–285.
69. Straus C, Trang H, Becquemin MH, Touraine P, Similowski T. Chemosensitivity recovery in Ondine's curse syndrome under treatment with desogestrel. *Respir Physiol Neurobiol.* 2010; Epub ahead of print.
70. Julu POO, Kerr AM, Apartopoulos F, et al. Characterization of breathing and associated central autonomic dysfunction in the RETT disorder. *Arch Dis Child.* 2001;85:29–37.
71. d'Orsi G, Demaio V, Scarpelli F, et al. Central sleep apnoea in Rett syndrome. *Neurol Sci.* 2009; 30:389–391.
72. Marcus CL, Carroll JL, McColley SA, et al. Polysomnographic characteristics of patients with Rett syndrome. *J Pediatr.* 1994;125:218–224.
73. Anzai Y, Ohya T. A case of effective gastrostomy for severe abdominal distention due to breathing dysfunction of Rett's syndrome: a treatment of autonomic disorder. *Brain Dev.* 2001;23: S240–S241.
74. Kerr AM, Julu POO, Hansen S, Apartopoulos F. Serotonin and breathing dysrhythmia in Rett syndrome. In: Perat MV, ed. *New Developments in Child Neurology.* Bologna: Monduzzi Editore; 1998:191–195.
75. Priano L, Grugni G, Miscio G, et al. Sleep cycling alternating pattern (CAP) expression is associated with hypersomnia and GH secretory pattern in Prader-Willi syndrome. *Sleep Med.* 2006;7:627–633.
76. Cotton S, Richdale A. Brief report: parental descriptions of sleep problems in children with autism, Down syndrome, and Prader-Willi syndrome. *Res Dev Disabil.* 2003;27(2):151–161.
77. Hertz G, Cataletto M, Feinsilver SH, Angulo M. Sleep and breathing patterns in patients with Prader-Willi syndrome (PWS): effects of age and gender. *Sleep.* 1993;16:366–371.
78. Hertz G, Cataletto M, Feinsilver SH, Angulo M. Developmental trends of sleep-disordered breathing in Prader-Willi syndrome. *Am J Med Gen.* 1995;56:188–190.
79. Harris JC, Allen RP. Is excessive daytime sleepiness characteristic of Prader-Willi syndrome? The effects of weight change. *Arch Pediatr Adolesc Med.* 1996;150(12):1288–1293.
80. Nevsimalova S, Vankova J, Stepanova I, et al. Hypocretin deficiency in Prader-Willi syndrome. *Eur J Neurol.* 2005;12:70–72.
81. O'Donoghue F, Camfferman D, Kennedy J, et al. Sleep-disordered breathing in Prader-Willi syndrome and its associations with neurobehavioral abnormalities. *J Pediatr.* 2005;147:823–829.
82. Festen DAM, Wevers M, de Weerd AW, et al. Psychomotor development in infants with Prader-Willi syndrome and associations with sleep-related breathing disorders. *Pediatr Res.* 2007;62: 221–224.
83. Schluter B, Buschatz D, Trowitzsch E, et al. Respiratory control in children with Prader-Willi syndrome. *Eur J Pediatr.* 1997;156:65–68.
84. Festen DAM, de Weerd AW, van den Bossche RAS, J et al. Sleep-related breathing disorders in prepubertal children with Prader-Willi syndrome and effects of growth hormone treatment. *J Clin Endocrinol Metab.* 2006;91(12):4911–4915.
85. Arens R, Gozal D, Burrell BC, et al. Arousal and cardiorespiratory responses to hypoxia in Prader-Willi syndrome. *Am J Respir Crit Care Med.* 1996;153(1):283–287.
86. Miller J, Silverstein J, Shuster J, et al. Short-Term Effects of Growth Hormone on Sleep Abnormalities in Prader-Willi syndrome. *J Clin Endocrinol Metab.* 2006;91(2):413–417.
87. Smith IE, King MA, Siklos PWL, Shneerson JM. Treatment of ventilatory failure in the Prader-Willi syndrome. *Eur Respir J.* 1998;11:1150–1152.
88. Vgontzas AN, Bixler EO, Kales A, Vela-Bueno A. Prader-Willi syndrome: effects of weight loss on sleep-disordered breathing, daytime sleepiness and REM sleep disturbance. *Acta Pediatr.* 1995;84:813–814.
89. Clift S, Dahlitz M, Parkes JD. Sleep apnoea in the Prader-Willi syndrome. *J Sleep Res.* 1994;3:121–126.
90. Carrel AL, Myers SE, Whitman BY, Allen DB. Growth hormone improves body composition, fat utilization, physical strength and agility, and growth in Prader-Willi syndrome: a controlled study. *J Pediatr.* 1999;134:215–221.
91. Lindgren AC, Hellstrom LG, Ritzen EM, Milerad J. Growth hormone treatment increases CO2 response, ventilation and central inspiratory drive in children with Prader-Willi syndrome. *Eur J Pediatr.* 1999;158:936–940.
92. Eiholzer U, Nordmann Y, L'Allemand D. Fatal outcome of sleep apnoea in PWS during the initial phase of growth hormone treatment. A case report. *Horm Res.* 2002;58:24–26.
93. Haqq AM, Stadler DD, Jackson RH, et al. Effects of growth hormone on pulmonary function, sleep quality, behavior, cognition, growth velocity, body composition, and resting energy expenditure in Prader-Willi syndrome. *J Clin Endocrinol Metab.* 2003;88(5):2206–2212.

94. Goldstone AP, Holland AJ, Hauffa BP, et al. On behalf of speakers contributors at the second expert meeting of the comprehensive care of patients with PWS. Recommendations for the diagnosis and management of Prader-Willi syndrome. *J Clin Endocrinol Metab*. 2008;93(11):4183–4197.
95. Martinot A, Hue V, Leclerc F, Vallee L, Closset M, Pruvo JP. Sudden death revealing chiari type 1 malformation in two children. *Intensive Care Med*. 1993;19:73–74.
96. Dauilliers Y, Stal V, Abril B, et al. Chiari malformation and sleep related breathing disorders. *J Neurol Neurosurg Psychiatry*. 2007;78:1344–1348.
97. Waters KA, Forbes P, Morielli A, et al. Sleep-disordered breathing in children with myelomeningocele. *J Pediatr*. 1998;132:672–681.
98. Ward SLD, Jacobs RA, Gates EP, et al. Abnormal ventilatory patterns during sleep in infants with myelomeningocele. *J Pediatr*. 1986;109:631–634.
99. Cochrane DD, Adderley R, White CP, Norman M, Steinbok P, et al. Apnea in patients with myelomeningocele. *Pediatr Neurosurg*. 1990;16:232–239.
100. Murray C, Seton C, Prelog K, Fitzgerald DA. Arnold Chiari type 1 malformation presenting with sleep disordered breathing in well children. *Arch Dis Child*. 2006;91:342–343.
101. Park TS, Hoffman HJ, Hendrick EB, Humpheys RP. Experience with surgical decompression of the Arnold-Chiari malformation in young infants with myelomeningocele. *Neurosurgery*. 1983;13:147–152.
102. Pollack IF, Kinnunen D, Albright AL. The effect of early craniocervical decompression on functional outcome in neonates and young infants with myelodysplasia and symptomatic Chiari II malformations: results from a prospective series. *Neurosurgery*. 1996;38:703–710.
103. Bell WO, Charney EB, Bruce DA, Sutton LN, Schut L. Symptomatic Arnold-Chiari malformation: review of experience with 22 cases. *J Neurosurg*. 1987; 66:812–816.
104. Gagnadoux F, Meslier N, Svab I, Menei P, Racineux JL. Sleep-disordered breathing in patients with Chiari malformation: improvement after surgery. *Neurology*. 2006;66:136–138.
105. Zolty P, Sanders MH, Pollack IF. Chiari malformation and sleep-disordered breathing: a review of diagnostic and management issues. *Sleep*. 2000;23:1–7.
106. Tomita T, Mclone DG. Acute respiratory arrest: a complication of malformation of the shunt in children with myelomeningocele and Arnold-Chiari malformation. *Am J Dis Child*. 1983;137: 142–144.
107. Newman CJ, O'Regan M, Hensey O. Sleep disorders in children with cerebral palsy. *Dev Med Child Neurol*. 2006;48(07):564–568.
108. Kotogal S, Gibbons VP, Stith JA. Sleep abnormalities in patients with severe cerebral palsy. *Dev Med Child Neurol*. 1994;36:304–311.
109. Hemmingsson H, Stenhammar AM, Paulsson K. Sleep problems and the need for parental night-time attention in children with physical disabilities. *Child Care, Health Dev*. 2008;35(1):89–95.
110. Hsiao KH, Nixon GM. The effect of treatment of obstructive sleep apnea on quality of life in children with cerebral palsy. *Res Dev Disabil*. 2003;29(2):133–140.
111. Stebbens VA, Dennis J, Samuels MP, Croft CB, Southall DP. Sleep related upper airway obstruction in a cohort with Down's syndrome. *Arch Dis Child*. 1991;66:1333–1338.
112. Marcus CL, Keens TG, Bautista DB, von Pechmann WS, Ward SL. Obstructive sleep apnea in children with down syndrome. *Pediatrics*. 1991;88:132–139.
113. Trois MS, Capone GT, Lutz JA, et al. Obstructive sleep apnea in adults with down syndrome. *J Clin Sleep Med*. 2009;5(4):317–323.
114. Fitzgerald DA, Paul A, Richmond C. Severity of obstructive apnoea in children with down syndrome who snore. *Arch Dis Child*. 2007; 92(5):423–425.
115. Ng DK, Hui HN, Chan CH, et al. Obstructive sleep apnoea in children with down syndrome. *Singapore Med J*. 2006;47(9):774–779.
116. Dyken ME, Lin-Dyken DC, Poulton S, Zimmerman MB, Sedars E. Prospective polysomnographic analysis of obstructive sleep apnea in down syndrome. *Arch Pediatr Adolesc Med*. 2003;157:655–660.
117. Jacobs IN, Gray RF, Todd NW. Upper airway obstruction in children with down syndrome. *Arch Otolaryngol Head Neck Surg*. 1996;122:945–950.
118. Shete MM, Stocks RM, Sebelik ME, Schoumacher RA. Effects of adeno-tonsillectomy on polysomnography patterns in down syndrome children with obstructive sleep apnea: a comparative study with children without down syndrome. *Int J Pediatr Otolaryngol*. 2010;74:241–244.
119. Donaldson JD, Redmond WM. Surgical management of obstructive sleep apnea in children with down syndrome. *J Otolaryngol*. 1988;17:398–403.
120. Donnelly LF, Shott SR, LaRose CR, et al. Causes of persistent obstructive sleep apnea despite previous tonsillectomy and adenoidectomy in children with down syndrome as depicted on static and dynamic cine MRI. *AJR Am J Roentgenol*. 2004;183(1):175–181.
121. Shott SR, Donnelly LF. Cine magnetic resonance imaging: evaluation of persistent airway obstruction after tonsil and adenoidectomy in children with down syndrome. *Laryngoscope*. 2004;114:1724–1729.
122. Goldstein NA, Armfield DR, Kingsley LA, Borland LM, Allen GC, Post JC. Postoperative complications after tonsillectomy and adenoidectomy in children with down syndrome. *Arch Otolaryngol Head Neck Surg*. 1998;124:171–176.
123. de Moura CP, Andrade D, Cunha LM, et al. Down syndrome: otolaryngological effects of rapid maxillary expansion. *J Laryngol Otolaryngol*. 2008;122:1318–1324.
124. Mitchell RB, Call E, Kelly J. Diagnosis and therapy for airway obstruction in children with down

syndrome. *Arch Otolaryngol Head Neck Surg.* 2003;129(6):642–645.
125. Suresh S, Wales P, Dakin C, Harris MA, Cooper DG. Sleep-related breathing disorder in Duchenne muscular dystrophy: disease spectrum in the paediatric population. *J Paediatr Child Health.* 2005;41:500–503.
126. Barbe F, Quera-Salva MA, McCann C, et al. Sleep-related respiratory disturbances in patients with Duchenne muscular dystrophy. *Eur Respir J.* 1994;7:1403–1408.
127. Manni R, Ottolini A, Cerveri I, et al. Breathing patterns and HbSaO2 changes during nocturnal sleep in patients with Duchenne muscular dystrophy. *J Neurol.* 1989;236:391–394.
128. Smith PEM, Calverley PMA, Edwards RHT. Hypoxemia during sleep in Duchenne muscular dystrophy. *Am Rev Respir Dis.* 1988;137:884–888.
129. Smith PEM, Edwards RHT, Calverley PMA. Oxygen treatment of sleep hypoxaemia in Duchenne muscular dystrophy. *Thorax.* 1989; 44:997–1001.
130. Simonds AK, Muntoni F, Heather S, Fielding S. Impact of nasal ventilation on survival in hypercapnic Duchenne muscular dystrophy. *Thorax.* 1998;53:949–952.
131. Raphael JC. Home mechanical ventilation and Duchenne's muscular dystrophy. In: Cornelio F, Lanzi G, Fedrizzi E, eds. *Neuromuscular Diseases During Development.* London, UK: John Libbey & Company Ltd; 1997:113–122.
132. Mohr CH, Hill NS. Long-tern follow-up of nocturnal ventilatory assistance in patients with respiratory failure due to Duchenne-type muscular dystrophy. *Chest.* 1990;97:91–96.
133. Mellies U, Dohna-Schwake C, Stehling F, Voit T. Sleep disordered breathing in spinal muscular atrophy. *Neuromusc Disord.* 2004;14(12): 797–803.
134. Mellies U, Ragette R, Dohna Schwake C, Boehm H, Voit T, Teschler H. Long-term noninvasive ventilation in children and adolescents with neuromuscular disorders. *Eur Respir J.* 2003;22(4):631–636.
135. Bull MJ, Givan DC, Sadove M, Bixler D, Hearn D. Improved outcome in Pierre Robin sequence: effect of multidisciplinary evaluation and management. *Pediatrics.* 1990;86:294–301.
136. Shprintzen RJ. The implications of the diagnosis of Robin sequence. *Cleft Palate Craniofacial J.* 1992;29:205–209.
137. Perkins JA, Sie KC, Milczuk H, Richardson MA. Airway management in children with craniofacial anomalies. *Cleft Palate Craniofacial J.* 1997; 34:135–140.
138. Sher AE. Mechanisms of airway obstruction in Robin sequence: implications for treatment. *Cleft Palate Craniofacial J.* 1992;29:224–231.
139. Sher AE, Shprintzen RJ, Thorpy MJ. Endoscopic observations of obstructive sleep apnea in children with anomalous upper airways: predictive and therapeutic value. *Int J Pediatr Otorhinolaryngol.* 1986;11:135–146.
140. Spier S, Rivlin J, Rowe RD, Egan T. Sleep in Pierre Robin syndrome. *Chest.* 1986;90:711–715.
141. Freed G, Pearlman MA, Brown AS, Barot LR. Polysomnographic indications for surgical intervention in Pierre Robin sequence: acute airway management and follow-up studies after repair and take-down of tongue-lip adhesion. *Cleft Palate J.* 1998;25:151–155.
142. Tomaski SM, Zalzal GH, Saal HM. Airway obstruction in the Pierre Robin sequence. *Laryngoscope.* 1995;105:111–114.
143. Miller SD, Glynn SF, Kiely JL, McNicholas WT. The role of nasal CPAP in obstructive sleep apnoea syndrome due to mandibular hypoplasia. *Respirology.* 2010;15(2):377–379.
144. Deegan PC, McGlone B, McNicholas WT. Treatment of Robin sequence with nasal CPAP. *J Laryngol Otolaryngol.* 1995;109:328–330.
145. Heaf DP, Helms PJ, Dinwiddie R, Matthew DJ. Nasopharyngeal airways in Pierre Robin syndrome. *J Pediatr.* 1982;100:698–703.
146. Denny AD, Talisman R, Hanson PR, Recinos RF. Mandibular distraction osteogenesis in very young patients to correct airway obstruction. *Plast Reconstr Surg.* 2001;108:302–311.
147. Genecov DG, Barcelo CR, Steinberg D, Trone T, Sperry E. Clinical experience with the application of distraction osteogenesis for airway obstruction. *J Craniofac Surg.* 2009;20(suppl 2):1817–1821.
148. Kiely JL, Deegan PC, McNicholas WT. Resolution of obstructive sleep apnea with growth in the Robin sequence. *Eur Respir J.* 1998;12:499–501.
149. Moore MH. Upper airway obstruction in the syndromal craniosynostoses. *Br J Plast Surg.* 1993; 46:355–362.
150. Kakitsuba N, Sadaoka T, Motoyama S, et al. Sleep apnea and sleep-related breathing disorders in patients with craniofacial synostosis. *Acta Otolaryngol.* 1994;17(suppl 5):6–10.
151. Sculerati N, Gottlieb MD, Zimbler MS, et al. Airway management in children with craniofacial anomalies. *Laryngoscope.* 1998;108:1806–1812.
152. Hui S, Wing YK, Kew J, Chan YL, Abdullah V, Fok TF. Obstructive sleep apnea syndrome in a family with Crouzon's syndrome. *Sleep.* 1998;21:298–303.
153. Li KK, Riley RW, Guilleminault C. An unreported risk in the use of home nasal continuous positive airway pressure and home nasal ventilation in children. *Chest.* 2000;117:916–918.
154. Lauritzen C, lilja J, Jarlstedt J. Airway obstruction and sleep apnoea in children craniofacial anomalies. *Plast Reconstr Surg.* 1986;77:1–5.
155. McCarthy JG, Glasberg SB, Cutting CB, et al. Twenty-year experience with early surgery for craniosynostosis:II. The craniofacial synostosis syndromes and pansynostosis—results and unsolved problems. *Plast Reconstr Surg.* 1995;96: 284–295.
156. Mitsukawa N, Satoh K. Midfacial distraction using a transfacial pinning technique for Syndromic craniosynostosis with obstructive respiratory disorders. *J Plast Reconstr Aesthet Surg.* In Press.

CHAPTER 17

Congenital Central Hypoventilation Syndrome

Debra E. Weese-Mayer, Pallavi P. Patwari, Michael S. Carroll, and Casey M. Rand

Introduction

Congenital Central Hypoventilation Syndrome (CCHS) is characterized by alveolar hypoventilation, disordered respiratory control, and anatomic and physiologic autonomic nervous system (ANS) dysregulation. Recall that the ANS is a multisystem regulatory branch of the peripheral nervous system, primarily functioning outside of conscious control (see Figure 17.1). CCHS is diagnosed in the absence of primary lung, cardiac, or neuromuscular disease or an identifiable brainstem lesion that might account for the *entire* phenotype inclusive of the ANS dysregulation (ANSD) [1]. Individuals with CCHS have diminutive tidal volumes and monotonous respiratory rates during asleep, and during wakefulness and sleep in more severe cases [1]. The hypoventilation during sleep is more severe than that which occurs during wakefulness. Consequently, individuals with CCHS become hypoxemic and hypercarbic; yet they lack ventilatory and arousal responsiveness to these endogenous ventilatory derangements during sleep as well as the perception of asphyxia during wakefulness at rest and with exercise [1]. The ANSD present in CCHS includes anatomic disorders (Hirschsprung Disease and tumors of neural crest origin) as well as physiologic dysfunction (diminished pupillary light response, esophageal dysmotility, severe breath-holding spells, reduced basal body temperature, sporadic profuse sweating, lack of

Key Points

- A *PHOX2B* mutation is required to make the diagnosis of CCHS. Knowledge of the specific *PHOX2B* mutation aids in the anticipated phenotype, including severity of the ventilatory control disorder, risk of sudden cardiac death, and risk of associated disorders, such as Hirschsprung disease, neural crest tumors as well as other adverse consequences.
- Parents of CCHS patients should be tested for the *PHOX2B* mutation to determine the risk of passing the *PHOX2B* mutation and CCHS on to their children (future siblings of the CCHS patient) and to assess their own risk of ANSD, possibly requiring medical intervention.
- While considerable evidence exists indicating that specific *PHOX2B* mutations dictate the severity of the disease, future studies to better understand how the *PHOX2B* genotype/mutation dictates and correlates with the CCHS phenotype are warranted.
- Because the biology of CCHS is not completely understood, it is hoped that families of the few CCHS patients who die will agree to autopsy, which can provide tissues to further identify and delineate biologic abnormalities. These tissues would include frozen (not fixed) brain, brainstem, carotid and aortic bodies, adrenal glands, autonomic plexus, sympathetic chain, and the entire gut.

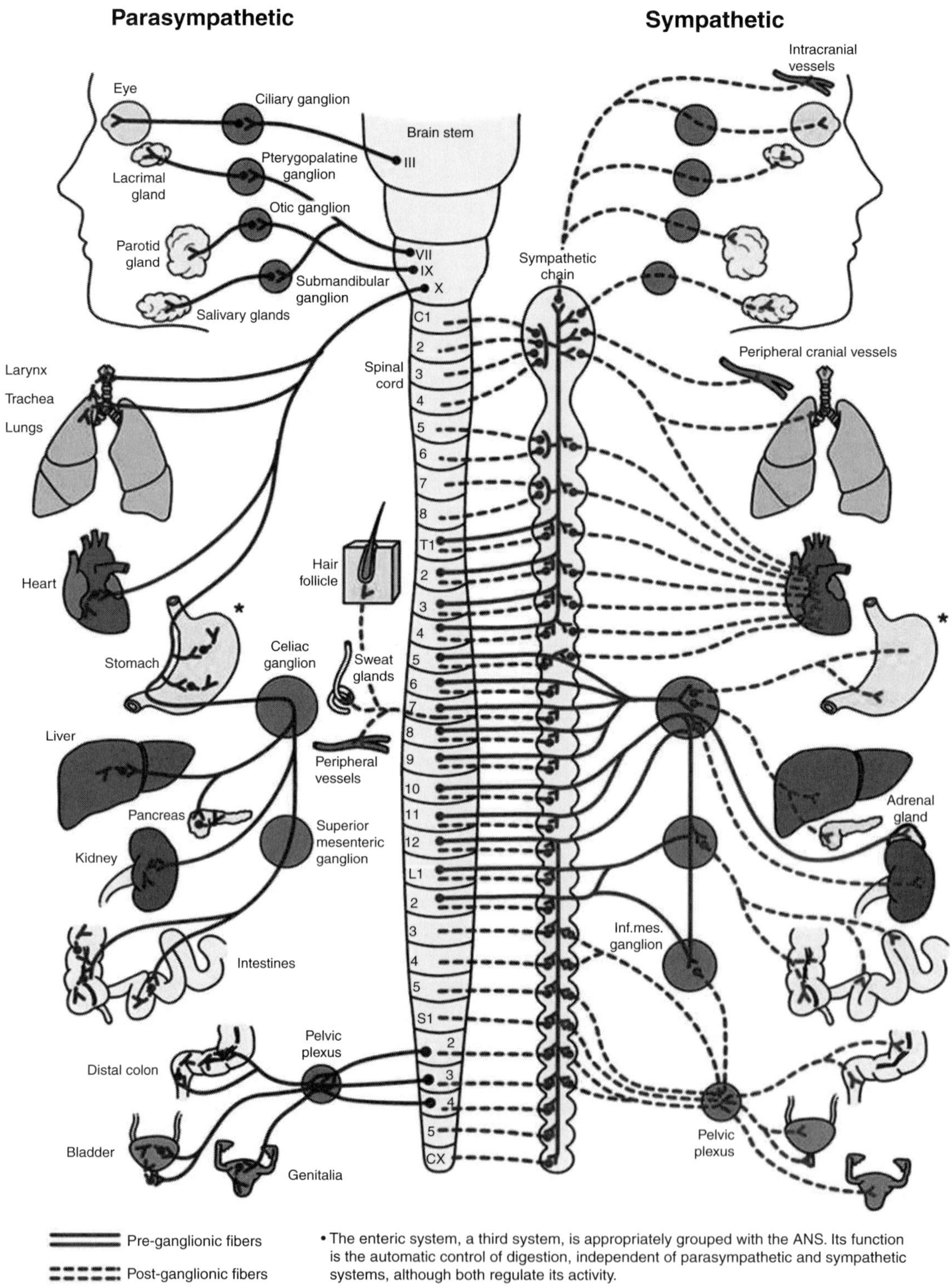

Figure 17.1 The ANS is part of the peripheral nervous system that functions "automatically" (involuntarily) to control various systems of the body and is subdivided into the parasympathetic, sympathetic, and enteric nervous systems. Detailed here are some of the targets specific to the parasympathetic nervous system and the sympathetic nervous system. Reproduced with permission from Ref. [36].

perception to dyspnea, altered perception of anxiety, and lack of adequate respiratory and cardiac physiologic responsiveness to the challenges of exercise and environmental stressors) [1–15].

Dr. Robert Mellins and colleagues described what we now identify as the first reported case of CCHS in 1970 [16]. By 1999, the year of the first American Thoracic Society (ATS) Statement on CCHS, we estimated 160 to 180 living children with CCHS worldwide, though anticipated that this was an underestimate [1]. The extent of this underestimate has since been confirmed with the 2010 ATS statement on CCHS reporting nearly 1000 cases of genetically confirmed CCHS worldwide [17]. However, the actual incidence of CCHS in the general population remains unknown.

PHOX2B: The Disease-Defining Gene for CCHS

A few publications between the 1980s and 2001 identified recurrence of the CCHS phenotype within families: monozygotic female twins [18], sisters [19], male-female siblings [2,20], and male-female half siblings [21]. Soon thereafter, reports of women diagnosed with CCHS, giving birth to infants with CCHS, suggested an autosomal dominant inheritance pattern [22,23]. Also reported was a case of a woman diagnosed with neuroblastoma in her own childhood who gave birth to a child with CCHS [24], supporting the likelihood of a transmitted genetic component. Subsequently, additional evidence for a genetic basis to CCHS and ANSD was provided by segregation analysis studied in a case-control family design [3,4], implicating CCHS as the most severe manifestation of a general ANSD [1,20]. Early genetic studies were restricted to genes related to Hirschsprung disease (HSCR) with limited significant findings. However, a breakthrough occurred when candidate gene research turned toward genes involved with ANS development. In 2003 and 2004 several groups undertaking autonomic-focused, CCHS candidate gene analysis reported variations in the paired-like homeobox 2B (*PHOX2B*) gene as associated with the disease [25–28].

PHOX2B encodes a highly conserved homeodomain transcription factor; it plays a key role in early embryologic development of ANS reflex circuits in mice [29,30] and has expression in both central autonomic neuron circuits and peripheral neural crest derivatives in the human embryo [25]. There are 2 polyalanine repeat regions in the *PHOX2B* gene. The second region, normally occurring with 20 alanines in exon 3 of *PHOX2B*, is the site of most of the CCHS-related mutations. In 2003, Amiel et al reported in-frame expansions of 25 to 29 alanines on the affected allele in 18 of 29 (62%) French CCHS cases and frameshift mutations in 2 of the 29 cases (7%); taken together, 69% of the 29 French patients were heterozygous for a *PHOX2B* mutation [25]. None of the identified *PHOX2B* mutations were found in matched controls [25]. Also in 2003, Weese-Mayer et al [28] reported on genes critical to the early embryology of the ANS in CCHS. Among the 67 CCHS cases studied, 100% of cases were heterozygous for a mutation in the *PHOX2B* gene [28]: 65 cases had polyalanine repeat expansion mutations (PARMs) in exon 3 that included 25 to 33 alanine repeats, 1 child had a *PHOX2B* non-PARM (NPARM) nonsense mutation (premature stop codon), and 1 child was later found to have a PARM, after resolution of a sample mix-up at the lab of origin [31]. Again, none of the control subjects had a mutation in the *PHOX2B* gene. This study identified *PHOX2B* as the disease-defining gene in CCHS. However, a subsequent report by Sasaki et al [27] in 2003 identified only 4 PARMs and 1 NPARM among 10 CCHS cases in Japan (50%).

The discrepancy in the proportion of CCHS cases caused by mutations in the *PHOX2B* gene would be clarified the next year. In 2004, Matera et al in Italy [26] confirmed the heterozygous *PHOX2B* PARM of 25 to 33 alanines in 21 of 24 CCHS cases and an NPARM frameshift mutation in 2 of the 3 remaining CCHS cases from Italy, Germany, and the Netherlands (23/24 cases, 96%). Matera et al were also able to explain the lower identification rate with the methodology used in the 2003 studies by Amiel et al and Sasaki et al. Specifically, they demonstrated the problem of amplification-induced allele drop out; in standard PCR reactions, the expanded allele with the greater number of alanines can remain undetected because of the difficulty in amplifying the expanded, guanine–cytosine (GC)-rich polyalanine region of the *PHOX2B* gene. This was confirmed when the French and Japanese cohorts were restudied with a new assay designed to amplify GC-rich regions; Horiuchi et al [32] identified a *PHOX2B* mutation in 90% of

10 Japanese cases (identifying *PHOX2B* mutations in 4/5 samples previously reported as *PHOX2B* mutation-negative [27]), and Trochet et al [33] identified a *PHOX2B* mutation in 93% of 174 subjects with CCHS from multiple nationalities (identifying *PHOX2B* mutations in 7/9 samples previously reported as *PHOX2B* mutation-negative [25]).

Berry-Kravis et al [31] and Weese-Mayer et al [34] later reported *PHOX2B* mutations in 184 subjects (in 2006) and collectively more than 350 subjects (in 2008) with CCHS, respectively, (100% sensitivity and specificity of detection), in a cohort primarily from the United States, with 10% of patients from abroad. Collectively, these studies show that *PHOX2B* is the disease-defining gene in CCHS. No novel disease-causing mutations have been found specific to CCHS in any of the other studied genes. Further, Weese-Mayer et al [28] established the first clinically available assay for the diagnosis of CCHS using a simple and accurate method for detecting and sizing the repeat sequence associated with the polyalanine tract expansion (patented; *PHOX2B* Screening Test proceeds support CCHS research), which could also be used for prenatal diagnosis, family testing, and diagnosis of individuals with relevant symptoms.

At the time of this writing, and as we recently summarized [17,35,36], there are approximately 1000 *PHOX2B* mutation-confirmed cases of CCHS worldwide. The range for number of repeats in the *PHOX2B* PARMs on the affected allele is 24 to 33 [25–28,31,33,37–47], producing genotypes of 20/24 to 20/33 (the normal genotype would be referred to as 20/20). PARMs account for the *PHOX2B* mutation in over 90% of CCHS cases. The 20/25, 20/26, and 20/27 genotypes remain the most common of the *PHOX2B* mutations (see Figure 17.2)[17,36]. The remaining patients, typically with the most severe CCHS phenotype, will be heterozygous for an NPARM, including missense, nonsense, and frameshift mutations in the *PHOX2B* gene (~10% of cases). NPARMs have been reported in the United States [28,31,34,36,48], Italy [26,43,49], Japan [27], France [25,33,44,50], Germany [41,51,52], Australia [53], the Netherlands [54], Taiwan [39,55], and China [56]. The 76 reported NPARMs include frame-shift 59/76, 78%), nonsense (3/76, 4%), missense (12/76, 16%), and missense with stop codon alteration (2/76, 3%) mutations (see Figure 17.3). The majority of CCHS-associated NPARMs are found at the end of exon 2 or in exon 3 (see Figure 17.3). Identified CCHS-causing mutations were not found in any of 482 controls reported in the literature, nor among 1520 healthy individuals in Taiwan [39].

PHOX2B Genotype/CCHS Phenotype

A growing body of literature supports a graded relationship between the *PHOX2B* mutation/genotype and the CCHS phenotype. Consequently, it is essential for all future publications to confirm the diagnosis of CCHS with *PHOX2B* testing and to analyze the data stratified by mutation/genotype. Data as of this writing are provided in the following section.

Continuous Ventilatory Dependence and Other Studies Pertinent to Respiratory Control

A relationship has been reported between the genotype for PARMs and the need for continuous

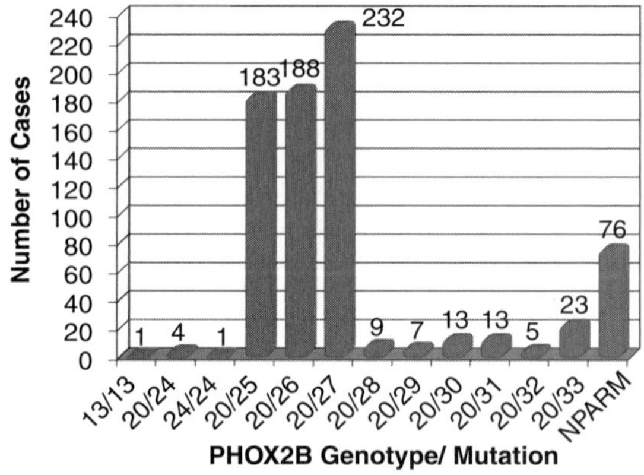

Figure 17.2 Frequency of *PHOX2B* mutations by genotype. Polyalanine repeat mutations (PARMs) in the *PHOX2B* gene range from 24 to 33 repeats (normal number of repeats is 20) with the most common mutation occurring as heterozygous PARMs with genotypes 20/25, 20/26, and 20/27. Nonpolyalanine repeats (NPARMs) are less common and include frameshift, nonsense, and missense mutations. Only one case of a homozygous PARM has been reported (homozygous 24/24 genotype) [37]. And only one case of a homozygous contraction has been reported (homozygous 13/13 genotype). Reproduced with permission from Refs. [36,17].

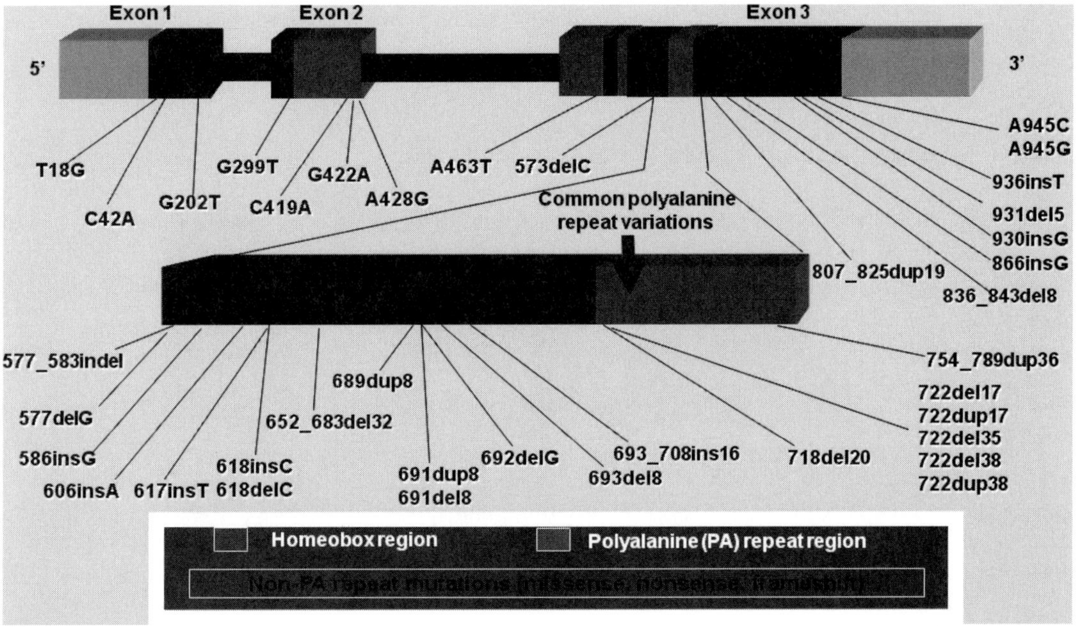

Figure 17.3 Schematic of the *PHOX2B* gene with location of all CCHS-associated mutations described to date in PHOX2B. All polyalanine repeat mutations (PARMs) are located within the second polyalanine expansion regions of exon 3. Nearly all NPARMs identified so far have been found at the extreme 3′ end of exon 2 or in exon 3. Reproduced with permission from Ref. [36].

ventilatory dependence [26,28,31]. Individuals with the 20/25 genotype rarely require 24 h/d ventilatory support; children with the 20/26 genotype have variable awake needs depending on activity level. Children with genotypes from 20/27 to 20/33 typically require continuous ventilatory support, though the paucity of cases in the 20/30 to 20/33 genotype group prevents rigorous analysis. Individuals with the later presentation of CCHS (please see section that follows) and the 20/24 or 20/25 genotype [45,57,58] appear to have the mildest hypoventilation; they present typically after exposure to respiratory depressants or severe pneumonia and may be managed successfully with only nocturnal ventilatory support. Ventilatory management of individuals with the NPARMs will be mutation-specific, although individuals with these mutations typically require continuous ventilatory support [31] (see Figure 17.4).

Reports describing awake and asleep ventilatory and arousal responses [59–62], mental concentration [10], respiratory sensations related to the physiologic compromise [11,12], physiologic response to exercise and leg motion [8–11,63,64], and focal abnormalities on functional MRI [65–68] likely reflect results for only the mildest affected CCHS patients. Unintended bias in these studies may be because of the following: (1) small sample size, (2) reporting in the pre-*PHOX2B* era, (3) inclusion of subjects with other causes of hypoventilation [60] or without documentation of a specific *PHOX2B* mutation confirming diagnosis of CCHS in all subjects, and (4) inclusion of children who were able to sustain adequate ventilation during wakefulness at rest suggesting that subjects likely had the 20/25 genotype (based on described phenotype and protocols).

Hirschsprung Disease (HSCR)

Previously, the incidence of HSCR in CCHS was thought to be 20%, though it is now possible to further refine that figure. HSCR is more prevalent among individuals with NPARMs than PARMs. Current analysis indicates that HSCR is reported in 87% to 100% of NPARMs in contrast to 13% to 20% of PARMs [31,33] (see Figure 17.4). To date, there are no reports of HSCR occurring in individuals with the 20/25 genotype and only rarely with the

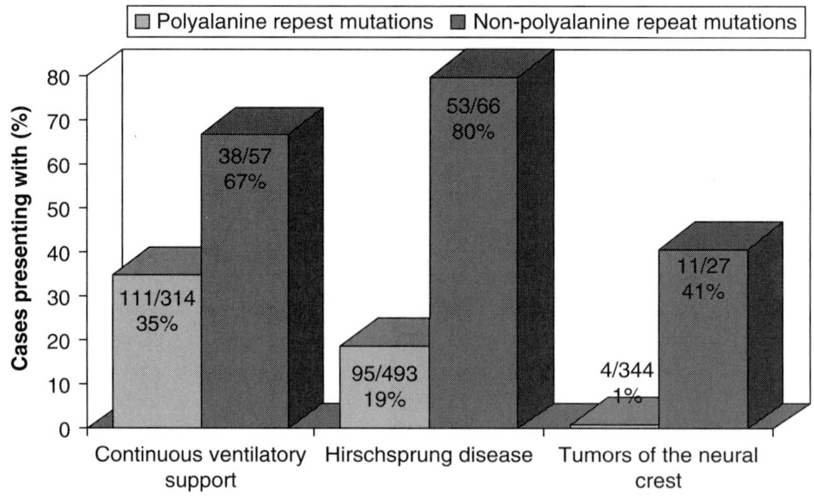

Figure 17.4 Phenotypic features in CCHS cases with polyalanine repeat mutations (PARMs) compared to Nonpolyalanine repeat mutations (NPARMs) in *PHOX2B*. As shown here, the rate of continuous ventilatory dependence (awake and asleep), Hirschsprung disease, and tumors of the neural crest in CCHS cases with NPARMs is higher than for PARMs, reflecting the more severe phenotype that is often seen (though variable depending on specific type of NPARM). The frequencies shown here comprise coincident features in all CCHS cases reported to date (with adequate clinical detail), including reports from groups in the United States, Italy, France, Japan, Germany, Taiwan, China, Australia, and the Netherlands as well as current information reported by the ATS Statement authors. *Neural crest tumor data derived from cases in which information was available and the child had survived at least the first year of life.* *All PARM cases with tumors had large (29–33 repeats) expansion mutations. Reproduced with permission from Refs. [36,17].

20/26 genotype. A high occurrence of HSCR in individuals with the 20/27 genotype was reported in one cohort [33], and also anecdotally recognized to occur in ~30% of individuals with the 20/27 to 20/33 genotype. Recent studies further suggest that the *RET* gene may have a pivotal role as a modifier gene for the HSCR phenotype in patients with CCHS [69,70].

Tumors of Neural Crest Origin

Extracranial solid tumors have been reported in individuals with CCHS, which include neuroblastomas, ganglioneuromas, and ganglio-neuroblastomas that may be found in the chest and abdomen in paraspinal ganglia, adrenal gland, and among other locations in which sympathetic nervous tissue is found. Neuroblastomas in CCHS have been found exclusively in ~50% of individuals with NPARMs. Other tumors of neural crest origin have been found with low frequency among individuals with PARMs (1%) [31,33] (see Figure 17.5). Even then, the only subjects with a PARM described thus far with a neural crest tumor (ganglioneuromas or ganglioneuroblastomas) have the 20/29 and 20/33 genotypes [25,28,31,33].

Cardiac Asystoles

Gronli et al [71] identified a correlation between the most common PARMs (genotypes 20/25–20/27) and length of R-R intervals on Holter monitoring. None of the children with the 20/25 genotype had sinus pauses of 3 seconds or longer. Yet, 19% of individuals with the 20/26 genotype and 83% of individuals with the 20/27 genotype had 3-second or longer pauses. Cardiac pacemakers were not indicated in children with the 20/25 genotype, but 25% of subjects with the 20/26 genotype and 67% of subjects with the 20/27 geno-type were implanted with a cardiac pacemaker. Of 3 individuals who did not receive a cardiac pacemaker and had prolonged cardiac pauses (20/26 and 20/27 genotypes), 2 died suddenly and 1 had severe neurocognitive compromise. One adult

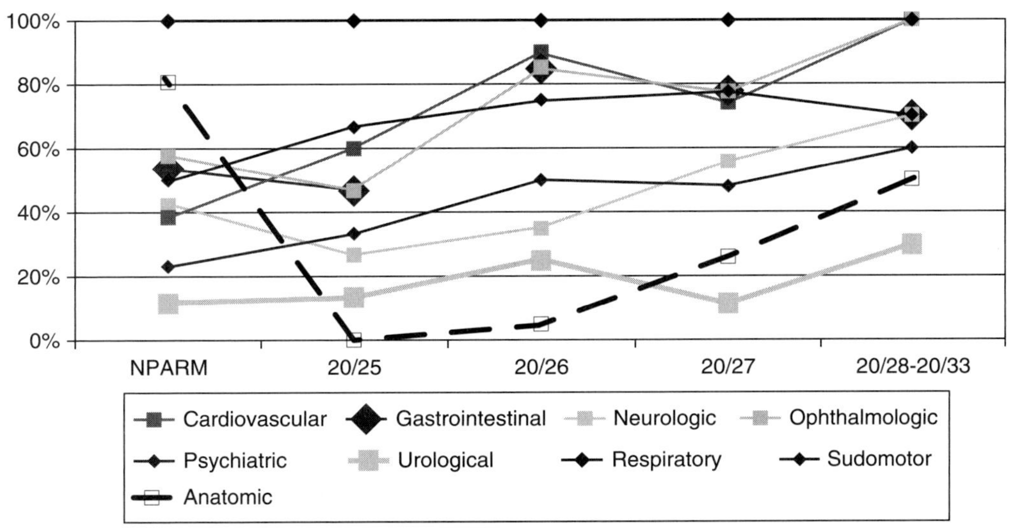

Figure 17.5 Frequency of autonomic nervous system dysregulation (ANSD) symptoms in CCHS cases versus *PHOX2B* genotype/mutation among 97 children. On chart and autonomic questionnaire review of various systems involved (listed at the bottom of the figure) in a pilot cohort of individuals with CCHS, there is a trend toward increasing percentage of physiologic and anatomic ANSD symptoms within each system as polyalanine size increases. There is a distinct difference with predominance of anatomic (Hirschsprung disease and/or tumors of neural crest origin) ANSD in NPARMs as compared to PARMs [72].

with the 20/25 genotype who was diagnosed in adulthood (LO-CCHS, later-onset congenital central hypoventilation syndrome) has documented pauses of 8 seconds and longer [58]. Thus individuals with the 20/25 genotype may be unaffected during childhood, but may demonstrate prolonged asystoles in adulthood if not adequately managed or promptly diagnosed. Risk of cardiac asystoles in individuals with NPARMs remainsunascertained.

Symptoms of ANSD

Weese-Mayer et al and Patwari et al [28,72] demonstrated that an increased number of polyalanine repeats among PARMs was associated with an increased number of symptoms of physiologic ANSD (see Figure 17.5). It should be noted that these measures of ANSD were identified from medical record review, questionnaires, and physiologic assessment, rather than from pediatric-specific tests of autonomic function.

Facial Dysmorphology

Todd et al [73] described a characteristic facies among children between the ages of 2 years and early adulthood with CCHS and primarily individuals with PARMs. The characteristic facies in CCHS is generally shorter and flatter, and with an inferior inflection of the lateral 1/3 of the upper vermilion border (lip trait). The face is not dysmorphic, but it is short relative to its width; the resulting effect is the characteristic boxy-shaped face observed in CCHS. Using 5 variables to characterize facies (upper lip height, biocular width, upper facial height, nasal tip protrusion, and the lip trait), Todd et al were able to correctly predict 86% of the CCHS cases and 82% of the controls. The limited number of cases with the 20/28 to 20/33 genotypes may have precluded identification of a significant correlation between *PHOX2B* genotype and measures of the CCHS facial phenotype in those children.

Dermatoglyphics

Todd et al [74] assessed dermatoglyphic pattern type frequency, left/right symmetry, and genotype/phenotype correlation in CCHS. Dermatoglyphic pattern type frequencies were altered in CCHS cases versus controls. Increased frequency of arches in females, and ulnar loops in males, with the largest differences for the left hand and for individuals with both CCHS and HSCR, was reported.No significant association was found between the number of polyalanine repeats in the *PHOX2B* genotypic category and dermatoglyphic pattern frequencies in the CCHS study groups.

Phenotype Specific to the NPARMs

While there is overlap in all areas of the phenotypic profile of PARMs and NPARMs, disease tends to be more severe in cases with NPARMs. However, severity of the NPARM phenotype will be mutation-specific and vary greatly as the effects of different NPARMs (eg, frameshift vs missense) on protein function will vary greatly. NPARMs generally occur *de novo* producing severe respiratory and autonomic dysfunction with HSCR and extensive gut involvement, need for continuous ventilatory support, and an increased tumor risk in those over 1 year of age [31,33]. The presence of extensive HSCR and a CCHS phenotype should act as a strong indicator of a possible *PHOX2B* NPARM. Thirty-eight- and 35-base pair deletions, leading to protein frameshift, produce very severe disease and have been identified by several research groups in different countries. A subset of more rarely identified NPARMs are associated with a very high incidence of HSCR but a milder physiologic CCHS phenotype and incomplete penetrance [31]. A few frameshift mutations located early in exon 3 of *PHOX2B* (618 delC, 577 delG) have been inherited and are variably penetrant [26,31], suggesting that frameshifts in this area may produce a milder cellular deficit than other frameshift mutations. The c.422G>A and c.428A>G mutations, leading missense mutations near the end of exon 2, have also been found in several unrelated cases of CCHS and, together with the c.299G>T (p.R100L) mutation [48], are the only missense mutations yet identified as causative in CCHS. Thec.419C>A (p.A140E) has recently been reported in later onset CCHS, both isolated and associated with HSCR [44,75].

Later-Onset CCHS

Individuals who present with symptoms compatible with CCHS but who are older than 1 month of age, and who have a *PHOX2B* mutation, are termed later-onset CCHS (LO-CCHS) [26,33,38,42–45,47,57,58,76–79]. LO-CCHS thus far appears to reflect the variable penetrance of the *PHOX2B* genotypes 20/24 and 20/25 or rarely an NPARM; and these mutations may require an environmental cofactor to elicit the phenotype. Individuals with the 20/24 genotype are likely "missed" because the hypoventilation is so subtle and the manifestation of the phenotype may require environmental cofactors [45] or the homozygous condition [37].

A careful medical history in infants, children, and adults "presenting" with alveolar hypoventilation after the first month of life will often identify symptoms compatible with prior hypoventilation and other disorders of ANSD. LO-CCHS should be considered in the event of centrally mediated alveolar hypoventilation and/or cyanosis or seizures reported following: (1) anesthetics or CNS depressants, (2) severe pulmonic infection, or (3) obstructive sleep apnea intervention. The physician who maintains a heightened level of suspicion for potential LO-CCHS can expedite the diagnosis by promptly testing for a *PHOX2B* mutation, avert potentially life-threatening decompensation, and minimize the risk of further neurocognitive compromise. The suggested evaluation would include the following: *PHOX2B* testing with both the Screening Test (targeted mutation fragment analysis) and the Sequencing Test (both available at www.genetests.org; both tests are needed to rule out *PHOX2B* mutations and mosaicism especially in the LO-CCHS cases [80]), review of digital AP and lateral photographs (to evaluate for facies consistent with CCHS; a moustache in adult males may conceal the "lip trait,") electrocardiographic assessment for prolonged sinus pauses (ideally via 72 hour Holter monitoring), sleep and awake physiologic evaluation inclusive of end tidal carbon dioxide monitoring and pulse oximetry (for ascertainment of hypoventilation, hypercarbia and/or hypoxemia), a hematocrit and reticulocyte count (for polycythemia and response to hypoxemia), a bicarbonate level (for signs of compensated respiratory acidosis), and chest x-ray, echocardiogram, or electrocardiogram (for signs of right chamber enlargement or pulmonary hypertension). A barium enema or manometry may be considered, in cases of intermittent chronic constipation, to exclude short segment HSCR. In so doing, other yet unidentified environmental or genetic factors that might impact the variable penetrance of the 20/24 and

20/25 mutations as well as the most recently described novel missense mutation [75] may be determined.

Distinction From Rapid-onset Obesity With Hypothalamic Dysfunction, Hypoventilation, and Autonomic Dysregulation (ROHHAD)

Practitioners will need to distinguish LO-CCHS from rapid-onset obesity, with hypothala-mic dysfunction, hypoventilation, and autonomic dysregulation (ROHHAD) [81,82], a rare disorder first described in 1965 [83]. ROHHAD was initially termed Late Onset Central Hypoventilation Syndrome with Hypo-thalamic Dysfunction [84], but was renamed in 2007 [81] to provide early recognition and increased awareness by alerting the physician to the typical sequence of presenting symptoms. Ize-Ludlow et al distinguished ROHHAD from CCHS and LO-CCHS by careful history and *PHOX2B* testing. With 75 cases reported in the literature [81–86], it is essential to recognize the phenotype as distinct from CCHS. The ROHHAD cases typically present between the ages of 1.5 and 7 years with the herald of rapid-onset obesity (20–40 pound gain over 4–6 months), then hypothalamic dysfunction including water imbalance, elevated prolactin levels, and altere-donset of puberty. Subsequently, a subset of cases of ROHHAD will experience a cardio-respiratory arrest after an intercurrent illness followed by obstructive sleep apnea and hypoventilation, autonomic dysregulation, and also, in a subset of cases, ganglioneuromas and ganglioneuroblastomas (often with accompanying scoliosis). The symptoms of autonomic dysregulation may include low body temperature, cold hands and feet, severe bradycardia, decreased pain perception, abnormal pupillary responses, among others. Also reported are disruptive behavioral and mood disorders. These children can often be supported with mask ventilation only at night; however, a subset will require 24 h/d ventilation via tracheostomy. The diagnosis of ROHHAD is based on the clinical presentation, the related clinical features, and documented absence of other potentially confounding diagnoses, including ruling out CCHS with clinically available *PHOX2B* testing (documenting an absence of PARMs and NPARMs), though efforts are underway to identify a genetic or epigenetic basis for ROHHAD.

Mosaicism in Subset of Parents With CCHS Children

Somatic mosaicism for a PARM was first reported in 2003 by Weese-Mayer et al [28] in 4 parents out of 54 available families (7.4%). In 2005, Trochet et al [33] identified somatic mosaicism in 1 parent of each of 10 CCHS patients, confirming that roughly 10% of chil-dren with CCHS will inherit the mutation from a mosaic parent. In both studies, mosai-cism was detected in DNA extracted from parents' peripheral leukocytes by observing a lighter signal from the expanded allele than from the normal allele, in contrast to the pattern seen in subjects with CCHS. The somatic mosaicism would be because of postzygotic mutations in the *PHOX2B* gene.

A quantitative estimate of somatic mosaicism in unaffected parents has been reported by study of DNA amplification products from asymptomatic parents of CCHS probands with alanine expansions and with genotypes ranging from 20/25 to 20/31 [43,44,80], ascertained by variation in mutant peak relative to control peak. In the case of an individual with CCHS, the amplitude of the mutant peak would be expected to be at 50% of the amplitude of the control peak. However, among the mosaic individuals, the range was reported from 9% to 35% in DNA from parental leukocytes, values confirmed in studies of fibroblast and saliva DNA from a subset of mosaic parents [44]; in another study, mosaic individuals were identified by less signal in the peak corresponding to the expanded allele [43].

Thus far, it appears that though most expansion mutations occur *de novo* in CCHS, 5% to 10% are inherited from a mosaic typically unaffected parent, and only for PARMs larger than the 20/25 genotype. These would be examples of somatic mosaicism because of postzygotic mutations [28,31,33,43]. Incomplete penetrance is demonstrated when certain *PHOX2B* mutations (20/24, 20/25, and a few NPARMs) are present in all the cells (including the reproductive cells of the germline) of individuals thought to be unaffected [26,28,45], but when studied may be found to have mild features of the CCHS phenotype.

Inheritance of CCHS and the *PHOX2B* Mutation

Though Amiel et al initially proposed, based on the absence of *PHOX2B* mutations in 8 sets of parents of CCHS probands, that the *PHOX2B* expansions appeared to be *de novo* [25], in 2003, Weese-Mayer et al reported the autosomal dominant inheritance of the same *PHOX2B* mutation and the CCHS phenotype from CCHS parent-child pairs and from unaffected mosaic parents for the same mutation observed in their affected child [28]. The findings of the autosomal dominant inheritance were later confirmed by Trochet et al [44]. Despite the inheritance pattern, most parents of affected children with CCHS do not carry a mutation at all; thus a high *de novo* mutation rate occurs in affected individuals. As noted above, the 20/24 and 20/25 genotype PARMs and some of the NPARMs may be found in the germline of asymptomatic parents of children with CCHS and even other family members, suggesting inheritance as dominant with incomplete penetrance [26,31,42,44,45,57,58]. Though family members who carry such mutations do not have CCHS, they may show other ANSD phenotypes, including HSCR or neuroblastoma [24,31], or they may be presymptomatic, presenting in later childhood or adulthood.

Genetic counseling is crucial for individuals diagnosed with CCHS, their parents and,in some cases, particular family members. Speci-fically for an individual with CCHS, there is a 50% chance of transmitting the mutation and therefore the disease phenotype, to each offspring. If an unaffected parent is mosaic for a *PHOX2B* mutation (identified because of an affected child), there will be up to a 50% chance of recurrence in any subsequent child. The mosaic mutation cannot be inherited as a mosaic mutation. If unaffected parents do carry a germline mutation (ie, a 20/25 genotype PARM), there may be numerous other family members who can carry the same mutation without having obvious symptoms. Consequently, genetic testing is indicated for all persons in position in the pedigree to inherit the mutation, which can often be traced back until the individual in whom the mutation originated is identified. To assess recurrence risk in a family, both parents of children with CCHS should have the *PHOX2B* Screening Test (targeted mutation fragment analysis) done to rule out mosaicism [80] (PARMs of genotypes 20/26 to 20/33 and severe NPARMs) or a nonpenetrant carrier state (genotypes 20/24 and 20/25 PARMs and mild NPARMs). Prenatal testing is available for families in which the *PHOX2B* mutation is known. Despite negative testing of parents of a CCHS child, germline mosaicism cannot be ruled out, and prenatal testing for subsequent pregnancies should be considered. Prenatal testing affords parents the information to make an informed decision with a range of possibilities from elective abortion to a fully prepared delivery room to optimize the baby's chance for a smooth transition to extrauterine life.

Steps Toward the Diagnosis of the Individual With CCHS

As soon as the diagnosis of CCHS is considered, blood should be sent for the clinically available *PHOX2B* Screening Test. If the Screening Test is negative, the sequel *PHOX2B* Sequencing Test should be performed. The ATS Statement on CCHS advises the 2-step *PHOX2B* testing which is the most cost-efficient approach (the mutation in 95% of CCHS cases will be identified with the inexpensive *PHOX2B* Screening Test; only a subset of the NPARMs will require the *PHOX2B* Sequencing Test to be identified). Simultaneous to the *PHOX2B* testing, other causes of hypoventilation should be considered to expedite proper intervention and facilitate treatment strategies for home care. Tests that will help to rule out primary lung disease, ventilatory muscle weakness, and cardiac disease would include chest x-ray and potentially chest CT, comprehensive neurological evaluation and potentially muscle biopsy, and echocardiogram, respectively. Causative gross anatomic brain/brainstem lesions should be ruled out with an MRI and/or CT scan of the brain and brainstem [87,88]. Likewise, inborn errors of metabolism should be considered and a metabolic screen should be performed.

Clinical Evaluation of the Individual With PHOX2B Mutation-Confirmed CCHS

To ascertain each child's needs, the ATS Statement on CCHS recommends annual in-hospital comprehensive physiologic studies awake and asleep. The aim is to assess ventilatory needs during varying levels of activity and concentration and all stages of sleep, with spontaneous breathing and with artificial ventilation, and ventilatory responsivity to endogenous and exogenous physiologic challenges awake and asleep. Performed over the course of a several day hospitalization in a center with extensive CCHS experience, these studies will allow for an understanding of a child's spontaneous breathing and artificial ventilation needs [17]. It is essential that these physiologic studies include constant supervision by highly trained personnel and continuous audiovisual surveillance with continuousrecording (at a minimum) of the follow-ing variables: respiratory inductance plethysmography (chest, abdomen, and sum), ECG, hemoglobin saturation with pulse waveform, end tidal carbon dioxide with waveform, sleep state staging, blood pressure, and temperature. Other recommended testing for individuals with *PHOX2B* mutation-confirmed CCHS is provided in Table 17.1.

Independent of the respiratory control abnormalities, children with CCHS have other evidence for diffuse autonomic dysregulation [3,4,72], and specific testing is therefore required. In the event of constipation symptoms, a barium enema or manometry and potentially full thickness rectal biopsy should be performed to diagnose or rule out presence of HSCR. For neural crest tumor surveillance, serial chest and abdominal imaging is essential among children with the NPARMs and those children with the 20/29 to the 20/33 genotype (neuroblastoma in NPARMs and ganglioneuroblastoma/ganglioneuromas in PARMs). Because no children with genotypes 20/24 to 20/28 have been identified with tumors of neural crest origin, the value of serial imaging in these cases is unknown. Seventy-two-hour Holter monitoring performed annually may determine aberrant cardiac rhythms, sinus pauses that will necessitate bipolar cardiac pacemaker implantation [89], and the frequency of shorter pauses (ie, less than 3 seconds) that may have physiologic and neurocognitive impact—especially in light of the decreased beat-to-beat heart rate variability, reduced respiratory sinus arrhythmia, and transient abrupt asystoles that have been described [71,90,91]. Echocardiograms, hematocrits, and reticulocyte counts performed every 12 months will provide information regarding potential cor pulmonale and polycythemia—essential as

Table 17.1 Recommended testing to characterize CCHS phenotype

	Annual in-hospital comprehensive physiologic testing (awake and asleep), exogenous and endogenous gas challenges, autonomic testing*	Assessment for Hirschsprung disease	Annual neuro-cognitive assessment	Annual 72-hour Holter recording and echocardiogram	Annual imaging to assess for tumors of neural crest origin
PHOX2B Genotype					
PARM					
20/24 and 20/25	X		X	X	
20/26	X	X	X	X	
20/27	X	X	X	X	
20/28–20/33	X	X	X	X	X+
NPARM	X	X	X	X	X++

Abbreviations: PARM, polyalanine repeat expansion mutation; NPARM, non-polyalanine repeat expansion mutation (missense, nonsense, frameshift).
*Infants under the age of 3 years should undergo comprehensive evaluations every 6 months.
+Annual chest and abdominal imaging to identify ganglioneuromas and ganglioneuroblastomas.
++Abdominal imaging and urine cathecholamines every 3 months in first 2 years, then every 6 months until 7 years of age to identify neuroblastomas.
Reproduced with permission from Ref. [17].

children with CCHS are at risk for progressive pulmonary hypertension and cor pulmonale, as a result of recurrent hypoxemia because of inadequate ventilator settings or tracheostomy caliber, unrecognized hypoventilation during spontaneous breathing while awake, excessive exercise with resultant physiologic compromise, or suboptimal compliance with artificial ventilation. Testing more frequently may be warranted if clinically indicated, especially in the child below 3 years of age (see Table 17.1). Comprehensive ophthalmologic testing as well as independent pupillometry are advisable as CCHS patients frequently exhibit ophthalmologic abnormalities reflecting the role of *PHOX2B* on the cranial nerves controlling pupillary function [2,5]. The aim is to determine the nature of ophthalmologic involvement and allow for intervention strategies to avoid interference with learning. Anecdotal reports of poor heat tolerance and profuse sweating have been described [1] though not yet studied comprehensively. Comprehensive autonomic testing as clinically indicated to assess syncope and to assess ANS function may include tilt testing, heart-rate-deep-breathing response, Valsalva maneuver, thermal stressors, pupillometry and others as new measures of autonomic testing are developed for infants and children.

Though suboptimal school performance and/or decreased intellectual function have been observed in CCHS patients [2,92–95], it is unclear whether this is because of hypoxemia from inadequate ventilatory support or a direct result of the primary neurologic problem associated with CCHS. With earlier identification and conservative standardized management for children with CCHS, improved neurocognitive performance is anticipated with distinction between sequelae of hypoxemia (because of hypoventilation or asystoles) and innate disease specific to CCHS. As recommended in the 2010 ATS Statement, comprehensive neurocognitive testing performed annually in a controlled setting will assess the child's progress relative to intervention, management, and compliance and may identify areas for intervention (see Table 17.1). At present, the oldest neonatally identified patients with CCHS are graduating from college, getting married, and maintaining employment. It behooves the family and medical personnel to provide optimal ventilation and oxygenation to assure maximization of neurocognitive potential. Aggressive educational intervention coupled with careful ventilatory and cardiovascular management is essential to optimize neurocognitive and quality of life outcome [2,93–95].

The 2010 ATS Statement advises that care of individuals with CCHS would be ideally provided through centers with extensive expertise in CCHS, working in close partnership with regional pediatric pulmonologists and pediatricians. As a result, the patients will experience consistency of management, education which can become a tool to promote advocacy for the child and family with CCHS, and ideally improved outcome for individuals. The rationale for the centers is an understanding that management of children with CCHS is more time-intensive than the care of other ventilator-dependent children. Because of the range of phenotype based on the *PHOX2B* mutations, experience with well over 30 to 40 patients only begins to provide the scope of experience necessary for understanding the needs of the child with CCHS.

Ventilatory Management of the Individual With *PHOX2B* Mutation-Confirmed CCHS

CCHS is a lifelong disease that does not resolve spontaneously or improve with advancing age except in rare anecdotal cases. Consequently, chronic home ventilatory support is essential for these children to leave the hospital and grow up in the family home. Ventilatory management options include the following: positive pressure ventilators via tracheostomy [1,96–98], bi-level positive airway pressure [1,99–107], negative pressure ventilators [108,109], or diaphragm pacing [110–121]. Oxygen administration without artificial ventilation is inadequate as hypoventilation persists and pulmonary hypertension ensues.

The authors of the 2010 ATS Statement on CCHS recommend positive pressure ventilation via a tracheostomy for the first several years of life. In conservative management, noninvasive ventilation should not be considered until 6 to 8 years of age, at the absolute earliest, in very stable CCHS patients requiring ventilatory support only during sleep because of the concerns of development of mid-face hypoplasia and safety of noninvasive ventilation as life-sustaining support. Weaning from the ventilator is not a realistic goal in children with CCHS. Ventilators and/or diaphragm pacers are adjusted to completely meet the ventilatory demands of each child, with settings determined specific to varying levels of activity, leaving much of their energy available for other activities. A reasonable range for PETco2 is 30 to 50 mm Hg (though ideally 35 to 40 mm Hg) and SpO2 of 95% or higher. Some centers use "ventilator ladders" in conjunction with pulse oximetry and PETco2 monitoring to maintain precise control of gas exchange within a narrow normal range. Home monitoring of oxygen saturation and end tidal carbon dioxide levels allows for early recognition of respiratory illness in the child with CCHS who will lack overt symptoms of fever and tachypnea. It is important to maintain normal oxygenation to avoid risk for development of deficits in cognition.

Because individuals with CCHS may experience respiratory arrest or severe hypoventilation at sleep onset, it is essential that mechanical ventilation is initiated before sleep in preparation for bedtime. Because the child with CCHS will not respond to physiologic compromise nor perceive a sense of shortness of breath, continuous monitoring with a home pulse oximeter (with visible pulse waveform) and end tidal carbon dioxide monitor (with visible waveform) in addition to attendance by an experienced registered nurse (RN) during all sleep time is advised to optimize management and safety. For those children requiring ventilatory support during wakefulness and sleep, the ATS Statement recommendation advises hourly checks of the pulse oximetry and end tidal carbon dioxide during the day as well as continuous care by the RN skilled in ventilator management. There is no role for the apnea/bradycardia transthoracic impedance monitor in the care of a child with CCHS. These monitors will not detect hypoventilation or tracheal obstruction [122], they will not detect the sinus pauses characteristic of children with CCHS (the pauses are abrupt, and may be hidden by the averaging algorithm in the monitor), and they may inadvertently demonstrate an elevated heart rate in the child with diaphragm pacers (from pacer artifact) [122].

Sedative medications and central nervous system depressants will worsen the hypoventilation, so they should be avoided in the individual with CCHS. In the event that an individual with CCHS requires sedation, full mechanical ventilator support must be readily available along with close monitoring and supervision. Swimming presents a serious danger for the child with CCHS, and underwater swimming contests present an even greater danger. Children with CCHS will not perceive the asphyxia that occurs with drowning and breath-holding and therefore will swim longer and farther than children without CCHS—thereby heightening the risk of drowning.

Long-term Prognosis

With modern technology for home ventilation, most children with CCHS can have prolonged survival with a good quality of life. The mortality rate for CCHS is low in patients who are aggressively managed and followed in CCHS centers, though continuous vigilance is necessary in terms of physiologic monitoring, equipment maintenance, and battery replacement in diaphragm and cardiac pacemakers. As children with CCHS are advancing into adulthood, the development of transitional medicine programs in these centers already caring for children with CCHS is essential.

Clinical Pearls

- Confirmation of a PHOX2B mutation is requisite to making a diagnosis of CCHS. Further, the nature of the PHOX2B mutation allows for anticipatory management in terms of ventilator dependence (awake and asleep vs asleep only), risk for Hirschsprung Disease, and risk for a tumor of neural crest origin.
- Hypoventilation in individuals with CCHS is often more apparent during activities of daily living. While an individual with CCHS may appear to have adequate awake ventilation at rest, he or she may demonstrate variable degrees of hypoventilation during age-appropriate activities (playing, eating, exercise, concentration, etc). Therefore, comprehensive physiologic testing at a center with expertise in CCHS is valuable in determining the degree of hypoventilation and optimal ventilatory sup-port required during these age-appropriate activities.
- Patients with CCHS require life-long mechanical assisted ventilation. They do not outgrow the disorder or the need for ventilatory support.

- Because CCHS patients have minimal to no lung disease, they have the widest option of ventilatory support techniques available. Positive pressure ventilation via tracheostomy in the first several years of life, when brain growth and development requiring normoxia occurs, is the recommendation of the ATS Statement on CCHS.
- Maintaining a high index of suspicion in cases of unexplained alveolar hypoventilation, delayed recovery of spontaneous breathing after sedation or anesthesia or in the event of severe respiratory infection, and seizures or neurocognitive delay will likely identify milder cases of LO-CCHS, thereby allowing for successful intervention.
- During sleep in individuals with CCHS, the respiratory rate is monotonous and may seem normal, but will occur commensurate with very low tidal volumes. Therefore, both pulse oximetry and carbondioxide monitoring are essential for diagnosis and prevention of physiologic compromise from hypoventilation.

Directions for Future Research in CCHS

As outlined in the 2010 ATS Statement (http://www.thoracic.org/newsroom/press-releases/resources/cchs-statement.pdf), our understanding of CCHS is rapidly expanding. By concentrating the care of individuals with CCHS in a limited number of centers worldwide, answers to current questions will be attainable in the lifetime of current children with CCHS. Many of these studies are already underway in a U.S.-led international cohort of CCHS patients. For the complete list of suggested future directions please access http://www.thoracic.org/newsroom/press-releases/resources/cchs-statement.pdf. An abbreviated list is provided below:

1. What is the populational incidence of *PHOX2B* mutations?
2. What is the incidence of *PHOX2B* mutations in patients referred to adult sleep labs or who have adverse reactions to anesthesia?
3. Is there any reason to think that the 3rd generation subjects with CCHS will have a change in phenotype especially for the 20/24 and 20/25 genotypes as well as a subset of the NPARMs?
4. What features of ANSD will be detectable *in utero* for fetuses known to have a *PHOX2B* mutation?
5. What is the incidence of mosaicism in the general population and in an expanded cohort of parents of children with *PHOX2B* mutation-confirmed CCHS?
6. Is there a CCHS phenotype of mosaic individuals?
7. How clear will the *PHOX2B* mutation-CCHS phenotype relationship be in largely expanded cohorts studied with pediatric-specific measures of respiratory control and autonomic testing?

References

1. Weese-Mayer DE, Shannon DC, Keens TG, Silvestri JM. Idiopathic congenital central hypoventilation syndrome: diagnosis and management. American Thoracic Society. *Am J Respir Crit Care Med.* 1999;160(1):368–373.
2. Weese-Mayer DE, Silvestri JM, Menzies LJ, Morrow-Kenny AS, Hunt CE, Hauptman SA. Congenital central hypoventilation syndrome: diagnosis, management, and long-term outcome in thirty-two children. *J Pediatr.* 1992;120(3):381–387.
3. Weese-Mayer DE, Silvestri JM, Huffman AD, et al. Case/control family study of autonomic nervous system dysfunction in idiopathic congenital central hypoventilation syndrome. *Am J Med Genet.* 2001;100(3):237–245.
4. Marazita ML, Maher BS, Cooper ME, et al. Genetic segregation analysis of autonomic nervous system dysfunction in families of probands with idiopathic congenital central hypoventilation syndrome. *Am J Med Genet.* 2001;100(3):229–236.
5. Goldberg DS, Ludwig IH Congenital central hypoventilation syndrome: ocular findings in 37 children. *J Pediatr Ophthalmol Strabismus.* 1996;33(3) 175–180.
6. Faure C, Viarme F, Cargill G, Navarro J, Gaultier C, Trang H. Abnormal esophageal motility in children with congenital central hypoventilation syndrome. *Gastroenterology.* 2002;122(5):1258–1263.
7. Pine DS, Weese-Mayer DE, Silvestri JM, et al. Anxiety and congenital central hypoventilation syndrome. *Am J Psychiatry.* 1994;151(6):864–870.
8. Silvestri JM, Weese-Mayer DE, Flanagan EA. Congenital central hypoventilation syndrome: cardiorespiratory responses to moderate exercise, simulating daily activity. *Pediatric Pulmonol.* 1995;20(2):89–93.
9. Paton JY, Swaminathan S, Sargent CW, Hawksworth A, Keens TG. Ventilatory response to exercise in children with congeni-tal central hypoventilation syndrome. *Am Rev Respir Dis.* 1993;147(5):1185–1191.
10. Shea SA, Andres LP, Paydarfar D, Banzett RB, Shannon DC. Effect of mental activity on breathing in congenital central hypoventilation syndrome. *Respir Physiol.* 1993;94(3):251–263.

11. Spengler CM, Banzett RB, Systrom DM, Shannon DC, Shea SA. Respiratory sensations during heavy exercise in subjects without respiratory chemosensitivity. *Respir Physiol.* 1998;114(1):65–74.
12. Shea SA, Andres LP, Shannon DC, Guz A, Banzett RB. Respiratory sensations in subjects who lack a ventilatory response to CO2. *Respir Physiol.* 1993;93(2):203–219.
13. Trang H, Girard A, Laude D, Elghozi JL. Short-term blood pressure and heart rate variability in congenital central hypoventilation syndrome (Ondine's curse). *Clin Sci (Lond).* 2005;108(3): 225–230.
14. Shea SA, Andres LP, Shannon DC, Banzett RB. Ventilatory responses to exercise in humans lacking ventilatory chemosensitivity. *J Physiol.* 1993;468:623–640.
15. O'Brien LM, Holbrook CR, Vanderlaan M, Amiel J, Gozal D. Autonomic function in children with congenital central hypoventilation syndrome and their families. *Chest.* 2005;128(4): 2478–2484.
16. Mellins RB, Balfour HH Jr, Turino GM, Winters RW. Failure of automatic control of ventilation (Ondine's curse). Report of an infant born with this syndrome and review of the literature. *Medicine (Baltimore).* 1970;49(6):487–504.
17. Weese-Mayer DE, Berry-Kravis EM, Ceccherini I, et al. An official ATS clinical policy statement: congenital central hypoventilation syndrome: genetic basis, diagnosis, and management. *Am J Respir Crit Care Med.* 2010;181(6):626–644.
18. Khalifa MM, Flavin MA, Wherrett BA Congenital central hypoventilation syndrome in monozygotic twins. *J Pediatr.* 1988;113(5):853–855.
19. Haddad GG, Mazza NM, Defendini R, et al. Congenital failure of automatic control of ventilation, gastrointestinal motility and heart rate. *Medicine (Baltimore).* 1978;57(6):517–526.
20. Weese-Mayer DE, Silvestri JM, Marazita ML, Hoo JJ. Congenital central hypoventilationsyndrome: inheritance and relation to sudden infant death syndrome. *Am J Med Genet.* 1993;47(3):360–367.
21. Hamilton J, Bodurtha JN. Congenital central hypoventilation syndrome and Hirschsprung's disease in half sibs. *J Med Genet.* 1989;26(4): 272–274.
22. Silvestri JM, Chen ML, Weese-Mayer DE, et al. Idiopathic congenital central hypoventilation syndrome: the next generation. *Am J Med Genet.* 2002;112(1):46–50.
23. Sritippayawan S, Hamutcu R, Kun SS, Ner Z, Ponce M, Keens TG. Mother-daughter transmission of congenital central hypoventilation syndrome. *Am J Respir Crit Care Med.* 2002; 166(3):367–369.
24. Devriendt K, Fryns JP, Naulaers G, Devlieger H, Alliet P. Neuroblastoma in a mother and congenital central hypoventilation in her daughter: variable expression of the same genetic disorder? *Am J Med Genet.* 2000;90(5):430–431.
25. Amiel J, Laudier B, Attie-Bitach T, et al. Polyalanine expansion and frameshift mutations of the paired-like homeobox gene PHOX2B in congenital central hypoventilation syndrome. *Nat Genet.* 2003;33(4):459–461.
26. Matera I, Bachetti T, Puppo F, et al. PHOX2B mutations and polyalanine expansions correlate with the severity of the respiratory phenotype and associated symptoms in both congenital and late onset Central Hypoventilation syndrome. *J Med Genet.* 2004;41(5):373–380.
27. Sasaki A, Kanai M, Kijima K, et al. Molecular analysis of congenital central hypoventilation syndrome. *Hum Genet.* 2003;114(1):22–26.
28. Weese-Mayer DE, Berry-Kravis EM, Zhou L, et al. Idiopathic congenital central hypoventilation syndrome: analysis of genes pertinent to early autonomic nervous system embryologic development and identification of mutations in PHOX2B. *Am J Med Genet A.* 2003;123A(3):267–278.
29. Pattyn A, Morin X, Cremer H, Goridis C, Brunet JF. Expression and interactions of the two closely related homeobox genes Phox2a and Phox2b during neurogenesis. *Development.* 1997;124(20):4065–4075.
30. Pattyn A, Morin X, Cremer H, Goridis C, Brunet JF. The homeobox gene Phox2b is essential for the development of autonomic neural crest derivatives. *Nature.* 1999;399(6734):366–370.
31. Berry-Kravis EM, Zhou L, Rand CM, Weese-Mayer DE. Congenital central hypoventilation syndrome: PHOX2B mutations and phenotype. *Am J Respir Crit Care Med.* 2006;174(10): 1139–1144.
32. Horiuchi H, Sasaki A, Osawa M, et al. Sensitive detection of polyalanine expansions in PHOX2B by polymerase chain reaction using bisulfite-converted DNA. *J Mol Diagn.* 2005;7(5):638–640.
33. Trochet D, Hong SJ, Lim JK, et al. Molecular consequences of PHOX2B missense, frameshift and alanine expansion mutations leading to autonomic dysfunction. *Hum Mol Genet.* 2005; 14(23):3697–3708.
34. Weese-Mayer DE, Rand CM, Loghmanee DA, et al. Congenital central hypoventilation syndrome: distribution of *PHOX2B* mutations in a large cohort. *Clin Autonom Res J.* 2008;18:241.
35. Weese-Mayer DE, Marazita M., Berry-Kravis L, M E. Congenital Central Hypoventilation Syndrome. GeneReviews at GeneTests: Medical Genetics Information Resource (database online). 2008.
36. Weese-Mayer DE, Rand CM, Berry-Kravis EM, et al. Congenital central hypoventilation syndrome from past to future: model for translational and transitional autonomic medicine. *Pediatr Pulmonol.* 2009;44(6):521–535.
37. Trochet D, de Pontual L, Estevao MH, et al. Homozygous mutation of the PHOX2B gene in congenital central hypoventilation syndrome (Ondine's Curse). *Hum Mutat.* 2008;29(5):770.
38. Barratt S, Kendrick AH, Buchanan F, Whittle AT. Central hypoventilation with PHOX2B expansion mutation presenting in adulthood. *Thorax.* 2007;62(10):919–920.

39. Hung CC, Su YN, Tsao PN, et al. Unequal crossover recombination—population screening for PHOX2B gene polyalanine polymorphism using CE. *Electrophoresis.* 2007;28(6):894–899.
40. Chen LR, Tsao PN, Su YN, et al. Congenital central hypoventilation syndrome with PHOX2B gene mutation in a Taiwanese infant. *J Formos Med Assoc.* 2007; 106(1): 69–73.
41. Fitze G, Konig IR, Paditz E, et al. Compound effect of PHOX2B and RET gene variants in congenital central hypoventilation syndrome combined with Hirschsprung disease. *Am J Med Genet A.* 2008;146A(11):1486–1489.
42. Lee P, Su YN, Yu CJ, Yang PC, Wu HD. PHOX2B mutation-confirmed congenital central hypoventilation syndrome in a chinese family: presentation from newborn to adulthood. *Chest.* 2009;135(2):537–544.
43. Parodi S, Bachetti T, Lantieri F, et al. Parental origin and somatic mosaicism of PHOX2B mutations in Congenital Central Hypoventilation Syndrome. *Hum Mutat.* 2008;29(1):206.
44. Trochet D, de Pontual L, Straus C, et al. PHOX2B germline and somatic mutations in late-onset central hypoventilation syndrome. *Am J Respir Crit Care Med.* 2008;177(8):906–911.
45. Repetto GM, Corrales RJ, Abara SG, et al. Later-onset congenital central hypoventilation syndrome due to a heterozygous 24-polyalanine repeat expansion mutation in the PHOX2B gene. *Acta Paediatr.* 2009;98(1):192–195.
46. Arai H, Otagiri T, Sasaki A, Umetsu K, Hayasaka K. Polyalanine expansion of PHOX2B in congenital central hypoventilation syndrome: rs17884724: A>C isassociated with 7-alanine expansion. *J Hum Genet.* 2009;55(1) 4–7.
47. Fine-Goulden MR, Manna S, Durward A. Cor pulmonale due to congenital central hypoventilation syndrome presenting in adolescence. *Pediatr Crit Care Med.* 2009;10(4):e41–e42.
48. Raabe EH, Laudenslager M, Winter C, et al. Prevalence and functional consequence of PHOX2B mutations in neuroblastoma. *Oncogene.* 2008; 27(4):469–476.
49. Bachetti T, Matera I, Borghini S, Di Duca M, Ravazzolo R, Ceccherini I. Distinct pathogenetic mechanisms for PHOX2B associated polyalanine expansions and frameshift mutations in congenital central hypoventilation syndrome. *Hum Mol Genet.* 2005;14(13):1815–1824.
50. Trochet D, Mathieu Y, Pontual L, et al. In Vitro studies of non poly alanine PHOX2B mutations argue against a loss-of-function mechanism for congenital central hypoventilation. *Hum Mutat.* 2009;30(2):E421–E431.
51. Fitze G, Paditz E, Schlafke M, Kuhlisch E, Roesner D, Schackert HK. Association of germline mutations and polymorphisms of the RET proto-oncogene with idiopathic congenital central hypoventilation syndrome in 33 patients. *J Med Genet.* 2003;40(2):E10.
52. Hennewig U, Hadzik B, Vogel M, et al. Congenital central hypoventilation syndrome with hyperinsulinism in a preterm infant. *J Hum Genet.* 2008;53:573–577.
53. Bajaj R, Smith J, Trochet D, et al. Congenital central hypoventilation syndrome and Hirschsprung's disease in an extremely preterm infant. *Pediatrics.* 2005;115(6):e737–738.
54. van Limpt V, Schramm A, van Lakeman A, et al. The Phox2B homeobox gene is mutated in sporadic neuroblastomas. *Oncogene.* 2004;23(57):9280–9288.
55. Ou-Yang MC, Yang SN, Hsu YM, et al. Concomitant existence of total bowel aganglionosis and congenital central hypoventilation syndrome in a neonate with PHOX2B gene mutation. *J Pediatr Surg.* 2007;42(2):e9–e11.
56. Or SF, Tong MF, Lo FM, et al. PHOX2B mutations in three Chinese patients with congenital central hypoventilation syndrome. *Chin Med J (Engl).* 2006;119(20):1749–1752.
57. Weese-Mayer DE, Berry-Kravis EM, and Zhou L Adult identified with congenital central hypoventilation syndrome–mutation in PHOX2B gene and late-onset CHS.[comment]. *Am J Respir Crit Care Med.* 2005; 171(1): 88.
58. Antic NA, Malow BA, Lange N, et al. PHOX2B mutation-confirmed congenital central hypoventilation syndrome: presentation in adulthood. *Am J Respir Crit Care Med.* 2006;174(8):923–927.
59. Marcus CL, Bautista DB, Amihyia A, Ward SL, Keens TG. Hypercapneic arousal responses in children with congenital central hypoventilation syndrome. *Pediatrics.* 1991;88(5):993–998.
60. Huang J, Colrain IM, Panitch HB, et al. Effect of sleep stage on breathing in children with central hypoventilation. *J Appl Physiol.* 2008;105(1):44–53.
61. Paton JY, Swaminathan S, Sargent CW, Keens TG. Hypoxic and hypercapnic ventilatory responses in awake children with congenital central hypoventilation syndrome. *Am Rev Respir Dis.* 1989;140(2):368–372.
62. Gozal D, Marcus CL, Shoseyov D, Keens TG. Peripheral chemoreceptor function in children with the congenital central hypoventilation syndrome. *J Appl Physiol.* 1993;74(1):379–387.
63. Gozal D, Marcus CL, Ward SL, Keens TG. Ventilatory responses to passive leg motion in children with congenital central hypoventilation syndrome. *Am J Respir Crit Care Med.* 1996;153(2):761–768.
64. Gozal D, Simakajornboon N. Passive motion of the extremities modifies alveolar ventilation during sleep in patients with congenital central hypoventilation syndrome. *Am J Respir Crit Care Med.* 2000;162(5):1747–1751.
65. Macey PM, Woo MA, Macey KE, et al. Hypoxia reveals posterior thalamic, cerebellar, midbrain, and limbic deficits in congenital central hypoventilation syndrome. *J Appl Physiol.* 2005;98(3):958–969.
66. Harper RM, Macey PM, Woo MA, et al. Hypercapnic exposure in congenital central hypoventilation syndrome reveals CNS respiratory control mechanisms. *J Neurophysiol.* 2005;93(3):1647–1658.
67. Woo MA, Macey PM, Macey KE, et al. FMRI responses to hyperoxia in congenital central hypoventilation syndrome. *Pediatr Res.* 005;57(4): 510–518.

68. Kumar R, Macey PM, Woo MA, Alger JR, Harper RM. Diffusion tensor imaging demonstrates brainstem and cerebellar abnormalities in congenital central hypoventilation syndrome. *Pediatr Res.* 2008;64(3):275–280.
69. de Pontual L, Pelet A, Trochet D, et al. Mutations of the RET gene in isolated and syndromic Hirschsprung's disease in human disclose major and modifier alleles at a single locus. *J Med Genet.* 2006;43(5):419–423.
70. de Pontual L, Pelet A, Clement-Ziza M, et al. Epistatic interactions with a common hypomorphic RET allele in syndromic Hirschsprung disease. *Hum Mutat.* 2007;28(8):790–796.
71. Gronli JO, Santucci BA, Leurgans SE, Berry-Kravis EM, Weese-Mayer DE. Congenital central hypoventilation syndrome: PHOX2B genotype determines risk for sudden death. *Pediatr Pulmonol.* 2008;43(1):77–86.
72. Patwari PP, Loghmanee DA, Rand CM, et al. Paired-like homeobox 2B *(PHOX2B)* gene and autonomic nervous system dysregulation (ANSD): comprehensive genotype/phenotype correlation in cohort of 98 congenital central hypoventilation syndrome (CCHS) cases. *Am J Respir Crit Care Med.* 2009;179(A):1745.
73. Todd ES, Weinberg SM, Berry-Kravis EM, et al. Facial phenotype in children and young adults with PHOX2B-determined congenital central hypoventilation syndrome: quantitative pattern of dysmorphology. *Pediatric Research.* 2006;59(1):39–45.
74. Todd ES, Scott NM, Weese-Mayer DE, et al. Characterization of dermatoglyphics in PHOX2B-confirmed congenital central hypoventilation syndrome. *Pediatrics.* 2006;118(2):e408–e414.
75. Parodi S, Baglietto MP, Pini Prato A, et al. A novel missense mutation in the PHOX2B gene is associated with late onset central hypoventilation syndrome. *Pediatr Pulmonol.* 2008;43(10): 1036–1039.
76. Diedrich A, Malow BA, Antic NA, et al. Vagal and sympathetic heart rate and blood pressure control in adult onset PHOX2B mutation-confirmed congenital central hypoventilation syndrome. *Clin Auton Res.* 2007;17(3):177–185.
77. Doherty LS, Kiely JL, Deegan PC, et al. Late-onset central hypoventilation syndrome: a family genetic study. *Eur Respir J.* 2007;29(2):312–316.
78. Trang H, Laudier B, Trochet D, et al. PHOX2B gene mutation in a patient with late-onset central hypoventilation. *Pediatr Pulmonol.* 2004;38(4): 349–351.
79. Mahmoud M, Bryan Y, Gunter J, Kreeger RN, Sadhasivam S. Anesthetic implications of undiagnosed late onset central hypoventilation syndrome in a child: from elective tonsillectomy to tracheostomy. *Paediatr Anaesth.* 2007;17(10):1001–1005.
80. Jennings LJ, Yu M, Zhou L, et al. Comparison of *PHOX2B* testing methods in the diagnosis of congenital central hypoventilation syndrome and mosaic carriers. *Diagnostic Molecular Pathology.* 2010;In Press.
81. Ize-Ludlow D, Gray JA, Sperling MA, et al. Rapid-onset obesity with hypothalamic dysfunction, hypoventilation, and autonomic dysregulation presenting in childhood. *Pediatrics.* 2007;120(1): e179–e188.
82. Carroll MS, Patwari PP, Weese-Mayer DE.Carbon dioxide chemoreception and hypoventilation syndromes with autonomic dysregulation. *J Appl Physiol.* 2010;108(4):976–988.
83. Fishman LS, Samson JH, Sperling DR Primary alveolar hypoventilation syndrome (ondine's curse). *Am J Dis Child.* 1965;110:155–161.
84. Katz ES, McGrath S, Marcus CL. Late-onset central hypoventilation with hypothalamic dysfunction: a distinct clinical syndrome. *Pediatric Pulmonol.* 2000;29(1):62–68.
85. De Pontual L, Trochet D, Caillat-Zucman S, et al. Delineation of late onset hypoventilation associated with hypothalamic dysfunction syndrome. *Pediatr Res.* 2008;64(6):689–694.
86. Bougneres P, Pantalone L, Linglart A, Rothenbühler A, Le Stunff C. Endocrine manifestations of the rapid-onset obesity with hypoventilation, hypothalamic, autonomic dysregulation and neural tumor (ROHHADNET) syndrome in early childhood. *J Clin Endocrinol Metab.* 2008;93(10):3971–3980.
87. Weese-Mayer DE, Brouillette RT, Naidich TP, McLone DG, Hunt CE. Magnetic resonance imaging and computerized tomography in central hypoventilation. *Am Rev Respir Dis.* 1988; 137(2):393–398.
88. Bachetti T, Robbiano A, Parodi S, et al. Brainstem anomalies in two patients affected by congenital central hypoventilation syndrome. *Am J Respir Crit Care Med.* 2006;174(6):706–709.
89. Epstein AE, DiMarco JP, Ellenbogen KA, et al. ACC/AHA/HRS 2008 Guidelines for Device-Based Therapy of Cardiac Rhythm Abnormalities: a report of the American College of Cardiology/ American Heart Association Task Force on Practice Guidelines (Writing Committee to Revise the ACC/AHA/NASPE 2002 Guideline Update for Implantation of Cardiac Pacemakers and Antiarrhythmia Devices) developed in collaboration with the American Association for Thoracic Surgery and Society of Thoracic Surgeons. *J Am Coll Cardiol.* 2008;51(21):e1–e62.
90. Woo MS, Woo MA, Gozal D, Jansen MT, Keens TG, Harper RM. Heart rate variability in congenital central hypoventilation syndrome. *Pediatr Res.* 1992;31(3):291–296.
91. Silvestri JM, Hanna BD, Volgman AS, Jones PJ, Barnes SD, Weese-Mayer DE. Cardiac rhythm disturbances among children with idiopathic congenital central hypoventilation syndrome. *Pediatr Pulmonol.* 2000;29(5):351–358.
92. Zelko FA, Nelson MN, Leurgans SE, Berry-Kravis EM, Weese-Mayer DE. Congenital central hypoventilation syndrome: neurocognitive functioning in school age children. *Pediatr Pulmonol.* 2010;45(1):92–98.
93. Oren J, Kelly DH, Shannon DC. Long-term follow-up of children with congenital central hypoventilation syndrome. *Pediatrics.* 1987;80(3): 375–380.

94. Marcus CL, Livingston FR, Wood SE, Keens TG. Hypercapnic and hypoxic ventilatory responses in parents and siblings of children with congenital central hypoventilation syndrome. *Am Rev Respir Dis.* 1991;144(1):136–140.
95. Silvestri JM, Weese-Mayer DE, Nelson MN. Neuropsychologic abnormalities in children with congenital central hypoventilation syndrome. *J Pediatr.* 1992;120(3):388–393.
96. Keens T, ed. *Syndromes Affecting Respiratory Control During Sleep.* New York, NY: Marcel Dekker, Inc; 2000.
97. Beckerman RC. Home positive pressure ventilation in congenital central hypoventilation syndrome: more than twenty years of experience. *Pediatr Pulmonol.* 1997;23:154–155.
98. Witmans MB, Chen ML, Davidson Ward SL, et al. *Congenital Syndromes Affecting Respiratory Control During Sleep.* Hoboken, NJ: John Wiley and Sons; 2006.
99. Marcus CL. *Ventilator Management of Abnormal Breathing During Seep: Continuous Positive Airway Pressure and Nocturnal Noninvasive Intermittent Positive Pressure Ventilation.* New York, NY: Marcel Dekker, Inc; 2000.
100. Kerbl R, Litscher H, Grubbauer HM, et al. Congenital central hypoventilation syndrome (Ondine's curse syndrome) in two siblings: delayed diagnosis and successful noninvasive treatment. *Eur J Pediatr.* 1996;155(11):977–980.
101. Costa Orvay JA, Pons Odena M, Jordan Garcia I, et al. Non-invasive ventilation in neonates with Ondine syndrome: a real indication?. *An Pediatr (Barc).* 2005;63(5):441–443.
102. Fauroux B, Boffa C, Desguerre I, Estournet B, Trang H. Long-term noninvasive mechanical ventilation for children at home: a national survey. *Pediatr Pulmonol.* 2003;35(2):119–125.
103. Paditz E. Nocturnal nasal mask ventilation in childhood. *Pneumologie.* 1994;48(10):744–749.
104. Simonds AK, Ward S, Heather S, Bush A, Muntoni F. Outcome of paediatric domiciliary mask ventilation in neuromuscular and skeletal disease. *Eur Respir J.* 2000;16(3):476–481.
105. Teague WG. Non-invasive positive pressure ventilation: current status in paediatric patients. *Paediatr Respir Rev.* 2005;6(1):52–60.
106. Tibballs J Henning RD. Noninvasive ventilatory strategies in the management of a newborn infant and three children with congenital central hypoventilation syndrome. *Pediatr Pulmonol.* 2003;36(6):544–548.
107. Villa MP, Dotta A, Castello D, et al. Bi-level positive airway pressure (BiPAP) ventilation in an infant with central hypoventilation syndrome. *Pediatr Pulmonol.* 1997;24(1):66–69.
108. Kajiura Y, Maeda H, Nishimura Y, et al. A case of primary alveolar hypoventilation syndrome with a good response to nocturnal low-flow oxygen inhalation and negative pressure ventilation. *Nihon Kyobu Shikkan Gakkai Zasshi.* 1992;30(12): 2151–2157.
109. Hartmann H, Jawad MH, Noyes J, Samuels MP, Southall DP. Negative extrathoracic pressure ventilation in central hypoventilation syndrome. *Arch Dis Child.* 1994;70(5):418–423.
110. Weese-Mayer DE, Hunt CE, Brouillette RT, Silvestri JM. Diaphragm pacing in infants and children. *J Pediatr.* 1992;120(1):1–8.
111. Weese-Mayer DE, Silvestri JM, Kenny AS, et al. Diaphragm pacing with a quadripolar phrenic nerve electrode: an international study. *Pacing Clin Electrophysiol.* 1996;19(9):1311–1319.
112. Weese-Mayer DE, Morrow AS, Brouillette RT, Ilbawi MN, Hunt CE. Diaphragm pacing in infants and children. A life-table analysis of implanted components. *Am Rev Respir Dis.* 1989;139(4):974–979.
113. Chen ML, Tablizo MA, Kun S, Keens TG. Diaphragm pacers as a treatment for congenital central hypoventilation syndrome. *Expert Rev Med Devices.* 2005;2(5):577–585.
114. Glenn WW, Phelps ML. Diaphragm pacing by electrical stimulation of the phrenic nerve. *Neurosurgery.* 1985;17(6):974–984.
115. Glenn WW, Brouillette RT, Dentz B, et al. Fundamental considerations in pacing of the diaphragm for chronic ventilatory insufficiency: a multi-center study. *Pacing Clin Electrophysiol.* 1988;11(11, pt 2):2121–2127.
116. Hunt CE, Brouillette RT, Weese-Mayer DE, et al. Diaphragm pacing in infants and children. *Pacing Clin Electrophysiol.* 1988;11(11, pt 2): 2135–2141.
117. Alonso Calderon JL, Garrido Garcia H,Perez Dominguez T, Mazaira J. Simultaneous, bilateral and permanent ventilation with a diaphragm pacing in childhood: the implantation technique and indications. *Cir Pediatr.* 1994;7(1):3–7.
118. Shaul DB, Danielson PD, McComb JG, Keens TG. Thoracoscopic placement of phrenic nerve electrodes for diaphragmatic pacing in children. *J Pediatr Surg.* 2002;37(7):974–978, discussion 974–978.
119. Hyland RH, Hutcheon MA, Perl A, et al. Upper airway occlusion induced by diaphragm pacing for primary alveolar hypoventilation: implications for the pathogenesis of obstructive sleep apnea. *Am Rev Respir Dis.* 1981;124(2):180–185.
120. Movahed MR, Jalili M, Kiciman N Absence of device-device interaction (DDI) in a patient with cardiac and diaphragmatic pacemakers for congenital central hypoventilation syndrome. *Pacing Clin Electrophysiol.* 2005;28(11):1238–1239.
121. Kolb C, Eicken A, Zrenner B, Schmitt C. Cardiac pacing in a patient with diaphragm pacing for congenital central hypoventilation syndrome (Ondine's curse). *J Cardiovasc Electrophysiol.* 2006;17(7):789–791.
122. Marzocchi M, Brouillette RT, Weese-Mayer DE, Morrow AS, Conway LP. Comparison of transthoracic impedance/heart rate monitoring and pulse oximetry for patients using diaphragm pacemakers. *Pediatric Pulmonol.* 1990;8(1):29–32.

CHAPTER 18

Assessment of Sleep Fragmentation

Shalini Paruthi and Ronald D. Chervin

Introduction

Sleep fragmentation can have significant nighttime and daytime consequences for children and their families. Sleep fragmentation, arousals, and awakenings equate to a large extent with sleep deprivation and lead to daytime sleepiness in children. This chapter will review sleep fragmentation, including definitions and surrogate markers, clinical utility, research methodologies, clinical tools, resultant effects, and recovery.

Key Points

- Polysomnography and actigraphy are used to quantify sleep fragmentation.
- Some sleep fragmentation is normal; sleep fragmentation quantified as an arousal index less than 14 cortical arousals per hour on an in-lab sleep study, including an initial night in a sleep lab environment, is within accepted normal limits in children.
- Rates of cortical arousals (arousal indices), sleep efficiency, sleep stage percentages, and nighttime awakenings can reflect sleep fragmentation in standard clinical sleep studies, whereas cyclic alternating pattern, respiratory cycle–related EEG changes, sleep pressure score, or mean durations of individual sleep or sleep stage bouts are examples of analyses that show potential to improve standard evaluations of sleep fragmentation.
- Quantification of subcortical, autonomic activity or arousals—through techniques such as peripheral arterial tonometry, pulse transit time, or heart rate variability—may help to assess subtle sleep fragmentation in a manner that could provide clinical utility.

Defining Sleep Fragmentation

Fragmentation of sleep can be quantified by the number of brief electroencephalographic (EEG) arousals, awakenings, stage shifts (between stages, to stage N1, or to wake), or by the percentage of stage N1 sleep [1]. The rates and durations of arousals and awakenings are most often taken to reflect the intensity of sleep fragmentation [2]. Reduced total sleep time or poor overall sleep efficiency on a polysomnogram can also reflect sleep fragmentation, though in a less specific manner because both measures are affected as much by delayed sleep latency or long awakenings as by shorter interruptions in sleep that better characterize the concept of sleep fragmentation. Depending on the type of recording available, sleep fragmentation may also be reflected in other ways. For example, a cardiopulmonary monitor may give clues to likely sleep fragmentation, if not definitive evidence, through identification of recurrent apneas, hypopneas, discrete oxygen desaturations, transient increases in otherwise stable heart rate, or movement artifact. Movement in fact is the only clue to sleep fragmentation in an actigraphic study (as discussed later in the chapter).

Sleep fragmentation can be assessed in many other ways that are not yet routinely used in the United States, though they show promise for clinical utility. Analysis of the cyclic alternating pattern (CAP) provides a standardized classification of types of arousals and cortical activations and seeks to quantify sleep stability (Figure 18.1). Respiratory cycle–related EEG changes (RCREC) highlight changes in cortical activity that are too subtle to see by eye, but can be shown by computer to occur on average with each respiratory cycle, worsen in sleep apnea, improve after sleep apnea is treated, and predict subsequent daytime sleepiness [3,4]. Arousals that follow apneas or hypopneas can be contrasted to those that occur spontaneously, using the sleep pressure score [5]. Patterns, timing, and contiguous lengths of uninterrupted sleep as summarized in analyses of sleep dynamics also show promise for clinical utility [6,7].

Nonetheless, the most commonly used and recognized measure of sleep fragmentation, in clinical practice, involves quantification of arousals or arousals per hour of sleep (an arousal index). The 1992 American Sleep Disorders Association (ASDA) consensus criteria defined an arousal as an increase in EEG frequency lasting at least 3-seconds duration [8]. If the arousal occurred in rapid eye movement (REM) sleep, an increase in submental muscle tone was also required. The recommendations did not discuss applicability of the definition at different ages of life. The 1992 ASDA definition for arousals was largely preserved in the 2007 American Academy of Sleep Medicine (AASM) Manual for the Scoring of Sleep and Associated Events (AASM Scoring Manual) [9]. Again applicable ages are not specified, and the task force for pediatric scoring rules did not find enough published evidence to recommend an arousal definition different from that used for adults. The new recommendations permit scoring of an arousal when at least 10 seconds of stable sleep is followed by an abrupt shift of EEG frequency to theta, alpha, or frequencies equal to or greater than 16 Hertz (but not spindles), for at least 3 seconds. In REM sleep, a concomitant increase in submental muscle tone is required for at least 1 second [9]. The AASM Scoring Manual also provides recommendations for scoring stage W, representing the waking state and awakenings from sleep. Stage W is scored when more than 50% of the epoch has alpha activity over the occipital region such as in a state of drowsiness. Stage W can also be scored when no alpha activity is noted, and eye blinks at a frequency of 0.5 to 2 Hz, reading eye movements, or irregular conjugate rapid eye movements associated with increased submental muscle tone are present such as in a state of full alertness [9].

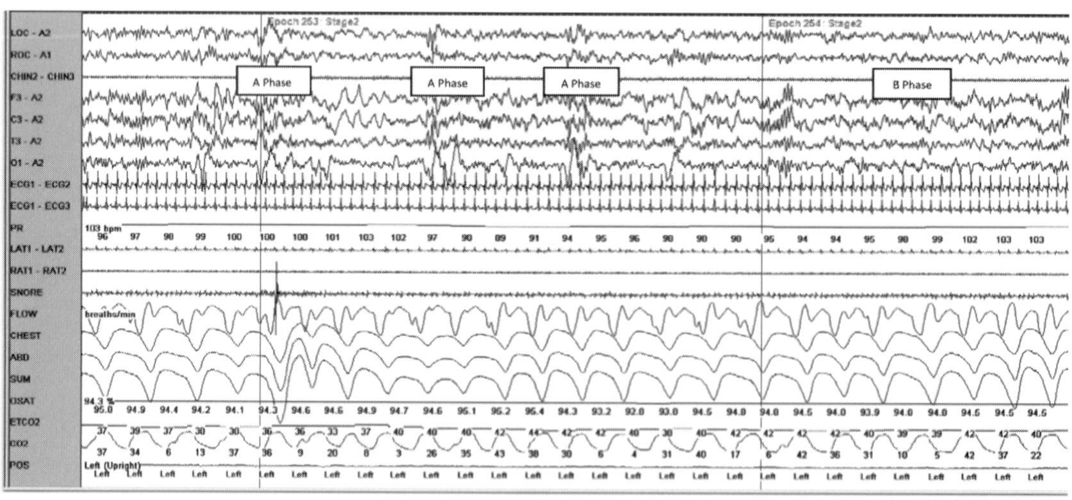

Figure 18.1 Cyclic alternating pattern. In this 60-second epoch, cyclic alternating pattern is seen with distinct transient increases in frequency and amplitude (A phase of the cycle, A1 subtype), which stands out from the background (B phase of the cycle).

Clinical Utility of Sleep Fragmentation Measures

In clinical practice, when parents bring their children in for awakenings at night, the challenge lies in determining whether an underlying medical cause or a behavioral cause is a problem. Depending on the age of the child, some sleep fragmentation may well be a normal, developmental phenomenon. To identify an organic cause of excessive awakenings at night, clinicians may order a polysomnogram, during which the arousal index is routinely scored, calculated, and reported. Most sleep laboratories do not differentiate spontaneous, respiratory-related, periodic limb movement–related, and technician-induced arousals. The AASM Pediatric Task Force considered an arousal index less than 14 events per hour of sleep to be normal for a prepubertal child in a sleep laboratory setting, taking first-night effect into account [10]. Discussing the arousal index can provide children and their parents with an estimate of sleep fragmentation in understandable terms. When polysomnograms are performed before and after procedures or other interventions, the arousal index may be useful to estimate treatment effect [11].

Tools to Quantify Sleep Fragmentation in Research and Clinical Settings

Animal Studies

Several animal models have been used to investigate effects of induced sleep fragmentation on sleep stages, cognition, and even mood disorders. These studies employed techniques such as shaker platforms or treadmill floors to disrupt sleep. For example, an oscillating orbital shaker platform was used to induce arousals for 30 seconds every 2 minutes in 5 mice over a total experiment time of 48 hours [12]. Some adaptation to sleep deprivation was noted during the second 24-hour period. The percentage of non-rapid eye movement (NREM) sleep time decreased, and REM sleep time also decreased, but the number of REM sleep episodes did not change [12]. Additional studies have used a treadmill floor cage, in which treadmill motion intermittently induces arousals from sleep. For example, investigators programmed a treadmill floor belt to move at a rate of 0.02 m/s for 30 seconds, followed by no movement for 90 seconds over 24 hours. Rats exposed to this paradigm and then tested in open fields showed behavior suggestive of decreased anxiety and locomotor hyperactivity [13]. Another study that also induced sleep fragmentation through the same treadmill floor movement protocol found subsequent impairment of spatial reference (memory of platform location) in 63 rats [14]. In a slightly modified protocol of 3-seconds movement followed by 30 seconds of rest, sleep fragmentation was induced for 7 days in 6 rats [15]. During measurements performed 4 and 7 days after sustained sleep fragmentation, there was a reduction in dentate gyrus cell proliferation. Interestingly, reduction in duration of NREM sleep bouts was achieved as evidence of sleep fragmentation, without change in total percentage of NREM sleep as compared with control rats [15]. Taken together, animal experiments such as these, which would be difficult to replicate for any prolonged periods in children, strongly suggest that frequent, brief arousals from sleep have important consequences for the brain and neurobehavioral functioning.

Human Studies

Research protocols in adults have either induced sleep fragmentation and examined the downstream effects or evaluated the tendency for a medical or sleep disorder to produce sleep fragmentation and its associated outcomes. When sleep fragmentation has been induced experimentally, several variables have been tested including type of audible or mechanical stimulus; duration, frequency, and timing of the stimulus; and number of sequential nights of disrupted sleep, all in relation to outcomes such as sleepiness on the multiple sleep latency test (MSLT), maintenance of wakefulness test (MWT), or Stanford Sleepiness Scale; neurocognitive functioning; or hormonal consequences [16–18]. To the authors' knowledge, however, no studies have been published in which sleep fragmentation was induced in healthy children to determine outcomes on the MSLT, MWT, or sleepiness questionnaire scales.

Actigraphy

Actigraphy has been used in research since the 1970s, and AASM practice parameters now help to clarify its role in clinical practice. Actigraphs are small devices, usually worn on the wrist, that monitor motion, thus providing information on nocturnal activity and sleeping positions. The actigraph specifically measures limb movement. A decrease or absence of movement provides an estimate of sleep periods, sleep onset latency, and wake after sleep onset time, to assist with calculation of sleep efficiency.

Actigraphy can be used as a diagnostic tool, as per the International Classification of Sleep Disorders, 2nd edition [19], primarily when polysomnography is impractical or a measure of sleep patterns over a prolonged period is desired. Actigraphy is a valid technique to determine sleep patterns in normal, healthy adult populations, and for estimation of total sleep time in patients with sleep-disordered breathing (SDB), circadian rhythm disorders, or hypersomnia [20]. Actigraphy can also assist in evaluation of response to treatment for insomnia and circadian rhythm disorders. This testing is also indicated in special populations such as nursing home residents and children [20]. Actigraphy can be particularly helpful in research and clinical settings to objectively evaluate a child's baseline sleep patterns, timing and duration of sleep, and frequency and duration of awakenings in a familiar, home environment. The device is minimally disruptive compared with in-lab sleep testing. Hence, in research protocols, up to a week of actigraphy recordings may be completed before in-lab sleep testing to provide more comprehensive data. In the 23 studies cited to support use of actigraphy in pediatric settings, actigraphy was used to quantify night awakenings, nocturnal activity, and sleeping position [20]. Commercially available analysis software can provide fragmentation indices, but clear clinical correlates are not yet well described [20].

Sleep fragmentation defined on actigraphy as estimated sleep percentage lower than 90% or 3 or more awakenings per night on average, with each awakening being 5 minutes or longer, was noted in up to 18% of 140 healthy children aged 7 to 12 years [21]. In another protocol that used actigraphy, the length of continuous sleep periods served as a surrogate for sleep fragmentation, which differed between control infants and those whose mothers had used substances during pregnancy (alcohol, tobacco, cocaine, marijuana, or methamphetamine) [22].

Nocturnal Polysomnography

For polysomnography, use of the AASM Scoring Manual [9] rather than previous scoring recommendations may improve detection of sleep fragmentation. In a comparison study between Rechtschaffen and Kales criteria and the AASM Scoring Manual, visual scoring of sleep was conducted on 10 control healthy children, 26 primary snorers (with an apnea-hypopnea index [AHI] <1) and 39 children with obstructive sleep apnea syndrome (OSAS; AHI >1). Using the AASM Scoring Manual recommendations, the authors were able to identify additional arousals from sleep, when compared with Rechtschaffen and Kales criteria, finding an increase in stage shifts and a higher percentage of stage N1 sleep in children with sleep apnea compared with the other 2 groups of children [23]. Additionally, primary snoring children also showed higher percentages of stage N1 sleep than did control subjects [23]. In the AASM Scoring Manual, nonarousal K-complexes or spindles can signal a stage shift (surrogate for sleep fragmentation) from REM sleep to stage N2, when a K-complex or spindle occurs in the first half of an epoch in the absence of REMs, even when chin tone remains low. These K-complexes are maximal over the prefrontal and frontal regions, with improved detection since the addition of bilateral frontal leads as recommended in the 2007 AASM Scoring Manual.

As mentioned earlier, sleep fragmentation is frequently quantified on polysomnography through the arousal index. For example, an increased arousal index was noted in snoring infants living in smoking households and was hypothesized to contribute to developmental problems [24]. Polysomnography has also shown increased duration of arousals and number of arousals that convert to wakefulness in infants exposed to opiates in utero [25]. Polysomnography allows measurements of sleep fragmentation with direct observation of the patient to further correlate sleep fragmentation with possible respiratory events, movements, or condition-specific phenomena such as scratching from atopic dermatitis [26].

In addition to the arousal index, clinically useful markers of fragmentation such as sleep stage percentages, sleep stage bouts, and stage shifts are also available through polysomnography. Quantification of stage percentages revealed an increase in percent stage N1 sleep in depressed adolescent males [27]. Comparison of 16 children with juvenile rheumatoid arthritis (JRA) to control subjects showed that the median length of stages N2, N3, and REM bouts of sleep was shorter in the JRA subjects [28]. Additionally, shifts from deeper to lighter stages of NREM sleep were more numerous, by 80%, in the JRA group. A subset of these children (all with JRA) underwent 5-nap MSLTs, and a shortened mean sleep latency (11.3 ± 3.2 minutes), as compared with generally accepted values in normal preadolescent children, was attributed to sleep fragmentation [28]. Standard sleep stage analyses have not always shown prominent differences between children with and without obstructive sleep apnea (OSA) [29]. In general, sleep stage percentages remain relatively stable, even in children with significant sleep disorders [29]. Sleep fragmentation may be better characterized with analysis of stage shifts or stage bout durations. For example, in a study of 68 children (5–12 years), the arousal index was 14.6 ± 7.3 for those with SDB (n = 48) vs 8.7 ± 2.5 for control children (n = 20), with $P < .0001$ [30]. The SDB children also had increased sleep stage changes, a higher percentage of stage N1 sleep, and shorter contiguous stage N2 durations. Stage N2 durations seemed to be the single best variable to characterize sleep fragmentation in SDB children vs control children. One year after treatment with adenotonsillectomy, children had longer sleep stage N2 sleep durations, and no sleep stage variable still differentiated the original SDB children from the control children [30]. Furthermore, an early research study provided information on the "first-night effect" and how it can overestimate sleep fragmentation. Over 4 consecutive nights in the sleep lab, the investigators found a significant difference between the first night compared with the second through fourth nights in stage occurrences, stage bouts, and stage shifts. They described the "first-night effect" as characterized by more stage N1, less stage REM, and more stage shifts [31].

Analyses That May Augment Utility of Standard Polysomnography

Cyclic alternating pattern (CAP), an EEG finding on polysomnograms in children and adults, is created by periodic arousals or brain activations that characterize unstable sleep. Cyclic alternating pattern has been investigated in sleep disorders such as OSA, insomnia, epilepsy, and narcolepsy. The CAPs reflect spontaneous, nonrandom sequences of transient increases in frequency or amplitude of EEG (phase A of the cycle) that stand out from background theta or delta EEG activity (phase B interval of the cycle). Three or more A phases are separated from each other by at least 2 seconds, up to 60 seconds, with the last A phase needed to end a sequence, but not included in the sequence. The percentage of CAP time in NREM sleep to total time spent in NREM sleep, known as the CAP rate, allows estimation of sleep instability [32–40]. An atlas of rules was published in 2001 [32], and recent investigations suggest that children, in comparison to adults may exhibit specific, age-dependent CAP differences [32,37–40].

The CAP A phases can be further subdivided as A1, A2, or A3. Subtype A1 describes synchronized EEG patterns such as high-voltage slow waves, with minimal variation, typically seen in the build-up of and maintenance of deep NREM sleep. The A1 phases may represent brain activation rather than arousal and may assist in preservation of sleep in the face of an internal or external stimulus. Thus, A1 phases may have a protective role for sleep continuity, and they have been positively correlated with higher cognitive functioning [33]. The A1 sequences are best visualized in the frontal or prefrontal recording areas. The A2 and A3 subtypes are strongly correlated with cortical arousals defined by the AASM Scoring Manual and often occur before REM sleep, a desynchronized state. The A2 subtype combines elements of A1 and A3 subtypes, including slow, high-voltage K waves but also desynchronized low-amplitude, fast waves; alpha activity; increased muscle tone; or increased cardiorespiratory rates. The A3 subtype represents desynchronized EEG patterns with remarkable enhancement of heart and muscle tone. Frequently measured CAP parameters include CAP time, CAP rate, number and duration of CAP cycles, and number and duration of continuous CAP sequences [33–36].

CAPs that characterize children's sleep have been described. For example, among children younger than 6 years, in comparison to older children and adults, CAP presents with more rhythmic theta or alpha activity in stage N1 and a frequency slower than 16 Hz in A2 and A3 CAP subtypes [34]. Children aged 8 to 12 years (Tanner stages 2–3) as compared with children aged 6 to 10 years have longer CAP rates in stage N3 as opposed to stage N1 or N2, longer mean CAP duration in stage N2, and the number of CAP cycles is greater in stage N2 [37]. Increased CAP rates may correlate with behavioral complaints including hyperactivity, inattentiveness, and mood irritability [33].

Normative pediatric data on CAP come from small studies and suggest a CAP rate of 6.8% to 12.9% in infants up to age 5 months [33], 25.9% in 3- to 6-year-old children [38], 33% in 6- to 10-year-old children [39], 62% in 8- to 12-year-old children [40], and 43% in 10- to 19-year-old children [41]. In summary, CAP analysis may provide systematized arousal analysis, a gauge of sleep instability in NREM sleep, and insight into sleep changes associated with common medical disorders, including but not limited to Down syndrome, autism, and dyslexia [33].

Respiratory Cycle-Related EEG Changes (RCREC) have also been used to improve insight into mechanisms by which SDB may fragment sleep in children. Computer analysis of RCREC occurs on a breath-to-breath basis for sleep recorded between any apneas or hypopneas [3]. The algorithm quantifies the extent to which EEG power changes, for each of several specified frequency ranges, in synchrony with the average respiratory cycle. The RCREC distinguish children with and without SDB [4]. Following adenotonsillectomy in children with SDB, RCREC tends to improve. One study of more than 100 children scheduled to undergo adenotonsillectomy or unrelated surgical care found that parent-rated subjective sleepiness was predicted by RCREC, even after the AHI was taken into account [42]. The RCREC may represent subtle inspiratory microarousals that are more prominent with labored breathing, but cannot be recognized by eye and yet contribute strongly to daytime sleepiness [43].

Sleep microarchitecture can be assessed using *EEG spectral analysis*. The basic concept for spectral analysis is that any signal (commonly in the delta, theta, alpha or beta range) can be broken down into subharmonic frequencies. The amplitude of the EEG signal or its square root (defined as power) can be quantified. The technique of spectral analysis allows for study of slower or faster rhythms that may be filtered out in the conventional EEG. The approach may allow identification of EEG changes that are too subtle to detect by eye. For example, spectral analysis of EEG just after apneic events that are not followed by visible arousals can still detect changes in cortical activity likely to represent subthreshold arousals [44]. This observation is important in children, long observed to have apneic events without scorable arousals, but now understood to have more subtle EEG changes in some cases when computers are used to detect them.

Furthermore, the *sleep pressure score* provides an additional tool to assess cortical arousals. The score can be derived from the equation: $SPS = R/T(1 - (S/T))$, where R is the rate of respiratory arousals, S is the rate of spontaneous arousals, and T is the total rate of arousals. It has been noted that spontaneous arousals decrease when respiratory-related arousals increase. This observation may help to explain why cortical arousals overall may not predict sleep apnea–related morbidity [5].

Many other approaches to the assessment of arousals in children have been investigated. These have focused, for example, on heart rate variability, pulse transit time (PTT), peripheral arterial tonometry (PAT), and pulse wave amplitude. These approaches may also provide useful information on sleep fragmentation in research settings, and perhaps clinical settings in the future.

Heart Rate Variability

Heart rate and beat-to-beat variability have been studied as alternative markers of arousal or sleep fragmentation in children. Small studies have shown conflicting evidence, with either modest heart rate variability in children with OSA [45] or significant differences in R-R intervals between children with and without SDB [46]. The 7 children with OSAS had reduced R-R intervals (faster heart rate) beginning a few seconds after initiation of obstruction, followed by slower heart rate, and then variable heart rates when breathing resumed [46]. For each recording, dispersion of next-intervals was determined for short, long, and intermediate R-R intervals and plotted onto scattergrams. These Poincare plots showed much greater next-interval dispersion (marker for beat-to-beat variability) following slower heart rates in OSAS children than in control children. This variation was less noticeable at intermediate and fast heart rates in OSAS children. The authors note importance of beat-to-beat evaluation because of noticeable oscillations, which become indiscernible in overall heart rate variability analysis [46].

In another study of 25 children (aged 1–18 years) with moderate to severe OSA, who underwent adenotonsillectomy, the mean pulse rate decreased in 21 of 25 children from 99.7 ± 11.2 to 90.1 ± 10.7 beats per minute following adenotonsillectomy. Furthermore, pulse rate variability decreased in 23 of 25 children [47].

Pulse Transit Time

Pulse transit time (PTT) is measured as the time delay between the EKG R wave and the arrival of the pulse wave at the finger, detected through an oximeter probe (Figure 18.2) [48]. PTT is noninvasive, varies inversely with blood pressure, and may also reflect stiffness of arterial walls at rest, as modulated by the autonomic nervous system. The use of PTT improved detection of respiratory events and microarousals especially during REM sleep and slow-wave sleep in children [49]. More apneas, hypopneas, and respiratory effort–related arousals terminated in PTT-defined arousals than in visible EEG arousals in a group of children who underwent sleep studies with esophageal manometry [50].

Peripheral Arterial Tonometry

Peripheral arterial tonometry (PAT) uses finger plethysmography to provide noninvasive beat-to-beat assessment of sympathetic tone and to detect changes in peripheral vascular cutaneous perfusion. In 40 children with SDB, 35% of respiratory events were associated with visible EEG arousals, whereas 92% were associated with PAT attenuation [51]. As movement can be a marker for sleep fragmentation, the inclusion of movement artifact increased sensitivity to 95% and specificity to 35% to detect arousals by PAT.

Further evidence for the potential clinical usefulness of PAT and PTT was provided by a study in which 10 healthy children underwent overnight polysomnography with PAT and PTT [52]. Increases in sensitivity and specificity were again noted with inclusion of movement artifact. When movement artifact events were included as markers for arousals, the sensitivity of PTT to recognize arousals rose to

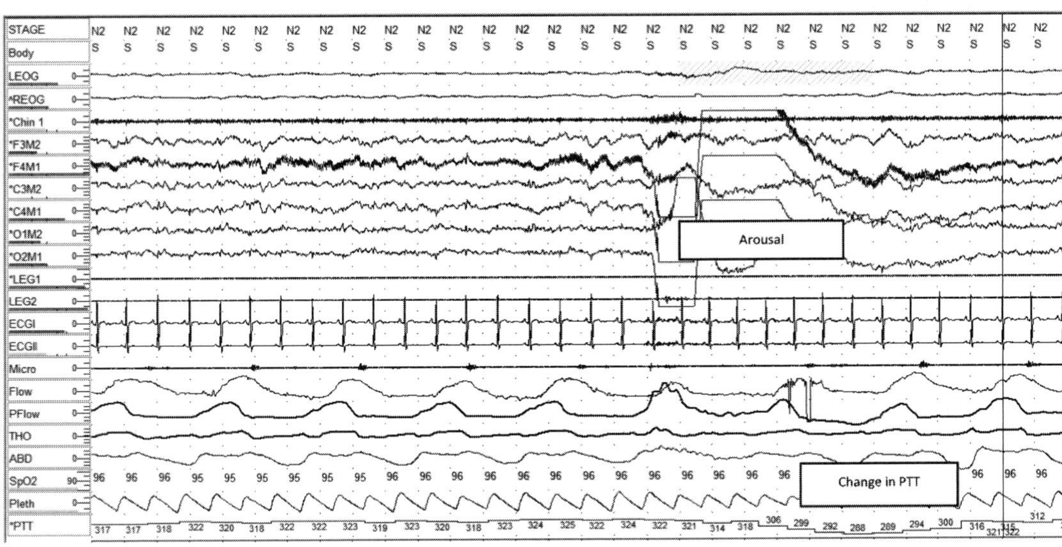

Figure 18.2 Pulse transit time (PTT). Note the change in PTT values associated with the arousal on electroencephalogram and electromyogram channels on a 30-second epoch.

0.96 (from 0.74), sensitivity of PAT rose to 0.92 (from 0.57), specificity of PTT rose to 0.30 (from 0.25), and specificity of PAT rose to 0.19 (from 0.13) [52].

Pulse Wave Amplitude

Pulse wave amplitude measures the difference between the peak and nadir values of corresponding photoplethysmogram pulse waveform for each cardiac cycle. A criterion 30% or more drop in the waveform improved detection of hypopneas and cortical arousals. Concordance between 2 trained scorers in identification of respiratory events was also achieved. This technique has yet to be applied to children [53].

Objective and Subjective Consequences of Sleep Fragmentation

The MSLT, MWT, and Sleepiness Scales

To objectively quantify daytime sleepiness as a consequence of sleep fragmentation, several studies had adults undergo multiple sleep latency testing following overnight polysomnography. Studies in young adults have also been performed. For example, in 36 healthy adults aged 21 to 35 years, the patients were screened for sleep disorders and a baseline mean sleep latency was measured. They then returned to the sleep laboratory for 2 consecutive nights and days of polysomnography and MSLTs. Each night fragmentation was induced by audible tones with an arousal rate of 1 arousal every 4 to 5 minutes. Mean sleep latency on the MSLT decreased from 14.3 ± 3.6 minutes at baseline to 9.8 ± 5.1 and 9.5 ± 5.0 minutes following fragmentation nights [16].

Further measures of sleepiness have also been studied in adults, including the MWT and Stanford Sleepiness Scale [54]. Among 12 healthy student volunteers (25 years of age), subjects underwent induced sleep fragmentation with audible tones. The 2-night study protocol was designed to investigate sleepiness following sleep fragmentation without visible cortical arousal. The first night allowed for acclimatization; during the second night, half the students were allowed uninterrupted sleep, while the other half received audible tones causing sleep disruption. The investigators defined fragmentation in their study as a transient increase in arterial blood pressure or increase in heart rate without visible EEG arousal, and thus, the measured cortical arousal frequency on polysomnography did not differ between the 2 groups of students on the second night. Of note, the audible tone did induce cortical arousal 44% of times it was administered. Mean sleep latency on the MSLT diminished from 8.0 ± 3.1 minutes (baseline) to 6.2 ± 2.1 minutes (following fragmentation), and the MWT results diminished from 29.0 ± 10.0 minutes (baseline) to 25.7 ± 9.7 minutes (following fragmentation). No significant difference emerged between groups in subjective daytime sleepiness as measured by the Stanford Sleepiness Scale [17].

In a study that assessed sleepiness, 45 children diagnosed with OSAS (apnea index >1) were given the modified (pediatric version) Epworth Sleepiness Scales (ESS) [55]. Scores averaged 8.3 ± 5.6, similar to those of other children diagnosed with primary snoring. No difference emerged between children diagnosed with mild, moderate, or severe OSA. The modified ESS also did not correlate with the polysomnogram arousal index [55]. These results suggest that the modified ESS may not be sensitive to sleep fragmentation in children, to the extent that standard polysomnographic measures do capture salient sleep fragmentation expected in the setting of pediatric OSA. In contrast, the Sleepiness Subscale of the Pediatric Sleep Questionnaire Sleep Related Breathing Disorder Scale [56] did correlate with several polysomnographic measures among 103 children with suspected OSA and controls [43].

In adults, investigators have found a linear relationship between the rate of arousal and subsequent sleepiness. Subjects in the study underwent a night of induced arousals, followed by 100 minutes of recovery sleep. Sleepiness was more pronounced if the arousal rate was more frequent (1 arousal per minute vs 1 arousal every 3 or 5 minutes of sleep) [1]. In a study of 5 adults, investigators found the greatest performance decrements when awakenings occurred on a disruption schedule of less than every 10 minutes, which implies that consolidated sleep of at least more than 10 minutes is necessary for the restorative properties of sleep [57].

Neurocognitive, Behavioral, and Hormonal Outcomes

Sleep fragmentation may impact daytime functioning. In 87 children (5–7 years) found to be primary snorers by parental report and polysomnography (obstructive apnea index <1 and AHI <5), a higher respiratory arousal index was found in comparison to that observed among 31 control children [58]. The primary snoring children were more likely to have difficulties with attention, anxious/depressive symptoms, and social problems than their control counterparts. Furthermore, lower levels of language and visuospatial ability and overall lower levels of cognitive ability in children with primary snoring were suggested by the authors as possibly related to increased sleep fragmentation and reduction in REM sleep [58]. In another study of twenty 14-month-old toddlers undergoing actigraphy and polysomnography, toddlers with greater sleep fragmentation during the polysomnography were noted to score significantly worse on the Behavior Rating Scale Emotional Regulation subscale [59].

In a study of 15 adults aged 20 to 28 years of age, sleep fragmentation caused a 2-fold increase in the total CAP rate, with increased length of CAP sequences and duration. This further resulted in decreased slow-wave sleep, increased number of A1 subtypes per hour of sleep, and increased power spectrum at all frequencies including slow-wave activity range. Subjects maintained or improved reaction times with stable error rates [36].

No pediatric studies have investigated hormonal consequences of sleep fragmentation in children. In 11 healthy adult men (18–29 years), polysomnography was performed on 3 consecutive nights, with the first night of nonfragmented sleep and the second and third nights with induced sleep fragmentation, through audible stimulus 12 inches from the subjects' heads and mechanical stimulus with vibrating devices placed beneath the mattresses. Mean arousal frequency was 5.5 arousals per hour on nonfragmented nights compared with 31.4 arousals per hour and 28.8 arousals per hour on fragmented nights. Insulin sensitivity decreased by 25% after sleep fragmentation and glucose effectiveness decreased by 21% after sleep fragmentation. Acute insulin response to glucose increased with fragmented sleep. Increased vagal tone and increased resting average heart rare were noted through heart rate variability analysis following fragmented sleep. The mean serum values for high-sensitivity C-reactive protein, interleukin-6, leptin, adiponectin, and resistin were unchanged despite 2 nights of fragmented sleep. Conversely, cortisol values were 12.5% higher after 2 days of fragmented sleep [18]. Taken together, the above studies, though not performed in children, suggest that increased sleep fragmentation can have significant consequences on hormonal levels and function.

Recovery From Sleep Fragmentation

A few studies have attempted to identify methods to decrease sleep fragmentation or better delineate adaptation responses to sleep fragmentation.

Reduction of sleep fragmentation was observed by actigraphy among 37 children (9–12 years) who underwent sleep restriction, to an average of 41 minutes less than usual sleep duration. However, these children also exhibited worsening performance on a simple reaction time test [60]. Conversely, sleep fragmentation increased in 40 children (9–12 years) who underwent sleep extension by an average of 35 minutes longer than usual. These children improved their performance in a digit forward memory test and reaction time on a continuous performance task [60].

Surgical weight loss by laparoscopic Roux-en-Y gastric bypass may also improve sleep fragmentation. Nineteen children (mean age 16 years) underwent polysomnographic assessments before and approximately 1 year after surgery. Fourteen children were found to have OSA on the initial polysomnogram. For the total group, the mean AHI improved from 20.5 ± 6.9 to 1.9 ± 0.6 respiratory events per hour. Surgical weight loss resulted in reduced stage N1 sleep time and a reduced arousal index overall in the total cohort [61]. Based on the data provided, it is unknown whether the improvement in sleep apnea or weight loss, or a combination of both, improved the sleep fragmentation.

Nasal occlusion, induced experimentally through the use of a petrolatum-impregnated gauze, seems to fragment sleep as reflected by the increased percentage of stage N1 and arousal index in 45 children (11–15 years). AHI and mean length of apneas also increased, and conversely, the oxygen saturation nadir decreased [62]. This study suggests that comprehensive treatment of nasal occlusion and nasal congestion may be important to reduce sleep fragmentation in patients.

Many of the above adult study designs employed a 2-night approach to investigate sleep fragmentation. By the second night, adaptation begins to occur; many of the subjects had higher arousal thresholds, as louder or longer application of stimuli was required to arouse the subjects from sleep. For example, in the study with 36 healthy young men, nearly the same average number of audible tone series were delivered on 2 subsequent nights (115 vs 118 series); however, on night 1, arousals occurred in 78% of the series, whereas on night 2, arousals only occurred in only 68% of the series. Additionally, the authors found a greater percentage of stage changes on night 1 compared with night 2 [16].

Similar plasticity of arousal responses has been reported in sleep-deprived infants. Fourteen 8-week-old infants with regular bedtimes and naptimes were subjected to a mean 120 minutes of sleep deprivation before the morning or afternoon nap period. With sleep deprivation, increased duration of napping was noted and more intense auditory stimuli were required to arouse the sleeping infants [63].

Clinical Pearls

1. Some sleep fragmentation is a normal, partly age-dependent phenomenon.
2. Sleep fragmentation can be caused by medical or sleep conditions such as pain, sleep apnea, many disorders associated with insomnia, or epilepsy.
3. Evaluation often includes polysomnography or actigraphy, in addition to clinical history and physical examination.
4. Treatment should be determined by an appropriate diagnosis, and symptom severity, rather than the complaint or phenomenon of sleep fragmentation itself.
5. Measures of sleep fragmentation can be used to estimate treatment effect if performed before and after the procedure or intervention.

Summary and Future Directions

Sleep fragmentation is common in many medical and primary sleep disorders. The assessment of sleep fragmentation is necessary to understand pathophysiologic consequences of the sleep disturbance. Measures commonly reported after standard nocturnal polysomnograms include arousal indices, awakenings, sleep stage shifts, and total sleep stage durations. Measures that have been used in research, applied in some clinical settings, and suggested to improve clinical utility of sleep studies include CAP, RCREC, EEG spectral analysis, sleep pressure score, PAT, PTT, and heart rate variability. Actigraphy can also be a valuable tool, especially when several days of data are desired to assess sleep fragmentation. Sleep fragmentation is likely to have clinically significant consequences, especially when arousals are frequent and brief. Sleep fragmentation has been studied in several specific medical sleep disorders, but significant work remains to be done to further characterize consequences and clarify what physiologic patterns and aspects of arousals are most consequential with respect to specific outcomes. Among children in particular, additional data are required to improve understanding of the extent to which sleep fragmentation, as opposed to other aspects of sleep disorders, results in important consequences such as impairment of daytime alertness, academic performance, behavior, mood disturbances, physical performance, or immune responses.

References

1. Levine B, Roehrs T, Stepanski E, Zorick F, Roth T. Fragmenting Sleep Diminishes its recuperative value. *Sleep*. 1987;10(6):590–599.
2. Stepanski EJ. The effect of sleep fragmentation on daytime function. *Sleep*. 2002;25(3):268–276.
3. Chervin RD, Burns JW, Subotic NS, Roussi C, Thelen B, Ruzicka DL. Method for detection of respiratory cycle-related EEG changes in sleep-disordered breathing. *Sleep*. 2004;27(1):110–115.
4. Chervin RD, Burns JW, Subotic NS, Roussi C, Thelen B, Ruzicka DL. Correlates of respiratory cycle-related EEG changes in children with sleep-disordered breathing. *Sleep*. 2004;27(1):116–121.

5. Tauman R, O'Brien LM, Holbrook CR, Gozal D. Sleep pressure score: a new index of sleep disruption in snoring children. *Sleep*. 2004;27(2): 274–278.
6. Chervin RD, Fetterolf JL, Ruzicka DL, Thelen BJ, Burns JW. Sleep stage dynamics differ between children with and without obstructive sleep apnea. *Sleep*. 2009;32(10):1325–1332.
7. Burns JW, Crofford LJ, Chervin RD. Sleep stage dynamics in fibromyalgia patients and controls. *Sleep Med*. 2008;6:689–696.
8. American Sleep Disorders Association. EEG arousals: scoring rules and examples. *Sleep*. 1992; 15:173–184.
9. Iber, C, Ancoli-Israel, S, Chesson, AL, Quan S. *The AASM Manual for the Scoring of Sleep and Associated Events*. West Chester, IL: American Academy of Sleep Medicine; 2007.
10. Grigg-Damberger M, Gozal D, Marcus CL, et al. The visual scoring of sleep and arousal in infants and children; development of polygraphic features, reliability, validity, and alternative methods. *J Clin Sleep Med*. 2007:3(2):201–240.
11. Scholle S, Zwacka G. Arousals and obstructive sleep apnea syndrome in children. *Clin Neurophysiol*. 2001;112(6):984–991.
12. Sinton CM, Kovakkattu D, Friese RS. Validation of a novel method to interrupt sleep in the mouse. *J Neuroscience Methods*. 2009;184:71–78.
13. Tartar JL, Ward CP, Cordeira JW, et al. Experimental sleep fragmentation and sleep deprivation in rats increases exploration in an open field test of anxiety while increasing plasma corticosterone levels. *Behavioural Brain Research*. 2009;197:450–453.
14. Ward CP, McCarley RW, Strecker RE. Experimental sleep fragmentation impairs spatial reference but not working memory in Fischer/Brown Norway rats. *J Sleep Res*. 2009;18:238–244.
15. Guzman-Marin R, Bashir T, Suntsova N, Szymusiak R, McGinty D. Hippocampal neurogenesis is reduced by sleep fragmentation in the adult rat. *Neuroscience*. 2007;148(1):325–333.
16. Roehrs R, Merlotti L, Petrucelli N, Stepanski E, Roth, T. Experimental sleep fragmentation. *Sleep*. 1994;5:438–443.
17. Martin SE, Wraith PK, Deary IJ, Douglas NJ. The effect of nonvisible sleep fragmentation on daytime function. *Am J Respir Crit Care Med*. 1997;155:1596–1601.
18. Stamatakis KA, Punjabi NM. Effects of sleep fragmentation on glucose metabolism in normal subjects. *Chest*. 2010;137(1):95–101.
19. American Academy of Sleep Medicine. *International Classification of Sleep Disorders: Diagnostic and Coding Manual*. 2nd ed. Westchester, IL: American Academy of Sleep Medicine; 2005.
20. Morgenthaler T, Alessi C, Friedman L, et al. Practice parameters for the use of actigraphy in the assessment of sleep and sleep disorders: an update for 2007. *Sleep*. 2007;30(4):519–529.
21. Sadeh A, Raviv A, Gruber R. Sleep patterns and sleep disruptions in school-age children. *Dev Psychol*. 2000;36(3):291–301.
22. Hanft A, Burnham M, Goodlin-Jones B, Anders TF. Sleep architecture in infants of substance-abusing mothers. *Infant Mental Health Journal*. 2006;27(2):141–151.
23. Miano S, Paolino MC, Castaldo R, Villa MP. Visual scoring of sleep: a comparison between the Rechtschaffen and Kales criteria and the American Academy of Sleep Medicine criteria in a pediatric population with obstructive sleep apnea syndrome. *Clin Neurophysiol*. 2010;121(1): 39–42.
24. Montgomery-Downs HE, Gozal D. Snore-associated sleep fragmentation in infancy: mental development effects and the contribution of secondhand cigarette smoke exposure. *Pediatrics*. 2006;117(3):e496-e502.
25. O'Brien CM, Jeffery HE. Sleep deprivation, disorganization and fragmentation during opiate withdrawal in newborns. *J Paediatr Child Health*. 2002;38:66–71.
26. Reuveni H, Chapnick G, Tal A, Tarasiuk A. Sleep fragmentation in children with atopic dermatitis. *Arch Pediatr Adolesc Med*. 1999;153:249–253.
27. Robert JJT, Hoffmann RF, Emslie GJ, et al. Sex and age differences in sleep macroarchitecture in childhood and adolescent depression. *Sleep*. 2006;29(3):351–358.
28. Zamir G, Press J, Tal A, Tarasiuk A. Sleep fragmentation in children with juvenile rheumatoid arthritis. *The Journal of Rheumatology*. 1998;25: 1191–1197.
29. Goh DY, Galster P, Marcus CL. Sleep architecture and respiratory disturbances in children with obstructive sleep apnea. *Am J Respir Crit Care Med*. 2000;162(2, pt1):682–686.
30. Chervin RD, Fetterolf JL, Ruzicka DL, Thelen BJ, Burns JW. Sleep stage dynamics differ between children with and without obstructive sleep apnea. *Sleep*. 2009;30(10):1325–1332.
31. Agnew HW Jr, Webb WB, Williams RL. The first night effect: an EEG study of sleep. *Psychophysiology*. 1996;2(3):263–266.
32. Terzano MG, Parrino L, Sherieri A, et al. Atlas, rules and recording techniques for the scoring of cyclic alternating pattern (CAP) in human sleep. *Sleep Med*. 2001;2(6):537–553.
33. Bruni O, Novelli L, Miano S, Parrino L, Terzano MG, Ferri R. Cyclic alternating pattern: A window into pediatric sleep. *Sleep Med*. 2010 Aug; 11(7):628–836.
34. Lopes MC, Rosa A, Roizenblatt S et al. Cyclic alternating pattern in peripubertal children. *Sleep*. 2005;28(2):215–219.
35. Ferri R, Bruni O, Miano S, Plazzi G, Spruyt K, Gozal D, Terzano MG. The time structure of the cyclic alternating pattern during sleep. *Sleep*. 2006;29(5):693–699.
36. Ferri R, Drago V, Arico D, et al. The effects of experimental sleep fragmentation on cognitive processing. *Sleep Med*. 2010;11(4):378–385.
37. Lopes MC, Rosa A, Roizenblatt S, et al. Cyclic alternating pattern in peripubertal children. *Sleep*. 2005;28(2):215–219.

38. Bruni O, Ferri R, Miano S, et al. Sleep cyclic alternating pattern in normal preschool-aged children. *Sleep*. 2005;28(2):220–230.
39. Bruni O, Ferri R. Miano S, et al. Sleep cyclic alternating pattern in normal school-age children. *Clin Neurophysiol*. 2002;113:1806–1814.
40. Lopes MC, Rosa A, Roizenblatt S, et al. Cyclic alternating pattern in peripubertal children. *Sleep*. 2005;28(2):215–219.
41. Parrino L, Boselli M, Spaggiari MC, Smerieri A, Terzano MG. Cyclic alternating pattern (CAP) in normal sleep: polysomnographic parameters in different age groups. *Electroencephalogr clin Neurophysiol*. 1998;107:439–450.
42. Chervin RD, Weatherly RA, Ruzicka DL, et al. Subjective sleepiness and polysomnographic correlates in children scheduled for adenotonsillectomy vs other surgical care. *Sleep*. 2006;29:495–503.
43. Chervin RD, Burns JW, Ruzicka DL. Electroencephalographic changes during respiratory cycles predict sleepiness in sleep apnea. *Am J Resp Crit Care Med*. 2005;171:652–658.
44. Bandla HP, Gozal D. Dynamic changes in EEG spectra during obstructive apnea in children. *Pediatr Pulmonol*. 2000;29(5):359–365.
45. D'Andrea LA, Rosen CL, Haddad GG. Severe hypoxemia in children with upper airway obstruction during sleep does not lead to significant changes in heart rate. *Pediatr Pulmonol*. 1993;16:362–369.
46. Aljadeff G, Gozal D, Schechtman VL, Burrell B, Harper RM, Ward SL. Heart rate variability in children with obstructive sleep apnea. *Sleep*. 1997;20(2):151–157.
47. Constantin E, McGregor CD, Cote V, Brouillette RT. Pulse Rate and Pulse Rate Variability Decrease After Adenotonsillectomy for Obstructive Sleep Apnea. *Pediatr Pulmonol*. 2008;43:498–504.
48. Stradling JR, Barbour C, Glennon J, Langford BA, Crosby JH. Prevalence of sleepiness and its relation to autonomic evidence of arousals and increased inspiratory effort in a community based population of men and women. *J Sleep Res*. 2000;9:381–388.
49. Pepin JL, Delavie N, Pin I, et al. Pulse transit time improves detection of sleep respiratory events and microarousals in children. *Chest*. 2005;127: 722–730.
50. Katz ES, Lutz J, Black C, Marcus CL. Pulse transit time as a measure of arousal and respiratory effort in children with sleep disordered breathing. *Pediatr Res*. 2003;53:580–588.
51. Tauman R, O'Brien LM, Mast BT, Holbrook CR, Gozal D. Peripheral arterial tonometry events and electroencephalographic arousals in children. *Sleep*. 2004;27(3):502–506.
52. O'Brien LM, Gozal D. Potential usefulness of noninvasive autonomic monitoring in recognition of arousals in normal healthy children. *J Clin Sleep Med*. 2007;3(1):41–47.
53. Zacharia A, Haba-Rubio J, Simon R, et al. Sleep apnea syndrome: improved detection of respiratory events and cortical arousals using oximetry pulse wave amplitude during polysomnography. *Sleep Breath*. 2008;12:33–38.
54. Hoddes E, Dement WC, Zarcone V. The history and use of the Stanford Sleepiness Scale. *Psychophysiology*. 1972;9:150.
55. Melendres MC, Lutz JM, Rubin ED, Marcus CL. Daytime sleepiness and hyperactivity in children with suspected sleep-disordered breathing. *Pediatrics*. 2004;114(3):768–775.
56. Chervin RD, Hedger K, Dillon JE, Pituch KJ. Pediatric sleep questionnaire (PSQ): validity and reliability of scales for sleep-disordered breathing, snoring, sleepiness, and behavioral problems. *Sleep Med*. 2000;1:21–32.
57. Downey R, Bonnet MH. Performance during frequent sleep disruption. *Sleep*. 1987;10(4): 354–363.
58. O'Brien LM, Mervis CB, Holbrook CR, et al. Neurobehavioral implications of habitual snoring in children. *Pediatrics*. 2004;114:44–49.
59. Montgomery-Downs HE, Gozal D. Toddler behavior following polysomnography: effects of unintended sleep disturbance. *Sleep*. 2006;29(10): 1282–1287.
60. Sadeh A, Gruber R, Raviv A. The effects of sleep restriction and extension on school-age children: what a difference an hour makes. *Child Dev*. 2003;74(2):444–455.
61. Kalra M, Mannaa M, Fitz K, et al. Effect of surgical weight loss on sleep architecture in adolescents with severe obesity. *Obes Surg*. 2008;18:675–679.
62. Millman RP, Acebo C, Rosenberg C, Carskadon MA. Response to nasal occlusion. *Chest*. 1996; 109(3):673–679.
63. Franco P, Seret N, Van Hees JN, et al. Decreased arousals among healthy infants after short-term sleep deprivation. *Pediatrics*. 2004;114(2): e192–e197.

CHAPTER 19

Imaging Modalities in Pediatric Sleep Medicine

Robert Joseph Thomas

Imaging modalities can have a major impact on the management of pediatric sleep-wake disorders. A role for imaging the brain itself is yet to be defined—but the potential exists. The rapidly developing brain in the pediatric age group is vulnerable to a range of stressors including that related to sleep [1] This chapter will make a case for assessing brain structure and function in disorders of sleep in children to complement the data already available in adults [2,3]. Once radiation risk is factored in, magnetic resonance imaging (MRI) techniques are the obvious choice. These techniques include structural, functional, and diffusion-weighted imaging. Structural scans can be subjected to sophisticated analysis such as voxel-based, tensor-based, and cortex-based analysis. Thickness of cortical areas can be computed (Figure 19.1). Functional magnetic resonance imaging (fMRI) traditionally uses the blood oxygen level–dependent (BOLD) signal for task-related activation, but resting state and connectivity analysis can add important new dimensions. The data presented will make a case for neuroimaging to better understand the impact of sleep pathology on the developing and maturing brain.

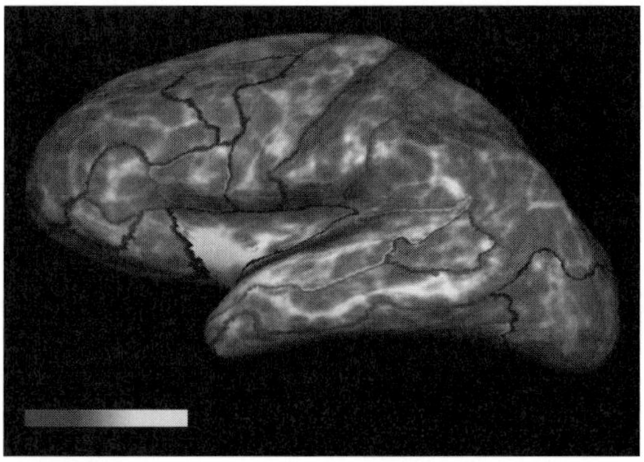

Figure 19.1 Cortical thickness map in a healthy adult. This map is generated from high-resolution anatomical MRI at 3 Tesla and analyzed using FreeSurfer, a freely available analysis suite. Cross-sectional analysis can relate pathology to structure, and changes can be readily tracked across time. Courtesy of Doug Greve, PhD, Martinos Center for Biomedical Imaging, Charlestown, Massachusetts.

Sleep Is Critical for Brain Health

There is increasing evidence that sleep is a state that is important for normal brain function. There are extensive changes in gene expression between behavioral states of sleep and wake [4–6] and after sleep deprivation [7–10]. Functions of sleep may be to maintain synaptic homeostasis and promote macromolecule biosynthesis [11]. There is also upregulation during sleep of genes involved in synthesis of proteins, heme, and maintenance of vesicle pools, as well as antioxidant enzymes and genes encoding proteins of energy-regulating pathways [11]. Wakefulness is an energetic challenge to the brain including the unfolded protein response, the electron transport chain, neuronal PAS (Period-Arnt-Sim) domain–containing protein 2, 5-adenosine monophosphate–activated protein kinase, the astrocyte-neuron lactate shuttle, production of reactive oxygen species, and uncoupling proteins [12,13]. In all species studied to date, there is upregulation of the molecular chaperone binding immunoglobulin protein with extended wakefulness [14,15].

Sleep seems to have an important role for normal synaptic function and maintenance [16–19]. Wakefulness appears to be associated with net synaptic potentiation, whereas sleep may favor global synaptic depression, thereby preserving an overall balance of synaptic strength. In rat cortex and hippocampus, changes in the phosphorylation states of α-amino-3-hydroxy-5-methylisoxazole-4-propionic acid receptors, calmodulin kinase II, and glycogen synthase kinase 3 beta are consistent with synaptic potentiation during wakefulness and depression during sleep [16]. Furthermore, the slope and amplitude of cortical evoked responses increase after wakefulness, decrease after sleep, and correlate with changes in slow-wave activity, a marker of sleep pressure [16–19]. Sleep is an important modulator of cortical plasticity that has strong developmental influences [20,21].

Sleep disorders in adults and children are characterized by a uniform set of abnormalities that vary only in proportion. These are sleep deprivation (reduction in the total amount of sleep), sleep fragmentation (loss of the continuity of sleep), sleep hypoxia (reduced oxygenation during sleep), sleep hypercapnia (reduced ventilation during sleep), sleep hypertension (increased sympathetic activation during sleep), and sleep metabolic dysfunction (a host of metabolic and cytokine alterations). All these abnormalities have the potential to cause brain injury. There are some differences in the expression of these abnormalities in adults vs children, but there is continuum and all patterns are seen in both groups. As examples, hypercapnia from obstructive hypoventilation is a typical feature of pediatric obstructive sleep apnea (OSA), sleep deprivation is rarely a feature of pediatric sleep apnea, and sleep fragmentation has different signatures [22,23]. Specifically, loss of "macro-continuity" of sleep is not typical of disturbed pediatric sleep, likely because of the high homeostatic sleep drive in younger individuals. Thus, conventional polysomnographic sleep quality metrics may be within normal limits yet other measures, such as autonomic [24–26] and cytokine or metabolic profiles [27–29], may be abnormal.

Vulnerability of the Pediatric Brain in Pediatric Sleep Disorders

High-resolution MRI can map the cortical changes associated with brain maturation [30–32]. Frontal cortical growth is prominent in the prepubertal years [33]. The rapid growth and subsequent pruning of synapses reflect in parallel changes in sleep delta power [34,35]. Several areas of the brain are sensitive to hypoxia, such as the hippocampus [36–38], basal ganglia [39], and cerebellum [40]. Thus, the pediatric brain has numerous vulnerabilities to injury mediated by sleep pathology.

OSA in children is an important public health problem that remains to be fully defined in pathophysiology, prevalence, and consequences [41–43]. Breathing patterns because of airway narrowing are highly variable, including obstructive cycling, increased respiratory effort, flow limitation, tachypnea, and/or gas exchange abnormalities [41]. Current approaches to quantification of respiratory abnormality during pediatric polysomnography may underestimate the severity of disordered breathing [44]. Disease phenotypes have been proposed, based primarily on the association of obesity or adenotonsillar hypertrophy [45]. Clinical neurocognitive associations have included learning difficulties and executive dysfunction [46,47], attention deficit hyperactivity problems [48–50], and behavioral difficulties [51]. Cognitive dysfunction in multiple domains of attention, executive functions, and mood regulation is a major clinical problem associated with sleep-disordered breathing in adults [46,52–60] and children [47,61–64]. Evidence suggests a pathophysiological association between intermittent hypoxia and sleep fragmentation with alterations in memory, attention, and intelligence in children [65]. Research has also identified a link between sleep disorders and problematic hyperactive behaviors and mood disturbances [47,66–69]. Furthermore, there is considerable interindividual variability in the presence and magnitude of neurobehavioral morbidity at any given level of disease severity. This further suggests that, in addition to the disease per se, both genetic [70] and environmental modifiers play a role in determining morbidity.

Removal of enlarged tonsils and adenoids is a standard for management of pediatric OSA. There is increasing concern that residual abnormalities may be frequent, with the potential to contribute to adverse long-term cognitive outcomes [71–73]. However, the impact of these residual respiratory abnormalities on cognitive function has not been determined. Major abnormalities in oxygenation typically resolve after adenotonsillectomy, but residual upper airway flow limitation or increased negative esophageal pressures may persist. The time course of changes (if any) in brain structure and function following treatment in the pediatric age group has not been determined.

Potential Mediators of Brain Injury in Sleep Disorders

Hypoxia

Exposure to intermittent hypoxia in rodents results in impaired executive function, excessive sleepiness, and sensitivity to sleep deprivation [74–77]. There is evidence of neuronal injury in the hippocampus [78,79] and basal forebrain [80] and neuronal loss in wake-promoting catecholaminergic systems [81]. Suggested mediating mechanisms include free radical–mediated injury, lipid peroxidation, induction of nitric oxide synthase, platelet activation factor, and apoptosis [82–84]. Mitochondrial dysfunction [85] can amplify these effects. Long-term potentiation (LTP) mechanisms are impaired [86]. Rats exposed to intermittent hypoxia during early postnatal development exhibited heightened behavioral activation when placed into a novel environment. These same rats also demonstrate reduced levels of extracellular dopamine during both the dark and light phases of the circadian cycle [87]. However, sleep architecture can be altered by hypoxia exposure [88].

Hypoxia-cognition models in humans include exposure to altitude [89,90] (although several studies have been inconclusive, for example, those by Anooshiravani et al [91], Merz et al [92], Pavlicek et al [93], and Thomas et al [94]) and in patients with chronic obstructive airway disease [95,96] and sleep apnea [46,52,53,56,97–102]. Executive dysfunction and some slowing in information processing are the primary domain impairments. A significant increase in amplitude and a delay in the evening decline in core body temperature raises the possibility of circadian effects [103]. A magnetic resonance spectroscopic assessment in severe adult sleep apnea reported reduced frontal white matter N-acetyl-aspartate and choline [104]. A different study reported hippocampal spectroscopic abnormalities [105].

Hypoxia at altitude and in those with chronic obstructive lung disease is associated with alterations in cerebral phosphate metabolism and blood flow as assessed by magnetic resonance spectroscopy and positron emission tomography (PET) [106–108]. PET and [(18)F]-2-deoxy-2-fluro-d-glucose imaging techniques were used to assess regional cerebral glucose metabolic rates in six U.S. marines (Caucasian lineage) before and after a 63-day training program for operations at high altitudes ranging from 10,500 to 20,320 feet [106]. Significant decreases in absolute cerebral glucose metabolism after high-altitude exposure were found in 5 regions: 3 frontal, the left occipital lobe, and the right thalamus; for the right and left cerebellum, significant increases in metabolism were found. The magnitudes of these differences, in terms of absolute metabolism, were large, ranging from 10% to 18%. In a study of 17 chronic obstructive lung disease vs 21 matched controls, magnetic resonance spectra were obtained from localized regions of parietal white matter and occipital gray matter. Absolute levels of N-acetyl aspartate, creatinine, choline, and myo-inositol were all lower in patients [108].

Sleep Deprivation and Fragmentation Effects: Assessment Using Slow-Wave/ Delta Power Analysis

The most consistent biological consequences of experimental sleep deprivation or restriction are attentional impairment and lapses, executive dysfunction, and affective change [109–115]. Sleep duration is curtailed in modern day society, resulting in population-level sleep restriction

[116–118]. Stimuli that fragment sleep in controlled experimental situations, such as auditory stimuli, reliably induce sleepiness, executive dysfunction, and depressed mood [119–122].

Delta power dynamics across a night is thought to reflect the behavior of the sleep homeostatic process [123,124]. Following sleep deprivation, recovery sleep is consistently characterized by an increase in delta power that is usually maximal in the anterior (frontal) measuring sites [125,126]. In the cerebral cortex, deep non-rapid eye movement (NREM) sleep manifests with low-frequency variations in surface potentials that characterize slow-wave activity electroencephalogram (EEG). At the neuronal unit level, these events reflect synchronization (<1 Hz) of cortical neuronal units between sustained firing (ON periods, which likely correspond to conditions of persistent membrane depolarization—"UP" states) and silent states (OFF periods, corresponding to membrane hyperpolarizations and "DOWN" states) [127–132]. During early NREM sleep after sustained wakefulness, periods of population activity (ON) are short, frequent, and associated with synchronous firing, whereas periods of neuronal silence are long and frequent. After sustained sleep, firing rates and synchrony decrease, whereas the duration of ON periods increases [133].

Delta power is a key homeostatic sleep drive marker [123,124]. Slow-wave activity in cortical areas that have had increased activity during the daytime, for example, after daytime repetitive tasks, generates more slow waves locally [134,135]. Declarative learning tasks significantly increase the density of sleep spindles relative to nonlearning control subjects [136,137]. The surface-positive half-waves of the <1 Hz NREM low oscillation [130,131,138–141] result from widespread cortical depolarization and are associated with distinctly enhanced coherence after learning in the slow-oscillatory, delta, slow-spindle, and gamma bands [142]. Rat barrel somatosensory cortex demonstrates increased delta power during subsequent sleep in models of asymmetric stimulation [134]. Using PET, several brain areas activated during the execution of a serial reaction time task during wakefulness are significantly more active during rapid eye movement sleep in subjects previously trained on the task than in nontrained subjects [143]. Experience and learning associated with a rotation adaptation task increase focal delta power during subsequent sleep [135].

In the synaptic homeostasis model of NREM sleep, wake is associated with learning, leading to LTP and strengthening of glutamatergic synapses, a process that eventually becomes unsustainable as the energy requirement for maintaining connections and associated firing increases. Sleep then occurs, leading to a proportional synaptic downscaling, leaving only the most robust connections intact. Synaptic downscaling during sleep would increase signal-to-noise ratio for the remaining connections, improving performance [17–19,144]. *Sleep fragmenting stimuli inhibit the slow oscillation* [145] and the synaptic downscaling function and could impair the coordinated interactions between hippocampal ripples and cortical spindles during slow-wave sleep [146–149]. In rodents, sleep fragmentation impairs hippocampal LTP [150]. Fragmenting stimuli may also have indirect effects, such as activation of glucocorticoid-related stress responses [151]. Sleep-dependent learning could be inhibited by ineffective sleep, similar to that reported with motor learning in schizophrenia, cocaine users, and insomnia [152–154]. Although the precise role of normal sleep in memory consolidation remains under investigation, sleep fragmentation may disrupt this function.

Neurogenesis

The 2 sites for neurogenesis in the adult brain are the subventricular region and the dentate gyrus of the hippocampus [155]. That this neurogenesis is functionally important is consistent with the evidence that hippocampal neurogenesis is critical for the therapeutic effects of antidepressant therapies (drugs, electroconvulsive therapy, and transcranial magnetic stimulation) [156–167]. Prevention of neurogenesis by irradiation can prevent antidepressant efficacy [168]. Hippocampal neurogenesis is reduced by sleep deprivation and fragmentation [169–172]. Relatively mild abnormalities of the cortisol circadian profile is well documented in states of deprived or fragmented sleep [173–177]; obesity may be a stronger influence in patients with sleep-disordered breathing [178]. Pediatric sleep disorders have the potential to impair hippocampal neurogenesis. There have been no direct studies of imaging of neurogenesis in pediatric or adult sleep disorders. Magnetic resonance spectroscopy can reportedly identify signals from neural stem and progenitor cells in the hippocampus [179,180]. If feasibility is established, pediatric sleep apnea can usefully be evaluated.

Hemodynamic Function

Sleep fragmentation is associated with daytime hypertension [181]. Sleep deprivation causes mild blood pressure increases [182]. Repetitive surges of blood pressure is an invariant biological response to sleep fragmentation [183,184]. Sleep apnea is a well-defined risk factor for secondary hypertension and blood pressure nondipping [185,186]. Sleep with the EEG morphology of cyclic alternating pattern (dominance of phasic EEG activity) is associated with nondipping of nocturnal blood pressure [187]. This sleep state is readily induced by a range of sleep-fragmenting stimuli. Sleep apnea is associated with an increased risk of strokes in adults [188,189], while data from the pediatric age group are lacking. Sleep hypertension is also a feature of sleep apnea and arousals from sleep in children [190].

Inflammation

Activation of innate systemic and nervous system inflammatory pathways occurs in sleep-deprived conditions [191]. Sleep apnea is associated with activation of a number of inflammatory pathways, possibly mediated by hypoxia [192–198]. Inflammation is also associated with the neuropathogenesis and clinical risk for Alzheimer disease and cognitive decline [199–203]. Pediatric sleep apnea is associated with increases in a number of inflammatory markers, including C-reactive protein and tumor necrosis factor-alpha [204–206].

Vascular Function

Sleep apnea is associated with carotid artery intimal thickening [207,208]. Endothelial dysfunction, a known risk factor for vascular dementia [209–212], is a well-defined association of sleep apnea [213], and the mediator is probably nocturnal hypoxia. Desaturation-oxygenation cycles seen in sleep apnea result in a significant oxidative stress [214] and generation of free radicals that can injure neurons [215–217]. Endothelial functional abnormalities similar to adults have been reported in pediatric sleep apnea [218–221].

Metabolic Function

Diabetes is a risk factor for cognitive decline [222–225]; a major role in Alzheimer disease has been suggested and is still being explored [226–228]. Sleep deprivation [229], sleep apnea [230–232], and experimental sleep fragmentation [233] are associated with impaired glucose tolerance and the metabolic syndrome. Hypoxia induces insulin resistance [234–236]. Oxidative stress may be important in vascular dementia and Alzheimer disease [237]. Sleep apnea–related hypoxia induces a massive increase in sympathetic activation [238–241], with downstream vascular effects that increase the risk of vascular dementia. Although the data in adults in terms of sleep apnea and metabolic syndrome are relatively mature, the pediatric data are similar [242,243].

Gene-Environment Interactions

Sleep has numerous heritable components, including the EEG, sleep duration, propensity for sleep fragmentation, and circadian preference. The *apolipoprotein ε4* genotype is a risk factor for Alzheimer disease [244]. The presence of ε4 may also increase the risk of adverse effects of sleep apnea and hypoxia on cognition in humans and mutant mice [70,245–247]. Other single-nucleotide polymorphisms that result in major alterations of gene function have been described for period 3 variable number of tandem repeats, brain-derived neurotrophic factor (BDNF) Met/Val, catechol-O-methyl transferase (COMT) Met/Val, and adenosine deaminase 22 G to A. These polymorphisms alter the sleep EEG (adenosine deaminase) [248], sensitivity to sleep deprivation (adenosine deaminase) [249], or the response to stimulants (COMT) [250]. Sleep pathology could interact with these genetic factors and common variable genomic markers, to modify cognition.

The BDNF effect may be particularly important for pediatric sleep medicine. BDNF is a critical factor for synaptic health [251–254] and is a regulator of sleep homeostasis [255–257]. Polymorphisms that reduce the function or availability of BDNF could amplify stress effects of sleep deprivation, fragmentation, hypoxia, or metabolic/cytokine stressors. Such interactions have been shown in animal models [258].

Potential for Imaging Brain Structure and Function in Pediatric Sleep Disorders

Structural Neuroimaging

OSA increases the risk of stroke in adults [259,260]. Such an association is yet to be reported in children, but is biologically plausible. Other than stroke, a steady stream of neuroimaging reports in adult sleep disorders have shown the power and pitfalls of current approaches. In a study of 21 OSA patients vs 21 control subjects assessed using high-resolution T1-weighted MRI and voxel-based morphometry, diminished regional and often unilateral gray matter loss were seen in multiple sites of the brain in patients, including the frontal and parietal cortex, temporal lobe, anterior cingulate, hippocampus, and cerebellum [261]. Reduced mammillary body volume was reported by the same group [262]; they also used whole-brain maps of T2 relaxation time and showed apparent injury in depressed OSA subjects. The areas with abnormal signal included the mid-cingulate and anterior cingulate, anterior insular, medial prefrontal, parietal, and left ventrolateral temporal cortices, left caudate nucleus, and bilateral hippocampus [263]. Heart failure patients, where sleep apnea is exceedingly common, reportedly showed significant and largely lateralized gray matter loss in autonomic and respiratory-related areas as well as regions not classically associated with such control, including the insula and basal ganglia, right cingulate gyrus, parahippocampal/fusiform gyrus, dorsal midbrain extending to the thalamus, ventral and superior lateral frontal cortex, bilateral cerebellar quadrangular lobules and right fastigial and neighboring nuclei, and bilateral deep parietal and lateral parietal-occipital cortex [264]. In a comparison of 39 severe sleep apnea patients vs 64 controls, reduction in cortical thickness using FreeSurfer was noted in bilateral mid-parahippocampal gyrus, right amygdala, right medial prefrontal cortex, left posterior cingulate, and isolated areas in the right temporal cortex and left postcentral gyrus [265].

Chronic high-altitude exposure is one model to assess the effects of hypoxia on brain development. One study obtained multimodal MRI data from 28 immigrant "high-altitude" young adults who were born and grew up at the Qinghai-Tibetan plateau matched with 28 matched "sea-level" controls [266]. The regional gray matter volumes using voxel-based morphometry, white matter integrity using diffusion-weighted imaging, and resting state BOLD fMRI were evaluated. Those who had grown up (to the age of 18 years at least) at altitude decreased gray matter volume at bilateral anterior insula, bilateral prefrontal cortex, the left precentral, the left cingulate, and the right lingual cortex. The connecting fiber tracts showed altered fractional anisotropy. Other reports of magnetic resonance abnormality after chronic altitude exposure suggest that this model can be usefully explored further [267–269].

An assessment of white matter integrity using diffusion-weighted imaging in OSA patients showed multiple regions of lower fractional anisotropy in the anterior corpus callosum; anterior and posterior cingulate cortex and cingulum bundle; right column of the fornix; and in portions of the frontal, ventral prefrontal, parietal and insular cortices, bilateral internal capsule, left cerebral peduncle, middle cerebellar peduncle and corticospinal tract, and deep cerebellar nuclei [270]. Factors that can modify structural neuroimaging outcomes include the technique used, statistical assumptions and methods, individual differences in anatomy and susceptibility to injury, disease severity and duration, and comorbid conditions such as hypertension.

There are now several reports of the use of structural neuroimaging to identify putative changes in neurons and synaptic density in the pediatric age group. These include gray matter correlations of intelligence quotient (IQ) in a normal pediatric population [271], reduced gray matter volume in the left dorsolateral prefrontal cortex in pediatric bipolar disorder [272], reductions in amygdala volume in pediatric anxiety disorder [273], decreased bilateral gray matter in frontal and cingulate regions in pediatric obsessive compulsive disorder [274], thalamic gray matter loss in pediatric multiple sclerosis [275], and left superior temporal gyrus and the left medial temporal lobe as the most consistent abnormalities in schizophrenia [276–279]. Cortical thickness measurements based on high-resolution MRI is another approach to determine gray matter distribution and change with disease states [280,281]. The technique has been applied, as examples, to Huntington disease [282], multiple sclerosis [283], schizophrenia [284–288], and Alzheimer disease [289,290]. In children, thickness-functional (neurobehavioral) correlates have been described [291]; translation to pediatric sleep disorders is an obvious next step.

Diffusion tensor mapping allows estimation of white matter development and health. This technique has been applied to the study of fiber tract development in the pediatric age group, including health [292,293] and white matter disease states [294–296]. The neuroanatomy of human pediatric sleep apnea remains unknown.

A plausible mechanism for any association between sleep fragmentation and white matter injury [297] is sleep blood pressure [181,183,298]. Blood pressure dipping during sleep is a normal physiological response that could reduce the exposure of the cerebrovascular circulation to hypertensive effects [299]. Dipping has been associated with the amount of conventional slow-wave sleep [299] and only occurs during a sleep state relatively devoid of phasic EEG complexes [187]. Nondipping is associated with brain atrophy and cognitive decline in elderly hypertensives [300]. Experimental sleep fragmentation can also induce insulin resistance [233], a feature of the metabolic syndrome, which has been in turn associated with insulin resistance silent brain infarction, periventricular hyperintensities, and subcortical white matter lesions [301,302].

Functional Neuroimaging

In humans, sleep loss seems to disproportionately impair prefrontal-based cortical functions [303–305]. Sleep is associated with a disproportionate reduction of metabolism in the high-order associative cortices [3]. Sleep deprivation and fragmentation, and sleep apnea, alter task-related activation in the executive network [306,307]. Both increases and decreases in fMRI activation within the executive network (lateral and medial prefrontal, posterior parietal cortex), or lateral temporal cortex in a navigation task, have been reported [308–315]. Our experience supports reductions rather than increases in activation in sleep apnea [307], narcolepsy [316], and following sleep deprivation [317]. The type and duration of task, circadian time, and degree of sleep deprivation can explain some of the differences between reports.

In pediatric disorders [318,319] characterized by language dysfunction [320], bipolar disorder [321], and executive dysfunction, including attention-deficit/hyperactivity disorder (ADHD), fMRI has been used [322–324]. A link between sleep fragmentation/sleep apnea and pediatric ADHD makes biological sense [325,326]. Structural and functional neuroimaging has the potential to map, in a unique dynamic way, brain anatomy and function in pediatric OSA over time, including the effects of treatment and any impact on development.

Specific Disorders

Sleep Apnea

This is an area of enquiry remarkably devoid of data. A PubMed search revealed no publication describing brain structure in pediatric sleep apnea. A cross-sectional study used proton magnetic resonance spectroscopic imaging in children has been reported. Neuropsychological test scores and mean neuronal metabolite ratios of target brain areas were compared. Relative to controls, children with severe sleep apnea had significant deficits in IQ and executive functions. Children with sleep apnea demonstrated decreases of the mean neuronal metabolite ratio N-acetyl aspartate/choline in the left hippocampus and right frontal cortex [327]. This is similar to that described in adults with severe OSA [104].

Narcolepsy

Structural (voxel-based morphometry) and functional brain imaging studies have suggested the involvement of the hypothalamus in narcolepsy, but the data are not all consistent [328]. The described changes have been none to relatively focal (hypothalamic) to widespread, such as the prefrontal cortex, limbic areas, and occipital areas [329–334]; a definitive study is awaited.

PET has shown hypermetabolism while awake in the anterior and mid-cingulate cortex, in the right cuneus and lingual gyrus [335]. Other PET studies have reported hypothalamic and thalamic hypometabolism [336,337]. Treatment-related changes can be demonstrated using fMRI [316]. In a magnetic resonance spectroscopy study, the neuronal marker N-acetyl-aspartate was reduced in the hypothalamus of narcolepsy with cataplexy patients compared with controls [338]. Secondary narcolepsy syndromes may show evidence of neuropathology in the hypothalamus/brainstem, ranging from neurocysticercosis [339], tumors [340–342], limbic/brainstem paraneoplastic encephalitis [343,344], and neuromyelitis optica with anti-aquaporin antibodies [345].

Kleine-Levin Syndrome

The clinical features of this syndrome of intermittent hypersomnia and associated features have been well described [346]. Hypothalamic disease can cause the syndrome in rare instances, such as sarcoidosis [347]. Single photon emission computed tomography has shown diencephalic hypoperfusion during episodes [348,349], which may not resolve fully each time.

Congenital Central Hypoventilation Syndrome

This "classic" syndrome is associated with sleep hypoventilation in NREM sleep. The paired-like homeobox 2B gene (PHOX2B) is the disease-defining gene [350–353]. Individuals with congenital central hypoventilation syndrome (CCHS) typically present in the newborn period with alveolar hypoventilation during sleep and often during wakefulness, altered respiratory control including reduced or absent ventilatory responses to hypercarbia and hypoxemia, and autonomic nervous system dysregulation. Thermoregulation is altered and perception of shortness of breath is absent, but voluntary breathing is retained. MRI abnormalities are seen in numerous brain areas, including the hypothalamus, posterior thalamus, midbrain, caudal raphe and locus coeruleus, the lateral medulla, parabrachial pons, cerebellum, and insular and cingulate cortices [354–357].

Diffusion tensor imaging [358–360] reveals increased radial diffusivity, primarily indicative of myelin injury, in fibers of the corona radiata, internal capsule, corpus callosum, hippocampus through the fornix, cingulum bundle, and temporal and parietal lobes. Increased axial diffusivity, suggestive of axonal injury, is seen in the internal capsule, thalamus, corona radiata, and occipital and temporal lobes. Multiple brain regions showed both higher axial and radial diffusivity, indicative of loss of tissue integrity with a combination of myelin and axonal injury, including basal ganglia, bed nucleus, and limbic, occipital, and temporal areas.

The PHOX2B mutation–confirmed CCHS confers risk for adverse neurocognitive outcome, though the range of functioning observed raises questions about factors that may contribute to neurocognitive variability. Visuoperceptual reasoning and visuographic speed appear particularly vulnerable [352].

Arnold-Chiari Malformation and Syringobulbia

The radiological features of these syndromes are available in standard textbooks. From a pediatric sleep perspective, sleep-disordered breathing, especially central, is a common association [361–363].

Circadian Rhythm Disorders

Hypothalamic or pineal pathology can cause delayed, advanced, or irregular circadian rhythms [364–367].

Summary

Neuroimaging in pediatric sleep medicine research is underused, as evidenced by the paucity of information in pediatric sleep disorders relative to the potential for sleep pathology to cause direct neural and neurovascular injury. Pediatric sleep apnea syndromes would seem a logical target for neuroimaging studies, using approaches similar to those in adult sleep and neurological disorders.

References

1. Jan JE, Reiter RJ, Bax MC, Ribary U, Freeman RD, Wasdell MB. Long-term sleep disturbances in children: a cause of neuronal loss. *Eur J Paediatr Neurol.* 2010:14:380–390.

2. Dang-Vu TT, Desseilles M, Petit D, Mazza S, Montplaisir J, Maquet P. Neuroimaging in sleep medicine. *Sleep Med.* 2007;8:349–372.
3. Desseilles M, Dang-Vu T, Schabus M, Sterpenich V, Maquet P, Schwartz S. Neuroimaging insights into the pathophysiology of sleep disorders. *Sleep.* 2008;31:777–794.
4. Mackiewicz M, Shockley KR, Romer MA, et al. Macromolecule biosynthesis: a key function of sleep. *Physiol Genomics.* 2007;31:441–457.
5. Cirelli C, LaVaute TM, Tononi G. Sleep and wakefulness modulate gene expression in Drosophila. *J Neurochem.* 2005;94:1411–1419.
6. Cirelli C, Bushey D. Sleep and wakefulness in Drosophila melanogaster. *Ann N Y Acad Sci.* 2008;1129:323–329.
7. Cirelli C, Faraguna U, Tononi G. Changes in brain gene expression after long-term sleep deprivation. *J Neurochem.* 2006;98:1632–1645.
8. Guindalini C, Andersen ML, Alvarenga T, Lee K, Tufik S. To what extent is sleep rebound effective in reversing the effects of paradoxical sleep deprivation on gene expression in the brain? *Behav Brain Res.* 2009;201:53–58.
9. Terao A, Wisor JP, Peyron C, et al. Gene expression in the rat brain during sleep deprivation and recovery sleep: an Affymetrix GeneChip study. *Neuroscience.* 2006;137:593–605.
10. Wisor JP, Pasumarthi RK, Gerashchenko D, et al. Sleep deprivation effects on circadian clock gene expression in the cerebral cortex parallel electroencephalographic differences among mouse strains. *J Neurosci.* 2008;28:7193–201.
11. Mackiewicz M, Zimmerman JE, Shockley KR, Churchill GA, Pack AI. What are microarrays teaching us about sleep? *Trends Mol Med.* 2009;15:79–87.
12. Naidoo N. Cellular stress/the unfolded protein response: Relevance to sleep and sleep disorders. *Sleep Med Rev.* 2009;13:195–204.
13. Scharf MT, Naidoo N, Zimmerman JE, Pack AI. The energy hypothesis of sleep revisited. *Prog Neurobiol.* 2008;86:264–280.
14. Mackiewicz M, Naidoo N, Zimmerman JE, Pack AI. Molecular mechanisms of sleep and wakefulness. *Ann N Y Acad Sci.* 2008;1129:335–349.
15. Naidoo N, Casiano V, Cater J, Zimmerman J, Pack AI. A role for the molecular chaperone protein BiP/GRP78 in Drosophila sleep homeostasis. *Sleep.* 2007;30:557–565.
16. Vyazovskiy VV, Cirelli C, Pfister-Genskow M, Faraguna U, Tononi G. Molecular and electrophysiological evidence for net synaptic potentiation in wake and depression in sleep. *Nat Neurosci.* 2008;11:200–208.
17. Esser SK, Hill SL, Tononi G. Sleep homeostasis and cortical synchronization: I. Modeling the effects of synaptic strength on sleep slow waves. *Sleep.* 2007;30:1617–1630.
18. Vyazovskiy VV, Riedner BA, Cirelli C, Tononi G. Sleep homeostasis and cortical synchronization: II. A local field potential study of sleep slow waves in the rat. *Sleep.* 2007;30:1631–1642.
19. Riedner BA, Vyazovskiy VV, Huber R, et al. Sleep homeostasis and cortical synchronization: III. A high-density EEG study of sleep slow waves in humans. *Sleep.* 2007;30:1643–157.
20. Aton SJ, Seibt J, Dumoulin M, et al. Mechanisms of sleep-dependent consolidation of cortical plasticity. *Neuron.* 2009;61:454–466.
21. Jha SK, Jones BE, Coleman T, et al. Sleep-dependent plasticity requires cortical activity. *J Neurosci.* 2005;25:9266–9274.
22. Grigg-Damberger M, Gozal D, Marcus CL, et al. The visual scoring of sleep and arousal in infants and children. *J Clin Sleep Med.* 2007;3:201–240.
23. O'Brien LM, Gozal D. Potential usefulness of noninvasive autonomic monitoring in recognition of arousals in normal healthy children. *J Clin Sleep Med.* 2007;3:41–47.
24. O'Brien LM, Gozal D. Autonomic dysfunction in children with sleep-disordered breathing. *Sleep.* 2005;28:747–752.
25. Pepin JL, Delavie N, Pin I, et al. Pulse transit time improves detection of sleep respiratory events and microarousals in children. *Chest.* 2005;127:722–730.
26. Tauman R, O'Brien LM, Mast BT, Holbrook CR, Gozal D. Peripheral arterial tonometry events and electroencephalographic arousals in children. *Sleep.* 2004; 27:502–506.
27. Gozal D, Capdevila OS, Kheirandish-Gozal L. Metabolic alterations and systemic inflammation in obstructive sleep apnea among nonobese and obese prepubertal children. *Am J Respir Crit Care Med.* 2008;177:1142–1149.
28. Tauman R, Serpero LD, Capdevila OS, et al. Adipokines in children with sleep disordered breathing. *Sleep.* 2007;30:443–449.
29. Gozal D, Serpero LD, Kheirandish-Gozal L, Capdevila OS, Khalyfa A, Tauman R. Sleep measures and morning plasma TNF-alpha levels in children with sleep-disordered breathing. *Sleep.* 2010;33:319–325.
30. Toga AW, Thompson PM, Sowell ER. Mapping brain maturation. *Trends Neurosci.* 2006;29:148–159.
31. Sowell ER, Trauner DA, Gamst A, Jernigan TL. Development of cortical and subcortical brain structures in childhood and adolescence: a structural MRI study. *Dev Med Child Neurol.* 2002;44:4–16.
32. Sowell ER, Peterson BS, Thompson PM, Welcome SE, Henkenius AL, Toga AW. Mapping cortical change across the human life span. *Nat Neurosci.* 2003;6:309–315.
33. Sowell ER, Thompson PM, Leonard CM, Welcome SE, Kan E, Toga AW. Longitudinal mapping of cortical thickness and brain growth in normal children. *J Neurosci.* 2004;24:8223–8231.
34. Campbell IG, Darchia N, Khaw WY, Higgins LM, Feinberg I. Sleep EEG evidence of sex differences in adolescent brain maturation. *Sleep.* 2005;28:637–643.
35. Feinberg I, Campbell IG. Sleep EEG changes during adolescence: an index of a fundamental brain reorganization. *Brain Cogn.* 2010;72:56–65.

36. Huchzermeyer C, Albus K, Gabriel HJ, et al. Gamma oscillations and spontaneous network activity in the hippocampus are highly sensitive to decreases in pO2 and concomitant changes in mitochondrial redox state. *J Neurosci.* 2008;28:1153–1162.
37. Lukyanetz EA, Shkryl VM, Kravchuk OV, Kostyuk PG. Action of hypoxia on different types of calcium channels in hippocampal neurons. *Biochim Biophys Acta.* 2003;1618:33–38.
38. Lukyanetz EA, Shkryl VM, Kravchuk OV, Kostyuk PG. Effect of hypoxia on calcium channels depends on extracellular calcium in CA1 hippocampal neurons. *Brain Res.* 2003;980:128–134.
39. Murray RS, Stensaas SS, Anderson RE, Matsuo F. Bilateral basal ganglia necrosis following diffuse hypoxic-ischemic injury. *Arch Neurol.* 1987; 44:897.
40. Wartenberg KE, Patsalides A, Yepes MS. Is magnetic resonance spectroscopy superior to conventional diagnostic tools in hypoxic-ischemic encephalopathy? *J Neuroimaging.* 2004;14:180–186.
41. Katz ES, D'Ambrosio CM. Pathophysiology of pediatric obstructive sleep apnea. *Proc Am Thorac Soc.* 2008;5:253–262.
42. Lumeng JC, Chervin RD. Epidemiology of pediatric obstructive sleep apnea. *Proc Am Thorac Soc.* 2008;5:242–252.
43. Muzumdar H, Arens R. Diagnostic issues in pediatric obstructive sleep apnea. *Proc Am Thorac Soc.* 2008;5:263–273.
44. Halbower AC, Ishman SL, McGinley BM. Childhood obstructive sleep-disordered breathing: a clinical update and discussion of technological innovations and challenges. *Chest.* 2007;132: 2030–2041.
45. Dayyat E, Kheirandish-Gozal L, Gozal D. Childhood obstructive sleep apnea: one or two distinct disease entities? *Sleep Med Clin.* 2007;2: 433–444.
46. Beebe DW, Gozal D. Obstructive sleep apnea and the prefrontal cortex: towards a comprehensive model linking nocturnal upper airway obstruction to daytime cognitive and behavioral deficits. *J Sleep Res.* 2002;11:1–16.
47. O'Brien LM, Mervis CB, Holbrook CR, et al. Neurobehavioral correlates of sleep-disordered breathing in children. *J Sleep Res.* 2004;13: 165–172.
48. Chervin RD, Dillon JE, Bassetti C, Ganoczy DA, Pituch KJ. Symptoms of sleep disorders, inattention, and hyperactivity in children. *Sleep.* 1997;20:1185–1192.
49. Surman CB, Thomas RJ, Aleardi M, Pagano C, Biederman J. Adults with ADHD and sleep complaints: a pilot study identifying sleep-disordered breathing using polysomnography and sleep quality assessment. *J Atten Disord.* 2006;9:550–555.
50. Wei JL, Mayo MS, Smith HJ, Reese M, Weatherly RA. Improved behavior and sleep after adenotonsillectomy in children with sleep-disordered breathing. *Arch Otolaryngol Head Neck Surg.* 2007;133:974–979.
51. Garetz SL. Behavior, cognition, and quality of life after adenotonsillectomy for pediatric sleep-disordered breathing: summary of the literature. *Otolaryngol Head Neck Surg.* 2008;138:S19–S26.
52. Bedard MA, Montplaisir J, Malo J, Richer F, Rouleau I. Persistent neuropsychological deficits and vigilance impairment in sleep apnea syndrome after treatment with continuous positive airways pressure (CPAP). *J Clin Exp Neuropsychol.* 1993; 15:330–341.
53. Bedard MA, Montplaisir J, Richer F, Rouleau I, Malo J. Obstructive sleep apnea syndrome: pathogenesis of neuropsychological deficits. *J Clin Exp Neuropsychol.* 1991;13:950–964.
54. Beebe DW, Groesz L, Wells C, Nichols A, McGee K. The neuropsychological effects of obstructive sleep apnea: a meta-analysis of norm-referenced and case-controlled data. *Sleep.* 2003;26:298–307.
55. Decary A, Rouleau I, Montplaisir J. Cognitive deficits associated with sleep apnea syndrome: a proposed neuropsychological test battery. *Sleep.* 2000;23:369–381.
56. Feuerstein C, Naegele B, Pepin JL, Levy P. Frontal lobe-related cognitive functions in patients with sleep apnea syndrome before and after treatment. *Acta Neurol Belg.* 1997;97:96–107.
57. Salorio CF, White DA, Piccirillo J, Duntley SP, Uhles ML. Learning, memory, and executive control in individuals with obstructive sleep apnea syndrome. *J Clin Exp Neuropsychol.* 2002;24:93–100.
58. Sateia MJ. Neuropsychological impairment and quality of life in obstructive sleep apnea. *Clin Chest Med.* 2003;24:249–259.
59. Verstraeten E, Cluydts R. Executive control of attention in sleep apnea patients: theoretical concepts and methodological considerations. *Sleep Med Rev.* 2004;8:257–267.
60. Verstraeten E, Cluydts R, Pevernagie D, Hoffmann G. Executive function in sleep apnea: controlling for attentional capacity in assessing executive attention. *Sleep.* 2004;27:685–693.
61. Beebe DW. Neurobehavioral morbidity associated with disordered breathing during sleep in children: a comprehensive review. *Sleep.* 2006;29: 1115–1134.
62. Gottlieb DJ, Chase C, Vezina RM, et al. Sleep-disordered breathing symptoms are associated with poorer cognitive function in 5-year-old children. *J Pediatr.* 2004;145:458–464.
63. Kurnatowski P, Putynski L, Lapienis M, Kowalska B. Neurocognitive abilities in children with adenotonsillar hypertrophy. *Int J Pediatr Otorhinolaryngol.* 2006;70:419–424.
64. Bass JL, Corwin M, Gozal D, et al. The effect of chronic or intermittent hypoxia on cognition in childhood: a review of the evidence. *Pediatrics.* 2004;114:805–816.
65. Gozal D, Kheirandish-Gozal L. Neurocognitive and behavioral morbidity in children with sleep disorders. *Curr Opin Pulm Med.* 2007;13:505–509.
66. Mehl RC, O'Brien LM, Jones JH, Dreisbach JK, Mervis CB, Gozal D. Correlates of sleep and pediatric bipolar disorder. *Sleep.* 2006;29:193–197.

67. O'Brien LM, Holbrook CR, Mervis CB, et al. Sleep and neurobehavioral characteristics of 5- to 7-year-old children with parentally reported symptoms of attention-deficit/hyperactivity disorder. *Pediatrics*. 2003;111:554–563.
68. O'Brien LM, Mervis CB, Holbrook CR, et al. Neurobehavioral implications of habitual snoring in children. *Pediatrics*. 2004;114:44–49.
69. O'Brien LM, Tauman R, Gozal D. Sleep pressure correlates of cognitive and behavioral morbidity in snoring children. *Sleep*. 2004;27:279–282.
70. Gozal D, Capdevila OS, Kheirandish-Gozal L, Crabtree VM. APOE epsilon 4 allele, cognitive dysfunction, and obstructive sleep apnea in children. *Neurology*. 2007;69:243–249.
71. Guilleminault C, Li K, Quo S, Inouye RN. A prospective study on the surgical outcomes of children with sleep-disordered breathing. *Sleep*. 2004;27:95–100.
72. Shine NP, Lannigan FJ, Coates HL, Wilson A. Adenotonsillectomy for obstructive sleep apnea in obese children: effects on respiratory parameters and clinical outcome. *Arch Otolaryngol Head Neck Surg*. 2006;132:1123–1127.
73. Guilleminault C, Huang YS, Glamann C, Li K, Chan A. Adenotonsillectomy and obstructive sleep apnea in children: a prospective survey. *Otolaryngol Head Neck Surg*. 2007;136:169–175.
74. Sanfilippo-Cohn B, Lai S, Zhan G, et al. Sex differences in susceptibility to oxidative injury and sleepiness from intermittent hypoxia. *Sleep*. 2006;29:152–159.
75. Veasey SC, Davis CW, Fenik P, et al. Long-term intermittent hypoxia in mice: protracted hypersomnolence with oxidative injury to sleep-wake brain regions. *Sleep*. 2004;27:194–201.
76. Zhan G, Fenik P, Pratico D, Veasey SC. Inducible nitric oxide synthase in long-term intermittent hypoxia: hypersomnolence and brain injury. *Am J Respir Crit Care Med*. 2005;171:1414–1420.
77. Morrell MJ. Residual sleepiness in patients with optimally treated sleep apnea: a case for hypoxia-induced oxidative brain injury. *Sleep*. 2004;27:186–187.
78. Gozal E, Gozal D, Pierce WM, et al. Proteomic analysis of CA1 and CA3 regions of rat hippocampus and differential susceptibility to intermittent hypoxia. *J Neurochem*. 2002;83:331–345.
79. Hambrecht VS, Vlisides PE, Row BW, Gozal D, Baghdoyan HA, Lydic R. Hypoxia modulates cholinergic but not opioid activation of G proteins in rat hippocampus. *Hippocampus*. 2007;17:934–942.
80. Row BW, Kheirandish L, Cheng Y, Rowell PP, Gozal D. Impaired spatial working memory and altered choline acetyltransferase (CHAT) immunoreactivity and nicotinic receptor binding in rats exposed to intermittent hypoxia during sleep. *Behav Brain Res*. 2007;177:308–314.
81. Zhu Y, Fenik P, Zhan G, et al. Selective loss of catecholaminergic wake active neurons in a murine sleep apnea model. *J Neurosci*. 2007;27:10060–10071.
82. Row BW, Liu R, Xu W, Kheirandish L, Gozal D. Intermittent hypoxia is associated with oxidative stress and spatial learning deficits in the rat. *Am J Respir Crit Care Med*. 2003;167:1548–1553.
83. Xu W, Chi L, Row BW, et al. Increased oxidative stress is associated with chronic intermittent hypoxia-mediated brain cortical neuronal cell apoptosis in a mouse model of sleep apnea. *Neuroscience*. 2004;126:313–323.
84. Li RC, Row BW, Kheirandish L, et al. Nitric oxide synthase and intermittent hypoxia-induced spatial learning deficits in the rat. *Neurobiol Dis*. 2004;17:44–53.
85. Douglas RM, Ryu J, Kanaan A, et al. Neuronal death during combined intermittent hypoxia/hypercapnia is due to mitochondrial dysfunction. *Am J Physiol Cell Physiol*. 2010;298:C1594–C1602.
86. Payne RS, Goldbart A, Gozal D, Schurr A. Effect of intermittent hypoxia on long-term potentiation in rat hippocampal slices. *Brain Res*. 2004;1029:195–199.
87. Decker MJ, Jones KA, Solomon IG, Keating GL, Rye DB. Reduced extracellular dopamine and increased responsiveness to novelty: neurochemical and behavioral sequelae of intermittent hypoxia. *Sleep*. 2005;28:169–176.
88. Polotsky VY, Rubin AE, Balbir A, et al. Intermittent hypoxia causes REM sleep deficits and decreases EEG delta power in NREM sleep in the C57BL/6J mouse. *Sleep Med*. 2006;7:7–16.
89. Hornbein TF, Townes BD, Schoene RB, Sutton JR, Houston CS. The cost to the central nervous system of climbing to extremely high altitude. *N Engl J Med*. 1989;321:1714–1719.
90. Virues-Ortega J, Buela-Casal G, Garrido E, Alcazar B. Neuropsychological functioning associated with high-altitude exposure. *Neuropsychol Rev*. 2004;14:197–224.
91. Anooshiravani M, Dumont L, Mardirosoff C, Soto-Debeuf G, Delavelle J. Brain magnetic resonance imaging (MRI) and neurological changes after a single high altitude climb. *Med Sci Sports Exerc*. 1999;31:969–972.
92. Merz TM, Treyer V, Hefti U, et al. Changes in cerebral glucose metabolism after an expedition to high altitudes. *High Alt Med Biol*. 2006;7:28–38.
93. Pavlicek V, Schirlo C, Nebel A, Regard M, Koller EA, Brugger P. Cognitive and emotional processing at high altitude. *Aviat Space Environ Med*. 2005;76:28–33.
94. Thomas RJ, Tamisier R, Boucher J, et al. Nocturnal hypoxia exposure with simulated altitude for 14 days does not significantly alter working memory or vigilance in humans. *Sleep*. 2007;30:1195–1203.
95. Antonelli Incalzi R, Marra C, Giordano A, et al. Cognitive impairment in chronic obstructive pulmonary disease—a neuropsychological and spect study. *J Neurol*. 2003;250:325–32.
96. Hjalmarsen A, Waterloo K, Dahl A, Jorde R, Viitanen M. Effect of long-term oxygen therapy on cognitive and neurological dysfunction

in chronic obstructive pulmonary disease. *Eur Neurol.* 1999;42:27–35.

97. Morrell MJ, Twigg G. Neural consequences of sleep disordered breathing: the role of intermittent hypoxia. *Adv Exp Med Biol.* 2006;588:75–88.
98. Naismith S, Winter V, Gotsopoulos H, Hickie I, Cistulli P. Neurobehavioral functioning in obstructive sleep apnea: differential effects of sleep quality, hypoxemia and subjective sleepiness. *J Clin Exp Neuropsychol.* 2004;26:43–54.
99. Ferini-Strambi L, Baietto C, Di Gioia MR, et al. Cognitive dysfunction in patients with obstructive sleep apnea (OSA): partial reversibility after continuous positive airway pressure (CPAP). *Brain Res Bull.* 2003;61:87–92.
100. Montplaisir J, Bedard MA, Richer F, Rouleau I. Neurobehavioral manifestations in obstructive sleep apnea syndrome before and after treatment with continuous positive airway pressure. *Sleep.* 1992;15:S17-S19.
101. Naegele B, Thouvard V, Pepin JL, et al. Deficits of cognitive executive functions in patients with sleep apnea syndrome. *Sleep.* 1995;18:43–52.
102. Saunamaki T, Jehkonen M. A review of executive functions in obstructive sleep apnea syndrome. *Acta Neurol Scand.* 2007;115:1–11.
103. Coste O, Beaumont M, Batejat D, Beers PV, Touitou Y. Prolonged mild hypoxia modifies human circadian core body temperature and may be associated with sleep disturbances. *Chronobiol Int.* 2004;21:419–433.
104. Alchanatis M, Deligiorgis N, Zias N, et al. Frontal brain lobe impairment in obstructive sleep apnoea: a proton MR spectroscopy study. *Eur Respir J.* 2004;24:980–986.
105. Bartlett DJ, Rae C, Thompson CH, et al. Hippocampal area metabolites relate to severity and cognitive function in obstructive sleep apnea. *Sleep Med.* 2004;5:593–596.
106. Hochachka PW, Clark CM, Matheson GO, et al. Effects on regional brain metabolism of high-altitude hypoxia: a study of six US marines. *Am J Physiol.* 1999;277:R314–R319.
107. Hamilton G, Mathur R, Allsop JM, et al. Changes in brain intracellular pH and membrane phospholipids on oxygen therapy in hypoxic patients with chronic obstructive pulmonary disease. *Metab Brain Dis.* 2003;18:95–109.
108. Shim TS, Lee JH, Kim SY, et al. Cerebral metabolic abnormalities in COPD patients detected by localized proton magnetic resonance spectroscopy. *Chest.* 2001;120:1506–1513.
109. Boonstra TW, Stins JF, Daffertshofer A, Beek PJ. Effects of sleep deprivation on neural functioning: an integrative review. *Cell Mol Life Sci.* 2007; 64:934–946.
110. Harrison Y, Horne JA. The impact of sleep deprivation on decision making: a review. *J Exp Psychol Appl.* 2000;6:236–249.
111. Thomas RJ, Kwong K. Modafinil activates cortical and subcortical sites in the sleep-deprived state. *Sleep.* 2006;29:1471–1481.
112. Huck NO, McBride SA, Kendall AP, Grugle NL, Killgore WD. The effects of modafinil, caffeine, and dextroamphetamine on judgments of simple versus complex emotional expressions following sleep deprivation. *Int J Neurosci.* 2008;118: 487–502.
113. Sagaspe P, Sanchez-Ortuno M, Charles A, et al. Effects of sleep deprivation on Color-Word, Emotional, and Specific Stroop interference and on self-reported anxiety. *Brain Cogn.* 2006;60: 76–87.
114. Franzen PL, Buysse DJ, Dahl RE, Thompson W, Siegle GJ. Sleep deprivation alters pupillary reactivity to emotional stimuli in healthy young adults. *Biol Psychol.* 2009;80:300–305.
115. Killgore WD, Kahn-Greene ET, Lipizzi EL, Newman RA, Kamimori GH, Balkin TJ. Sleep deprivation reduces perceived emotional intelligence and constructive thinking skills. *Sleep Med.* 2008;9:517–526.
116. Ikehara S, Iso H, Date C, et al. Association of sleep duration with mortality from cardiovascular disease and other causes for Japanese men and women: the JACC study. *Sleep.* 2009;32:295–301.
117. Nunes J, Jean-Louis G, Zizi F, et al. Sleep duration among black and white Americans: results of the National Health Interview Survey. *J Natl Med Assoc.* 2008;100:317–322.
118. Gangwisch JE, Heymsfield SB, Boden-Albala B, et al. Sleep duration associated with mortality in elderly, but not middle-aged, adults in a large US sample. *Sleep.* 2008;31:1087–1096.
119. Stepanski EJ. The effect of sleep fragmentation on daytime function. *Sleep.* 2002;25:268–276.
120. Bonnet MH, Arand DL. Clinical effects of sleep fragmentation versus sleep deprivation. *Sleep Med Rev.* 2003;7:297–310.
121. Bonnet MH. Cognitive effects of sleep and sleep fragmentation. *Sleep.* 1993;16:S65–S67.
122. Bonnet MH. The effect of sleep fragmentation on sleep and performance in younger and older subjects. *Neurobiol Aging.* 1989;10:21–25.
123. Dijk DJ. EEG slow waves and sleep spindles: windows on the sleeping brain. *Behav Brain Res.* 1995;69:109–116.
124. Achermann P. The two-process model of sleep regulation revisited. *Aviat Space Environ Med.* 2004;75:A37–A43.
125. Munch M, Knoblauch V, Blatter K, et al. The frontal predominance in human EEG delta activity after sleep loss decreases with age. *Eur J Neurosci.* 2004;20:1402–1410.
126. Knoblauch V, Krauchi K, Renz C, Wirz-Justice A, Cajochen C. Homeostatic control of slow-wave and spindle frequency activity during human sleep: effect of differential sleep pressure and brain topography. *Cereb Cortex.* 2002;12:1092–1100.
127. Steriade M. Sleep oscillations and their blockage by activating systems. *J Psychiatry Neurosci.* 1994;19:354–358.
128. Steriade M. Synchronized activities of coupled oscillators in the cerebral cortex and thalamus

at different levels of vigilance. *Cereb Cortex.* 1997;7:583–604.
129. Steriade M. Coherent oscillations and short-term plasticity in corticothalamic networks. *Trends Neurosci.* 1999;22:337–345.
130. Steriade M. The corticothalamic system in sleep. *Front Biosci.* 2003;8:d878-d899.
131. Steriade M. Grouping of brain rhythms in corticothalamic systems. *Neuroscience.* 2006;137: 1087–1106.
132. Steriade M, Amzica F. Slow sleep oscillation, rhythmic K-complexes, and their paroxysmal developments. *J Sleep Res.* 1998;7(suppl 1):30–35.
133. Vyazovskiy VV, Olcese U, Lazimy YM, et al. Cortical firing and sleep homeostasis. *Neuron.* 2009;63:865–878.
134. Vyazovskiy V, Borbely AA, Tobler I. Unilateral vibrissae stimulation during waking induces interhemispheric EEG asymmetry during subsequent sleep in the rat. *J Sleep Res.* 2000;9:367–371.
135. Huber R, Ghilardi MF, Massimini M, Tononi G. Local sleep and learning. *Nature.* 2004;430: 78–81.
136. Gais S, Molle M, Helms K, Born J. Learning-dependent increases in sleep spindle density. *J Neurosci.* 2002;22:6830–6834.
137. Schmidt C, Peigneux P, Muto V, et al. Encoding difficulty promotes postlearning changes in sleep spindle activity during napping. *J Neurosci.* 2006;26:8976–8982.
138. Amzica F, Steriade M. Electrophysiological correlates of sleep delta waves. *Electroencephalogr Clin Neurophysiol.* 1998;107:69–83.
139. Amzica F, Steriade M. Integration of low-frequency sleep oscillations in corticothalamic networks. *Acta Neurobiol Exp (Wars).* 2000;60:229–245.
140. Lewandowski MH, Blasiak T. Slow oscillation circuit of the intergeniculate leaflet. *Acta Neurobiol Exp (Wars).* 2004;64:277–288.
141. Steriade M. Active neocortical processes during quiescent sleep. *Arch Ital Biol.* 2001;139:37–51.
142. Molle M, Marshall L, Gais S, Born J. Learning increases human electroencephalographic coherence during subsequent slow sleep oscillations. *Proc Natl Acad Sci U S A.* 2004;101:13963–13968.
143. Maquet P, Laureys S, Peigneux P, et al. Experience-dependent changes in cerebral activation during human REM sleep. *Nat Neurosci.* 2000;3:831–836.
144. Kurth S, Jenni OG, Riedner BA, Tononi G, Carskadon MA, Huber R. Characteristics of sleep slow waves in children and adolescents. *Sleep.* 2010;33:475–480.
145. Bazhenov M, Timofeev I, Steriade M, Sejnowski TJ. Model of thalamocortical slow-wave sleep oscillations and transitions to activated States. *J Neurosci.* 2002;22:8691–704.
146. Siapas AG, Wilson MA. Coordinated interactions between hippocampal ripples and cortical spindles during slow-wave sleep. *Neuron.* 1998;21: 1123–1128.
147. Molle M, Yeshenko O, Marshall L, Sara SJ, Born J. Hippocampal sharp wave-ripples linked to slow oscillations in rat slow-wave sleep. *J Neurophysiol.* 2006;96:62–70.
148. Isomura Y, Sirota A, Ozen S, et al. Integration and segregation of activity in entorhinal-hippocampal subregions by neocortical slow oscillations. *Neuron.* 2006;52:871–882.
149. Clemens Z, Molle M, Eross L, Barsi P, Halasz P, Born J. Temporal coupling of parahippocampal ripples, sleep spindles and slow oscillations in humans. *Brain.* 2007;130:2868–2878.
150. Tartar JL, Ward CP, McKenna JT, et al. Hippocampal synaptic plasticity and spatial learning are impaired in a rat model of sleep fragmentation. *Eur J Neurosci.* 2006;23:2739–2748.
151. Plihal W, Born J. Memory consolidation in human sleep depends on inhibition of glucocorticoid release. *Neuroreport.* 1999;10:2741–2747.
152. Manoach DS, Cain MS, Vangel MG, Khurana A, Goff DC, Stickgold R. A failure of sleep-dependent procedural learning in chronic, medicated schizophrenia. *Biol Psychiatry.* 2004;56:951–956.
153. Morgan PT, Pace-Schott EF, Sahul ZH, Coric V, Stickgold R, Malison RT. Sleep, sleep-dependent procedural learning and vigilance in chronic cocaine users: Evidence for occult insomnia. *Drug Alcohol Depend.* 2006;82:238–249.
154. Nissen C, Kloepfer C, Nofzinger EA, Feige B, Voderholzer U, Riemann D. Impaired sleep-related memory consolidation in primary insomnia—a pilot study. *Sleep.* 2006;29:1068–1073.
155. Liu YW, Mee EW, Bergin P, et al. Adult neurogenesis in mesial temporal lobe epilepsy: a review of recent animal and human studies. *Curr Pharm Biotechnol.* 2007;8:187–194.
156. Warner-Schmidt JL, Duman RS. Hippocampal neurogenesis: opposing effects of stress and antidepressant treatment. *Hippocampus.* 2006;16: 239–249.
157. Thakker-Varia S, Krol JJ, Nettleton J, et al. The neuropeptide VGF produces antidepressant-like behavioral effects and enhances proliferation in the hippocampus. *J Neurosci.* 2007;27:12156–12167.
158. Schmidt HD, Duman RS. The role of neurotrophic factors in adult hippocampal neurogenesis, antidepressant treatments and animal models of depressive-like behavior. *Behav Pharmacol.* 2007;18:391–418.
159. Perera TD, Coplan JD, Lisanby SH, et al. Antidepressant-induced neurogenesis in the hippocampus of adult nonhuman primates. *J Neurosci.* 2007;27:4894–4901.
160. Paizanis E, Hamon M, Lanfumey L. Hippocampal neurogenesis, depressive disorders, and antidepressant therapy. *Neural Plast.* 2007:73754.
161. Hitoshi S, Maruta N, Higashi M, Kumar A, Kato N, Ikenaka K. Antidepressant drugs reverse the loss of adult neural stem cells following chronic stress. *J Neurosci Res.* 2007;85:3574–3585.
162. Ernst C, Olson AK, Pinel JP, Lam RW, Christie BR. Antidepressant effects of exercise: evidence for an adult-neurogenesis hypothesis? *J Psychiatry Neurosci.* 2006;31:84–92.

163. Duman RS, Nakagawa S, Malberg J. Regulation of adult neurogenesis by antidepressant treatment. *Neuropsychopharmacology*. 2001;25:836–844.
164. Banasr M, Duman RS. Regulation of neurogenesis and gliogenesis by stress and antidepressant treatment. *CNS Neurol Disord Drug Targets*. 2007;6:311–320.
165. Arias-Carrion O, Verdugo-Diaz L, Feria-Velasco A, et al. Neurogenesis in the subventricular zone following transcranial magnetic field stimulation and nigrostriatal lesions. *J Neurosci Res*. 2004;78:16–28.
166. Madsen TM, Treschow A, Bengzon J, Bolwig TG, Lindvall O, Tingstrom A. Increased neurogenesis in a model of electroconvulsive therapy. *Biol Psychiatry*. 2000;47:1043–1049.
167. Bolwig TG, Madsen TM. Electroconvulsive therapy in melancholia: the role of hippocampal neurogenesis. *Acta Psychiatr Scand Suppl*. 2007;433:130–135.
168. Santarelli L, Saxe M, Gross C, et al. Requirement of hippocampal neurogenesis for the behavioral effects of antidepressants. *Science*. 2003;301:805–809.
169. Guzman-Marin R, Bashir T, Suntsova N, Szymusiak R, McGinty D. Hippocampal neurogenesis is reduced by sleep fragmentation in the adult rat. *Neuroscience*. 2007;148:325–333.
170. Roman V, Van der Borght K, Leemburg SA, Van der Zee EA, Meerlo P. Sleep restriction by forced activity reduces hippocampal cell proliferation. *Brain Res*. 2005;1065:53–59.
171. Guzman-Marin R, Suntsova N, Stewart DR, Gong H, Szymusiak R, McGinty D. Sleep deprivation reduces proliferation of cells in the dentate gyrus of the hippocampus in rats. *J Physiol*. 2003;549:563–571.
172. Guzman-Marin R, Suntsova N, Methippara M, Greiffenstein R, Szymusiak R, McGinty D. Sleep deprivation suppresses neurogenesis in the adult hippocampus of rats. *Eur J Neurosci*. 2005;22:2111–2116.
173. Buckley TM, Schatzberg AF. On the interactions of the hypothalamic-pituitary-adrenal (HPA) axis and sleep: normal HPA axis activity and circadian rhythm, exemplary sleep disorders. *J Clin Endocrinol Metab*. 2005;90:3106–3114.
174. Parlapiano C, Borgia MC, Minni A, Alessandri N, Basal I, Saponara M. Cortisol circadian rhythm and 24-hour Holter arterial pressure in OSAS patients. *Endocr Res*. 2005;31:371–374.
175. McEwen BS. Sleep deprivation as a neurobiologic and physiologic stressor: allostasis and allostatic load. *Metabolism*. 2006;55:S20–S23.
176. Leproult R, Copinschi G, Buxton O, Van Cauter E. Sleep loss results in an elevation of cortisol levels the next evening. *Sleep*. 1997;20:865–870.
177. Alexander A. Elevated salivary cortisol due to sleep deprivation. *Occup Med (Lond)*. 2003;53:409; author reply 10.
178. Dadoun F, Darmon P, Achard V, et al. Effect of sleep apnea syndrome on the circadian profile of cortisol in obese men. *Am J Physiol Endocrinol Metab*. 2007;293:E466–E474.
179. Manganas LN, Zhang X, Li Y, et al. Magnetic resonance spectroscopy identifies neural progenitor cells in the live human brain. *Science*. 2007;318:980–985.
180. Dong Z, Dreher W, Leibfritz D, Peterson BS. Challenges of using MR spectroscopy to detect neural progenitor cells in vivo. *AJNR Am J Neuroradiol*. 2009;30:1096–1101.
181. Morrell MJ, Finn L, Kim H, Peppard PE, Badr MS, Young T. Sleep fragmentation, awake blood pressure, and sleep-disordered breathing in a population-based study. *Am J Respir Crit Care Med*. 2000;162:2091–2096.
182. Ogawa Y, Kanbayashi T, Saito Y, et al. Total sleep deprivation elevates blood pressure through arterial baroreflex resetting: a study with microneurographic technique. *Sleep*. 2003;26:986–989.
183. Carrington MJ, Trinder J. Blood pressure and heart rate during continuous experimental sleep fragmentation in healthy adults. *Sleep*. 2008;31:1701–1712.
184. Davies RJ, Belt PJ, Roberts SJ, Ali NJ, Stradling JR. Arterial blood pressure responses to graded transient arousal from sleep in normal humans. *J Appl Physiol*. 1993;74:1123–1130.
185. Suzuki M, Guilleminault C, Otsuka K, Shiomi T. Blood pressure "dipping" and "non-dipping" in obstructive sleep apnea syndrome patients. *Sleep*. 1996;19:382–387.
186. Ziegler MG. Sleep disorders and the failure to lower nocturnal blood pressure. *Curr Opin Nephrol Hypertens*. 2003;12:97–102.
187. Iellamo F, Placidi F, Marciani MG, et al. Baroreflex buffering of sympathetic activation during sleep: evidence from autonomic assessment of sleep macroarchitecture and microarchitecture. *Hypertension*. 2004;43:814–819.
188. Godoy J, Mellado P, Tapia J, Santin J. Obstructive sleep apnea as an independent stroke risk factor: possible mechanisms. *Curr Mol Med*. 2009;9:203–209.
189. Yaggi HK, Concato J, Kernan WN, Lichtman JH, Brass LM, Mohsenin V. Obstructive sleep apnea as a risk factor for stroke and death. *N Engl J Med*. 2005;353:2034–2041.
190. O'Driscoll DM, Foster AM, Ng ML, et al. Acute cardiovascular changes with obstructive events in children with sleep disordered breathing. *Sleep*. 2009;32:1265–1271.
191. Krueger JM. The role of cytokines in sleep regulation. *Curr Pharm Des*. 2008;14:3408–3416.
192. Kapsimalis F, Basta M, Varouchakis G, Gourgoulianis K, Vgontzas A, Kryger M. Cytokines and pathological sleep. *Sleep Med*. 2008;9:603–614.
193. Li AM, Lam HS, Chan MH, et al. Inflammatory cytokines and childhood obstructive sleep apnoea. *Ann Acad Med Singapore*. 2008;37:649–654.
194. McNicholas WT. Obstructive sleep apnea and inflammation. *Prog Cardiovasc Dis*. 2009;51:392–399.
195. Mehra R, Storfer-Isser A, Kirchner HL, et al. Soluble interleukin 6 receptor: A novel marker of

moderate to severe sleep-related breathing disorder. *Arch Intern Med.* 2006;166:1725–1731.
196. Ryan S, McNicholas WT. Intermittent hypoxia and activation of inflammatory molecular pathways in OSAS. *Arch Physiol Biochem.* 2008;114:261–266.
197. Thomopoulos C, Tsioufis C, Dimitriadis K, et al. Obstructive sleep apnoea syndrome is associated with enhanced sub-clinical inflammation and asymmetric dimethyl-arginine levels in hypertensives. *J Hum Hypertens.* 2009;23:65–67.
198. Yue HJ, Mills PJ, Ancoli-Israel S, Loredo JS, Ziegler MG, Dimsdale JE. The roles of TNF-alpha and the soluble TNF receptor I on sleep architecture in OSA. *Sleep Breath.* 2009 Aug;13(3): 263–269.
199. Bossu P, Ciaramella A, Salani F, et al. Interleukin-18 produced by peripheral blood cells is increased in Alzheimer's disease and correlates with cognitive impairment. *Brain Behav Immun.* 2008;22: 487–492.
200. Guerreiro RJ, Santana I, Bras JM, Santiago B, Paiva A, Oliveira C. Peripheral inflammatory cytokines as biomarkers in Alzheimer's disease and mild cognitive impairment. *Neurodegener Dis.* 2007;4:406–412.
201. Lee JW, Lee YK, Yuk DY, et al. Neuro-inflammation induced by lipopolysaccharide causes cognitive impairment through enhancement of beta-amyloid generation. *J Neuroinflammation.* 2008;5:37.
202. Holmes C, Cunningham C, Zotova E, et al. Systemic inflammation and disease progression in Alzheimer disease. *Neurology.* 2009;73:768–774.
203. Licastro F, Porcellini E, Caruso C, Lio D, Corder EH. Genetic risk profiles for Alzheimer's disease: integration of APOE genotype and variants that up-regulate inflammation. *Neurobiol Aging.* 2007; 28:1637–1643.
204. Goldbart AD, Tal A. Inflammation and sleep disordered breathing in children: a state-of-the-art review. *Pediatr Pulmonol.* 2008;43:1151–1160.
205. Tauman R, Ivanenko A, O'Brien LM, Gozal D. Plasma C-reactive protein levels among children with sleep-disordered breathing. *Pediatrics.* 2004;113:e564–e569.
206. Gozal D, Serpero LD, Sans Capdevila O, Kheirandish-Gozal L. Systemic inflammation in non-obese children with obstructive sleep apnea. *Sleep Med.* 2008;9:254–259.
207. Li C, Zhang XL, Liu H, Wang ZG, Yin KS. Association among plasma interleukin-18 levels, carotid intima-media thickness and severity of obstructive sleep apnea. *Chin Med J (Engl).* 2009;122:24–29.
208. Minoguchi K, Yokoe T, Tazaki T, et al. Increased carotid intima-media thickness and serum inflammatory markers in obstructive sleep apnea. *Am J Respir Crit Care Med.* 2005;172:625–630.
209. Abbatecola AM, Barbieri M, Rizzo MR, et al. Arterial stiffness and cognition in elderly persons with impaired glucose tolerance and microalbuminuria. *J Gerontol A Biol Sci Med Sci.* 2008;63:991–996.
210. Kearney-Schwartz A, Rossignol P, Bracard S, et al. Vascular structure and function is correlated to cognitive performance and white matter hyperintensities in older hypertensive patients with subjective memory complaints. *Stroke.* 2009;40: 1229–1236.
211. Provias J, Jeynes B. Neurofibrillary tangles and senile plaques in Alzheimer's brains are associated with reduced capillary expression of vascular endothelial growth factor and endothelial nitric oxide synthase. *Curr Neurovasc Res.* 2008;5:199–205.
212. Zuliani G, Cavalieri M, Galvani M, et al. Markers of endothelial dysfunction in older subjects with late onset Alzheimer's disease or vascular dementia. *J Neurol Sci.* 2008;272:164–170.
213. Budhiraja R, Parthasarathy S, Quan SF. Endothelial dysfunction in obstructive sleep apnea. *J Clin Sleep Med.* 2007;3:409–415.
214. Lavie L. Oxidative stress—a unifying paradigm in obstructive sleep apnea and comorbidities. *Prog Cardiovasc Dis.* 2009;51:303–312.
215. Gella A, Durany N. Oxidative stress in Alzheimer disease. *Cell Adh Migr.* 2009;3.
216. Zhu X, Smith MA, Honda K, et al. Vascular oxidative stress in Alzheimer disease. *J Neurol Sci.* 2007;257:240–246.
217. Zhu X, Su B, Wang X, Smith MA, Perry G. Causes of oxidative stress in Alzheimer disease. *Cell Mol Life Sci.* 2007;64:2202–2210.
218. Dubern B, Aggoun Y, Boule M, Fauroux B, Bonnet D, Tounian P. Arterial alterations in severely obese children with obstructive sleep apnoea. *Int J Pediatr Obes.* 2010;5:230–236.
219. Bhattacharjee R, Alotaibi WH, Kheirandish-Gozal L, Capdevila OS, Gozal D. Endothelial dysfunction in obese non-hypertensive children without evidence of sleep disordered breathing. *BMC Pediatr.* 2010;10:8.
220. Kheirandish-Gozal L, Bhattacharjee R, Kim J, Clair HB, Gozal D. Endothelial progenitor cells and vascular dysfunction in children with obstructive sleep apnea. *Am J Respir Crit Care Med.* 2010;182:92–97.
221. Gozal D, Kheirandish-Gozal L, Serpero LD, Sans Capdevila O, Dayyat E. Obstructive sleep apnea and endothelial function in school-aged nonobese children: effect of adenotonsillectomy. *Circulation.* 2007;116:2307–2314.
222. Bruce DG, Davis WA, Casey GP, et al. Predictors of cognitive decline in older individuals with diabetes. *Diabetes Care.* 2008;31:2103–2107.
223. Hassing LB, Grant MD, Hofer SM, et al. Type 2 diabetes mellitus contributes to cognitive decline in old age: a longitudinal population-based study. *J Int Neuropsychol Soc.* 2004;10:599–607.
224. Maggi S, Limongi F, Noale M, et al. Diabetes as a risk factor for cognitive decline in older patients. *Dement Geriatr Cogn Disord.* 2009;27:24–33.
225. Okereke OI, Kang JH, Cook NR, et al. Type 2 diabetes mellitus and cognitive decline in two large cohorts of community-dwelling older adults. *J Am Geriatr Soc.* 2008;56:1028–1036.
226. Akomolafe A, Beiser A, Meigs JB, et al. Diabetes mellitus and risk of developing Alzheimer disease: results from the Framingham Study. *Arch Neurol.* 2006;63:1551–1555.

227. Moroz N, Tong M, Longato L, Xu H, de la Monte SM. Limited Alzheimer-type neurodegeneration in experimental obesity and type 2 diabetes mellitus. *J Alzheimers Dis*. 2008;15:29–44.
228. Irie F, Fitzpatrick AL, Lopez OL, et al. Enhanced risk for Alzheimer disease in persons with type 2 diabetes and APOE epsilon4: the cardiovascular health study cognition study. *Arch Neurol*. 2008;65: 89–93.
229. Knutson KL, Spiegel K, Penev P, Van Cauter E. The metabolic consequences of sleep deprivation. *Sleep Med Rev*. 2007;11:163–178.
230. Calvin AD, Albuquerque FN, Lopez-Jimenez F, Somers VK. Obstructive Sleep Apnea, Inflammation, and the Metabolic Syndrome. *Metab Syndr Relat Disord*. 2009;17:245–257.
231. Kostoglou-Athanassiou I, Athanassiou P. Metabolic syndrome and sleep apnea. *Hippokratia*. 2008;12: 81–86.
232. Vgontzas AN, Bixler EO, Chrousos GP. Sleep apnea is a manifestation of the metabolic syndrome. *Sleep Med Rev*. 2005;9:211–224.
233. Tasali E, Leproult R, Ehrmann DA, Van Cauter E. Slow-wave sleep and the risk of type 2 diabetes in humans. *Proc Natl Acad Sci U S A*. 2008;105:1044–1049.
234. Iiyori N, Alonso LC, Li J, et al. Intermittent hypoxia causes insulin resistance in lean mice independent of autonomic activity. *Am J Respir Crit Care Med*. 2007;175:851–857.
235. Polotsky VY, Li J, Punjabi NM, et al. Intermittent hypoxia increases insulin resistance in genetically obese mice. *J Physiol*. 2003;552:253–264.
236. Ye J. Emerging role of adipose tissue hypoxia in obesity and insulin resistance. *Int J Obes (Lond)*. 2009;33:54–66.
237. Bennett S, Grant MM, Aldred S. Oxidative stress in vascular dementia and Alzheimer's disease: a common pathology. *J Alzheimers Dis*. 2009;17:245–257.
238. Fletcher EC. Sympathetic over activity in the etiology of hypertension of obstructive sleep apnea. *Sleep*. 2003;26:15–19.
239. Gilmartin GS, Tamisier R, Curley M, Weiss JW. Ventilatory, hemodynamic, sympathetic nervous system, and vascular reactivity changes after recurrent nocturnal sustained hypoxia in humans. *Am J Physiol Heart Circ Physiol*. 2008;295: H778–H785.
240. Imadojemu VA, Mawji Z, Kunselman A, Gray KS, Hogeman CS, Leuenberger UA. Sympathetic chemoreflex responses in obstructive sleep apnea and effects of continuous positive airway pressure therapy. *Chest*. 2007;131:1406–1413.
241. Leuenberger UA, Brubaker D, Quraishi S, Hogeman CS, Imadojemu VA, Gray KS. Effects of intermittent hypoxia on sympathetic activity and blood pressure in humans. *Auton Neurosci*. 2005;121:87–93.
242. Katz ES, D'Ambrosio CM. Pediatric obstructive sleep apnea syndrome. *Clin Chest Med*. 2010;31: 221–234.
243. Waters KA, Mast BT, Vella S, et al. Structural equation modeling of sleep apnea, inflammation, and metabolic dysfunction in children. *J Sleep Res*. 2007;16:388–395.
244. Bu G. Apolipoprotein E and its receptors in Alzheimer's disease: pathways, pathogenesis and therapy. *Nat Rev Neurosci*. 2009;10:333–344.
245. Kheirandish L, Row BW, Li RC, Brittian KR, Gozal D. Apolipoprotein E-deficient mice exhibit increased vulnerability to intermittent hypoxia-induced spatial learning deficits. *Sleep*. 2005;28: 1412–1417.
246. Cosentino FI, Bosco P, Drago V, et al. The APOE epsilon4 allele increases the risk of impaired spatial working memory in obstructive sleep apnea. *Sleep Med*. 2008;9:831–839.
247. Spira AP, Blackwell T, Stone KL, et al. Sleep-disordered breathing and cognition in older women. *J Am Geriatr Soc*. 2008;56:45–50.
248. Retey JV, Adam M, Honegger E, et al. A functional genetic variation of adenosine deaminase affects the duration and intensity of deep sleep in humans. *Proc Natl Acad Sci U S A*. 2005;102:15676–15681.
249. Landolt HP. Sleep homeostasis: a role for adenosine in humans? *Biochem Pharmacol*. 2008;75:2070–2079.
250. Dauvilliers Y, Neidhart E, Billiard M, Tafti M. Sexual dimorphism of the catechol-O-methyltransferase gene in narcolepsy is associated with response to modafinil. *Pharmacogenomics J*. 2002;2:65–68.
251. Lu B. BDNF and activity-dependent synaptic modulation. *Learn Mem*. 2003;10:86–98.
252. Kuipers SD, Bramham CR. Brain-derived neurotrophic factor mechanisms and function in adult synaptic plasticity: new insights and implications for therapy. *Curr Opin Drug Discov Devel*. 2006;9:580–586.
253. Martinowich K, Lu B. Interaction between BDNF and serotonin: role in mood disorders. *Neuropsychopharmacology*. 2008;33:73–83.
254. Lu B, Wang KH, Nose A. Molecular mechanisms underlying neural circuit formation. *Curr Opin Neurobiol*. 2009;19:162–167.
255. Faraguna U, Vyazovskiy VV, Nelson AB, Tononi G, Cirelli C. A causal role for brain-derived neurotrophic factor in the homeostatic regulation of sleep. *J Neurosci*. 2008;28:4088–4095.
256. Huber R, Tononi G, Cirelli C. Exploratory behavior, cortical BDNF expression, and sleep homeostasis. *Sleep*. 2007;30:129–139.
257. Faraguna U, Nelson A, Vyazovskiy VV, Cirelli C, Tononi G. Unilateral cortical spreading depression affects sleep need and induces molecular and electrophysiological signs of synaptic potentiation in vivo. *Cereb Cortex*. 2010 (E-pub ahead of print).
258. Xie H, Leung KL, Chen L, et al. Brain-derived neurotrophic factor rescues and prevents chronic intermittent hypoxia-induced impairment of hippocampal long-term synaptic plasticity. *Neurobiol Dis*. 2010;40:155–162.
259. Redline S, Yenokyan G, Gottlieb DJ, et al. Obstructive sleep apnea hypopnea and incident

stroke: the sleep heart health study. *Am J Respir Crit Care Med*. 2010;182:269–277.
260. Minoguchi K, Yokoe T, Tazaki T, et al. Silent brain infarction and platelet activation in obstructive sleep apnea. *Am J Respir Crit Care Med*. 2007;175:612–617.
261. Macey PM, Henderson LA, Macey KE, et al. Brain morphology associated with obstructive sleep apnea. *Am J Respir Crit Care Med*. 2002;166:1382–1387.
262. Kumar R, Birrer BV, Macey PM, et al. Reduced mammillary body volume in patients with obstructive sleep apnea. *Neurosci Lett*. 2008;438: 330–334.
263. Cross RL, Kumar R, Macey PM, et al. Neural alterations and depressive symptoms in obstructive sleep apnea patients. *Sleep*. 2008;31:1103–1109.
264. Woo MA, Macey PM, Fonarow GC, Hamilton MA, Harper RM. Regional brain gray matter loss in heart failure. *J Appl Physiol*. 2003;95: 677–684.
265. Macey PM, Kumar R, Woo MA, Harper RM. Reduced cortical thickness in obstructive sleep apnea patients. *Sleep*. 2009;32:A229.
266. Yan X, Zhang J, Shi J, Gong Q, Weng X. Cerebral and functional adaptation with chronic hypoxia exposure: a multi-modal MRI study. *Brain Res*. 2010;1348:21–29.
267. Di Paola M, Bozzali M, Fadda L, Musicco M, Sabatini U, Caltagirone C. Reduced oxygen due to high-altitude exposure relates to atrophy in motor-function brain areas. *Eur J Neurol*. 2008;15:1050–1057.
268. Fayed N, Diaz L, Davila J, Medrano J. Hematological indices, mountain sickness and MRI brain abnormalities in professional and amateur mountain climbers after altitude exposure. *Neurol Res*. 2010;32:144–147.
269. Fayed N, Modrego PJ, Morales H. Evidence of brain damage after high-altitude climbing by means of magnetic resonance imaging. *Am J Med*. 2006;119:168e1–168e6.
270. Macey PM, Kumar R, Woo MA, Valladares EM, Yan-Go FL, Harper RM. Brain structural changes in obstructive sleep apnea. *Sleep*. 2008;31: 967–977.
271. Wilke M, Sohn JH, Byars AW, Holland SK. Bright spots: correlations of gray matter volume with IQ in a normal pediatric population. *Neuroimage*. 2003;20:202–215.
272. Dickstein DP, Milham MP, Nugent AC, et al. Frontotemporal alterations in pediatric bipolar disorder: results of a voxel-based morphometry study. *Arch Gen Psychiatry*. 2005;62:734–741.
273. Milham MP, Nugent AC, Drevets WC, et al. Selective reduction in amygdala volume in pediatric anxiety disorders: a voxel-based morphometry investigation. *Biol Psychiatry*. 2005;57:961–966.
274. Carmona S, Bassas N, Rovira M, et al. Pediatric OCD structural brain deficits in conflict monitoring circuits: a voxel-based morphometry study. *Neurosci Lett*. 2007;421:218–223.
275. Mesaros S, Rocca MA, Absinta M, et al. Evidence of thalamic gray matter loss in pediatric multiple sclerosis. *Neurology*. 2008;70:1107–1112.
276. Honea R, Crow TJ, Passingham D, Mackay CE. Regional deficits in brain volume in schizophrenia: a meta-analysis of voxel-based morphometry studies. *Am J Psychiatry*. 2005;162:2233–2245.
277. Jayakumar PN, Venkatasubramanian G, Gangadhar BN, Janakiramaiah N, Keshavan MS. Optimized voxel-based morphometry of gray matter volume in first-episode, antipsychotic-naive schizophrenia. *Prog Neuropsychopharmacol Biol Psychiatry*. 2005;29:587–591.
278. Job DE, Whalley HC, McConnell S, Glabus M, Johnstone EC, Lawrie SM. Voxel-based morphometry of grey matter densities in subjects at high risk of schizophrenia. *Schizophr Res*. 2003;64:1–13.
279. Kubicki M, Shenton ME, Salisbury DF, et al. Voxel-based morphometric analysis of gray matter in first episode schizophrenia. *Neuroimage*. 2002;17:1711–1719.
280. Dale AM, Fischl B, Sereno MI. Cortical surface-based analysis. I. Segmentation and surface reconstruction. *Neuroimage*. 1999;9:179–194.
281. Fischl B, Sereno MI, Dale AM. Cortical surface-based analysis. II: Inflation, flattening, and a surface-based coordinate system. *Neuroimage*. 1999;9:195–207.
282. Rosas HD, Liu AK, Hersch S, et al. Regional and progressive thinning of the cortical ribbon in Huntington's disease. *Neurology*. 2002;58: 695–701.
283. Calabrese M, Atzori M, Bernardi V, et al. Cortical atrophy is relevant in multiple sclerosis at clinical onset. *J Neurol*. 2007;254:1212–1220.
284. Wisco JJ, Kuperberg G, Manoach D, et al. Abnormal cortical folding patterns within Broca's area in schizophrenia: evidence from structural MRI. *Schizophr Res*. 2007;94:317–327.
285. Greenstein DK, Wolfe S, Gochman P, Rapoport JL, Gogtay N. Remission status and cortical thickness in childhood-onset schizophrenia. *J Am Acad Child Adolesc Psychiatry*. 2008;47:1133–1140.
286. Narr KL, Bilder RM, Toga AW, et al. Mapping cortical thickness and gray matter concentration in first episode schizophrenia. *Cereb Cortex*. 2005;15:708–719.
287. Qiu A, Vaillant M, Barta P, Ratnanather JT, Miller MI. Region-of-interest-based analysis with application of cortical thickness variation of left planum temporale in schizophrenia and psychotic bipolar disorder. *Hum Brain Mapp*. 2008;29: 973–985.
288. Thoma RJ, Hanlon FM, Sanchez N, et al. Auditory sensory gating deficit and cortical thickness in schizophrenia. *Neurol Clin Neurophysiol*. 2004;2004:62.
289. Dickerson BC, Bakkour A, Salat DH, et al. The cortical signature of Alzheimer's disease: regionally specific cortical thinning relates to symptom severity in very mild to mild AD dementia and is detectable in asymptomatic amyloid-positive individuals. *Cereb Cortex*. 2009;19:497–510.

290. Dickerson BC, Feczko E, Augustinack JC, et al. Differential effects of aging and Alzheimer's disease on medial temporal lobe cortical thickness and surface area. *Neurobiol Aging*. 2009;30: 432–440.
291. Walhovd KB, Moe V, Slinning K, et al. Volumetric cerebral characteristics of children exposed to opiates and other substances in utero. *Neuroimage*. 2007;36:1331–1344.
292. Hermoye L, Saint-Martin C, Cosnard G, et al. Pediatric diffusion tensor imaging: normal database and observation of the white matter maturation in early childhood. *Neuroimage*. 2006;29: 493–504.
293. Schmithorst VJ, Wilke M, Dardzinski BJ, Holland SK. Cognitive functions correlate with white matter architecture in a normal pediatric population: a diffusion tensor MRI study. *Hum Brain Mapp*. 2005;26:139–147.
294. Akpinar E, Koroglu M, Ptak T. Diffusion tensor MR imaging in pediatric head trauma. *J Comput Assist Tomogr*. 2007;31:657–661.
295. Kim MJ, Provenzale JM, Law M. Magnetic resonance and diffusion tensor imaging in pediatric white matter diseases. *Top Magn Reson Imaging*. 2006;17:265–274.
296. Wozniak JR, Krach L, Ward E, et al. Neurocognitive and neuroimaging correlates of pediatric traumatic brain injury: a diffusion tensor imaging (DTI) study. *Arch Clin Neuropsychol*. 2007;22: 555–568.
297. Robbins J, Redline S, Ervin A, Walsleben JA, Ding J, Nieto FJ. Associations of sleep-disordered breathing and cerebral changes on MRI. *J Clin Sleep Med*. 2005;1:159–165.
298. Lofaso F, Goldenberg F, d'Ortho MP, Coste A, Harf A. Arterial blood pressure response to transient arousals from NREM sleep in nonapneic snorers with sleep fragmentation. *Chest*. 1998;113: 985–991.
299. Loredo JS, Nelesen R, Ancoli-Israel S, Dimsdale JE. Sleep quality and blood pressure dipping in normal adults. *Sleep*. 2004;27:1097–1103.
300. Nagai M, Hoshide S, Ishikawa J, Shimada K, Kario K. Ambulatory blood pressure as an independent determinant of brain atrophy and cognitive function in elderly hypertension. *J Hypertens*. 2008;26:1636–1641.
301. Bokura H, Yamaguchi S, Iijima K, Nagai A, Oguro H. Metabolic syndrome is associated with silent ischemic brain lesions. *Stroke*. 2008;39: 1607–1609.
302. Enzinger C, Fazekas F, Matthews PM, et al. Risk factors for progression of brain atrophy in aging: six-year follow-up of normal subjects. *Neurology*. 2005;64:1704–1711.
303. Muzur A, Pace-Schott EF, Hobson JA. The prefrontal cortex in sleep. *Trends Cogn Sci*. 2002;6: 475–481.
304. Wu JC, Gillin JC, Buchsbaum MS, et al. The effect of sleep deprivation on cerebral glucose metabolic rate in normal humans assessed with positron emission tomography. *Sleep*. 1991;14:155–162.
305. Wu JC, Gillin JC, Buchsbaum MS, et al. Frontal lobe metabolic decreases with sleep deprivation not totally reversed by recovery sleep. *Neuropsychopharmacology*. 2006;31:2783–2792.
306. Chee MW, Chuah LY. Functional neuroimaging insights into how sleep and sleep deprivation affect memory and cognition. *Curr Opin Neurol*. 2008;21:417–423.
307. Thomas RJ, Rosen BR, Stern CE, Weiss JW, Kwong KK. Functional imaging of working memory in obstructive sleep-disordered breathing. *J Appl Physiol*. 2005;98:2226–2234.
308. Chee MW, Choo WC. Functional imaging of working memory after 24 hr of total sleep deprivation. *J Neurosci*. 2004;24:4560–4567.
309. Chee MW, Chuah LY, Venkatraman V, Chan WY, Philip P, Dinges DF. Functional imaging of working memory following normal sleep and after 24 and 35 h of sleep deprivation: Correlations of fronto-parietal activation with performance. *Neuroimage*. 2006;31:419–428.
310. Drummond SP, Brown GG. The effects of total sleep deprivation on cerebral responses to cognitive performance. *Neuropsychopharmacology*. 2001; 25:S68–S73.
311. Drummond SP, Brown GG, Salamat JS, Gillin JC. Increasing task difficulty facilitates the cerebral compensatory response to total sleep deprivation. *Sleep*. 2004;27:445–451.
312. Drummond SP, Meloy MJ, Yanagi MA, Orff HJ, Brown GG. Compensatory recruitment after sleep deprivation and the relationship with performance. *Psychiatry Res*. 2005;140:211–223.
313. Mu Q, Nahas Z, Johnson KA, et al. Decreased cortical response to verbal working memory following sleep deprivation. *Sleep*. 2005;28:55–67.
314. Strangman G, Thompson JH, Strauss MM, Marshburn TH, Sutton JP. Functional brain imaging of a complex navigation task following one night of total sleep deprivation: a preliminary study. *J Sleep Res*. 2005;14:369–375.
315. Ayalon L, Ancoli-Israel S, Klemfuss Z, Shalauta MD, Drummond SP. Increased brain activation during verbal learning in obstructive sleep apnea. *Neuroimage*. 2006;31:1817–1825.
316. Thomas RJ. Fatigue in the executive cortical network demonstrated in narcoleptics using functional magnetic resonance imaging—a preliminary study. *Sleep Med*. 2005;6:399–406.
317. Thomas R, Kwong KK. Modafinil activates cortical and subcortical sites in the sleep-deprived state. *Sleep*. 2006;29:1459–1469.
318. O'Shaughnessy ES, Berl MM, Moore EN, Gaillard WD. Pediatric functional magnetic resonance imaging (fMRI): issues and applications. *J Child Neurol*. 2008;23:791–801.
319. Kotsoni E, Byrd D, Casey BJ. Special considerations for functional magnetic resonance imaging of pediatric populations. *J Magn Reson Imaging*. 2006;23:877–886.
320. Wilke M, Lidzba K, Staudt M, Buchenau K, Grodd W, Krageloh-Mann I. Comprehensive language mapping in children, using functional

magnetic resonance imaging: what's missing counts. *Neuroreport*. 2005;16:915–919.
321. Chang K, Adleman NE, Dienes K, Simeonova DI, Menon V, Reiss A. Anomalous prefrontal-subcortical activation in familial pediatric bipolar disorder: a functional magnetic resonance imaging investigation. *Arch Gen Psychiatry*. 2004;61: 781–792.
322. Suskauer SJ, Simmonds DJ, Fotedar S, et al. Functional magnetic resonance imaging evidence for abnormalities in response selection in attention deficit hyperactivity disorder: differences in activation associated with response inhibition but not habitual motor response. *J Cogn Neurosci*. 2008;20:478–493.
323. Konrad K, Neufang S, Hanisch C, Fink GR, Herpertz-Dahlmann B. Dysfunctional attentional networks in children with attention deficit/hyperactivity disorder: evidence from an event-related functional magnetic resonance imaging study. *Biol Psychiatry*. 2006;59:643–651.
324. Vaidya CJ, Bunge SA, Dudukovic NM, Zalecki CA, Elliott GR, Gabrieli JD. Altered neural substrates of cognitive control in childhood ADHD: evidence from functional magnetic resonance imaging. *Am J Psychiatry*. 2005;162:1605–1613.
325. Huang YS, Guilleminault C, Li HY, Yang CM, Wu YY, Chen NH. Attention-deficit/hyperactivity disorder with obstructive sleep apnea: a treatment outcome study. *Sleep Med*. 2007;8:18–30.
326. Schredl M, Alm B, Sobanski E. Sleep quality in adult patients with attention deficit hyperactivity disorder (ADHD). *Eur Arch Psychiatry Clin Neurosci*. 2007;257:164–168.
327. Halbower AC, Degaonkar M, Barker PB, et al. Childhood obstructive sleep apnea associates with neuropsychological deficits and neuronal brain injury. *PLoS Med*. 2006;3:e301.
328. Dang-Vu TT, Desseilles M, Schwartz S, Maquet P. Neuroimaging of narcolepsy. *CNS Neurol Disord Drug Targets*. 2009;8:254–263.
329. Brenneis C, Brandauer E, Frauscher B, et al. Voxel-based morphometry in narcolepsy. *Sleep Med*. 2005;6:531–536.
330. Buskova J, Vaneckova M, Sonka K, Seidl Z, Nevsimalova S. Reduced hypothalamic gray matter in narcolepsy with cataplexy. *Neuro Endocrinol Lett*. 2006;27:769–772.
331. Joo EY, Tae WS, Kim ST, Hong SB. Gray matter concentration abnormality in brains of narcolepsy patients. *Korean J Radiol*. 2009;10:552–558.
332. Kaufmann C, Schuld A, Pollmacher T, Auer DP. Reduced cortical gray matter in narcolepsy: preliminary findings with voxel-based morphometry. *Neurology*. 2002;58:1852–1855.
333. Kim SJ, Lyoo IK, Lee YS, et al. Gray matter deficits in young adults with narcolepsy. *Acta Neurol Scand*. 2009;119:61–67.
334. Overeem S, Steens SC, Good CD, et al. Voxel-based morphometry in hypocretin-deficient narcolepsy. *Sleep*. 2003;26:44–46.
335. Dauvilliers Y, Comte F, Bayard S, Carlander B, Zanca M, Touchon J. A brain PET study in patients with narcolepsy-cataplexy. *J Neurol Neurosurg Psychiatry*. 2009;81:344–348.
336. Joo EY, Tae WS, Kim JH, Kim BT, Hong SB. Glucose hypometabolism of hypothalamus and thalamus in narcolepsy. *Ann Neurol*. 2004;56:437–440.
337. Kim YK, Yoon IY, Shin YK, Cho SS, Kim SE. Modafinil-induced hippocampal activation in narcolepsy. *Neurosci Lett*. 2007;422:91–96.
338. Tonon C, Franceschini C, Testa C, et al. Distribution of neurochemical abnormalities in patients with narcolepsy with cataplexy: an in vivo brain proton MR spectroscopy study. *Brain Res Bull*. 2009;80:147–150.
339. Watson NF, Doherty MJ, Zunt JR. Secondary narcolepsy following neurocysticercosis infection. *J Clin Sleep Med*. 2005;1:41–42.
340. Aldrich MS, Naylor MW. Narcolepsy associated with lesions of the diencephalon. *Neurology*. 1989;39:1505–1508.
341. Marcus CL, Trescher WH, Halbower AC, Lutz J. Secondary narcolepsy in children with brain tumors. *Sleep*. 2002;25:435–439.
342. Muller HL, Muller-Stover S, Gebhardt U, Kolb R, Sorensen N, Handwerker G. Secondary narcolepsy may be a causative factor of increased daytime sleepiness in obese childhood craniopharyngioma patients. *J Pediatr Endocrinol Metab*. 2006;19(suppl 1):423–429.
343. Landolfi JC, Nadkarni M. Paraneoplastic limbic encephalitis and possible narcolepsy in a patient with testicular cancer: case study. *Neuro Oncol*. 2003;5:214–216.
344. Overeem S, Dalmau J, Bataller L, et al. Hypocretin-1 CSF levels in anti-Ma2 associated encephalitis. *Neurology*. 2004;62:138–140.
345. Kanbayashi T, Shimohata T, Nakashima I, et al. Symptomatic narcolepsy in patients with neuromyelitis optica and multiple sclerosis: new neurochemical and immunological implications. *Arch Neurol*. 2009;66:1563–1566.
346. Huang YS, Lakkis C, Guilleminault C. Kleine-Levin syndrome: current status. *Med Clin North Am* 2010;94:557–562.
347. Afshar K, Engelfried K, Sharma OP. Sarcoidosis: a rare cause of Kleine-Levine-Critchley syndrome. *Sarcoidosis Vasc Diffuse Lung Dis*. 2008;25: 60–63.
348. Hong SB, Joo EY, Tae WS, Lee J, Han SJ, Lee HW. Episodic diencephalic hypoperfusion in Kleine-Levin syndrome. *Sleep*. 2006;29:1091–1093.
349. Huang YS, Guilleminault C, Kao PF, Liu FY. SPECT findings in the Kleine-Levin syndrome. *Sleep*. 2005;28:955–960.
350. Carroll MS, Patwari PP, Weese-Mayer DE. Carbon dioxide chemoreception and hypoventilation syndromes with autonomic dysregulation. *J Appl Physiol*. 2010;108:979–988.
351. Patwari PP, Carroll MS, Rand CM, Kumar R, Harper R, Weese-Mayer DE. Congenital central hypoventilation syndrome and the PHOX2B gene: a model of respiratory and autonomic dysregulation. *Respir Physiol Neurobiol*. 2010;173: 322–325.

352. Zelko FA, Nelson MN, Leurgans SE, Berry-Kravis EM, Weese-Mayer DE. Congenital central hypoventilation syndrome: neurocognitive functioning in school age children. *Pediatr Pulmonol* 2009;45:92–98.
353. Weese-Mayer DE, Berry-Kravis EM, Ceccherini I, Keens TG, Loghmanee DA, Trang H. An official ATS clinical policy statement: Congenital central hypoventilation syndrome: genetic basis, diagnosis, and management. *Am J Respir Crit Care Med.* 2010;181:626–644.
354. Macey PM, Richard CA, Kumar R, et al. Hippocampal volume reduction in congenital central hypoventilation syndrome. *PLoS One.* 2009;4:e6436.
355. Kumar R, Lee K, Macey PM, Woo MA, Harper RM. Mammillary body and fornix injury in congenital central hypoventilation syndrome. *Pediatr Res.* 2009;66:429–434.
356. Kumar R, Macey PM, Woo MA, Alger JR, Keens TG, Harper RM. Neuroanatomic deficits in congenital central hypoventilation syndrome. *J Comp Neurol.* 2005;487:361–371.
357. Kumar R, Ahdout R, Macey PM, et al. Reduced caudate nuclei volumes in patients with congenital central hypoventilation syndrome. *Neuroscience.* 2009;163:1373–1379.
358. Kumar R, Macey PM, Woo MA, Harper RM. Rostral brain axonal injury in congenital central hypoventilation syndrome. *J Neurosci Res.* 2010;88:2146–2154.
359. Kumar R, Macey PM, Woo MA, Alger JR, Harper RM. Diffusion tensor imaging demonstrates brainstem and cerebellar abnormalities in congenital central hypoventilation syndrome. *Pediatr Res.* 2008;64:275–280.
360. Kumar R, Macey PM, Woo MA, Alger JR, Harper RM. Elevated mean diffusivity in widespread brain regions in congenital central hypoventilation syndrome. *J Magn Reson Imaging.* 2006;24:1252–1258.
361. Arcaya J, Cacho J, Del Campo F, Grande J, Maillo A. Arnold-Chiari malformation associated with sleep apnea and central dysregulation of arterial pressure. *Acta Neurol Scand.* 1993;88:224–226.
362. Rabec C, Laurent G, Baudouin N, et al. Central sleep apnoea in Arnold-Chiari malformation: evidence of pathophysiological heterogeneity. *Eur Respir J.* 1998;12:1482–1485.
363. Keefover R, Sam M, Bodensteiner J, Nicholson A. Hypersomnolence and pure central sleep apnea associated with the Chiari I malformation. *J Child Neurol.* 1995;10:65–67.
364. Erlich SS, Apuzzo ML. The pineal gland: anatomy, physiology, and clinical significance. *J Neurosurg.* 1985;63:321–341.
365. Macchi MM, Bruce JN. Human pineal physiology and functional significance of melatonin. *Front Neuroendocrinol.* 2004;25:177–195.
366. Kubota M, Shinozaki M, Nagata J, Sasaki H. Circadian rhythm disturbance in patients with hypothalamic lesion. *Jpn J Psychiatry Neurol.* 1991;45:157–158.
367. Cohen RA, Albers EH. Disruption of human circadian and cognitive regulation following a discrete hypothalamic lesion: a case study. *Neurology.* 1991;41:726–729.

CHAPTER 20

Pediatric Sleep Pharmacology

Rafael Pelayo and Kin Yuen

Introduction

This chapter will review the most common pharmacological options in the treatment of sleep disorders in children. In the past, a discussion of the topic of pediatric sleep pharmacology centered on sedatives for insomnia [1–3]. Although insomnia is still an important area of consideration, the topic has broadened to include pharmacological treatment options in children for narcolepsy, parasomnias, restless legs syndrome (RLS), and sleep apnea. In this chapter, we will first review the general principles of pharmacology for pediatric sleep disorders, and a more detailed discussion of specific sleep disorders will follow.

General Principles of Pharmacological Treatment

All clinicians, whether they treat adults or children, learn pharmacological approaches the same way. First we learn physiology, then pathophysiology, and for the rest of our careers, we apply this knowledge to the pharmacological management of our patients. When we learn of new pharmacological treatment options, we try to place them within this framework of physiology and pathophysiology. Without knowledge of sleep physiology and pathophysiology, rational pharmacological management is not possible. Despite high prevalence in children, sleep disorders are not emphasized during typical medical school or pediatric residency education. This paucity of education may account for the relatively little information being available on the pharmacological management of sleep disorders in children. Most reviews are based on expert consensus rather than evidence based trials [3].

When medications are used to treat sleep disorders in children, they are typically neither FDA approved for the pediatric age range, nor for the intended sleep disorder. The antihypertensive agent clonidine, a centrally acting alpha agonist, is an example of the latter. Clonidine is not an indicated medication for insomnia in adults. However, clonidine is one of the most commonly prescribed medications for insomnia in children despite the absence of any randomized control trials supporting its use. Pediatricians prescribe clonidine for children of all ages, infants through teens [3–6]. There is no reason to suspect that the pathophysiology of chronic insomnia is that different between adults and children. It seems clearly problematic that an antihypertensive agent that is never considered in the modern medical management in adults with chronic insomnia is apparently, unquestionably, routinely used in children. It is important to place the most common pharmacological options within a framework of the pathophysiology of sleep disorders in children.

Parental Expectations

Before starting a discussion with parents of what to prescribe their child, first we must be certain that indeed there is pathology, and the pathology is found in the child, and not in another family member. Sleep disorders are very common among adults. A discussion with the parents of what constitutes normal sleep may be necessary. Although the need for sleep has a biological basis, the way we sleep is learned and influenced by the cultural environment. This is analogous to eating. All newborns first drink milk, but the diet of older children is different throughout the world. The child will learn or form associations with regard to sleep. As the child is readied for bed, the child may associate sleep onset with particular events. The child may associate this process with increased attention and activity rather than getting ready for bed. If continued, the child may then develop an association with parental activity that requires persistent parental involvement to fall asleep. The awakenings in the middle of night often necessitate similar actions. What initially were brief awakenings may develop into lengthy struggles. What wakes up the child may not be what is keeping the child awake. Now the parental actions became the focus of the problem. If returning the child to sleep requires frequent parental assistance, the parents' sleep may be very disturbed. The entire family may start to dread the nighttime instead of looking forward to going to sleep. The nighttime routines are no longer pleasurable, but become a source of frustration. A vicious cycle may form which is exacerbated by middle-of-the night awakenings. Parents may report the infant waking up crying every hour. The normal sleep cycle length in an infant is approximately 1 hour and is followed by a brief arousal before initiating the next sleep cycle. The parents may misidentify normal sleep behavior. We cannot overstate the importance of a review of parental expectations and understanding of normal sleep before discussing medication.

Other Roadblocks

Stojanovski and colleagues examined trends in physician prescribing of medications for children with sleep difficulties in outpatient settings in the United States [6]. The study used data from the National Ambulatory Medical Care Survey (NAMCS) collected from 1993 to 2004. During this time period, there were approximately 18.6 million patient visits for sleep related difficulty in children. The rate of medication prescriptions for children with sleep disorders appears to be increasing. The study found that approximately 18.6 million visits occurred for sleep related difficulty in children. In this 12-year study period, 81% of patients with pediatric insomnia were prescribed a sleep medication: 33% received antihistamines, and another 26% were prescribed alpha-2 agonists (presumably clonidine). The finding that 81% of children were prescribed a medication is particularly remarkable considering that only 48% of the adult patients suffering from insomnia were prescribed a medication [6]. For insomnia, the likelihood of a child being prescribed an off-label medication is greater than the likelihood of an adult receiving a labeled medication!

The paucity of information on the pharmacological treatment of sleep disorders in children may not be surprising given the inherent problems of the clinical situation. Most pharmacological guidelines were developed for sleep disorders in adults and must be empirically extrapolated to children. The physician is often forced to prescribe medications as an "off-label" indication. This may result in frustrating insurance reimbursement delays or denials for the family. These reimbursement problems may affect the availability of a specific medication, the family's compliance with the medication, or force the physician to prescribe a less desirable alternative. The medication may not be available commercially in an easily administered form. Younger children may not be able to swallow pills, or ingest chewable tablets, requiring the local pharmacist to compound the medication into a suspension. In addition, because of the natural aversion among both parents and physicians to use medications for pediatric sleep disorders, medications are usually prescribed as a last resort or in the most refractory situations. At times, a decision to use medication in a child may be made not necessarily to assist the child as much as to help the parents or other family members sleep better. It is not unusual that parents may finally seek help for a child's long-standing sleep problem when the parents feel they can no longer put up with interruptions to their own sleep. The clinician needs to be aware of this situation, which may cause guilty feelings to arise in the family members.

Further, complicating the pharmacological treatment of sleep disorders in children is the general lack of specialized training in sleep disorders available to all health care providers, not just pediatricians, who are working with these children. Failure to consider or properly apply nondrug treatments as part of the comprehensive management of the child may also lead to unsatisfactory results for the patient and the family. These factors result in children with sleep disorders that are not properly managed because of either under dosing or overdosing of medication or incorrect medication selection. Accelerated clearance of the hypnotics because of different pharmacokinetics in children may also be a factor [7].

Sedation Does Not Equate Sleep

A key principle in sleep pharmacology is not to equate sedation with normal refreshing sleep. Perhaps the simplest and best known example of this principle is alcohol. Consuming large amounts of alcohol can be very sedating, but we do not wake up feeling particularly refreshed after a night of excessive drinking. There may be an overreliance on the effects of the medication by both the parents and the healthcare provider, without adequate understanding of the cause of the poor sleep or the appropriate application of behavioral techniques to help improve the child's sleep.

A common scenario in clinical practice is a parent's complaint of a child's paradoxical reaction to a hypnotic medication. The parent may state, "He did not sleep at all" or "he became hyper." From a physiological point of view, how can we explain that a child did not get sleepy when given a hypnotic agent? Is the child's brain missing the usual gamma aminobutyric acid (GABA) receptors? Of course not, but the child's poor reaction to the medication is not typically questioned, and the medication is simply removed from the limited list of pharmacological options available to the patient.

Dosage and Timing

A more physiological approach would be to understand why the medication failed to achieve the desired result. In the authors' experience, the reason may not be because of the choice of medication per se. Insufficient doses or incorrect timing of administration is more likely the cause for the absence of efficacy and/or adverse reactions. Therefore, when performing an initial evaluation of a child's sleep complaints, we should not exclude a medication simply because the parent says that particular medication has already been tried and failed. We have a very limited number of medications available and cannot afford to summarily disregard the most common options. Instead, we must find out in detail how the "failed" medication was given, at what time, what dose, and had the child eaten immediately before the medication administration. For example, hypnotics are meant to be given on an empty stomach because food delays the absorption. If the medication is given too early in the evening, the child may simply not be sleepy enough for the medication to work.

When prescribing a medication for a child, there is a natural inclination to give the lowest dose possible. However, children may have faster hepatic metabolism of the medication resulting in faster elimination [7]. If the dose of the agent is too low, the medication may disinhibit a child, but not make the child actually fall asleep. The parents would report unusual behavior. If a child typically fights his/her bedtime, because of a fear of being alone in the dark for example, and the medication dose given to the child only makes that child drowsy but without falling asleep, then frightening hypnagogic hallucinations may occur. This might particularly be disturbing in children with an underlying psychiatric or neurological condition, for whom the outside world may already be confusing. With the resulting confusion or disorientation caused by too low dose of a sedating medication, it is not surprising that parents may report paradoxical reactions to the putative hypnotic.

Not only is the specific medication and dosage key, but the timing of administration is also very important. It is important because of the circadian modulation of alertness. Humans will typically experience an enhanced alertness in the evening, which is often referred to as a "second wind." During this circadian phase, it is harder to fall asleep. If the hypnotic medication is given during this circadian time window, it may not work. If the medication is given too early while the child is not ready to sleep, but rather has heightened alertness, dissociative phenomenon such as frightening hypnagogic hallucinations may occur [2]. In the case of children with neurological or psychiatric disorders, they may not understand that the medication was meant to help them sleep. Typically, hypnotics shorten the usual falling asleep time (sleep latency) at most by only 20 or 30 minutes compared to placebo. Giving a medication 2 or 3 hours before the usual falling asleep time could commonly elicit the aforementioned response. This same medication and dose given at a more appropriate circadian time could be effective.

This lack of proper management of the sleep problem may be particularly common among children with neurological, psychiatric, behavioral, or emotional disorders. The use of psychotropic medication in children has been increasing [8]. If the child cannot communicate what he or she feels is causing the sleep difficulty, incorrect assumptions may be made by the family and/or health care provider. In cases of insomnia, this can result in an escalating cycle of progressively more sedating agents with increasing likelihood of adverse effects. Concomitant daytime sedation may occur, which may interfere with the child's daytime therapeutic program and exacerbate the child's disabilities. In some situations, the fear of putative addiction may limit the physician or the family from using pharmacotherapy adequately to improve the child's sleep.

Social Environment

All discussions of pediatric sleep pharmacology need to take into account the cultural background of the family. The parents need to be in agreement about their expectations of the child's sleep, especially if the parents have different cultural backgrounds. The parents' own prior sleep experiences both in childhood and as adults should be explored. Also the influence of other family members, such as grandparents, in shaping the family's views should be considered. If the child lives in 2 separate households as typically can occur with divorce, is the sleep problem present in both homes or are there differences? Will any prescribed medication be given in both homes?

Given the paucity of evidence-based medicine in pediatric sleep pharmacotherapy, the reader should be particularly cautious when applying the information in this chapter to individual patients. There is a great need for double-blind, placebo-controlled trials.

Insomnia

The pharmacological treatment of insomnia was recently reviewed [3]. Insomnia is characterized in adults by difficulty falling asleep and/or staying asleep associated with subjective daytime impairment. In children, this same definition may be applied, but modified. Commonly, it is the parents' subjective impairment that leads the family to seek medical attention. The young child may awaken for a variety of reasons, but will often eventually fall back asleep. However, the parent's sleep schedule is disrupted. The medical history is incomplete without a discussion of what the parents' sleep was like before they were parents. If the parents had any prior sleep impairment, such as mild sleep apnea, they will have greater difficulty handling the typical sleep disruptions of parenthood. The amount and schedule of sleep each of the parents in the household preferred before they were parents should be reviewed before making any pharmacological decisions.

The sleepless child can be a challenging situation for both the family and the primary health care provider. The primary health care provider may have limited training in pediatric sleep disorders. The insomnia's manifestation and management will depend on the child's age. In general, behavior techniques should be the mainstay of treatment [9]. Medications may have a role as an adjunct in the insomnia management.

Infants

For infants, the pharmacological options for insomnia are limited. Insomnia in an otherwise healthy infant is typically because of behavioral problems such as behavioral insomnia of childhood, sleep onset association type, or nocturnal feeding [10]. The child can sleep well if the associations the child makes with sleep onset are present throughout the sleep period. If the associations, such as the presence of the parents, are absent during the sleep period, then the child usually has difficulty returning to sleep after awakening. It is important to keep in mind that what wakes up the infant may not be what is keeping the infant awake [9,11].

Parents often seek medical attention for their sleepless infant because of concerns that the infant may have a physical cause for the problem. In general, if the child's growth, development, and examination are normal, a physical cause for the poor sleep is less likely. One simple way to distinguish if the sleep problems in the infant are physical versus behavioral is to evaluate for any difference in the sleep pattern when the child sleeps alone or with a parent. This should be observed over several nights before reaching a conclusion. If the child sleeps much better when he or she is with the parent, the problem is more likely behavioral. If the infant sleeps as poorly with or without the parent, the problem may be physical. Gastroesophageal reflux and sleep disordered breathing should be part of the differential diagnosis. In some situations, a combination of both physical and behavioral factors may be playing a role.

The health care provider must specifically ask the parents if they have given the child any substance to improve the child's poor sleep. The parents may not volunteer that they have attempted to give the child a substance such as alcohol, or over the counter acetaminophen or antihistamines. In addition, ambiguities and differences among the parents about how the child should sleep may complicate the clinical situation. For example, one parent may prefer to co-sleep with the child, but the other parent may not.

Toddlers

Among toddlers, parental complaints of poor sleep are not uncommon. The most common situations are behavioral insomnia of childhood limit setting type and nocturnal fears [10]. The child may appear to be physiologically ready to sleep, but may either refuse to go to sleep or gets out of bed after the child has been tucked into bed. Once the child falls asleep, the sleep should be of normal quality. Difficulty falling back to sleep may occur if the child's sleep is disrupted. Medications are not typically given in these situations [9,11]. If the problem has reached such a magnitude that the child's poor sleep is causing a disruption of the household or the parents sleep, then medications may be requested by the family. Within the context of behavior modification program, a brief adjunctive trial of medication might be attempted.

Adolescents

The most common form of insomnia in adolescents is sleep onset insomnia typical of delayed sleep phase syndrome [12]. Delayed sleep phase syndrome is a condition in which the adolescent falls asleep later than expected and has normal sleep during the night but has difficulty waking up at the expected time. Typically, the children are described as preferring to stay up late at night. The children usually have a later sleep and wake up time on weekends and holidays. The treatment usually consists of behavioral changes when the child is motivated to change the behavior. These behavioral changes may also include progressive scheduled exposure to bright light at the desired wake up time. The use of bright light to influence a circadian sleep disorder is called phototherapy [13,14]. Children who are avoiding school may mimic this sleep disorder. To help the child fall asleep faster, different substances have been tried. Melatonin has been used with variable effect. Melatonin is further described below.

Prescription hypnotics do not have an FDA indication for adolescents younger than 18 years old. An "off-label" use as an adjunct to the behavioral modification of the circadian problem may be considered in certain clinical situations. Because these patients typically only have sleep onset insomnia without significant nocturnal disruption, a short acting hypnotic agent may be considered for a short period of time. Zaleplon, a nonbenzodiazepine hypnotic, may theoretically be used in adolescents with delayed sleep phase syndrome because it has fast onset of action, and its hypnotic effects should wear off well before the desired wake up time. Zaleplon has a short elimination half-life of approximately one hour. This short duration, unlike diphenhydramine, will minimize any next day sedation. Because the duration of medication treatment is expected to be of relatively a short time, zaleplon also has the additional benefit of minimal rebound insomnia. Rebound insomnia refers to an exacerbation of insomnia on abrupt cessation of a hypnotic. The degree of insomnia is more severe than the initial insomnia before starting hypnotics. Rebound insomnia is more typical of short acting benzodiazepine hypnotics such as triazolam. Gradual tapering is helpful to avoid a significant rebound effect.

A potential medication to consider in the treatment of delayed sleep phase syndrome in adolescents is ramelteon. Ramelteon is a selective melatonin type 1 and 2 receptor agonist that has been approved for sleep onset insomnia in patients 18 and older [15]. It lacks the potential for abuse commonly associated with hypnotics. Systematic trials in younger patients are not available. A case study did report efficacy in an 18 year old and a 7 year old with autism and insomnia [16].

Diphenhydramine

Diphenhydramine hydrochloride, 2-(diphenylmethoxy)-N, N-dimethylethylamine hydrochloride, is a competitive H1-histamine receptor blocker that has multiple effects on the central and peripheral nervous systems. Diphenhydramine is rapidly absorbed from the gastrointestinal tract without any gastric irritation. Peak blood and tissue levels are achieved within 2 hours of ingestion. It is an active ingredient in many over-the-counter (OTC) medications: anti-allergy, sedative, hypnotic, antitussive, and antiemetic preparations [17–23]. Diphenhydramine is characterized by ethylamine moieties, which make them highly lipophilic and hence penetrate the blood brain barrier more easily. A large number of H1-receptor sites are located on the frontal lobes and in the deep structures of the brain. Positron emission tomography studies conducted by Yanai et al have demonstrated that the first generation agents occupy approximately 75% of the H1-receptor sites in the brain [24]. Brain histamine is involved in a wide range of physiological functions such as regulation of the sleep–wake cycle, arousal, cognition, and memory mainly through interactions with histamine H1 receptors. Neurons producing histamine, histaminergic neurons, are exclusively located in the posterior hypothalamus and transmit histamine to almost all regions of the brain [25].

Various studies have been done to evaluate the usefulness of diphenhydramine in sleep disorders of both adults and children. When given shortly before bedtime, a significant decrease in sleep latency time and number of awakenings were observed. The duration of activity following an average dose of diphenhydramine is 4 to 6 hours [26]. A plasma diphenhydramine level exceeding 30 ng/ml produces drowsiness [26,27]. The recommended dosage for adults is 25 to 50 mg, whereas in children the lowest effective dose starts from 0.5 mg/kg to 25 mg maximum.

A randomized controlled trial of infant response to diphenhydramine was published called the Trial of Infant Response to Diphenhydramine ("TIRED study") [28]. This study recruited 44 infants aged 6 to 15 months with frequent parent-reported nighttime awakenings. The primary outcome was a parental report of improvement in the number of night awakenings requiring parental assistance. The trial was stopped early because of lack of effectiveness of diphenhydramine over placebo. Only 1 of 22 children receiving diphenhydramine showed improvement compared with 3 of 22 receiving placebo. The study concluded that during 1 week of therapy and at follow-up 2 and 4 weeks later, diphenhydramine was no more effective than placebo in reducing nighttime awakening or improving overall parental happiness with sleep for infants [28].

The most common adverse reaction to diphenhydramine at therapeutic doses is impaired consciousness. The predominant features in an overdose are anticholinergic effects, which include fever, mydriasis, blurred vision, dry mouth, constipation, urinary retention, tachycardia, dystonia, and confusion. Other common symptoms of diphenhydramine poisoning include catatonic stupor, anxiety, and visual hallucinations [17]. Rare presentations include respiratory insufficiency, rhabdomyolysis, and cardiac rhythm disturbances and seizures [17,29,30].

Fatal intoxications with diphenhydramine in 5 infants were reported in a case series by Baker et al [21]. The infants were 6, 8, 9, 12, and 12 weeks old. Postmortem blood diphenhydramine levels in the cases were 1.6, 1.5, 1.6, 1.1, and 1.1 mg/L, respectively. In one case, the child's father admitted giving the infant diphenhydramine in an attempt to induce the infant to sleep; in another case, a day care provider admitted putting diphenhydramine in the baby's bottle [21].

Chloral Hydrate

Chloral hydrate (CH) is a commonly used sedative hypnotic and prescribed to both children and adults. Usual dosing ranges between 25 to 50 mg/kg/dose up to a maximum of 1 g/dose PO or PR. Even at higher doses, 80 to 100 mg/kg has been given to children younger than 5 years with good effect and minimal toxicity [31]. However, neonatal dosing may need adjustment, particularly when used in a multidose fashion [31]. After it is absorbed from the GI tract, CH is converted by alcohol dehydrogenase to trichloroethanol (TCE), the active metabolite. TCE is slightly lipid soluble and therefore penetrates the blood-brain-barrier. A CNS depressant, TCE, causes drowsiness and sedation, then sleep within 1 hour. The plasma t ½ of TCE is 8 to12 hours in older children and adults, but for neonates and infants is 3 to 4 times longer [31].

Therapeutic doses normally reduce blood pressure minimally and suppress respirations slightly, but protective airway reflexes are not affected. However, children with obstructive sleep apnea (OSA), wheezing, Leigh's disease, or other encephalic white matter or brain stem disorders may be at increased risk for respiratory compromise [31]. Respiratory suppression may also occur in overdose situations, with deep stupor and coma. Furthermore, cardiovascular instability, in the form of decreased myocardial contractility, shortened refractory period, and changes in myocardial sensitivity to endogenous catecholamines, accounts for most of the mortality, which occurs when CH is given in toxic levels. Similarly, CH may be contraindicated in children who are also on stimulants, because of rare reports of malignant arrhythmias. While co-administration with other classes of sedatives always acts synergistically on the CNS, taking CH with fluoxetine has also been reported to cause prolonged sedation, but for unclear reasons [31]. Tolerance to its sedating effects may occur. Chronic use of CH for insomnia should be discouraged given the potential for side effects and tolerance. A study comparing the use of CH to music therapy in children undergoing EEG testing found music therapy to be an effective alternative [32].

Other Over-the-Counter Hypnotics

Besides diphenhydramine, other H1 antihistamines are also often used for their sedative effects, as they are lipid soluble and pass through the blood-brain-barrier [33]. Ethanolamines and phenothiazines have marked sedative effects, whereas ethylenediamines cause moderate sedation, and alkylamines mild sedation [34]. However, centrally acting H1 antagonists have also been shown to have convulsant effects, especially in young children, and over dosage has been associated with seizure and death [21]. Furthermore, these agents may worsen OSA, also may suppress REM sleep, and produce a marked compensatory rebound following withdrawal of these agents, resulting worsened sleep instability and fragmentation [35].

Melatonin

As its name is derived from its effect on melanin pigmentation in frogs, melatonin (N-acetyl-5-methoxytryptamine) is the main hormone secreted by the pineal gland. As the pineal gland lacks a blood-brain-barrier, it is sensitive to the influence of peripherally active drugs [36]. Melatonin is synthesized from its precursor tryptophan, which is hydroxylated to 5-hydroxytryptophan and then decarboxylated to serotonin. This is then *N*-acetylated and converted to melatonin by hydroxyindole-O-methyltransferase. Production by the pineal gland shows a high-amplitude circadian rhythm resulting in low plasma levels during the day and high levels at night. This rhythmicity is comparable in humans and in experimental animals (either diurnal or nocturnal), with daily dark phase levels 3 to 10 times higher than during the light phase [36]. It is believed that the physiologic increase in blood melatonin concentration by 10 to 15 fold, which occurs 1 to 2 hours before bedtime, may be the final trigger for inducing sleep [37]. The circadian rhythm of melatonin usually develops between the second and third month of life, and nighttime melatonin is low or undetectable at 2 to 3 months of age, then increases steadily. Neonates and infants depend on their mother's melatonin circadian rhythm through her milk [36].

Melatonin may possess a phase-setting effect instead of, or in addition to, a direct hypnotic effect [36]. While its role in circadian rhythm-based sleep disorders like jet lag and delayed sleep phase syndrome has been reported, the hypnotic effect of melatonin is less well demonstrated. Improved subjective sleep has been noted. Conflicting reports on the efficacy of melatonin have been attributed to possible differences in melatonin dosages, the timing of administration, experimental approaches, and diversity of subjects. A recent meta analysis published in the British Medical Journal concluded ". . . no evidence that melatonin is effective in treating secondary sleep disorders or sleep disorders accompanying sleep restriction, such as jet lag and shiftwork disorder"[38].

In adults, small physiologic doses of 0.1 to 0.3 mg of melatonin in the evening can generate serum concentrations that are within the normal nocturnal range (50–200 pg/mL). Melatonin is more effective when given 2 hours before bedtime, than when given immediately before bedtime, and dose ranges between 0.3 mg and 10 mg are used for short-term insomnia. While dosing guidelines have not yet been established, in adults doses starting between 0.3 to 1.0 mg may be used, and increased to effect.

Unfortunately, dosing in children is less clear, but in a case series of 15 neurologically impaired children with chronic sleep disturbances, including fragmented sleep and delayed sleep phase, 2 to 10 mg resulted in subjective improvement in their sleep [36].

However, the National Sleep Foundation has warned against using melatonin in patients with immune disorders, lymphoproliferative disorders, and in those taking corticosteroids or other immunosuppressants, given its ability to enhance immune function [36]. Finally, it must be kept in mind that melatonin is still considered a "diet supplement," and the Food and Drug Administration does not regulate its safety, purity, or efficacy [37].

The use of melatonin for children may be most effective in insomnia because of circadian factors. This would include children with delayed sleep phase syndrome and also blind children. Children with midline brain defects such as agenesis of corpus callosum sometimes seem to respond to melatonin treatment for insomnia. This may be due presumably to associated defects in the pineal region [39,40]. Smits et al conducted a double-blind, placebo-controlled trial of 5 mg of melatonin in children age 6 to 12 with sleep onset insomnia. The melatonin treated group reported falling asleep 63 minutes earlier and had an increased total sleep time of 41 minutes.

Weiss and colleagues reported on the use of sleep hygiene and melatonin treatment for initial insomnia in children with attention-deficit/hyperactivity disorder (ADHD) [41]. This is analogous to the use of combination of hypnotics and cognitive behavioral therapy for adults with insomnia. In this study, 27 stimulant-treated children (6–14 years of age) with ADHD and sleep onset of insomnia (>60 minutes) received sleep hygiene intervention. Nonresponders were randomized to a 30-day double-blind, placebo-controlled, crossover trial of 5-mg pharmaceutical-grade melatonin. The results showed a significant reduction in initial insomnia of 16 minutes with melatonin relative to placebo. Of note, the improved sleep had no demonstrable effect on ADHD symptoms [41]. A similar report by Van der Heijden and colleagues investigated the effect of melatonin treatment on sleep, behavior, cognition, and quality of life in children with ADHD and chronic sleep onset insomnia. A total of 105 medication-free children, ages 6 to 12 years, with ADHD and sleep onset insomnia participated in a randomized, double-blind, placebo-controlled trial using 3 or 6 mg melatonin, or placebo for 4 weeks. Melatonin advanced circadian rhythms of sleep–wake and endogenous melatonin and enhanced total time asleep in children with ADHD and chronic sleep onset insomnia. Similar to the Weiss study, they found that improved sleep with melatonin had no effect on problem behavior, cognitive performance, or quality of life [42].

A randomized double-blind, placebo-controlled crossover trial of controlled release melatonin (5 mg) in the treatment of delayed sleep phase syndrome and impaired sleep maintenance of children with neurodevelopmental disabilities including autistic spectrum disorders was published [43]. This was a 10-day trial with melatonin followed by a 3-month open-label component of the study. The dose was gradually increased to a maximum of 15 mg. Sleep characteristics were measured by caregiver using sleep logs and actigraphs. Clinician rating of severity of the sleep disorder and improvement from baseline, along with caregiver ratings of global functioning and family stress, was also obtained. Fifty children (average age of 7 years) completed the study. Sleep latency decreased from on average 72 to 32 minutes, an improvement of over 30 minutes. The sleep maintenance measures did not improve. There was additional improvement in sleep diaries measures of sleep efficiency and the longest sleep episode in the open-label phase. Perhaps most importantly the therapy was found to be effective in reducing family stress [43]. It is important to realize that in families with children with neurodevelopmental disabilities, even small improvements, may have a large impact in the family.

More recently a smaller randomized, double-blind, placebo-controlled of melatonin in children specifically with autism spectrum disorder and fragile X syndrome was published [44]. In this study, a 4-week trial of melatonin 3 mg or placebo was given to children with an average age of 5 (ranging 2–15 years). Data were successfully obtained from 12 subjects. The mean night sleep duration was longer on melatonin than placebo by 21 minutes, and the mean sleep onset latency was shorter by 28 minutes. The authors concluded melatonin was effective and tolerated by children with autism spectrum disorder and fragile X syndrome [44]. These results are similar to another randomized trial of melatonin in children with ADHD [42].

The results of a long-term trial of melatonin report that it is well tolerated [45]. A follow-up parental survey study of children with ADHD and chronic sleep onset insomnia report that in 3.7 years there were no serious adverse events or treatment related co-morbidities. The majority of children surveyed used melatonin daily. Parents also reported improved behavior and mood [45].

Clonidine

Clonidine was originally marketed for the treatment of hypertension under the trade name Catapres, but its sedating properties have led to its use as a soporific. Clonidine is a central alpha2-adrenergic receptor agonist, with a half-life of 6 to 24 hours. Onset of action is within 1 hour, with peak effects at 2 to 4 hours. At least 50% is excreted unchanged in the urine. Although it is known to stimulate receptors on the presynaptic terminals of noradrenergic neurons with a resultant decrease in NE release, the actual mechanism of sedation is not clear. Side effects include hypotension, bradycardia, irritability, anticholinergic effects (eg, dry mouth), and REM suppression. With abrupt discontinuation, rebound hypertension and REM rebound can occur. Although not used as a hypnotic in adults, clonidine is widely used for sedation in pediatrics for patients with sleep disturbances associated with neuro developmental disorders or ADHD. There is no manufacturer-recommended hypnotic dose but, in practice, the starting dose is usually 50 μg, increased in 50-μg increments [4,46].

Benzodiazepines

Benzodiazepines hypnotics have been used extensively in adults with insomnia. The mechanism of action is based on activation of the GABA receptor [47]. Benzodiazepines may have muscle relaxing properties and should be avoided in children with suspected OSA syndrome. On a polysomnogram, benzodiazepines may alter the normal sleep stages referred to as sleep architecture. There can be drug related artifacts such as atypical sleep spindles and suppression of slow wave sleep. Benzodiazepine hypnotics are not commonly used for children with sleep disorders. An important exception is clonazepam [48]. Clonazepam is rapidly and completely absorbed after oral administration. The bioavailability is about 90%. Maximum plasma concentrations are reached within 1 to 4 hours after oral administration. The half-life of clonazepam is typically 30 to 40 hours. Clonazepam can be used to prevent parasomnias associated with partial arousals such as sleep terrors or sleep walking. These parasomnias may decrease as the child gets older. When parasomnias are very frequent and disturbing to the patient and family, a low dose of clonazepam at 0.25 to 0.5 mg may be helpful. Clonazepam may increase the arousal threshold allowing the child to sleep without interruption. Clonazepam is available in thin wafers that dissolve on the tongue and therefore obviating the need for the child to swallow a pill.

Nonbenzodiazepine Hypnotics

There are 3 nonbenzodiazepine hypnotics (perhaps a more accurate term is selective benzodiazepine receptor agonists) currently available in the United States: zolpidem (both immediate release and extended release), eszopiclone, and zaleplon [49,50]. Their use in children is considered "off-label," and therefore no official dosing guidelines are available. None of these medications are available in liquid form, which makes them difficult to administer to small children. They arguably offer some advantages compared to older (nonselective) benzodiazepine hypnotics. These newer medications preserve the overall sleep architecture. At the recommended doses, they do not typically have the insomnia rebound effects experienced with benzodiazepine hypnotics when they are abruptly stopped.

The standard adult dose of immediate release zolpidem and zaleplon is 10 mg. They both have a rapid onset of action and shorten sleep latency. Zolpidem has a half-life of 2.5 hours, and zaleplon has a half-life of 1 hour. This difference in duration is clinically important. Zolpidem may help improve both sleep onset and to some degree sleep maintenance insomnia symptoms. Zaleplon typically only improves the sleep onset insomnia and is not expected to significantly increase the total sleep time. Zaleplon's shorter half-life may allow it to be administered after sleep disruption in some situations to help the patient to return to sleep, but this practice has not been studied in children [51].

Zolpidem, both in the immediate release and extended release forms, is widely prescribed for adults with insomnia. Although its use in children is off-label, some limited data are available. Blumer and colleagues studied the pharmacokinetic profile of zolpidem in children [52]. In this study of pharmacokinetics, zolpidem was assessed in an open-label protocol in children with insomnia. Twenty-one children were divided evenly into 3 groups: 2 to 6, above 6 to 12, and above 12 to 18 years. Overall, the authors concluded zolpidem was well tolerated, and a pediatric dose of 0.25 mg/kg was recommended for future efficacy studies with a maximum dose of 20 mg.

The standard adult dose of immediate release of zolpidem is 10 mg, and the extended release dose is 12.5 mg. The standard adult dose may be prescribed to older children who can swallow the pill. It is not absolutely necessary to lower the dose because these medications have short half-lives and minimal side effects. Clearance of zolpidem in children is 3 times higher than in young adults and is lower in elderly adults [49]. A 5 mg size of immediate release zolpidem and 6.25 mg of extended release are available and intended for use in the elderly or patients with decreased hepatic clearance. As described previously, in the authors' experience, giving a lower dosage to children may be either ineffective or results in frightening sleep epi phenomenon such as hypnagogic hallucinations. The medication is most effective when taken on an empty stomach.

An 8-week, multicenter, double-blind, placebo-controlled study of zolpidem in children with ADHD was published; it failed to find significant efficacy [53]. In this study in children 6 through 17 years of age, the dose of zolpidem was 0.25 mg/kg/d with a maximum of only 10 mg/d. The mean change in latency to persistent sleep did not differ significantly between zolpidem and placebo. Although there were no next-day residual effects associated with zolpidem, there were more complaints of dizziness, headache, and hallucinations with zolpidem [53]. Ten patients (7.4%) discontinued zolpidem because of adverse events. Of note, adverse events were reported in almost 50% of the placebo group. Possibly the lack of efficacy was because of dosage being too low given the faster clearance of zolpidem in children.

Eszolpiclone is a nonbenzodiazepine hypnotic that was more recently approved in the United States [54–56]. This medication has a longer half-life, 6 hours, than zolpidem and zaleplon. This may, theoretically, be helpful in children because they typically sleep longer than adults. To date, there are no published studies in children.

Prescription hypnotics do not have an FDA indication for adolescents younger than 18 years old. An "off-label" use as an adjunct to the behavioral modification of the circadian problem may be considered in certain clinical situations. Because these patients typically only have sleep onset insomnia without significant nocturnal disruption, a short acting hypnotic agent may be considered for a short period of time. Zaleplon, a nonbenzodiazepine hypnotic, may theoretically be used in adolescents with delayed sleep phase syndrome. Zaleplon has a short elimination half-life of approximately 1 hour. This short duration of action, unlike diphenhydramine, will minimize any next day sedation or risk of rebound insomnia. Rebound insomnia refers to an exacerbation of insomnia on abrupt cessation of a hypnotic. The degree of insomnia is more severe than the initial insomnia before starting hypnotics. Rebound insomnia is more typical of short acting benzodiazepine hypnotics such as triazolam. Gradual tapering may be helpful to avoid a significant rebound effect.

Neuroleptics

Neuroleptics such as risperidone aripiprazole and olanzapine are typically prescribed to treated psychiatric conditions. Their off-label use in children with psychiatric or developmental disorders is not uncommon [57–60]. Neuroleptics are also used off-label to treat insomnia in adults [61–63]. Given this situation, it is tempting to consider the use of neuroleptics in the treatment of sleep disorders such as insomnia in children. However, there are no published data on the use of neuroleptics in the treatment of otherwise healthy children with insomnia. Although these medications may facilitate sleep and have effects on sleep architecture such as increasing slow wave sleep, their routine use to treat sleep disorders in children is not recommended. In addition, excessive weight gain is a report side effect of some neuroleptics, which would exacerbate any sleep disordered breathing present in the child.

Narcolepsy

Successful treatment for narcolepsy needs to include both behavioral and pharmacological treatments. The situation is analogous to juvenile diabetes mellitus where a combination of diet with medication helps control the condition. With the discovery of a gene responsible for narcolepsy, novel potential therapeutic approaches may be discovered [64,65]. Absence of hypocretin in the spinal fluid is diagnostic for narcolepsy [66].

Drug therapy must take into account possible side effects, while being mindful that narcolepsy is a lifelong illness, and patients will have to receive medication for years. Tolerance or addiction may be seen with some compounds. Treatment of narcolepsy thus balances avoidance of side effects, including tolerance, with maintenance of an active life. Physicians need to monitor for the development of hypertension, abnormal liver function, depression, irritability, anorexia, insomnia, or psychosis associated with medications [67].

Given emerging evidence of its autoimmune underpinnings, there has been increased interest in early diagnosis of narcolepsy–cataplexy, which would allow for the possibility of immunomodulators that may reduce the destruction of hypocretin-producing hypothalamic neurons, and reduce or eliminate the burden of this disease. Case reports and series of steroids, plasmapheresis, and intravenous immunoglobulin therapy (IVIG) have shown limited or no success, though cataplexy or improved sleepiness has been reported with the latter treatment in some cases [68–73].

Pharmacotherapies targeted to treating daytime sleepiness and cataplexy are the mainstays of narcolepsy treatment. While more studies have been performed in adults, no double-blind, placebo-controlled trials of medication have been specifically conducted for children with narcolepsy. Nonetheless, as the disease commonly presents in childhood, useful drugs in younger population and the evidence as it stands are given.

Gamma Hydroxybutyrate/ Sodium Oxybate

Sodium oxybate (GHB) is the treatment of choice for narcolepsy with cataplexy and is FDA-approved for both the treatment of cataplexy and excessive daytime sleepiness (EDS). GHB is an endogenous central nervous system metabolite with highest concentrations in the hypothalamus and basal ganglia. It is considered a neuromodulator/neurotransmitter affecting dopamine, serotonin, gamma-aminobutyric acid, and endogenous opioids; it is also considered to be a GABA-B receptor agonist [1,74]. As a therapeutic agent in narcolepsy–cataplexy, its mechanisms of actions are incompletely understood, but clinically it has been shown to dramatically reduce cataplexy, as well as treat daytime sleepiness and improve sleep fragmentation/disturbed sleep typical of narcolepsy–cataplexy [75–78]. The improvement in cataplexy is much more rapid than the effect on daytime sleepiness, which may take up to 6 to 8 weeks. GHB has powerful central nervous system depressant effects, and it has been shown to increase slow wave sleep. It has a short half-life (90–120 minutes), so that the first dose is taken at bedtime, and a second dose is most commonly taken 2.5 to 4 hours later, though timing may vary between patients. The recommended starting dose in adults is 4.5 g/d divided into 2 equal doses of 2.25 g. Dosing may be gradually increased over 8 weeks or longer, with a typical adult dose goal of 6 to 9 g, which has been shown to be effective for improvements in EDS and nocturnal sleep [79]. Until the full alerting effects of GHB are fully manifested, other alerting agents may be used. Side effects include disorientation in the middle of the night, grogginess on awakening, enuresis, and nausea especially at initiation and at higher doses. Use of this medication also confers a significant sodium load, which may be limiting for those with fluid retention, congestive heart failure, or hypertension.

In a pediatric narcolepsy series reported from Stanford, 85% of children (similar rates for pre-, peri-, and postpubertal children) were treated with GHB with a reportedly high positive effect on daytime sleepiness, disturbed nighttime sleep, and cataplexy [80]. Irritability and nausea were commonly reported side effects, and the report found no impact of the use of GHB on the occurrence of subsequent puberty. The authors also reported that GHB alone, or in association with one other drug, modafinil, was sufficient treatment in half of prepubertal cases of narcolepsy-cataplexy [80].

Treatment of Daytime Sleepiness

Central nervous system stimulants have been the drugs most widely used in the treatment of narcolepsy, and amphetamines were first proposed in 1935 [81]. However, a number of side effects including irritability, anxiety, nervousness, headache, psychosis, tachycardia, hypertension, nocturnal sleep disturbances, tolerance, and drug dependence may arise. The use of methylphenidate was later encouraged because of a shorter half-life and lower incidence of similar side effects. Today, modafinil is considered first-line therapy for EDS associated with narcolepsy. The mechanism of this wake-promoting drug is unknown, but it is different from that of amphetamines and is hypothesized to work on hypothalamic wake-promoting circuits. The results of several multicenter trials have demonstrated improvements in objective measures of sleepiness and improved wakefulness in narcoleptic patients, and additive effects have been demonstrated when used with GHB [77,82,83]. Doses of 200 to 400 mg are typically used, with morning and noon-hour administration. Elimination half-life is 10 to 12 hours. Importantly, modafinil can reduce the effectiveness of oral contraceptives, and therefore patients should be advised to use additional forms of contraception. Abuse potential for this medication is low, and discontinuation of modafinil is not associated with rebound hypersomnolence; nor is there evidence of tolerance. Armodafinil is the R-enantiomer of modafinil with a longer duration of action, approved in 2007 for the treatment of EDS in narcolepsy. Armodafinil has been shown to improve EDS throughout the day in randomized double-blind, placebo-controlled trials, and improvements in multiple sleep latency test (MSLT) at doses of 150 to 250 mg. The MSLT is a series of 5 scheduled daytime naps, spaced 2 hours apart, to elicit standardized measures of daytime sleepiness. The use of armodafinil in children has not been recommended [84].

Modafinil has been reported in the treatment of EDS in narcoleptic children [85]. The possibility of significant drug reactions at high doses is a concern in children.

The toxicity of modafinil has been reviewed [86,87]. An adolescent attempted to commit suicide by ingesting 5000 mgs of modafinil. Approximately 2 hours following ingestion, the patient complained of headache, nausea, and abdominal pain. An electrocardiogram demonstrated prolonged QTc interval. Observation for 72 hours revealed 24 hours of inability to sleep, tachycardia, and dyskinesia. There was no deterioration of kidney or liver functions, and no change in complete blood count or blood pressure. The youngest unintentional modafinil ingestion was in a 1 year old [86].

Treatment of Cataplexy

GHB was originally FDA approved only for the treatment of cataplexy, and later the indication was expanded to include excessive sleepiness associated with narcolepsy. Before GHB was available, several other medications were found to be effective for cataplexy. Tricyclic antidepressants such as imipramine and clomipramine, which block presynaptic reuptake of catecholamines, were commonly used. However, anticholinergic side effects were also common. Selective serotonin reuptake inhibitors replaced tricyclics in popularity to treat cataplexy. Newer antidepressants with selective noradrenergic/serotonergic uptake inhibition remain good choices in adults, with respect to both side effect profile and efficacy for cataplexy. The most commonly used drug in this class is venlafaxine at typical doses of 75 to 150 mg once daily (as low as 37.5 mg in younger pediatric patients). Atomoxetine, a highly specific noradrenergic reuptake blocker, has also been effective for treatment of cataplexy as well as EDS in adults and children, and maybe useful in resistance cataplexy at doses of 18 to 100 mg in 1 or 2 divided doses [88].

Obstructive Sleep Apnea

The role of pharmaceuticals in the treatment of OSA has changed over time. In the past, oxygen and protriptyline (PROT) were advocated but were not considered mainline treatments [89]. Adenotonsillectomy and positive airway pressure therapy, CPAP, have been the mainstays of treatment. Newer concepts of possible inflammatory effects of OSA have led to exploration of new medications as treatment options [90–93]. While most children with OSA will respond clinically to surgery and CPAP, the possibility of residual symptoms or intolerance to the mainstream treatments requires us to seek other options. Recent studies indicate that obese children and adolescents with OSA were more likely to remain symptomatic despite adenotonsillectomy [94,95].

Pharmacologic agents such as PROT have been used in selected adult patients, but studies in children are lacking. A nonsedating tricyclic antidepressant, PROT, was initially found to improve OSA, by decreasing REM time [96]. As respiratory events tend to be worse during this stage of sleep and apneas tend to last the longest, oxygen saturation may improve with use of this medication, and thus PROT may theoretically prove most useful in those with events solely in or that significantly worsen in REM sleep [96,97]. However, severe anticholinergic side effects like dry mouth, constipation, urinary retention, and impotence occur in approximately 50% of patients taking this medication, with the last 2 side effects often limiting its use. Furthermore, the lack of controlled studies in children precludes its general use in this population.

Nasal steroids have been proposed as a treatment for OSA in children. Brouillette and colleagues proposed a 6-week course of a nasal glucocorticoid spray, fluticasone, would decrease the severity of OSA in children with adenotonsillar hypertrophy [98]. They conducted a randomized, triple-blind, placebo-controlled, parallel-group trial of nasal fluticasone versus placebo in children aged 1 to 10 years with OSA. Thirteen children received fluticasone and 12 received placebo. The mixed/obstructive apnea/hypopnea index decreased from 10.7 ± 2.6 (SE) to 5.8 ± 2.2 in the fluticasone group but increased from 10.9 ± 2.3 to 13.1 ± 3.6 in the placebo group. The frequencies of hemoglobin desaturation and respiratory movement/arousals also decreased more in the fluticasone group. Changes from baseline in tonsillar size, adenoidal size, and symptom score were not significantly different between groups. The authors concluded that nasal fluticasone decreased the frequency of mixed and obstructive apneas and hypopneas, suggesting that topical corticosteroids may be helpful in ameliorating pediatric OSA. However, despite the decrease in overall mixed/obstructive apnea/hypopnea index by almost 50%, the average index was still in the pathological range, and there was no improvement in the children's symptoms. The role of nasal steroids in the treatment of children with OSA is not entirely clear; however, further evidence supporting the use of the nasal steroids is emerging [99]. A 6-week treatment with intranasal budesonide effectively reduced the severity of mild OSA syndrome and the magnitude of the underlying adenoidal hypertrophy in double-blind, randomized, and crossover trial [93]. Steroids may play a temporizing role until surgery or CPAP is available.

More recently, the role of nasal steroids in conjunction with receptor antagonist montelukast was studied in children with residual OSA after adenotonsillectomy [92]. Residual SDB may be present in many children after surgery. In this study, children with residual SDB with apnea hypopnea index (AHI) greater than 1 were enrolled. Treatment with montelukast and intranasal budesonide aqueous solution was administered for a period of 12 weeks. Twenty-two children received treatment and were compared to 14 children with residual SDB who did not receive medication. The mean AHI after surgery was 3.9 ± 1.2/h, which improved to after treatment 0.3 ± 0.3/h. The arterial oxygen saturation nadir improved from 87.3% to 92.5%.

The role of a systemic inflammatory process in OSA is supported by findings of increased C-reactive protein levels in children with OSA. The authors suggested this may be a major determinant of increased risk for neurocognitive dysfunction [90]. This is further supported by a study showing corticosteroids reduced cellular proliferation and the production of pro-inflammatory cytokines in a tonsil/adenoid mixed-cell culture system [100]. The authors used whole tissue cell cultures of adenoids and tonsils from children with OSA to assess the inflammatory process. This same research group also found that using tonsillar tissue cell cultures and leukotriene antagonists such as montelukast reduced adenotonsillar cellular proliferation rates. The authors suggested that targeted pharmacologic disruption of the leukotriene pathways may provide nonsurgical alternatives for prevention and treatment OSA in children [101].

Although the use of medication to avoid surgery or CPAP for OSA is appealing in children, at this time there is insufficient clinical experience to recommend any medication as a long-term treatment. Reports of psychiatric adverse events have been reported in children using montelukast [102]. The possibility of medication adverse events must be weighed against the potential morbidity of surgery or difficulties with CPAP. Individual clinical decisions with close follow-up will have to be made in children who are CPAP intolerant or have residual symptoms of OSA despite surgery.

Restless Legs Syndrome/ Periodic Limb Movements in Sleep

RLS is an autosomal dominant chronic neurologic disorder [10]. It is characterized by leg discomfort that makes the patients wanting to move their legs. The leg discomfort may be hard to describe and in children may be characterized as "growing pains" [103–105]. The discomfort is relieved with movement and is more common in the evening. Periodic limb movements in sleep (PLMS) may occur alone without RLS. RLS/PLMS can result in significant daytime difficulty as a result of sleep disruption. RLS and PLMS are both associated with poor quality sleep. This effect on sleep may lead to daytime behavior that mimics ADHD [106–108].

Allen and colleagues have developed a theory for the pathophysiology of idiopathic RLS [109–113]. The pathophysiology of RLS has been associated with iron metabolism [108,111,114–118]. Patients have been found to improve with iron supplementation. Iron insufficiency in certain brain regions may occur in patients with RLS [111,112]. Iron is a co-factor for tyrosine hydroxylase in dopamine synthesis. Iron deficiency exacerbates RLS symptoms. Iron supplementation may be helpful in children with RLS [114]. Vitamin C may help improve iron absorption.

Carbidopa/Levodopa

Dopamine precursors and agonists have been effective in relieving both RLS and PLMS [119]. Levodopa (L-DOPA, LARODOPA, DOPAR, L-3, 4-dihydroxyphenylalanine), the metabolic precursor of dopamine, is used for treating Parkinson's disease. It is also used to treat RLS/PLM in sleep both in adults and pediatric population [120,121]. Levodopa in itself is largely inert. Its therapeutic as well as adverse effects result from the decarboxylation of levodopa to dopamine. In the brain, levodopa is converted to dopamine by decarboxylation. The dopamine produced is responsible for its therapeutic effects [17]. In modern practice, levodopa is almost always administered in combination with a peripherally acting inhibitor of aromatic L-amino acid decarboxylase such as carbidopa. In addition, dopamine released into the circulation by peripheral conversion of levodopa produces undesirable effects such as nausea. The main complication of levodopa therapy for RLS/PLM is the development of worsening symptoms during the afternoon or early evening, despite adequate control later at night. This phenomenon which has been termed "restless legs augmentation" may occur frequently sometimes within months after initiating therapy. Once augmentation has occurred, levodopa therapy should be discontinued, and a different agent should be used. Administering additional doses of levodopa earlier during the day usually results in further exacerbation of the augmentation phenomenon [107,122,123]. In addition to motor fluctuations and nausea, other adverse effects may be observed with levodopa therapy such as induction of hallucinations, confusion, and orthostatic hypotension. These other side effects are more typically seen in adult patients with Parkinson's disease using higher dosages than used in the treatment of PLMS and RLS. In the clinical practice of treating children with PLMS and RLS, nausea is by far the most common side effect. Sensitivity to side effects makes it necessary to initiate therapy at very low doses (one half of a 25/100 levodopa/carbidopa tablet daily) and increase as tolerated every few days. The therapeutic dose for relieve of PLMS and RLS symptoms will be lower than used in Parkinson's disease. The maximal dose is determined by side effects, but most adolescents require at least 75 mg carbidopa and up to 1.5 g of l-dopa [124].

Selective Dopamine Agonists

Selective dopamine agonists are potent treatments for periodic limb movements disorders (PLMD) and RLS. They tend to have less side effects than carbidopa/levodopa. Pramipexole, ropinirole, and pergolide are the most commonly used medication in this category [119]. Pramipexole and ropinirole were both FDA approved for the treatment of RLS in adults [125–127]. Selective dopaminergic agonists have similar side effects to carbidopa/levodopa but at a lower frequency. These agents are more potent and allow for lower dosages than with carbidopa/levodopa. Montplaisir and colleagues have found pramipexole to be effective in a double-blind, placebo-controlled study in adults [128]. The starting dose in adults in this study was 0.375 mg.

In children the lowest dose available is an empirical starting dose. Pramipexole is available in a 0.125 mg size tablet. This tablet is scored and can be halved if an even lower starting dosage is desired. There is a case report of an 11 years old girl with RLS and depressive symptoms that improved with 0.5 mg of ropinirole [129].

Regardless of which medication is used, it is important to make medication changes slowly because the symptoms of PLMS and RLS both seem to fluctuate independently of the medication. In addition, if the dosage is too high, significant side effects may occur. We advise parents to only adjust the medication once a week at most when they first start the medication. Once an effective dose is found, it does not typically have to be adjusted except to allow for the child's growth. In adults the dosage of RLS usually does not exceed 1.5 mg and is often effective at a much lower dose.

Parasomnias

There are no medications with a FDA indication for any of the 15 different parasomnias listed in the *International Classification of Sleep Disorders* [10]. Benzodiazepines, which have been used extensively in adults with insomnia, are the most commonly used agents for the off-label treatment of parasomnias. Benzodiazepines have been particularly useful for arousal parasomnias such as sleepwalking and Rapid Eye Movement sleep behavior disorder (RBD). The mechanism of action is based on activation of the GABA receptor complex [47]. Benzodiazepines may have muscle relaxing properties and should be used with caution if co-morbid sleep disordered breathing is suspected. On a polysomnogram, benzodiazepines may alter the normal sleep stages referred to as sleep architecture. There can be drug related artifacts such as atypical sleep spindles and suppression of slow wave sleep.

Among the benzodiazepine class, clonazepam is the most common medication used in the treatment of parasomnias [48,130,131]. The popularity of the clinical use of clonazepam in parasomnias may be because of familiarity with the drug along with the putative clinical efficacy. The exact mechanism of action is unknown. The principal mechanism of clonazepam seems to be enhancement of the activity of GABA complex, acting as an allosteric modulator of the major inhibitory neurotransmitter GABA A complex, which is a chloride channel. GABA independent mechanisms have been reported [132]. Clonazepam has also been reported to have antidopaminergic activity [133] and serotonergic properties [134,135]. Clonazepam specifically modulates the activity of thalamic reticular nucleus neurons, which may explain some of its anticonvulsant properties [136]. Clonazepam is rapidly and completely absorbed after oral administration. Onset of action is 20 to 60 minutes. The time to peak level is 1 to 3 hours. Duration of action is 6 to 8 hours in children and up to 12 hours in adults. The bioavailability is about 90%. Maximum plasma concentrations are reached within 1 to 4 hours after oral administration. The half-life of clonazepam is typically 30 to 40 hours. The half-life tends to be longer in adults compared with children. The metabolism is extensively hepatic and excreted in urine.

Benzodiazepines and Arousal Parasomnias

Clonazepam can be used to prevent parasomnias associated with partial arousals such as sleep terrors or sleepwalking. These parasomnias may decrease as the child gets older. When parasomnias are very frequent and disturbing to the patient and family, a low dose of clonazepam at 0.25 to 0.5 mg may be helpful. Clonazepam may increase the arousal threshold allowing the child to sleep without interruption. Clonazepam is available in thin wafers that dissolve on the tongue obviating the need for the child to swallow a pill.

Clonazepam is the drug of choice for arousal parasomnias such as sleep terrors and sleepwalking. For arousal parasomnias in children, most are managed with reassurance or timed awakening and making the environment safe for the child. The frequency of episodes tends to lessen with age. Studies for the pharmacologic treatment of parasomnias in children have been done with the use of imipramine and diazepam, but not clonazepam. There are very limited studies in children as most do not require pharmacological interventions. There has been a case report of a boy with Asperger's whose sleepwalking was successfully managed with melatonin [137]. For adults, treatment is recommended if the parasomnia is associated with injury or danger to the patient or others. Guilleminault et al looked at

84 children with sleep terrors with and without sleepwalking and found that 49 of these patients had sleep disordered breathing and with treatment, the parasomnias disappeared [138].

Clonazepam has been studied as pharmacotherapy for arousal parasomnias over the last 2 decades. It has predominantly been studied in adults and specifically in those who have had a sleep related injury. Schenck et al studied 100 patients who presented to their sleep center with nocturnal injuries and diagnosed them with polysomnography [139]. Of these patients, 54 were diagnosed with either sleep terrors or sleepwalking (age of onset ranging from 3 to 58 years old). Clonazepam was prescribed in 28 of these patients as well as 33 patients with RBD. Of the 61, 51 patients (83.6%) reportedly had significant improvement in sleep injury up to 6 years after starting treatment. Schenck and Mahowald went on to study a further 170 adults with sleep related injury between 1982 and 1994, of whom 69 had either sleepwalking or sleep terrors; other diagnoses include RBD, RLS, and chronic insomnia [140]. Of these patients, 146 (86%) had complete or near complete control of their symptoms. There have also been case reports of patients with behaviors such as driving and sleep violence who have been diagnosed with sleepwalking and have responded to clonazepam (Schenck and Mahawald) [140,141].

Benzodiazepines decrease sleep latency and episodes of wake after sleep onset. Clonazepam may therefore reduce arousability during slow wave sleep in arousal parasomnias [142]. In terms of dose, most studies have used doses ranging from 0.25 to 2 mg. Schenck and Mahowald started at 0.25 to 0.5 mg taken 1 to 2 hours before bedtime [140]. The dose was increased every few nights until symptoms were controlled or side effects occurred. Clonazepam is available in disintegrating wafers for children. Side effects reported with the use of clonazepam in this setting included daytime sleepiness (in morning) and memory dysfunction, as well as alopecia. The side effects resolve with a reduction of dose in most cases.

Pearls

1. Do not equate sedation with good quality sleep.
2. Adult dosing does not always apply to children; children may have faster hepatic clearance.
3. OSA may manifest as insomnia or parasomnias in children.
4. Behavioral treatment should be considered before initiating pharmacotherapy.

Conclusions

There is a great need for more information on the pharmacological management of sleep disorders in children. Pharmacological guidelines need to be developed specifically for sleep disorders in children. Ideally, these guidelines should be FDA approved for the specific sleep disorder and for the pediatric age range. Development of easy to swallow, chewable, or liquid forms of these medications are needed. Integration of behavioral and pharmacological treatments may yield better patient outcomes. This would require pediatricians to have a comprehensive understanding of clinical sleep disorders in children. Training programs should play lead roles in enhancing pediatricians' knowledge of the pharmacological treatment of sleep disorders in children.

References

1. Pelayo R, Dubik M. Pediatric sleep pharmacology. *Semin Pediatr Neurol*. 2008;15:79–90.
2. Pelayo R, Chen W, Monzon S, Guilleminault C. Pediatric sleep pharmacology: you want to give my kid sleeping pills? *Pediatr Clin North Am*. 2004;51:117–134.
3. Owens JA, Moturi S. Pharmacologic treatment of pediatric insomnia. *Child Adolesc Psychiatr Clin N Am*. 2009;18:1001–1016.
4. Schnoes CJ, Kuhn BR, Workman EF, Ellis CR. Pediatric prescribing practices for clonidine and other pharmacologic agents for children with sleep disturbance. *Clin Pediatr (Phila)*. 2006;45: 229–238.
5. Owens JA, Rosen CL, Mindell JA. Medication use in the treatment of pediatric insomnia: results of a survey of community-based pediatricians. *Pediatrics*. 2003;111:e628–e635.
6. Stojanovski SD, Rasu RS, Balkrishnan R, Nahata MC. Trends in medication prescribing for pediatric sleep difficulties in US outpatient settings. *Sleep*. 2007;30:1013–1017.
7. Blumer JL, Reed MD, Steinberg F, et al. Potential pharmacokinetic basis for zolpidem dosing in

children with sleep difficulties. *Clin Pharmacol Ther.* 2008 Apr;83:551–558. Epub 2007 Oct 24.

8. Zito JM, Safer DJ, dosReis S, Gardner JF, Boles M, Lynch F. Trends in the prescribing of psychotropic medications to preschoolers. *JAMA.* 2000;283:1025–1030.
9. Morgenthaler TI, Owens J, Alessi C, et al. Practice parameters for behavioral treatment of bedtime problems and night wakings in infants and young children. *Sleep.* 2006;29:1277–1281.
10. *International Classification of Sleep Disorders.* 2nd ed. Westchester, IL: American Academy of Sleep Medicine; 2005.
11. Morgenthaler T, Kramer M, Alessi C, et al. Practice parameters for the psychological and behavioral treatment of insomnia: an update. An american academy of sleep medicine report. *Sleep.* 2006;29:1415–1419.
12. Morgenthaler TI, Lee-Chiong T, Alessi C, et al. Practice parameters for the clinical evaluation and treatment of circadian rhythm sleep disorders. An American Academy of Sleep Medicine report. *Sleep.* 2007;30:1445–1459.
13. Wyatt JK. Delayed sleep phase syndrome: pathophysiology and treatment options. *Sleep.* 2004;27:1195–1203.
14. Chesson AL Jr, Littner M, Davila D, et al. Practice parameters for the use of light therapy in the treatment of sleep disorders. Standards of Practice Committee, American Academy of Sleep Medicine. *Sleep.* 1999;22:641–660.
15. Johnson MW, Suess PE, Griffiths RR. Ramelteon: a novel hypnotic lacking abuse liability and sedative adverse effects. *Arch Gen Psychiatry.* 2006; 63:1149–1157.
16. Stigler KA, Posey DJ, McDougle CJ. Ramelteon for insomnia in two youths with autistic disorder. *J Child Adolesc Psychopharmacol.* 2006;16: 631–636.
17. *Goodman and Gilman's the Pharmacologic Basis of Therapeutics.* 9th ed. New York, NY: Macmillan Publishing Co; 1996.
18. Kay GG. The effects of antihistamines on cognition and performance. *J Allergy Clin Immunol.* 2000;105:S622–S627.
19. Duke C, Rimsza M. Case 1 presentation of bizarre behaviors. *Pediatr Rev.* 1998;19:245–246.
20. Russo RM, Gururaj VJ, Allen JE. The effectiveness of diphenhydramine HCI in pediatric sleep disorders. *J Clin Pharmacol.* 1976;16:284–288.
21. Baker AM, Johnson DG, Levisky JA, et al. Fatal diphenhydramine intoxication in infants. *J Forensic Sci.* 2003;48:425–428.
22. Labeling of diphenhydramine-containing drug products for over-the- counter human use. Final rule. *Fed Regist.* 2002;67:72555–72559.
23. Bender BG, McCormick DR, Milgrom H. Children's school performance is not impaired by short-term administration of diphenhydramine or loratadine. *J Pediatr.* 2001;138:656–660.
24. Yanai K, Ryu JH, Watanabe T, et al. Histamine H1 receptor occupancy in human brains after single oral doses of histamine H1 antagonists measured by positron emission tomography. *Br J Pharmacol.* 1995;116:1649–1655.
25. Tashiro M, Mochizuki H, Iwabuchi K, et al. Roles of histamine in regulation of arousal and cognition: functional neuroimaging of histamine H1 receptors in human brain. *Life Sci.* 2002;72: 409–414.
26. Gengo F, Gabos C, Miller JK. The pharmacodynamics of diphenhydramine-induced drowsiness and changes in mental performance. *Clin Pharmacol Ther.* 1989;45:15–21.
27. Albert KS, Hallmark MR, Sakmar E, Weidler DJ, Wagner JG. Pharmacokinetics of diphenhydramine in man. *J Pharmacokinet Biopharm.* 1975;3: 159–170.
28. Merenstein D, Diener-West M, Halbower AC, Krist A, Rubin HR. The trial of infant response to diphenhydramine: the TIRED study—a randomized, controlled, patient-oriented trial. *Arch Pediatr Adolesc Med.* 2006;160:707–712.
29. Dinndorf PA, McCabe MA, Frierdich S. Risk of abuse of diphenhydramine in children and adolescents with chronic illnesses. *J Pediatr.* 1998; 133:293–295.
30. Nigro N, Eandi M. [Sleep: notes on pediatric pharmacotherapy (in the light of current knowledge of its principal characteristics)]. *Minerva Pediatr.* 1975;27:1999–2007.
31. Pershad J, Palmisano P, Nichols M. Chloral hydrate: the good and the bad. *Pediatr Emerg Care.* 1999;15:432–435.
32. Loewy J, Hallan C, Friedman E, Martinez C. Sleep/sedation in children undergoing EEG testing: a comparison of chloral hydrate and music therapy. *Am J Electroneurodiagnostic Technol.* 2006;46:343–355.
33. Haydon RC III. Are second-generation antihistamines appropriate for most children and adults? *Arch Otolaryngol Head Neck Surg.* 2001;127:1510–1513.
34. Meltzer EO. Comparative safety of H1 antihistamines. *Ann Allergy.* 1991;67:625–633.
35. Corey JP, Houser SM, Ng BA. Nasal congestion: a review of its etiology, evaluation, and treatment. *Ear Nose Throat J.* 2000;79:690–693, 6, 8 passim.
36. Touitou Y. Human aging and melatonin. Clinical relevance. *Exp Gerontol.* 2001;36:1083–1100.
37. Wagner J, Wagner ML, Hening WA. Beyond benzodiazepines: alternative pharmacologic agents for the treatment of insomnia. *Ann Pharmacother.* 1998;32:680–691.
38. Buscemi N, Vandermeer B, Hooton N, et al. Efficacy and safety of exogenous melatonin for secondary sleep disorders and sleep disorders accompanying sleep restriction: meta-analysis. *Bmj.* 2006;332:385–393.
39. Jan JE, Tai J, Hahn G, Rothstein RR. Melatonin replacement therapy in a child with a pineal tumor. *J Child Neurol.* 2001;16:139–140.
40. Smits MG, Nagtegaal EE, van der Heijden J, Coenen AM, Kerkhof GA. Melatonin for chronic sleep onset insomnia in children: a randomized

placebo-controlled trial. *J Child Neurol.* 2001; 16:86–92.
41. Weiss MD, Wasdell MB, Bomben MM, Rea KJ, Freeman RD. Sleep hygiene and melatonin treatment for children and adolescents with ADHD and initial insomnia. *J Am Acad Child Adolesc Psychiatry.* 2006;45:512–519.
42. Van der Heijden KB, Smits MG, Van Someren EJ, Ridderinkhof KR, Gunning WB. Effect of melatonin on sleep, behavior, and cognition in ADHD and chronic sleep onset insomnia. *J Am Acad Child Adolesc Psychiatry.* 2007;46:233–241.
43. Wasdell MB, Jan JE, Bomben MM, et al. A randomized, placebo-controlled trial of controlled release melatonin treatment of delayed sleep phase syndrome and impaired sleep maintenance in children with neurodevelopmental disabilities. *J Pineal Res.* 2008;44:57–64.
44. Wirojanan J, Jacquemont S, Diaz R, et al. The efficacy of melatonin for sleep problems in children with autism, fragile X syndrome, or autism and fragile X syndrome. *J Clin Sleep Med.* 2009;5:145–150.
45. Hoebert M, van der Heijden KB, van Geijlswijk IM, Smits MG. Long-term follow-up of melatonin treatment in children with ADHD and chronic sleep onset insomnia. *J Pineal Res.* 2009;47:1–7.
46. Ingrassia A, Turk J. The use of clonidine for severe and intractable sleep problems in children with neurodevelopmental disorders—a case series. *Eur Child Adolesc Psychiatry.* 2005;14:34–40.
47. Ashton H. Guidelines for the rational use of benzodiazepines. When and what to use. *Drugs.* 1994;48:25–40.
48. Wills L, Garcia J. Parasomnias: epidemiology and management. *CNS Drugs.* 2002;16:803–810.
49. Salva P, Costa J. Clinical pharmacokinetics and pharmacodynamics of zolpidem. Therapeutic implications. *Clin Pharmacokinet.* 1995;29:142–153.
50. Weitzel KW, Wickman JM, Augustin SG, Strom JG. Zaleplon: a pyrazolopyrimidine sedative-hypnotic agent for the treatment of insomnia. *Clin Ther.* 2000;22:1254–1267.
51. Zammit GK, Corser B, Doghramji K, et al. Sleep and residual sedation after administration of zaleplon, zolpidem, and placebo during experimental middle-of-the-night awakening. *J Clin Sleep Med.* 2006; 2:417–423.
52. Blumer JL, Reed MD, Steinberg F, et al. Potential pharmacokinetic basis for zolpidem dosing in children with sleep difficulties. *Clin Pharmacol Ther.* 2008;83:551–558.
53. Blumer JL, Findling RL, Shih WJ, Soubrane C, Reed MD. Controlled clinical trial of zolpidem for the treatment of insomnia associated with attention-deficit/ hyperactivity disorder in children 6 to 17 years of age. *Pediatrics.* 2009;123:e770–e776.
54. Najib J. Eszopiclone, a nonbenzodiazepine sedative-hypnotic agent for the treatment of transient and chronic insomnia. *Clin Ther.* 2006;28:491–516.
55. Roth T, Walsh JK, Krystal A, Wessel T, Roehrs TA. An evaluation of the efficacy and safety of eszopiclone over 12 months in patients with chronic primary insomnia. *Sleep Med.* 2005;6:487–495.
56. Walsh JK, Krystal AD, Amato DA, et al. Nightly treatment of primary insomnia with eszopiclone for six months: effect on sleep, quality of life, and work limitations. *Sleep.* 2007;30:959–968.
57. Masi G, Cosenza A, Millepiedi S, Muratori F, Pari C, Salvadori F. Aripiprazole monotherapy in children and young adolescents with pervasive developmental disorders: a retrospective study. *CNS Drugs.* 2009;23:511–521.
58. Valicenti-McDermott MR, Demb H. Clinical effects and adverse reactions of off-label use of aripiprazole in children and adolescents with developmental disabilities. *J Child Adolesc Psychopharmacol.* 2006;16:549–560.
59. Harrison-Woolrych M, Garcia-Quiroga J, Ashton J, Herbison P. Safety and usage of atypical antipsychotic medicines in children: a nationwide prospective cohort study. *Drug Saf.* 2007;30:569–579.
60. Capone GT, Goyal P, Grados M, Smith B, Kammann H. Risperidone use in children with down syndrome, severe intellectual disability, and comorbid autistic spectrum disorders: a naturalistic study. *J Dev Behav Pediatr.* 2008;29:106–116.
61. Sokolski KN, Brown BJ. Quetiapine for insomnia associated with refractory depression exacerbated by phenelzine. *Ann Pharmacother.* 2006;40:567–570.
62. Juri C, Chana P, Tapia J, Kunstmann C, Parrao T. Quetiapine for insomnia in Parkinson disease: results from an open-label trial. *Clin Neuropharmacol.* 2005;28:185–187.
63. Doan RJ. Risperidone for insomnia in PDDs. *Can J Psychiatry.* 1998;43:1050–1051.
64. Taheri S, Zeitzer JM, Mignot E. The role of hypocretins (orexins) in sleep regulation and narcolepsy. *Annu Rev Neurosci.* 2002;25:283–313.
65. Ripley B, Overeem S, Fujiki N, et al. CSF hypocretin/orexin levels in narcolepsy and other neurological conditions. *Neurology.* 2001;57: 2253–2258.
66. Mignot E, Lammers GJ, Ripley B, et al. The role of cerebrospinal fluid hypocretin measurement in the diagnosis of narcolepsy and other hypersomnias. *Arch Neurol.* 2002;59:1553–1562.
67. Guilleminault C, Pelayo R. Narcolepsy in children: a practical guide to its diagnosis, treatment and follow-up. *Paediatr Drugs.* 2000;2:1–9.
68. Lecendreux M, Maret S, Bassetti C, Mouren MC, Tafti M. Clinical efficacy of high-dose intravenous immunoglobulins near the onset of narcolepsy in a 10-year-old boy. *J Sleep Res.* 2003;12:347–348.
69. Dauvilliers Y, Carlander B, Rivier F, Touchon J, Tafti M. Successful management of cataplexy with intravenous immunoglobulins at narcolepsy onset. *Ann Neurol.* 2004;56:905–908.
70. Dauvilliers Y. Follow-up of four narcolepsy patients treated with intravenous immunoglobulins. *Ann Neurol.* 2006;60:153.
71. Fronczek R, Verschuuren J, Lammers GJ. Response to intravenous immunoglobulins and placebo in a patient with narcolepsy with cataplexy. *J Neurol.* 2007;254:1607–1608.
72. Plazzi G, Poli F, Franceschini C, et al. Intravenous high-dose immunoglobulin treatment in recent

onset childhood narcolepsy with cataplexy. *J Neurol.* 2008;255:1549–1554.
73. Dauvilliers Y, Abril B, Mas E, Michel F, Tafti M. Normalization of hypocretin-1 in narcolepsy after intravenous immunoglobulin treatment. *Neurology.* 2009;73:1333–1334.
74. Lammers GJ, Bassetti C, Billiard M, et al. Sodium oxybate is an effective and safe treatment for narcolepsy. *Sleep Med.* 2010;11:105–106; author reply 6–8.
75. Lammers GJ, Arends J, Declerck AC, Ferrari MD, Schouwink G, Troost J. Gammahydroxybutyrate and narcolepsy: a double-blind, placebo-controlled study. *Sleep.* 1993;16:216–220.
76. U.S. Xyrem Multicenter Study Group. Sodium oxybate demonstrates long-term efficacy for the treatment of cataplexy in patients with narcolepsy. *Sleep Med.* 2004;5:119–123.
77. Black J, Houghton WC. Sodium oxybate improves excessive daytime sleepiness in narcolepsy. *Sleep.* 2006;29:939–946.
78. A randomized, double blind, placebo-controlled multicenter trial comparing the effects of three doses of orally administered sodium oxybate with placebo for the treatment of narcolepsy. *Sleep.* 2002;25:42–49.
79. Scharf MB, Lai AA, Branigan B, Stover R, Berkowitz DB. Pharmacokinetics of gammahydroxybutyrate (GHB) in narcoleptic patients. *Sleep.* 1998;21:507–514.
80. Aran A E, E, Lin, Ling. Clinical Aspects and management issues in childhood narcolepsy-cataplexy. *Sleep.* 2010: In press.
81. Littner M, Johnson SF, McCall WV, et al. Practice parameters for the treatment of narcolepsy: an update for 2000. *Sleep.* 2001;24:451–466.
82. Randomized trial of modafinil as a treatment for the excessive daytime somnolence of narcolepsy: US Modafinil in Narcolepsy Multicenter Study Group. *Neurology.* 2000;54:1166–1175.
83. Broughton RJ, Fleming JA, George CF, et al. Randomized, double-blind, placebo-controlled crossover trial of modafinil in the treatment of excessive daytime sleepiness in narcolepsy. *Neurology.* 1997;49:444–451.
84. Lankford DA. Armodafinil: a new treatment for excessive sleepiness. *Expert Opin Investig Drugs.* 2008;17:565–573.
85. Ivanenko A, Tauman R, Gozal D. Modafinil in the treatment of excessive daytime sleepiness in children. *Sleep Med.* 2003;4:579–582.
86. Spiller HA, Borys D, Griffith JR, et al. Toxicity from modafinil ingestion. *Clin Toxicol (Phila).* 2009;47:153–156.
87. Neuman G, Shehadeh N, Pillar G. Unsuccessful suicide attempt of a 15 year old adolescent with ingestion of 5000 mg modafinil. *J Clin Sleep Med.* 2009;5:372–373.
88. Billiard M. Narcolepsy: current treatment options and future approaches. *Neuropsychiatr Dis Treat.* 2008;4:557–566.
89. Marcus CL, Carroll JL, Bamford O, Pyzik P, Loughlin GM. Supplemental oxygen during sleep in children with sleep-disordered breathing. *Am J Respir Crit Care Med.* 1995;152:1297–1301.
90. Gozal D, Crabtree VM, Sans Capdevila O, Witcher LA, Kheirandish-Gozal L. C-reactive protein, obstructive sleep apnea, and cognitive dysfunction in school-aged children. *Am J Respir Crit Care Med.* 2007;176:188–193.
91. Gozal D, Kheirandish L. Oxidant stress and inflammation in the snoring child: Confluent pathways to upper airway pathogenesis and end-organ morbidity. *Sleep Med. Rev.* 2006;10:83–96.
92. Kheirandish L, Goldbart AD, Gozal D. Intranasal steroids and oral leukotriene modifier therapy in residual sleep-disordered breathing after tonsillectomy and adenoidectomy in children. *Pediatrics.* 2006;117:e61–e66.
93. Kheirandish-Gozal L, Gozal D. Intranasal budesonide treatment for children with mild obstructive sleep apnea syndrome. *Pediatrics.* 2008;122:e149–e155.
94. Gozal D, Kheirandish-Gozal L. Obesity and excessive daytime sleepiness in prepubertal children with obstructive sleep apnea. *Pediatrics.* 2009;123:13–18.
95. Dayyat E, Kheirandish-Gozal L, Sans Capdevila O, Maarafeya MM, Gozal D. Obstructive sleep apnea in children: relative contributions of body mass index and adenotonsillar hypertrophy. *Chest.* 2009;136:137–144.
96. Hudgel DW, Thanakitcharu S. Pharmacologic treatment of sleep-disordered breathing. *Am J Respir Crit Care Med.* 1998;158:691–699.
97. Thornton WK, Roberts DH. Nonsurgical management of the obstructive sleep apnea patient. *J Oral Maxillofac Surg.* 1996;54:1103–1108.
98. Brouillette RT, Manoukian JJ, Ducharme FM, et al. Efficacy of fluticasone nasal spray for pediatric obstructive sleep apnea. *J Pediatr.* 2001;138: 838–844.
99. Marcus CL. Nasal steroids as treatment for obstructive sleep apnea: don't throw away the scalpel yet. *J Pediatr.* 2001;138:795–797.
100. Kheirandish-Gozal L, Serpero LD, Dayyat E, et al. Corticosteroids suppress in vitro tonsillar proliferation in children with obstructive sleep apnoea. *Eur Respir J.* 2009;33:1077–1084.
101. Dayyat E, Serpero LD, Kheirandish-Gozal L, et al. Leukotriene pathways and in vitro adenotonsillar cell proliferation in children with obstructive sleep apnea. *Chest.* 2009;135:1142–1149.
102. Wallerstedt SM, Brunlof G, Sundstrom A, Eriksson AL. Montelukast and psychiatric disorders in children. *Pharmacoepidemiol Drug Saf.* 2009;18:858–864.
103. Picchietti D, Allen RP, Walters AS, Davidson JE, Myers A, Ferini-Strambi L. Restless legs syndrome: prevalence and impact in children and adolescents–the Peds REST study. *Pediatrics.* 2007;120:253–266.
104. Picchietti DL, Stevens HE. Early manifestations of restless legs syndrome in childhood and adolescence. *Sleep Med.* 2008;9:770–781.
105. Mohri I, Kato-Nishimura K, Tachibana N, Ozono K, Taniike M. Restless legs syndrome (RLS): an

unrecognized cause for bedtime problems and insomnia in children. *Sleep Med.* 2008;9:701–702.
106. Picchietti DL, Underwood DJ, Farris WA, et al. Further studies on periodic limb movement disorder and restless legs syndrome in children with attention-deficit hyperactivity disorder. *Mov Disord.* 1999;14:1000–1007.
107. Hening W, Allen R, Earley C, Kushida C, Picchietti D, Silber M. The treatment of restless legs syndrome and periodic limb movement disorder. An American Academy of Sleep Medicine Review. *Sleep*. 1999;22:970–999.
108. Picchietti D. Is iron deficiency an underlying cause of pediatric restless legs syndrome and of attention-deficit/hyperactivity disorder? *Sleep Med.* 2007;8:693–694.
109. Allen RP, Earley CJ. Restless legs syndrome: a review of clinical and pathophysiologic features. *J Clin Neurophysiol.* 2001;18:128–147.
110. Earley CJ, Hyland K, Allen RP. CSF dopamine, serotonin, and biopterin metabolites in patients with restless legs syndrome. *Mov Disord.* 2001 16:144–149.
111. Allen RP, Barker PB, Wehrl F, Song HK, Earley CJ. MRI measurement of brain iron in patients with restless legs syndrome. *Neurology*. 2001;56: 263–265.
112. Earley CJ, Connor JR, Beard JL, Malecki EA, Epstein DK, Allen RP. Abnormalities in CSF concentrations of ferritin and transferrin in restless legs syndrome. *Neurology*. 2000;54:1698–1700.
113. Allen RP, Mignot E, Ripley B, Nishino S, Earley CJ. Increased CSF hypocretin-1 (orexin-A) in restless legs syndrome. *Neurology*. 2002;59:639–641.
114. Patrick LR. Restless legs syndrome: pathophysiology and the role of iron and folate. *Altern Med Rev*. 2007;12:101–112.
115. Konofal E, Cortese S, Marchand M, Mouren MC, Arnulf I, Lecendreux M. Impact of restless legs syndrome and iron deficiency on attention-deficit/hyperactivity disorder in children. *Sleep Med.* 2007;8:711–715.
116. Dosman CF, Brian JA, Drmic IE, et al. Children with autism: effect of iron supplementation on sleep and ferritin. *Pediatr Neurol.* 2007;36:152–158.
117. Beard JL. Iron status and periodic limb movements of sleep in children: a causal relationship? *Sleep Med.* 2004;5:89–90.
118. Simakajornboon N, Gozal D, Vlasic V, Mack C, Sharon D, McGinley BM. Periodic limb movements in sleep and iron status in children. *Sleep*. 2003;26:735–738.
119. Littner MR, Kushida C, Anderson WM, et al. Practice parameters for the dopaminergic treatment of restless legs syndrome and periodic limb movement disorder. *Sleep*. 2004;27:557–559.
120. Chesson AL Jr, Wise M, Davila D, et al. Practice parameters for the treatment of restless legs syndrome and periodic limb movement disorder. An American Academy of Sleep Medicine Report. Standards of Practice Committee of the American Academy of Sleep Medicine. *Sleep*. 1999;22: 961–968.
121. Walters AS, Mandelbaum DE, Lewin DS, Kugler S, England SJ, Miller M. Dopaminergic therapy in children with restless legs/periodic limb movements in sleep and ADHD. Dopaminergic Therapy Study Group. *Pediatr Neurol.* 2000;22: 182–186.
122. Earley CJ, Allen RP. Pergolide and carbidopa/levodopa treatment of the restless legs syndrome and periodic leg movements in sleep in a consecutive series of patients. *Sleep*. 1996;19:801–810.
123. Allen RP, Earley CJ. Augmentation of the restless legs syndrome with carbidopa/levodopa. *Sleep*. 1996; 19:205–213.
124. Burg FD, Ingelfinger JR, Polin R, Gershon A. *Gellis and Kagan`s Current Pediatric Therapy*. 17th ed. Orlando, FL: WB Saunders Company; 2002.
125. Oertel WH, Stiasny-Kolster K, Bergtholdt B, et al. Efficacy of pramipexole in restless legs syndrome: a six-week, multicenter, randomized, double-blind study (effect-RLS study). *Mov Disord.* 2007;22:213–219.
126. Allen RP, Ritchie SY. Clinical efficacy of ropinirole for restless legs syndrome is not affected by age at symptom onset. *Sleep Med.* 2008;9:899–902.
127. Quilici S, Abrams KR, Nicolas A, et al. Meta-analysis of the efficacy and tolerability of pramipexole versus ropinirole in the treatment of restless legs syndrome. *Sleep Med.* 2008;9:715–726.
128. Montplaisir J, Nicolas A, Denesle R, Gomez-Mancilla B. Restless legs syndrome improved by pramipexole: a double-blind randomized trial. *Neurology*. 1999;52:938–943.
129. Cortese S, Konofal E, Lecendreux M. Effectiveness of ropinirole for RLS and depressive symptoms in an 11-year-old girl. *Sleep Med.* 2009;10:259–261.
130. Mahowald MW, Schenck CH, Bornemann MA. Pathophysiologic mechanisms in REM sleep behavior disorder. *Curr Neurol Neurosci Rep.* 2007;7:167–172.
131. Schenck CH, Arnulf I, Mahowald MW. Sleep and sex: what can go wrong? A review of the literature on sleep related disorders and abnormal sexual behaviors and experiences. *Sleep*. 2007;30: 683–702.
132. Paul V, Krishnamoorthy MS. The antimyoclonic action of clonazepam through a GABA—independent mechanism. *Indian J Physiol Pharmacol.* 1989;33: 243–246.
133. Tenn CC, Niles LP. Mechanisms underlying the antidopaminergic effect of clonazepam and melatonin in striatum. *Neuropharmacology*. 1997;36: 1659–1663.
134. Jenner P, Pratt JA, Marsden CD. Mechanism of action of clonazepam in myoclonus in relation to effects on GABA and 5-HT. *Adv Neurol.* 1986;43:629–643.
135. Chadwick D, Hallett M, Harris R, Jenner P, Reynolds EH, Marsden CD. Clinical, biochemical, and physiological features distinguishing myoclonus responsive to 5-hydroxytryptophan, tryptophan with a monoamine oxidase inhibitor, and clonazepam. *Brain*. 1977;100:455–487.
136. Sohal VS, Keist R, Rudolph U, Huguenard JR. Dynamic GABA(A) receptor subtype-specific

modulation of the synchrony and duration of thalamic oscillations. *J Neurosci.* 2003;23: 3649–3657.
137. Jan JE, Freeman RD, Wasdell MB, Bomben MM. A child with severe night terrors and sleep-walking responds to melatonin therapy. *Dev Med Child Neurol.* 2004;46:789.
138. Guilleminault C, Palombini L, Pelayo R, Chervin RD. Sleepwalking and sleep terrors in prepubertal children: what triggers them? *Pediatrics.* 2003;111:e17–e25.
139. Schenck CH, Milner DM, Hurwitz TD, Bundlie SR, Mahowald MW. A polysomnographic and clinical report on sleep-related injury in 100 adult patients. *Am J Psychiatry.* 1989;146:1166–1173.
140. Schenck CH, Mahowald MW. Long-term, nightly benzodiazepine treatment of injurious parasomnias and other disorders of disrupted nocturnal sleep in 170 adults. *Am J Med.* 1996;100: 333–337.
141. Schenck CH, Mahowald MW. Two cases of premenstrual sleep terrors and injurious sleep-walking. *J Psychosom Obstet Gynaecol.* 1995;16: 79–84.
142. Remulla A, Guilleminault C. Somnambulism (sleepwalking). *Expert Opin Pharmacother.* 2004;5:2069–2074.

CHAPTER 21

Sleep and Headaches

Martina Vendrame and Sanjeev V. Kothare

Introduction

Although there is accumulating clinical evidence supporting the notion that sleep and headaches have an intimate association, the nature of this relationship appears complex and is yet not fully understood. It is generally observed that headaches may represent one of the symptoms of sleep disorders; on the other hand, disrupted sleep may be the consequence of a headache syndrome. Moreover, both sleep and headache disorders may share common anatomic and physiological substrates, and therefore, both may be the expression of common underlying pathogenic mechanisms (Table 21.1). Only the understanding of the pathophysiology of both conditions can elucidate this complex relationship and aid in a rational clinical and therapeutic approach.

In this chapter, we will present the available clinical observations associating different headache syndromes to sleep disorders, with attention to the scientific evidence explaining their shared pathophysiology. Current diagnostic tools to tackle both disorders will be illustrated, and present and future treatment strategies will be discussed (Clinical Pearls presented in Table 21.2).

Headache Syndromes and Their Relationship to Sleep

Headache Disorders Secondary to Disturbances of Sleep

Most headaches secondary to sleep disturbances are generally poorly defined and tend to be reported after extensive sleep disruption [1,2]. They occur more often on awakening, but are also described during nocturnal sleep periods [1,2]. Not only are patients affected by tension type of headache but also normal subjects suffer from a dull, frontal headache when they are deprived of sleep [2]. In patients with migraine, sleep deprivation poses as a known trigger, whereas sleep restoration resolves and prevents future attacks [3,4]. The association between sleep deprivation and/or poor sleep quality and headache has been recognized for centuries, but the mechanism by which one leads to the other is still unclear [5]. The early work by Paiva and colleagues has helped understand which sleep disorders causing sleep disruption are linked to worsening of headache syndromes [6,7]. Not only can sleep-disordered breathing (SDB), such as obstructive sleep apnea (OSA), but also periodic limb movement of sleep (PLMS), psychophysiologic insomnia, and fibromyalgia may be seen associated in patients with different headache syndromes [6,7].

Headaches in Sleep Disordered Breathing

In both adult and the pediatric patients with OSA, several reports have shown that early morning headaches are a common complaint, and headache itself may be the presenting feature of OSA [6–11]. The prevalence of OSA among groups of headache patients with headache has been reported to be between 54% and 89% [8,11].

Patients with nocturnal respiratory failure and chronic hypoxemia secondary to OSA report morning headaches, and they are generally alleviated with proper nocturnal oxygenation with

Table 21.1 Headache disorders related to sleep disturbances in childhood

1. Headache disorders secondary to disturbances of sleep
   a. Headaches in sleep-disordered breathing
   b. Headaches in periodic limb movement of sleep
   c. Headaches related to insomnia and other chronic disorders disturbing sleep
2. Headache disorders "causing" disturbances of sleep
   a. Chronic migraine
   b. Chronic tension-type headache
3. Headache disorders intrinsically related to sleep physiology
   a. Migraine
      Migraine and narcolepsy
      Migraine and parasomnias
   b. Cluster headache
      Cluster headache and narcolepsy
   c. Chronic paroxysmal hemicrania

Table 21.2 Clinical pearls

When a child presents with headaches, both nocturnal/morning headaches as well as migraine-like headache:

1. Consider OSA as causing/contributing factor
2. Obtain appropriate history with the aid of sleep logs and questionnaires. However, headache may be the sole presenting symptom.
3. Actigraphy may be of aid in children suspected to have circadian rhythm disorders and in young children unable to tolerate PSG.
4. Consider PSG as the gold standard to rule in/out primary sleep disorders.
5. PLMS and insomnias may also be causing/contributing factors.

When a child is affected by chronic headache syndromes (ie, chronic migraine and chronic tension-type of headache):

1. Inquire about sleep quality (length of sleep, night awakenings, sleep fragmentation), possibly with the aid of sleep logs and questionnaires.
2. Underlying mood disorder, such as anxiety/depression, should be ruled out. Referral to a psychiatrist may be warranted.

In a child with known diagnosis of sleep disorders (ie, OSA, PLMS, narcolepsy, parasomnias):

1. Appropriate history should include questioning on headaches.
2. Migraine and CH may be coexisting disorders also in narcolepsy and parasomnias.

CH, cluster headache; OSA, obstructive sleep apnea; PLMS, periodic limb movement of sleep; PSG, polysomnography.

continuous positive airway pressure (CPAP) [8,12]. This evidence indicates that the onset of headache in patients with OSA may be related to direct physiologic and hemodynamic effects of hypoxia or hypercapnia. In support of this hypothesis, a direct correlation between headache frequency and SDB parameters measured with polysomnography (PSG) has been reported by Rains and colleagues [13]. Of the 826 patients seen at a sleep center, 35% complained of morning headaches that were found to be related to their elevated apnea-hypopnea index, lower oxygen saturation peaks, and number of arousals from sleep [13]. In another study by Goder and colleagues, 432 patients with sleep disorders (age range 18–86 years) and 30 healthy subjects (age range 24–55 years) were studied prospectively with PSG [9]. The reported frequency of past headaches and the frequency of morning headache in the sleep laboratory were significantly increased in patients with OSA compared with healthy subjects [9]. The occurrence of morning headache was associated with a decrease in total sleep time, sleep efficiency, and amount of rapid eye movement (REM) sleep and with an increase in the wake time during the preceding night [9].

The role of decreased cerebral vasoactivity in OSA has been indicated by recent studies examining the direct effects of recurring apneas on cerebral circulation and their consequences on cerebrovascular reactivity and compliance [14]. Furtner and colleagues found severe disturbances of cerebrovascular reactivity in OSA patients, including loss of vasoreactivity and increase of arterial stiffness, especially during periods of high density of apneas [14]. The authors suggest that such changes are likely to impair cerebral circulation and may be detrimental to the endothelium [14].

Few studies have reported a correlation between prevalence of OSA and specific types of headache [11,15,16]. A retrospective analysis of PSG findings in children with headache showed that 49% of subjects (44 out of 90) were affected by SDB; migraine headache and chronic migraine headache were more common in children with SDB than other types of headache, such as tension type [11]. In particular, the sleep of children with severe migraine was characterized by a shorter duration of sleep time and higher sleep latency when compared with children with milder migraine [11]. Moreover, chronic migraine was associated with more disrupted sleep and with higher arousal index than in children with acute migraine [11]. Similar studies in children have also been reported by others [15,16]. Specifically, Bruni and colleagues administered a questionnaire to 164 children with migraine and found a higher prevalence of SDB in comparison with children with tension-type headache [15]. Another questionnaire-based study on a nonclinical population of children and adolescents has shown that childhood migraneurs show a tendency toward eveningness [17]. The increased prevalence of SDB in children with headache and the observed concurrent poor sleep efficiency with higher sleep fragmentation strongly indicate that SDB may be responsible for sleep disruption, and in turn to the onset of different headache syndromes, perhaps more commonly migraine and tension-type headaches.

An important risk factor for SDB in children is obesity. Obesity in children, as well as in the adult population, is associated with increased risk for OSA and, in turn, may lead to increased risk of headache disorders [11,18]. Pathophysiological mechanisms contributing to the association of obesity-OSA-headaches may include adenotonsillar hypertrophy, increased critical airway closing pressure, and altered chest wall mechanics causing hypoventilation [18]. Moreover, high body mass index (BMI) and OSA are both associated with the metabolic syndrome, which includes several features such as hypertension, insulin resistance, dyslipidemia, and proinflammatory states [19]. In support of this paradigm, a recent study has demonstrated that children with headaches and higher BMIs had a higher risk for SDB than children with headaches with normal BMIs [11]. Control of the SDB and obesity resulted in better control of their headaches and improved sleep.

Headaches in Periodic Limb Movement of Sleep

Early reports in the adult population have observed a high prevalence of PLMS in patients with headache in comparison with the general population [6,7]. In one study, 2 of the 25 subjects presenting with headache had a de novo diagnosis of PLMS on their PSG [7]. However, in a later study, the same group of investigators showed that treatment of an identifiable sleep disorder led to either an improvement or resolution of their headaches, but patients with PLMS reported only a marginal to no improvement of their headaches, even after treatment of their PLMS [6].

In the recent study by Vendrame and colleagues, 9% (10 of 90) of the children complaining of headache were diagnosed with PLMS by PSG [11]. Of those 9 children, 8 had episodic migraine headache, 1 had tension-type headache, and 1 had chronic migraine [11]. PSG did not show a correlation between headache frequency and periodic limb movement index, although the small number of the subjects limited the analysis [11].

Overall, there is some evidence to an association of PLMS with headaches. It can be speculated that, similar to SDB, PLMS may disrupt sleep and contribute to worsening headaches, yet treatment of the PLMS with improved sleep fragmentation does not improve headache severity or frequency, thus indicating that alternate and as yet unknown mechanisms may be involved.

Headaches Related to Insomnia and Other Chronic Disorders Disturbing Sleep

Other sleep disorders have also been considered as potential contributors to headache onset. Among these, psychophysiologic insomnia, insomnia secondary to chronic substance abuse, and insomnia secondary to chronic conditions such as fibromyalgia and chronic fatigue syndrome have been considered as contributing or associated with higher frequency and intensity of headaches [6,7,20]. Mood disorders such as anxiety have been linked to hyperarousals and consequent disrupted sleep and insomnia in both clinical and animal studies [21].

Both fibromyalgia and chronic fatigue syndrome have been associated with disrupted sleep in adults as well as in children [22,23]. Fibromyalgia is characterized by widespread musculoskeletal pain in association with fatigue, irritable bowel syndrome, chronic headaches, and nonrefreshing sleep [22]. Central nervous system sensitization is a major pathophysiologic aspect of fibromyalgia, and various external stimuli such as trauma and stress may also contribute to its development in young and older children [22]. Similarly, chronic fatigue syndrome is characterized by intense fatigue, in association with asthenia and easily induced tiredness and chronic headaches that is not reversed after a night's sleep [23].

Headache Disorders Causing Disturbances of Sleep

In both adult and children, specific headache syndromes have been related to disturbances in sleep. These include chronic headache syndromes such as chronic migraine and chronic tension-type headache occurring predominantly in the daytime, but may also occur during sleep.

Chronic Migraine and Chronic Tension-Type Headache

Chronic tension-type headache is frequently associated with subjective sleep complaints and objective disturbances in sleep quality, night awakening, and daytime sleepiness [15,24,25]. Carotenuto and colleagues have shown that chronic headache disorders were a cumulative risk factor for hypersomnia in school-aged children (odds ratio 15.061) [24]. These types of chronic headaches are thought to lead to sleep disturbances similar to those in patients with chronic pain and depression [26]. These alterations in sleep physiology include decreases in total sleep time, sleep efficiency, and slow-wave sleep (SWS), and excessive awakenings and nocturnal movements [11,27]. The mechanism by which the headache disorder would "cause" the sleep disturbance in these chronic headache syndromes has been attributed to a possible underlying mood disorder, such as anxiety or depression [5,20,28]. To this effect, Sahota and colleagues have pointed out that when "an individual complains of long periods of sleep loss because of headache, it is well to consider anxiety or depression as the dominant aspect of the illness" [5].

Several population-based studies and clinical investigations have found high rates of comorbidity between mood disorders and chronic headache, specifically tension type [29,30]. In a clinical population of children with headaches, tension-type headache has been specifically linked to nocturnal bruxism [11]. Of interest is the observation that high prevalence of bruxism has also been reported in patients affected by mood disorders per se, suggesting that mood disorders, chronic headache (specifically tension type), and bruxism may often coexist [31,32].

Headache Disorders Intrinsically Related to Sleep Physiology

Migraine, cluster headache (CH), chronic paroxysmal hemicrania (CPH), and, in the adult population, hypnic headache (HH) represent a group of primary headache disorders that often occur during specific sleep stages and therefore seem to be intimately related to the physiology of sleep itself.

Migraine

Migraine headaches tend to occur during the second part of the night, but do not appear to have a fixed association with a particular sleep stage, as studies on patients monitored during nocturnal migraine attacks have shown that they may awaken with a migraine attack out of REM sleep, or that attacks may occur in SWS. The seminal report of Dexter and Weitzman documented nocturnal migraine attacks specifically out of REM sleep in 6 patients monitored with PSG

[33]. Other observations suggesting a relationship between SWS and REM stages and arousals with migraine, and the fact that migraine attacks can arise out of a dream, are in agreement with this early evidence [34,35]. Others have investigated PSG findings preceding migraine attacks and found a significant decrease in the number of arousals, a decrease in REM density, a significant decrease of beta power in the SWS, and a decrease of alpha power during the first REM period, suggesting a decrease in cortical activation during sleep preceding migraine attacks [36]. According to these authors and others, alterations in the function of aminergic or cholinergic brainstem nuclei may be the underlying pathogenic mechanism of migraine and sleep dysfunction [36,37]. Others have pointed out that migraine attacks tend to occur with a circadian pattern and, when nocturnal, they occur during early morning with peaks between 4 and 9 AM [38,39]. This observation, in addition to the fact that patients with migraine report symptoms of hypothalamic dysfunction (such as irritability, depression, hunger, and thirst) 24 hours before the attack, has lead to the hypothesis that migraine pathogenesis may be related to hypothalamic and adaptive homeostatic mechanisms [20,38,40–42].

Given the strong evidence on the intimate association between migraine and sleep physiology, it is not surprising that migraine has been intrinsically linked to the pathogenesis of certain sleep disorders.

Narcolepsy has been related to dysfunction of REM sleep, and its relation with migraine should be intuitively expected. Dahmen and colleagues accordingly showed the coexistence of migraine in patients with proven narcolepsy [43,44]. Migraine prevalence was 2-fold to 4-fold increased in the narcoleptic patients and the onset of narcolepsy symptoms was 12.3 ± 11.4 years before the onset of migraine symptoms [44].

Parasomnias have also been associated with migraine headaches. Barabas and colleagues found a high prevalence of somnambulism in 222 children with migraines in comparison with the general population [45]. The same authors postulate that the strength of association between somnambulism and migraine raises the possibility of considering somnambulism as a minor diagnostic critèrion in the clinical diagnosis of childhood migraine [45]. Similar findings have been reported by others [11,15,27]. The association between migraine and parasomnias may be related to serotonin abnormalities known to underlie both disorders [45].

Cluster Headache

CH has been described in children as young as 1 year of age [46]. CH attacks can occur daily, with predilection during nocturnal sleep, and in cluster periods of 1 to 2 months. There is substantial clinical evidence relating CH to sleep and the biological clock. CH attacks follow a strict circadian rhythm, occurring at the same time for each individual, and when nocturnal, tend to peak around 1 to 3 AM [20,47]. Old and recent observations agree on the occurrence of CH at the onset of the first REM sleep, about 90 minutes after sleep onset [33,48]. There is also a yearly/biennial cycling nature of CH, with higher frequencies during the summer and winter solstices and lower frequencies during winter equinoxes [20]. These features highly suggest an association between CH and hypothalamic dysfunction. In support to this notion is the fact that several alterations in hormonal secretions have been related to CH, and the evidence that lithium, its most effective treatment, selectively accumulates in the hypothalamus modifying serotonergic transmission and decreasing REM sleep [49–51]. Similar to migraine, CH has also been associated with narcolepsy; their shared pathogenic mechanisms have been proven by the genetic association between a polymorphism of hypocretin receptor 2 gene, part of the hypocretin/orexin system implicated in narcolepsy, and the risk of CH [52].

Chronic Paroxysmal Hemicrania

CPH shares clinical and pathophysiological features with CH. Together with CH, it is classified as part of the trigeminal autonomic cephalalgias, a group of primary headache syndromes all marked by headache and associated autonomic features [53]. CPH attacks localize to the oculotemporal area, are briefer than CH attacks, and occur in clusters of 10 to 20 per day [53]. CPH has been described at any age, with a mean age of onset of 34 years, and the youngest patient described being 6 years old [54,55].

Similar to CH, CPH attacks tend to occur during nocturnal sleep, and they also appear to be strongly associated with REM sleep [56].

Hypnic Headache

Although not described in the pediatric population, HH is the only primary headache syndrome strictly associated with sleep, and as such it may help elucidate the intrinsic relationship between headache and sleep [57]. Patients with HH experience attacks only during diurnal and nocturnal sleep, and often at the same time of the night [57–59]. Most of the studies using PSG on HH patients have shown that the attacks occur only during REM stage sleep [60–63], and only few studies reported the association with non-REM (NREM) sleep stages [64,65]. From the meta-analysis of 71 published cases of HH presented by Evers and Goadsby, it appears that most of the HH attacks emerge out of REM sleep and that the same patient will experience the recurrent attacks out of the same stage of sleep [59]. An interesting observation on PSG data in 2 patients suffering from nocturnal headache showed that there were increases and irregularities of arterial pressure before awakening with headache, and these changes began during NREM sleep and lasted during REM sleep preceding the awakening with headache [66]. These findings may suggest that the real onset of the headache may be during NREM sleep, and the awakening occurs out of REM sleep when the arousal pain threshold is lowered [66].

The fact that HH is seen only in the elderly suggests that changes in the physiology of sleep that occur with aging and specifically not present during childhood may be pivotal contributing factors to the pathogenesis of HH. With aging, shorter nocturnal sleep time and shorter SWS stage are seen [20]. Furthermore, a decrease in cell number in the suprachiasmatic nucleus (SCN) is also observed, and this may be responsible for the reduced secretion of melatonin, subsequent disruption in circadian rhythms and sleep-wake cycles, and predisposition to HH [20].

Pathophysiology to Explain Headache and Sleep Disorders

There are several cerebral centers with shared function between regulation of sleep and headache/pain control. These include (1) the hypothalamus; (2) the brainstem aminergic nuclei, including the nuclei of raphe and the locus coeruleus; and (3) the SCN-pineal-melatonin axis. These areas are anatomically and functionally interconnected. The brainstem aminergic nuclei are connected to the lateral hypothalamus and the basal forebrain; lesions in their connections cause sleepiness and coma [67]. Within the hypothalamus, the SCN responds to light-dark changes and regulates the secretion of melatonin from the pineal gland, constituting the anatomic and functional SCN-pineal-melatonin axis [68]. Direct and indirect clinical evidence suggests that their interplay underlines the observed chronobiological features of certain headache syndromes.

Hypothalamic Regulation of Sleep and Headache

In the anterior hypothalamus the ventro lateral preoptic (VPLO) nucleus is mainly active during sleep, and its damage produces insomnia [67]. The VPLO and the ascending arousal pathways reciprocally control each other, whereby activity from one site inhibits the other, with the so-called "flip-flop" switch that forms the basis of awake/sleep transitions [67]. The hypothalamic control of circadian rhythms relates to the function of the SCN, the "master clock" regulating the 24-hour circadian rhythms, which act via the hypothalamic supraventricular zone and the dorsomedian nucleus to control the VPLO [67,68].

Anatomical/physiological and clinical evidence implicates the hypothalamus to the pathogenesis of headache, especially to migraine and CH syndromes. The hypothalamus receives and sends inputs to the limbic system and visceral relay nuclei, contributing to the affective, vegetative, as well as gastrointestinal and autonomic symptoms seen in migraine headache [20]. Moreover, the hypothalamus may have a direct role in pain control: nociceptive fibers connect directly the hypothalamus to the spinal cord, and to opioidergic centers within the brainstem [20]. In CH, there is an alteration of the circadian secretory rhythm of several hormones, including prolactin, growth hormone, and thyrotropin, supporting the idea of periodic hypothalamic dysfunction during the clusters of headaches [49]. A recent study using positron emission tomography (PET) scanning in patients with CH has documented a marked activation of the antero-ventral hypothalamus during the attacks, providing direct evidence of the hypothalamic role in CH pathogenesis [69].

The Brain Stem Aminergic Nuclei: Regulation of Sleep and Headaches by the Serotonergic System

The nuclei of the dorsal raphe and the locus coeruleus are the main producers of serotonin and norepinephrine, and as such, they regulate not only sleep-wake states, but also nociceptive information and cerebral blood flow and blood brain barrier permeability, thereby contributing to headache pathogenesis. The serotonergic system is under the direct control of the SCN and demonstrates circadian rhythmicity, likely taking part in regulation of circadian rhythms.

There is plenty of anatomical/physiological and clinical evidence suggesting the role of serotonin in migraine pathogenesis. During a migraine attack, the urinary excretion of the main metabolite of serotonin, 5-hydroxy-indoleacetic acid, increases; pharmacologic depletion of serotonin triggers migraine attacks; conversely, rapid delivery of serotonin ablates migraine attacks. Moreover, the serotonin receptor agonists, so-called "triptans," have been proven to be effective medications in the treatment of migraine headaches. Interestingly, during REM sleep, serotonin is decreased, and this in part explains the association between REM sleep and migraine [34]. In support of this evidence, data from PET studies have revealed strong activation of these brainstem aminergic nuclei during and after a migraine attack [70].

Role of the SCN-Pineal-Melatonin Axis in Sleep and Headache

The secretion of melatonin from the pineal gland is dictated by inputs from the SCN, and its role in controlling circadian rhythms is well established [67,68]. A more recent notion relating melatonin to headache pathogenesis is supported by overwhelming physiological and clinical evidence. Melatonin has several actions on the central nervous system and is known to possess a strong analgesic action in headache [71,72]. Melatonin potentiates the inhibitory action of gamma-aminobutyric acid; it controls membrane calcium transmission modulating tone and vasoactivity of cerebral blood vessels; and it is also known to inhibit prostaglandin synthesis [72]. Clinical evidence has shown decreased urinary and plasma levels of melatonin during headaches in both migraine and CH patients [50,73,74]. In summary then, and as proof of principle, Leone and colleagues have reported the efficacy of melatonin therapy in the prophylaxis of CH and chronic migraine [75].

Diagnostic Tools Addressing Relationship Between Headache and Sleep

Sleep Logs and Sleep Questionnaire Studies

Sleep logs, sleepiness scales, and sleep questionnaires are screening tools to help in identifying and quantifying the degree of sleepiness [76]. Most of the sleep questionnaires have the advantage of providing a comprehensive screening including diverse aspects of not only sleep quality but also daily function of the child and possible comorbidities. They are economic and easy to obtain; but in the case of young children, are biased by parents' perception and therefore not always reliable [77]. Questionnaires have been used in several studies addressing the prevalence of sleep disorders in populations of children with headaches (see Table 21.3) [15,26,27,78,79]. As such, they have been proven useful for identifying possible treatable sleep disorders in children referred for evaluation of headaches. In some studies, questionnaires have been customized, for example, to screen for all precipitating factors for headaches. In the study by Spierings and colleagues, the questionnaire inquired about different precipitating and aggravating headache factors, such as (1) physical activity, (2) straining, (3) bending over, (4) stress/tension, (5) coughing/sneezing, (6) fatigue, (7) reading, (8) driving, (9) lack of sleep, (10) specific foods/drinks, (11) alcohol, (12) not eating on time, (13) smoke, (14) smell, (15) light, (16) noise, (17) menstruation, and (18) weather and was able to specifically identify lack of sleep as one of the major factors contributing to headache onset [79].

We can hence conclude that sleep logs, sleep scales, and questionnaires are important screening tools for the coexistence of sleep and headache problems, and, given their affordability and

Table 21.3 Studies addressing headache and sleep disorders in the pediatric population

Reference	Used tools and study design	Population studied	Study conclusions
[15]	Customized questionnaire	283 subjects with headache (164 with migraine and 119 with tension-type headache); results compared with healthy norms.	The group with migraine had more "disturbed sleep" with increased symptoms of SDB and parasomnias than the group with tension-type headache and norms.
[26]	Customized questionnaire	113 subjects with headache and 110 controls.	The group with headache took longer to fall asleep (31.4 vs 21.1 min) and longer to fall back asleep after waking up at night (28.5 vs 14.6 min).
[79]	Customized questionnaire (interviewed by phone) on headache precipitating factors.	55 subjects with headache (38 with migraine and 17 with tension-type headache).	The most common precipitating factors were stress/tension, not eating on time, fatigue, and lack of sleep.
[27]	(1) Children's Sleep Habits Questionnaire, (2) standardized headache questionnaire.	118 subjects with headache; results compared with published control norms.	Sleep disturbances were sleeping too little (42%), bruxism (29%), child cosleeping with parents (25%), and snoring (23%).
[78]	(1) Child Sleep Habits Questionnaire, (2) migraine information questionnaire, (3) Behavior Assessment System for Children (BASC-2) Parent Rating Scales.	51 subjects with migraine, who had at least 10 sibling without migraine.	Group with migraine had higher total sleep, sleep delay, and daytime sleepiness scores than controls. More severe migraines had higher total sleep and sleep duration scores than those with milder headaches. Higher total sleep scores predicted greater behavior problems.
[25]	Actigraphy and diaries. Behavior problems were assessed by parental reports.	28 subjects with headache and 108 controls.	The group with headache had poorer sleep quality and more excessive daytime sleepiness. They also had higher levels of internalizing behavior problems.
[82]	Actigraphy and diaries.	18 subjects with migraine and 17 controls.	The group with migraine had longer sleep onset latency. Nocturnal motor activity had the lowest values on the night preceding the attack.
[11]	PSG PSG results were correlated with headache type and severity, BMI.	90 subjects headache with migraine [60], chronic migraine [11], tension headache [6], and nonspecific headache [13];	SDB was more frequent in migraine (56.6%) and nonspecific headache (54%) vs chronic migraine (27%). In the group with nonspecific headache, children with SDB had higher BMI. Severe and chronic migraine were associated with shorter sleep time, longer sleep latency, and shorter rapid eye movement and slow-wave sleep.

SDB, sleep-disordered breathing; PSG, polysomnography; BMI, body mass index.

easiness in use, should be used routinely in both sleep and headache clinics. When they raise a suspicion for a sleep disorder or headache syndrome, further testing should be obtained.

Actigraphy Studies

Actigraphy is a method mostly used to study sleep-wake patterns and circadian rhythms by assessing activity, most commonly at the wrist or the ankle [80]. Although actigraphy is not as reliable as PSG for determining some sleep measurements, studies are in general agreement that actigraphy, with its ability to record continuously for long time periods, is more reliable than information provided by parental reports with sleep logs and questionnaires [77]. In addition, actigraphy has been useful in evaluating sleep in individuals who are less likely to tolerate PSG, such as infants and young children, or certain populations such as autism. Actigraphy has been found highly appropriate for examining the sleep variability (ie, night-to-night variability) in patients with insomnia and in the evaluation of circadian rhythm disorders [81]. Of interest, results of actigraphic recordings correlate well with measurements of melatonin and core body temperature rhythms [81]. Actigraphy has been used for the evaluation of sleep disturbances in children with headaches in few studies (see Table 21.3) [25,82]. In these studies, actigraphy provided data regarding the quality of sleep in terms of sleep duration and fragmentation, and correlated well with questionnaire information on daytime sleepiness and daily function [25,82].

Actigraphy may thus become of important use in the evaluation of those children with headache complaints who (1) cannot tolerate PSG, for example, young age, or special populations such as in those with autism; or (2) have suspected comorbidities of insomnia, or other medical conditions causing sleep fragmentation and poor sleep; or (3) may be affected by a circadian rhythm disorder.

Polysomnography

PSG represents the gold standard for the diagnosis of most sleep disorders in both adults and children. Although usually limited to the length of 1 night, it is a reliable tool providing quantifiable and reproducible data in conclusively diagnosing SDB [76]. Very few studies in children and adults with sleep disorders and headache have used PSG with consistent results (see Table 21.3) [6–9,11,36]. In some early studies, PSG was employed for gathering direct information on the physiology of sleep during nocturnal headache attacks on a research basis [33,34].

In approaching a child with headache and suspected to have a sleep disorder, PSG should serve as a confirmatory tool for diagnosing SDB, PLMS, degree of nocturnal hypoxemia and hypercarbia, and sleep fragmentation, after appropriate screening tools such as sleep logs, sleepiness scales, and sleep questionnaires have been undertaken. However, it should be mentioned that PSG should also be considered in appropriate cases even with negative screening questionnaires, because the presence of disturbed sleep may not be obvious from the parent's history. When a child suffers from nocturnal headache attacks, PSG may help characterizing the nature of the headache disorder in specific sleep stages, confirming specific sleep disorders such as SDB, and tailoring adequate intervention for both the sleep disorder and the headache syndrome.

Treatment Strategies to Improve Both

The optimal treatment approach of a child with headaches and a sleep disturbance would be to comprehensively treat both disorders simultaneously. In general, the first step is to institute nonpharmacologic measures such as regulation of sleep (improved sleep hygiene), limitation to use of caffeine, regular exercise, and identification of provocative influences (eg, certain foods, social stressors) [83].

In cases where headache is presumed to be the result of a sleep disorder (as it may be in OSA, PLMS, insomnias; see Table 21.1), initial therapy should target toward the sleep disorder. Treatment of the underlying disorder may consolidate sleep and eliminate the headaches. To that extent, current clinical evidence has shown improvement of headaches after adequate treatment of OSA [8,12]. For obese children with OSA, treatment of adeno-tonsillar hypertrophy and possibly CPAP are considered the primary approaches [18]. Moreover, obese children with SDB may benefit from conservative interventions such as oral appliances, positional therapy, exercise programs, and weight reduction [18]. In obese children with SDB and headaches, pharmacological interventions targeting both weight loss and headaches may be warranted. For example, the use of topiramate in children with migraine has been found to be effective, safe, and well tolerated and, in light of its weight reduction effects, may represent the treatment of choice in these cases [84].

When the sleep disturbance is more likely the result of the headache syndrome, as in chronic headache syndromes (see Table 21.1), the headaches should be addressed first. In these cases, it is important to identify and address possible underlying mood disorders. Behavioral therapy should be the first line of approach, and referral to a psychiatrist may be warranted.

The therapeutic approach to cases in which headache and sleep disorders coexist and seem pathologically intrinsically related (as it may be in migraine, CH, and CPH, see Table 21.1), pharmacological strategies need to address both problems. For instance, the use of melatonin has been proven effective in the treatment of childhood migraine and in adults with headache specifically suffering from circadian rhythm disorders [85,86]. Melatonin is also a valuable treatment option in cases of both childhood and adult insomnia [87,88]. Ramelteon, a melatonin receptor agonist, has also been found to be effective and generally well-tolerated treatment for insomnia symptoms in adults [89]. Similarly, cyproheptadine, an anti-histaminic and anti-serotonergic drug, is commonly used for prophylaxis in migraine and CH [90]. Although not used as a sedative, it is known to cause drowsiness [90]. Animal studies have shown that it can improve quality of sleep in sleep-deprived rats, but clinical evidence is lacking [91].

In general, it is important to take into account that certain medications may be valuable for helping both headaches and the putative sleep disturbance, and these should be the first-line treatment when the disorders coexist. For example, tricyclic antidepressants, such as amitriptyline have sedative effects, and therefore can be useful for both prophylaxis against daily headaches and the insomnia [92]. Because amitryptyline causes weight gain, obese children should be treated with other tricyclic antidepressants not affecting the patient's weight, such as protriptyline [93]. Similar benefits may be obtained with the use of other sedating antidepressants such as mirtazapine, in light of its anti-histaminic activity [94]. Benzodiazepines and muscle relaxants may also be of complementary help [94].

On the other hand, it is also important to keep in mind that certain medications that may help one disorder but worsen the other. For example, several drugs used for both prophylactic and abortive therapy in headache may cause insomnia and disrupted sleep. For instance, selective serotonin reuptake inhibitors, and beta-blockers have been used in chronic headache syndromes, but are known to cause sleep disruption [95]. Caffeine-based abortive treatments of headaches may cause insomnia, especially when taken during the second half of the day [96]. Avoiding such approaches to treat headaches becomes essential in a child suffering from a coexisting sleep disturbance of any kind. Alternately, use of beta-blockers, which inhibit melatonin, may be used in the morning in an attempt to not disrupt sleep at night [97].

Recent studies have supported the use of cognitive behavioral therapy and in particular Internet-based programs for pediatric recurrent headache [98]. Two different self-help training programs (multimodal cognitive-behavioral training [CBT] and applied relaxation [AR]) presented via the Internet were compared with an educational intervention (EDU) in a population of 65 children and adolescents with recurrent headache [98]. Significant reduction in headache frequency, duration and pain catastrophizing was seen, in particular with CBT, indicating that Internet programs may be useful for pediatric recurrent headache, especially given their accessibility and suitability for children and adolescents [98]. Similarly, the efficacy of cognitive-behavioral therapy for insomnia (CBT-I) in children with nonmalignant chronic pain has provided significant improvements in sleep as well as daily functioning in relation to pain [99].

Future Research

Both basic and clinical research is of importance in further delineating the shared physiologic and pathological mechanisms between sleep physiology and headaches.

Imaging studies have yield interesting insights on the anatomical and physiological substrates of headache attacks. Using PET scanning and proton magnetic resonance spectroscopy, investigators have been able to identify hypothalamic and brainstem structures involved in sleep also involved in the generation of migraine and CH attacks [69,70,100]. The identification of these structures, and the possibility to gather information on their function through novel techniques, will allow further development of targeted treatment approaches for both sleep disorders and headache syndromes.

Clinical research addressing the co-morbidity of headache and sleep disorders and their burden on the child's life and society is still lacking. Most of the retrospective studies are limited by referral biases, and most of the analytical investigations have not included the systematic employment of reliable measures such as PSG. Moreover, the need for double-blind clinical studies aiming at the identification of the optimal pharmacological therapy to tackle both sleep and headache disorders are obvious.

Conclusions

Substantial evidence suggests that sleep disorders and headache are associated at both clinical and anatomical/physiological levels. Headaches may represent the symptoms of an underlying sleep disorder, and conversely, chronic headache syndromes may account for sleep disturbances. Evidence on comorbidities between primary headaches and sleep disorders has pointed out their shared pathogenic mechanisms, and as such, has indicated that (1) clinical attention to the coexistence of both pathologies is imperative, (2) appropriate sleep screening tools and sleep studies should be offered, and (3) bidirectional behavioral and pharmacological therapy are warranted. In general, most of the clinical evidence has come from studies on adult samples. Although still scant, information on the pediatric population is emerging and receiving increasing attention. Further analytical studies addressing diagnostic and therapeutic approaches of headache and sleep disorders in children and adolescent are needed.

References

1. Kayed K, Sjaastad O. Nocturnal and early morning headaches. *Ann Clin Res.* 1985;17(5):243–246.
2. Blau JN. Sleep deprivation headache. *Cephalalgia.* 1990;10(4):157–160.
3. Alstadhaug K, Salvesen R, Bekkelund S. Insomnia and circadian variation of attacks in episodic migraine. *Headache.* 2007;47(8):1184–1188.
4. Blau JN. Resolution of migraine attacks: sleep and the recovery phase. *J Neurol Neurosurg Psychiatry.* 1982;45(3):223–226.
5. Sahota PK, Dexter JD. Sleep and headache syndromes: a clinical review. *Headache.* 1990; 30(2):80–84.
6. Paiva T, Farinha A, Martins A, Batista A, Guilleminault C. Chronic headaches and sleep disorders. *Arch Intern Med.* 1997;157(15): 1701–1705.
7. Paiva T, Batista A, Martins P, Martins A. The relationship between headaches and sleep disturbances. *Headache.* 1995;35(10):590–596.
8. Poceta JS, Dalessio DJ. Identification and treatment of sleep apnea in patients with chronic headache. *Headache.* 1995;35(10):586–589.
9. Goder R, Friege L, Fritzer G, Strenge H, Aldenhoff JB, Hinze-Selch D. Morning headaches in patients with sleep disorders: a systematic polysomnographic study. *Sleep Med.* 2003;4(5):385–391.
10. Loh NK, Dinner DS, Foldvary N, Skobieranda F, Yew WW. Do patients with obstructive sleep apnea wake up with headaches? *Arch Intern Med.* 1999;159(15):1765–1768.
11. Vendrame M, Kaleyias J, Valencia I, Legido A, Kothare SV. Polysomnographic findings in children with headaches. *Pediatr Neurol.* 2008;39(1):6–11.
12. Biondi DM. Headaches and their relationship to sleep. *Dent Clin North Am.* 2001;45(4):685–700.
13. Rains J, Penzien D, Mohammed Y. Sleep and headache: morning headache associated with sleep disordered breathing (abstract). *Cephalalgia.* 2001;21:520.
14. Furtner M, Staudacher M, Frauscher B, et al. Cerebral vasoreactivity decreases overnight in severe obstructive sleep apnea syndrome: a study of cerebral hemodynamics. *Sleep Med.* 2009; 10(8):875–881.
15. Bruni O, Fabrizi P, Ottaviano S, Cortesi F, Giannotti F, Guidetti V. Prevalence of sleep disorders in childhood and adolescence with headache: a case-control study. *Cephalalgia.* 1997;17(4):492–498.
16. Isik U, Ersu RH, Ay P, et al. Prevalence of headache and its association with sleep disorders in children. *Pediatr Neurol.* 2007;36(3):146–151.
17. Bruni O, Russo PM, Ferri R, Novelli L, Galli F, Guidetti V. Relationships between headache and sleep in a non-clinical population of children and adolescents. *Sleep Med.* 2008;9(5):542–548.
18. Arens R, Muzumdar H. Childhood obesity and obstructive sleep apnea syndrome. *J Appl Physiol.* 2009;108(2):436–444.
19. Tsaoussoglou M, Bixler EO, Calhoun S, Chrousos GP, Sauder K, Vgontzas AN. Sleep-disordered breathing in obese children is associated with prevalent excessive daytime sleepiness, inflammation, and metabolic abnormalities. *J Clin Endocrinol Metab.* 2009;95(1):143–150.
20. Dodick DW, Eross EJ, Parish JM, Silber M. Clinical, anatomical, and physiologic relationship between sleep and headache. *Headache.* 2003;43(3):282–922.
21. Bonnet MH. Hyperarousal and Insomnia. *Sleep Med Rev.* 14(1):33.
22. Buskila D. Pediatric Fibromyalgia. *Rheum Dis Clin North Am.* 2009;35(2):253–261.

23. Avellaneda Fernandez A, Perez Martin A, Izquierdo Martinez M, et al. Chronic fatigue syndrome: aetiology, diagnosis and treatment. *BMC Psychiatry*. 2009;(9)(suppl 1):S1. PMCID: 2766938.
24. Carotenuto M, Guidetti V, Ruju F, Galli F, Tagliente FR, Pascotto A. Headache disorders as risk factors for sleep disturbances in school aged children. *J Headache Pain*. 2005;6(4):268–270.
25. Bursztein C, Steinberg T, Sadeh A. Sleep, sleepiness, and behavior problems in children with headache. *J Child Neurol*. 2006;21(12):1012–1019.
26. Spierings EL, van Hoof MJ. Fatigue and sleep in chronic headache sufferers: an age- and sex-controlled questionnaire study. *Headache*. 1997; 37(9):549–552.
27. Miller VA, Palermo TM, Powers SW, Scher MS, Hershey AD. Migraine headaches and sleep disturbances in children. *Headache*. 2003;43(4): 362–368.
28. Jennum P, Jensen R. Sleep and headache. *Sleep Med Rev*. 2002;6(6):471-479.
29. Baskin SM, Lipchik GL, Smitherman TA. Mood and anxiety disorders in chronic headache. *Headache*. 2006;46(suppl 3):S76–S87.
30. Seshia SS, Phillips DF, von Baeyer CL. Childhood chronic daily headache: a biopsychosocial perspective. *Dev Med Child Neurol*. 2008;50(7): 541–545.
31. Gungormus Z, Erciyas K. Evaluation of the relationship between anxiety and depression and bruxism. *J Int Med Res*. 2009;37(2):547–550.
32. Kampe T, Edman G, Bader G, Tagdae T, Karlsson S. Personality traits in a group of subjects with long-standing bruxing behaviour. *J Oral Rehabil*. 1997;24(8):588–593.
33. Dexter JD, Weitzman ED. The relationship of nocturnal headaches to sleep stage patterns. *Neurology*. 1970;20(5):513–518.
34. Dexter JD. The relationship between stage III + IV + REM sleep and arousals with migraine. *Headache*. 1979;19(7):364–369.
35. Heather-Greener GQ, Comstock D, Joyce R. An investigation of the manifest dream content associated with migraine headaches: a study of the dreams that precede nocturnal migraines. *Psychotherpsychosoma*. 1996;65(4):216–221.
36. Goder R, Fritzer G, Kapsokalyvas A, et al. Polysomnographic findings in nights preceding a migraine attack. *Cephalalgia*. 2001;21(1):31–37.
37. Sicuteri F. Hypothesis: migraine, a central biochemical dysnociception. *Headache*. 1976;16(4): 145–159.
38. Montagna P. Hypothalamus, sleep and headaches. *Neurol Sci*. 2006;27(suppl 2): S138–S143.
39. Alstadhaug K, Salvesen R, Bekkelund S. 24-hour distribution of migraine attacks. *Headache*. 2008;48(1):95–100.
40. Zurak N. Role of the suprachiasmatic nucleus in the pathogenesis of migraine attacks. *Cephalalgia*. 1997;17(7):723–728.
41. Blau JN. Migraine prodromes separated from the aura: complete migraine. *Br Medical Journal*. 1980;281(6241):658–660.
42. Craig AD. A new view of pain as a homeostatic emotion. *Trends Neurosci*. 2003;26(6):303–307.
43. Dahmen N, Querings K, Grun B, Bierbrauer J. Increased frequency of migraine in narcoleptic patients. *Neurology*. 1999;52(6):1291–1293.
44. Dahmen N, Kasten M, Wieczorek S, Gencik M, Epplen JT, Ullrich B. Increased frequency of migraine in narcoleptic patients: a confirmatory study. *Cephalalgia*. 2003;23(1):14–19.
45. Barabas G, Ferrari M, Matthews WS. Childhood migraine and somnambulism. *Neurology*. 1983; 33(7):948–949.
46. Kudrow L. Cluster headache: diagnosis and management. *Headache*. 1979;19(3):142–150.
47. Goadsby PJ. Pathophysiology of cluster headache: a trigeminal autonomic cephalgia. *Lancet Neurol*. 2002;1(4):251–257.
48. Kunkle EC, Wolff HG. Headache; an outline for diagnosis and treatment. *Med Clin North Am*. 1948;32:557–569.
49. Leone M, Bussone G. A review of hormonal findings in cluster headache. Evidence for hypothalamic involvement. *Cephalalgia*. 1993;13(5):309–17.
50. Leone M, Lucini V, D'Amico D, et al. Twenty-four-hour melatonin and cortisol plasma levels in relation to timing of cluster headache. *Cephalalgia*. 1995;15(3):224–229.
51. Treiser SL, Cascio CS, O'Donohue TL, Thoa NB, Jacobowitz DM, Kellar KJ. Lithium increases serotonin release and decreases serotonin receptors in the hippocampus. *Science*. 1981;213(4515): 1529–1531.
52. Rainero I, Gallone S, Valfre W, et al. A polymorphism of the hypocretin receptor 2 gene is associated with cluster headache. *Neurology*. 2004;63(7): 1286–1288.
53. Sjaastad O, Apfelbaum R, Caskey W, et al. Chronic paroxysmal hemicrania (CPH). The clinical manifestations. A review. *Ups J Med Sci Suppl*. 1980;31:27–33.
54. Kudrow DB, Kudrow L. Successful aspirin prophylaxis in a child with chronic paroxysmal hemicrania. *Headache*. 1989;29(5):280–281.
55. Gladstein J, Holden EW, Peralta L. Chronic paroxysmal hemicrania in a child. *Headache*. 1994;34(9):519–520.
56. Kayed K, Godtlibsen OB, Sjaastad O. Chronic paroxysmal hemicrania IV: "REM sleep locked" nocturnal headache attacks. *Sleep*. 1978;1(1):91–95.
57. Raskin NH. The hypnic headache syndrome. *Headache*. 1988;28(8):534–536.
58. Dodick DW, Mosek AC, Campbell JK. The hypnic ("alarm clock") headache syndrome. *Cephalalgia*. 1998;18(3):152–156.
59. Evers S, Goadsby PJ. Hypnic headache: clinical features, pathophysiology, and treatment. *Neurology*. 2003;60(6):905–909.
60. Dodick DW. Polysomnography in hypnic headache syndrome. *Headache*. 2000;40(9):748–752.
61. Evers S, Rahmann A, Schwaag S, Ludemann P, Husstedt IW. Hypnic headache - the first German cases including polysomnography. *Cephalalgia*. 2003;23(1):20–23.

62. Pinessi L, Rainero I, Cicolin A, Zibetti M, Gentile S, Mutani R. Hypnic headache syndrome: association of the attacks with REM sleep. *Cephalalgia*. 2003;23(2):150–154.
63. Patsouros N, Laloux P, Ossemann M. Hypnic headache: a case report with polysomnography. *Acta neurologica Belgica*. 2004;104(1):37–40.
64. Manni R, Sances G, Terzaghi M, Ghiotto N, Nappi G. Hypnic headache: PSG evidence of both REM- and NREM-related attacks. *Neurology*. 2004;62(8):1411–1413.
65. Arjona JA, Jimenez-Jimenez FJ, Vela-Bueno A, Tallon-Barranco A. Hypnic headache associated with stage 3 slow wave sleep. *Headache*. 2000; 40(9):753–754.
66. Cirignotta F, Coccagna G, Sacquegna T, et al. Nocturnal headache: systemic arterial pressure and heart rate during sleep. *Cephalalgia*. 1983; 3(suppl 1):54–57.
67. Saper CB, Scammell TE, Lu J. Hypothalamic regulation of sleep and circadian rhythms. *Nature*. 2005;437(7063):1257–1263.
68. Benarroch EE. Suprachiasmatic nucleus and melatonin: reciprocal interactions and clinical correlations. *Neurology*. 2008;71(8):594–598.
69. May A, Bahra A, Buchel C, Frackowiak RS, Goadsby PJ. Hypothalamic activation in cluster headache attacks. *Lancet*. 1998;352(9124): 275–278.
70. Weiller C, May A, Limmroth V, et al. Brain stem activation in spontaneous human migraine attacks. *Nat Med*. 1995;1(7):658–660.
71. Brzezinski A. Melatonin in humans. *N Engl jJ Med*. 1997;336(3):186–195.
72. Morgan PJ, Barrett P, Howell HE, Helliwell R. Melatonin receptors: localization, molecular pharmacology and physiological significance. *NeurochemInt*. 1994;24(2):101–146.
73. Brun J, Claustrat B, Saddier P, Chazot G. Nocturnal melatonin excretion is decreased in patients with migraine without aura attacks associated with menses. *Cephalalgia*. 1995;15(2):136–139; discussion 79.
74. Claustrat B, Brun J, Geoffriau M, Zaidan R, Mallo C, Chazot G. Nocturnal plasma melatonin profile and melatonin kinetics during infusion in status migrainosus. *Cephalalgia*. 1997;17(4):511–517; (discussion 487).
75. Leone M, D'Amico D, Moschiano F, Fraschini F, Bussone G. Melatonin versus placebo in the prophylaxis of cluster headache: a double-blind pilot study with parallel groups. *Cephalalgia*. 1996;16(7):494–496.
76. Kothare SV, Kaleyias J. The clinical and laboratory assessment of the sleepy child. *Semin Pediatr Neurol*. 2008;15(2):61–69.
77. Holley S, Hill CM, Stevenson J. A comparison of actigraphy and parental report of sleep habits in typically developing children aged 6 to 11 years. *Behav Sleep Med*. 8(1):16–27.
78. Heng K, Wirrell E. Sleep disturbance in children with migraine. *J Child Neurol*. 2006;21(9): 761–766.
79. Spierings EL, Ranke AH, Honkoop PC. Precipitating and aggravating factors of migraine versus tension-type headache. *Headache*. 2001; 41(6):554–558.
80. Sadeh A, Acebo C. The role of actigraphy in sleep medicine. *Sleep Med Rev*. 2002;6(2):113–124.
81. Ancoli-Israel S, Cole R, Alessi C, Chambers M, Moorcroft W, Pollak CP. The role of actigraphy in the study of sleep and circadian rhythms. *Sleep*. 2003;26(3):342–392.
82. Bruni O, Russo PM, Violani C, Guidetti V. Sleep and migraine: an actigraphic study. *Cephalalgia*. 2004;24(2):134–139.
83. Lewis D, Ashwal S, Hershey A, Hirtz D, Yonker M, Silberstein S. Practice parameter: pharmacological treatment of migraine headache in children and adolescents: report of the American Academy of Neurology Quality Standards Subcommittee and the Practice Committee of the Child Neurology Society. *Neurology*. 2004;63(12): 2215–2224.
84. Cruz MJ, Valencia I, Legido A, et al. Efficacy and tolerability of topiramate in pediatric migraine. *Pediatr Neurol*. 2009;41(3):167–170.
85. Miano S, Parisi P, Pelliccia A, Luchetti A, Paolino MC, Villa MP. Melatonin to prevent migraine or tension-type headache in children. *Neurol Sci*. 2008;29(4):285–287.
86. Nagtegaal JE, Smits MG, Swart AC, Kerkhof GA, van der Meer YG. Melatonin-responsive headache in delayed sleep phase syndrome: preliminary observations. *Headache*. 1998;38(4):303–307.
87. Owens JA. Pharmacotherapy of pediatric insomnia. *J Am Acad Child Adolesc Psychiatry*. 2009; 48(2):99–107.
88. Walsh JK. Pharmacologic management of insomnia. *J Clin Psychiatry*. 2004;65 Suppl 16:41–45.
89. Gross PK, Nourse R, Wasser TE. Ramelteon for insomnia symptoms in a community sample of adults with generalized anxiety disorder: an open label study. *J Clin Sleep Med*. 2009;5(1):28–33. PMCID: 2637163.
90. Lewis DW, Yonker M, Winner P, Sowell M. The treatment of pediatric migraine. *Pediatr Ann*. 2005;34(6):448–460.
91. Tokunaga S, Takeda Y, Shinomiya K, Hirase M, Kamei C. Effects of some H1-antagonists on the sleep-wake cycle in sleep-disturbed rats. *J Pharmacol Sci*. 2007;103(2):201–206.
92. Ware JC. Tricyclic antidepressants in the treatment of insomnia. *J Clin Psychiatry*. 1983;44(9, pt 2): 25–28.
93. Taylor FR. Weight change associated with the use of migraine-preventive medications. *Clin Ther*. 2008;30(6):1069–1080.
94. Redillas C, Solomon S. Prophylactic pharmacological treatment of chronic daily headache. *Headache*. 2000;40(2):83–102.
95. Safer DJ, Zito JM. Treatment-emergent adverse events from selective serotonin reuptake inhibitors by age group: children versus adolescents. *J Child Adolesc Psychopharmacol*. 2006; 16(1–2):159–169.

96. Bigal ME, Lipton RB. Overuse of acute migraine medications and migraine chronification. *Curr Pain Headache Rep*. 2009;13(4):301–307.
97. Stoschitzky K, Sakotnik A, Lercher P, et al. Influence of beta-blockers on melatonin release. *Eur J Clin Pharmacol*. 1999; 55(2):111–115.
98. Trautmann E, Kroner-Herwig B. A randomized controlled trial of internet-based self-help training for recurrent headache in childhood and adolescence. *Behav Res Ther*. 48(1):28–37.
99. Jungquist CR, O'Brien C, Matteson-Rusby S, et al. The efficacy of cognitive-behavioral therapy for insomnia in patients with chronic pain. *Sleep medicine*. 11(3):302–309. PMCID: 2830371.
100. Lodi R, Pierangeli G, Tonon C, et al. Study of hypothalamic metabolism in cluster headache by proton MR spectroscopy. *Neurology*. 2006;66(8): 1264–1266.

CHAPTER 22

Sleep in Traumatic Brain Injury in Children

Stephen H. Sheldon

Introduction

Difficulty sleep following head trauma and loss of consciousness and coma has been well documented. Relationships of traumatic head injuries with chronic sleep disturbances have only recently received attention in the medical literature [1]. Degrees of closed head trauma less than that resulting in initial clinical manifestations can also affect the sleep-wake cycle, affect degrees of alertness, and result in consequential manifestations after the immediate effects of the trauma have subsided.

Clinical Presentation

Following closed head injury, sleep disturbances may be particularly delayed, especially if the trauma was considerable enough to result in a prolonged period of unconsciousness. Nonetheless, excessive sleepiness may follow minor trauma subsequent to apparently minimal loss of consciousness. Regardless of the length of unconsciousness, sleep patterns following the injury, disrupted sleep, and/or the degree of daytime sleepiness considerably differ from patients' sleep patterns before the injury.

Excessive daytime sleepiness and increased total sleep time is a common manifestation following an initial period of postinjury unconsciousness [2]. Sleep attacks and/or unintentional sleep episodes may occur. Nocturnal sleep may or may not be prolonged. On the other hand, total sleep time within each 24-hour day may become extensive and true hypersomnia may occur. Other symptoms may include but are not limited to difficulty concentrating, attention span problems, irritability, mood changes, memory lapses, and general feeling of fatigue. Headache and minor neurological findings of central nervous system (CNS) dysfunction might occur but are not necessarily present.

Less commonly, initial head injury can be followed by difficulties falling to sleep and/or staying asleep. However, in a group of 182 children who had suffered traumatic injury in rural China, short sleep time and daytime sleepiness were commonly associated features [3]. This problem of sleeplessness may be associated with subjective daytime sleepiness and fatigue. Insomnia secondary to psychological causes following head injury is less common.

Narcolepsy with or without cataplexy is quite unusual following closed head injuries. Post-traumatic narcolepsy, although previously described, is more likely coincidental and unrelated. Because nomenclature has changed considerably over the years, the term narcolepsy is now only used for a specific complex of symptoms and the symptom of profound sleepiness following closed head trauma is now appropriately termed hypersomnia [4].

Increased focus on mild traumatic brain injury has focused on brain activation and neuropsychological sequelae [5,6]. Meta-analysis and prospective studies have revealed favorable outcomes in the first few weeks following minimal head injury with little or no permanent impairment on neuropsychological testing by 3 months after injury. On the other hand, functional magnetic resonance imaging (MRI) has been used to study neural mechanisms of cognitive function after mild head injury. Following mild brain trauma, there may be a mismatch of activation and allocation of working memory-processing resources. Nonetheless, cognitive function appears to be no different from normal controls [7].

Pathophysiology of Sleep Disorders Following Head Trauma

Two main mechanisms of injury may result in post-traumatic hypersomnia. CNS injury may result from direct trauma to the head or may be the result of acceleration or deceleration injury. Focal damage might include localized cerebral contusion or hematoma. Generalized injury can include diffuse axonal injury, generalized edema, or hypoxemic changes associated with alteration in blood flow [8,9]. Damage depends on the degree, direction, and duration of the acceleration or deceleration. Cerebral injury may be a primary result of direct trauma and may not respond to treatment. Lesions that are detected early enough are potentially preventable [10,11].

Sleep-related symptoms secondary to closed head trauma are also determined by the location of injury within areas of the CNS responsible for sleep-wake regulation. Brainstem reticular formation, posterior hypothalamus, and the region of the third ventricle are areas particularly responsible for maintaining wakefulness. Shearing injury can result in microhemorrhage in these areas. When affected, excessive sleepiness and hypersomnia often occur. Lesions high in the cervical portion of the spinal cord have also been reported to result in excessive sleepiness and sleep attacks [12,13]. Cervical cord injury may result in sleep-disordered breathing, and daytime sleepiness secondary to a sleep-related breathing abnormality can result [14].

Low CSF hypocretin-1 is highly specific and sensitive for narcolepsy syndrome with cataplexy. Hypocretin abnormalities that are similar to those seen in patients with narcolepsy with cataplexy do not appear to be the major cause of hypersomnia [12]. Nevertheless, there may be a continuum in the pathophysiology of narcolepsy with or without cataplexy and hypersomnia from other causes. The association of low hypocretin levels has been rarely found in children following head injury, and because of the infrequency of case reports, it is unclear of the association [15,16]. Indeed, because symptoms of narcolepsy can begin quite early in childhood, association between narcolepsy, cataplexy, and head trauma may be coincidental. Nonetheless, hypocretin-1 levels in CSF are rarely obtained following head injury, making epidemiological assessment difficult. Overlap between syndromes associated with excessive sleepiness suggests common hypothalamic, hypocretin-independent system dysfunction, which may be present in many patients with sleep difficulties and hypersomnolence following head trauma [17].

Injuries involving the base of the skull and sphenoid bone may consequently result in sleep-related difficulties because of damage to the base of the frontal lobes and the anterior medial hypothalamus region. Because basal forebrain is intimately involved with the initiation of sleep, dysfunction and deregulation of the sleep wake cycles may result. Dopaminergic pathways and hypothalamic dysfunction may also be involved [18].

Closed head injury can also affect the suprachiasmatic nucleus, subsequently resulting in circadian dysregulation of the sleep-wake cycle [19]. Problems of both sleeplessness and sleepiness associated with hypersomnia may result. Additionally, if significantly affected and if there is involvement of interconnections that help govern biological rhythms, complete sleep-wake rhythm reversal might occur [20].

Prevalence of sleep disorders following head trauma is unknown. Li and colleagues have shown that parasomnias and daytime sleepiness subscales of the Childhood Sleep Habits Questionnaire were significantly greater in school-age children who had suffered trauma than a comparison group. Sleep duration was also shorter in the group who had suffered trauma (23%) than the comparison group (12%) [20].

Diagnostic Evaluation and Assessment

Diagnostic evaluation begins with a comprehensive history, physical examination, and neurological evaluation. Temporal association of the head injury with the onset of symptoms is important. When symptoms appear shortly after the recovery from major head trauma, the association is clear. However, when symptoms are temporally distant from the original trauma, the association may not be as clear. Somnolence may be associated with occult or slowly developing pathology and might suggest the presence of increasing intracranial pressure, gradually enlarging subdural and/or epidural hematoma, arachnoid cysts, infection, or seizures. Additionally, consideration must be given to medication that might affect the CNS including but not limited to CNS depressants (particularly benzodiazepines) and anticonvulsant medication that might result in excessive daytime sleepiness, sleeplessness, or both. Patients with bilateral thalamic lesions may present with compulsive presleep behavior. Patients may be exhibit subjective sleepiness, but do not demonstrate manifest sleepiness during the day [21].

Evaluation

Historical and physical examination information are the most vital aspects of analysis. Preexisting sleep-related disorders require documentation as well as documentation of evolution of symptoms following the head injury. The presence and/or absence of focal neurological findings, sleep-related breathing disorders, and sleep-related movement disorders require assessment.

Polysomnography may help in the assessment of sleep-related disturbances or co-morbid conditions. Bradypnea might indicate the presence of injury to the medullary respiratory center and hypoventilation and that occurring particularly during rapid eye movement (REM) sleep might suggest phrenic nerve dysfunction secondary to cervical spine injury. Periodic breathing might also be present with injury to the medulla and might indicate the presence of increasing intracranial pressure.

Patients with post-traumatic hypersomnia generally reveal an increase in sleep duration with or without changes in sleep structure. Post-traumatic insomnia may reveal long sleep latency, considerable fragmentation of sleep continuity, poor sleep efficiency, and decrease in N2 sleep.

When daytime sleepiness, sleep attacks, or unintentional sleep episodes are present, a multiple sleep latency test may be helpful. Sleep latency may be markedly shortened, but REM sleep abnormalities are not typically present. If cataplexy is present, REM sleep abnormalities may be noted, and CSF may be evaluated for hypocretin levels.

Prolonged total sleep time and disruption of sleep wake cycles may also be assessed with actigraphy. Multiple sleep latency testing and actigraphy may be helpful tools in objectively determining the presence of pathology following head trauma.

New assessments such as functional MRI may be important in assessing patients with both major head trauma as well as minimal traumatic injury. Nevertheless, neither large-scale nor longitudinal studies are available to provide cogent information regarding the long-term prognosis and/or outcome of head injury in children [6].

Treatment

Sleep-related symptoms should be treated as they might otherwise be treated and based on clinical presentation. Hypersomnia is often treated with stimulant medication. Phenyethylamine stimulants are often required including, but not limited to, methylphenidate and amphetamines[1]. Although modafinil has become a common first-line medication for the treatment of excessive daytime sleepiness associated with narcolepsy, use of modafinil in the treatment of hypersomnia is still unclear. Additionally, use of modafinil for sleepiness in childhood is not well documented. Although side effects of modafinil are few, there are considerably less norepinephrine-like properties. Children who have hypersomnia subsequent to closed head trauma more often respond better to the more potent stimulant effect of methylphenidate. On the other hand, generalized effects of these stimulant medications may result in increased systemic blood pressure and with significant intracranial vascular injury may be contraindicated.

Current data have shown that facilitation or enhancement of neuroplasticity and brain repair in head trauma can be seen using novel algorithms [5]. Treatments should be tailored to each particular patient. Environmental influences can have a significant effect on neural plasticity.

In the presence of concurrent and/or comorbid sleep-related pathology, the primary underlying disorder must be addressed and required concurrent to management. Obstructive sleep apnea may require otolaryngological management or positive airway pressure. Central sleep apnea and complex sleep-disordered breathing resulting from the head trauma and/or increased intracranial pressure may require more complicated positive airway pressure management. This may be noninvasive mask ventilation. When better airway control and ventilatory management are essential, a tracheostomy and ventilator care might be warranted.

Problem of sleeplessness following head trauma in children is typically more difficult to treat. Insomnia is more recalcitrant to behavioral therapy and gradual extinction approaches. There is often a poor response to hypnotic therapy and those medications with hypnotic properties may significantly impact subtle clues regarding worsening of the patients' condition and/or the appearance of complications from the head injury.

Prognosis

There are few data available that have evaluated outcome in children with post-traumatic sleep disturbances. Prognosis often depends on the area and extent of the brain damaged and whether there are comorbid conditions present. In general, once symptoms have stabilized, sleep disturbances related to the traumatic brain injury show little further change, other than a reversible response to treatment.

Summary

Sleep-related disorders are common following both severe and milder forms of head trauma. Problem of sleepiness and problem of sleeplessness (sleep onset and sleep maintenance disorders) can be present. Sleep-related breathing disorders may be a sequela of the head injury, may occur as part of the intracranial injury, or may be left unrecognized before the injury and exist as a premorbid condition. Management may be difficult and should be part of a comprehensive plan of intervention following any form of head trauma.

References

1. Mahowald MW. Sleep in Traumatic Brain Injury and Other acquired CNS conditions. In: Culebras A, ed. *Sleep Disorders and Neurological Disease*. New York: Marcel Dekker; 2000:365–385.
2. Hooper SR, Alexander J, Moore D, et al. Caregiver reports of common symptoms in children following traumatic brain injury. *Neuro Rehabilitation*. 2004;19:175–189.
3. Li Y, Jin H, Owens JA, Hu C The association between sleep and injury among school-aged children in rural China: a case control study. *Sleep Med*. 2008;9:142–148.
4. American Academy of Sleep Medicine. *International Classification of Sleep Disorders*. 2nd ed. Westchester, IL: American Academy of Sleep Medicine; 2007.
5. McCrea M, Iverson GL, McAllister TW, et al. An integrated review of recovery after mild traumatic brain injury (MTBI): implications for clinical management. *Clinl Neuropsychol*. 2009;23:1368–1390.
6. DeFina P, Fellus J, Polito MZ, Thompson JW, Moser RS, DeLuca J. The new neuroscience frontier: promoting neuroplasticity and brain repair in traumatic brain injury. *Clin Neuropsychol*. 2009;23(8):1391–1399.
7. McAllister TW, Sparling MB, Flashman LA, Guerin SJ, Mamourian AC, Saykin AJ. Differential working memory load effects after mild traumatic brain injury. *Neuroimage*. 2001;14:1004–1012.
8. Adams JH, Graham DI, Gennarelli TA. Neuropathology of acceleration induced head injury in the subhuman primate. In: Grossman RG, Gildenberg PL, eds. *Head Injury: Basic and Clinical Aspects*. New York, NY: Raven; 1982:141–150.
9. Gennarelli TA, Thibault LE, Adams JH, Graham DI, Thompson CJ, Marcincin RP. Diffuse axonal injury and traumatic coma in the primate. *Ann Neurol*. 1982;12:564–574.
10. Adams JH. The neuropathology of head injuries. In: Vinken PJ, Bruyn GW, eds. *Handbook of Clinical Neurology:Injuries of the Brain and Skull. Part 1*. Amsterdam, NY: North Holland Publ; 1975:35–65.
11. Jennett B, Teasdale G. *The Management of Head Injuries*. Philadelphia, PA: FA Davis; 1981.
12. Adey W, Bors E, Porter RW. EEG patterns after high cervical lesions in man. *Arch Neurol*. 1968;19:377–383.
13. Hall CW, Danoff D. Sleep attacks—apparent relationship to atlantoaxial dislocation. *Arch Neurol*. 1975;32:57–58.
14. Guilleminault C, Yuen KM, Gulevich MG, Karadeniz D, Leger D, Philip P. Hypersomnia

after head-neck trauma: a medicolegal dilemma. *Neurology*. 2000;54:653–659.
15. Roth B. *Narcolepsy and Hypersomnia*. Basel: Karger, 1980.
16. Parkes JD. *Sleep and Its Disorders*. London, UK: WB Saunders; 1985.
17. Bassetti C, Gugger M, Bischof M, et al. The narcoleptic borderland: a multimodal diagnostic approach including cerebrospinal fluid levels of hypocretin-1 (orexin A). *Sleep Med*. 2003;4(1):7–12.
18. Rodrigues RN, Silva AA. [Excessive daytime sleepiness after traumatic brain injury: association with periodic limb movements and REM behavior disorder: case report]. *Arq NeuroPsiquiatr*. 2002;60:656–660.
19. Billiard M, Negri C, Baldy-Moulignier M, Roquefeuille B, Passouant P. Organisation du sommeil chz les sujets atteints d'inconscience post-traumatique chronique. *Rev Electroencephalogr Neurophysiol*. 1979;9:149–152.
20. Catsman-Berrevoets CE, Von Harskamp F. Compulsive pre sleep behavior and apathy due to bilateral thalamic stroke: response to bromocriptine. *Neurology*. 1988:38:647–649.
21. Guilleminault C, Faull KF, Miles L, van den Hoed. Post-traumatic excessive daytime sleepiness: a review of 20 cases. *Neurology*. 1983;33:1584–1589.
22. Guilleminault C, Quera-Salva MA, Goldberg MP. Pseudo-hypersomnia and pre-sleep behavior with bilateral paramedian thalamic lesions. *Brain*. 1993;116:1549–1563.
23. Dauvilliers Y, Baumann C, Carlander B, et al. CSF hypocretin-1 levels in narcolepsy, Kleine-Levin syndrome, and other hypersomnias and neurological conditions. *J Neurol Neurosurg Psychiatry*. 2003;74(12): 1667–1673.

CHAPTER 23

Craniofacial Disorders and Sleep

Tarig Ali-Dinar and Nalton F. Ferraro

Introduction: Exposition of the Anatomic and Physiologic Relationships in the Upper Airway

Patency of the upper airway during sleep is integrally related to craniofacial morphology, but craniofacial structure is only 1 element that defines airway patency. If a tube is narrow enough, its walls collapsible enough, and the transluminal pressure differential great enough, the tube will fail as a conduit. This happens in the obstructive sleep apnea (OSA) syndrome; but this tube, the upper airway, has daunting structural complexity and variability. There are 2 main intake ports in this tube; internally, it has recesses, multiple valves, moveable baffles, and glands that can swell or fill parts of the tube with mucus. The rigidity of the tube can change very quickly secondary to both internal and external control factors; parts of this tube can grow into the lumen (eg, tonsils), the tube carries multiple fluids, and it works better in certain positions than others. This is the normal human upper airway and it functions beautifully most of the time.

To fully understand the upper airway, it will be useful to examine the normal airway, the congenitally abnormal airway (nature's experiments), and therapeutic interventions that attempt to change the airway. In this way, one can gain insight into the impact that structure has on the function of this complex system. The patency is the result of anatomy and physiologic controls.

The insights into the physiologic controls of the upper airway are exciting and these new insights must be applied to the more obvious morphologic patterns [1–4]. It is this dual approach that ultimately will lead to the most predictable and efficacious care of children with craniofacial deformity and sleep-disordered breathing. It is understandable that an obvious mechanical or anatomic constriction in the upper airway draws attention, and it is correct and justifiable to address vigorously the anatomical issues. It is important, however, to remind oneself that craniofacial morphology is an important, but generally not the sole factor, in determining airway patency. Neuromuscular controls are always active [5].

Clearly, operations and devices that expand the upper airway column can be gratifyingly successful in treating OSA; conversely, operations that obstruct the airway column can induce OSA [6–11]. The deduction from these clinical operations is that anatomy and anatomical changes are very important. To deduce, however, that anatomy is the unequivocal determinant in airway patency is risky indeed [12]. To use an operation as the universal antidote to OSA has proven not to work. The uvulopalatopharyngoplasty has helped many people with OSA, but when it is applied universally and without discrimination regarding the clinical context, it fails significantly or helps only marginally. The very operation then is called into question, but what must be examined are the indications and the clinical context. If this is not done, then any treatment is no more than a hammer in search of nails. "What is your treatment for OSA?" is not much different from asking "What antibiotic do you use for infection?" Much more must be learned about the situation before the question can be answered. Even tracheostomy, which bypasses all the constrictions of the upper airway, may not be treatment enough. Mixter et al clearly demonstrated this in the paper that revealed tracheostomy failures in midface deficient children because of unrecognized tracheomalacia and bronchomalacia [13]. The approach must be kept expansive, and all possibilities must be considered.

This openness to a multifactorial approach to studying the upper airway assists in diagnosis and treatment. It allows sequencing of treatments and does not close the door on any rational combination of modalities. A child with syndromic midface deficiency may have a worsening of OSA secondary to adenotonsillar hypertrophy. Tonsillectomy and adenoidectomy may move the child back to an acceptable baseline in preparation for a midface operation at a more ideal time. In another example, a 5-year-old child with syndromic midface deficiency who is best treated with a midface operation at age 8 years may need an interval or bridging treatment. The child may not tolerate continuous positive airway pressure (CPAP) because the nasal resistance is so high. Operations can be considered (such as turbinoplasty, uvulopalatoplasty, and glossopexy) not for cure, but to decrease nasal resistance to allow CPAP to be used successfully. Perhaps a custom mask for CPAP could also help. If this does not work, a tracheostomy can be considered, weighted against an earlier midface advancement. The key is an interdisciplinary, broad overview of the clinical problem, not a narrow unifocal view.

These children with craniofacial abnormalities are still subject to central controls but structural abnormalities do place strict limitations on airway patency despite central mechanisms that might be at work to compensate or overcome these structural problems. A Children's Hospital series of 14 babies with Beckwith-Wiedmann syndrome and significant macroglossia revealed only 3 babies with significant obstructive sleep apnea syndrome (OSAS) (Figure 23.1). The lack of OSAS in this group is interesting. Is it simply that the whole airway is bigger in these large babies, or are there protective neuromuscular mechanisms in play? Is it a combination of

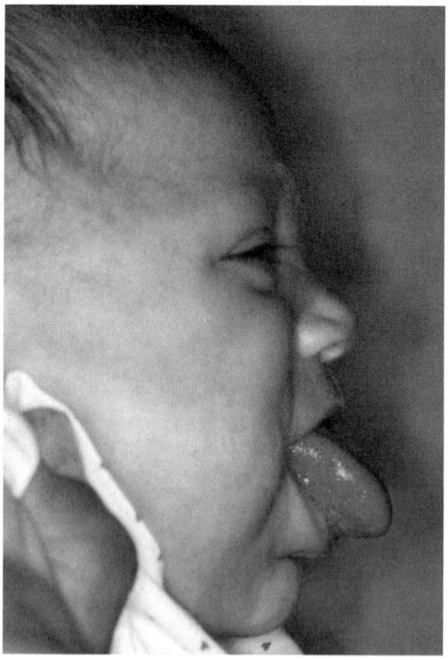

Figure 23.1 A baby with Beckwith-Wiedemann Syndrome, large tongue but no sleep apnea.

multiple factors? Conversely, in another series of children with lymphatic malformation of lingual based and floor of mouth, 58% require tracheostomy in infancy [14] (Figure 23.2). Is this a result of the sheer mass of the malformation or are there other factors in play? In lymphatic malformation, a mass threshold is reached for the oropharyngeal structures that cannot be overcome by any central neurologic compensatory mechanisms. Study of the converse situation is important for perspective also. When central and neuromuscular controls are malfunctioning, normal anatomic structures alone cannot maintain airway patency. A patient with normal craniofacial structures can develop worsening OSAS because of progressive myotonia. The literature is replete with reports of neuromuscular conditions that ultimately cause airway collapse. These examples include conditions such as cerebral palsy and muscular dystrophy [15]. A case report of OSAS improvement in a patient with muscular dystrophy after uvulopalatopharyngoplasty and tonsillectomy demonstrates the interplay between anatomy and neuromuscular tone. Even in a neuromuscular condition, improving the anatomy of the upper airway can shift the equation toward airway patency. This, of course, is a temporary improvement in a

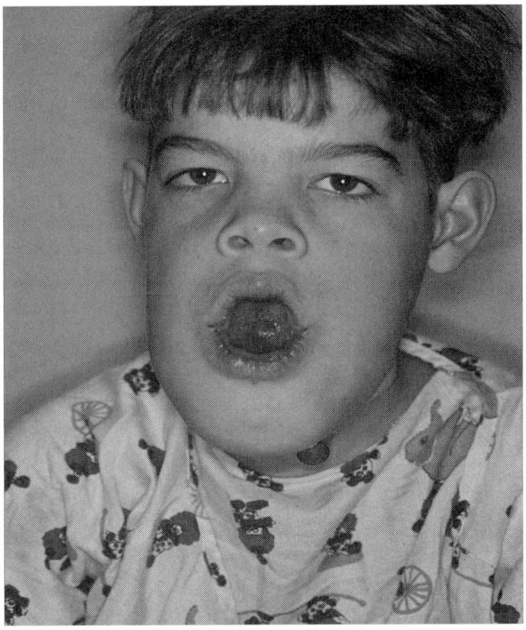

Figure 23.2 Patient with cervicofacial lymphatic malformation (cystic hygroma) and severe airway compromise. Tongue, floor of mouth, and neck are involved.

neuromuscular condition that is progressive [16]. Another anatomical approach for what is primarily a neuromuscular problem is noted in a study of children with cerebral palsy who underwent mandibular advancement with distraction devices to treat airway obstruction [17]. There can be a reasonable rationale for treating the anatomy in OSAS even if the fundamental etiology is neuromuscular (especially when it is not progressive). This, however, must be done with great caution and awareness. The decision is easier if the anatomical abnormalities that are contributing to the clinical presentation are clear-cut. If anatomical structures are normal, or near normal, changing anatomy to compensate for neuromuscular defects is a risk at best. If CPAP is not possible or if tracheostomy appears even riskier, then trying to surgically improve the airway may be reasonable. Interdisciplinary consultation is absolutely necessary.

This chapter deals primarily with the craniofacial syndromes and disorders that result in constrictions or obstructions in the upper airway. The separation of the anatomy from the neurophysiology is an artifice and is done for clarity of exposition. It is abundantly clear that one is intertwined with the other. In general, the anatomy is visible and apparent, whereas the neurophysiologic controls are hidden from view. Review of normal growth of the craniofacial structure and how it is changed in various disorders provide both perspective for understanding and rationale for treatment.

The general principles from this introduction that are of paramount importance in understanding the craniofacial disorders and their relation to sleep-disordered breathing include the following:

1. The upper airway is anatomically complex and there is interplay between anatomy and neurophysiologic controls.
2. Airway patency can be maintained by neural controls despite significantly abnormal facial structure.
3. Conversely, airways that appear normal in structure can lose patency because of physiological control problems.
4. As the upper airway develops from infancy to adulthood, changes include not only a larger framework but also other functional changes. For example, tonsils and adenoids can enlarge and then shrink, allergies can cause turbinates to enlarge, airway rigidity changes with medicines, and age and fat deposition can fluctuate dramatically. The craniofacial skeleton must always be considered with these dynamic changes in mind.
5. The skeletal framework and soft tissue envelope have a complex relationship, as we will see in subsequent sections.

Principles of Craniofacial Growth

Humans grow from the top-down—a cephalocaudal gradient of growth. The brain and cranium get big very quickly and dwarf a very little face. The structures of the face itself grow in a cephalocaudal direction. The maxilla requires more postnatal growth than the orbits and the mandible more postnatal growth than the maxilla [18].

The growth has vertical, anteroposterior and transverse vectors. Much but not all of the spatial growth is paced by the brain. The structures of the face widen, and they must also grow down and forward. The airway depends on this growth. A vertically short and posteriorly positioned face puts the airway at considerable disadvantage. The soft palate encroaches on the posterior pharyngeal wall, and the tongue encroaches on the soft palate and the pharyngeal wall. This is the infantile pattern, and it is remarkable that on the whole, babies breathe quite well considering the crowded airway. This is why the work cited above on the protective neuromuscular mechanisms in babies is so important and exciting.

The major facial segments grow by 2 interactive mechanisms. The first is strategic deposition and resorption of bone in a fieldlike fashion For example, bone is added to the posterior mandibular ramus and resorbs from the anterior ramus. Bone is added to the chin anteriorly while there is resorption taking place posteriorly. There are similar resorptive and depositional fields in the midface, the nose, and the zygomas. At the same time, these major structures translate in space anteriorly and inferiorly. This is by a mechanism that is not elucidated. The result is that the structures widen and are anteroinferiorly displaced, opening up the airway and increasing the capacity to accommodate the soft tissues. This 3-dimensional growth over the fourth dimension of time is extraordinarily complex, and the bony interactions with the soft tissue and with functional forces generate much discussion [18].

Growth of the brain controls calvarial and skull base growth, assuming that there is not a premature fusion of sutures as exists in some of the craniofacial syndromes. In the craniosynostotic midface deficient syndromes, cranial and skull-based sutures do not respond normally, affecting skull shape and therefore portions of the airway. In Crouzon and Apert syndromes for example, the coronal suture does not respond and the brain cannot grow forward and ultimately the midface cannot grow forward. The anterior cranial base is short and the airway from nasopharynx to oropharynx is shallow and AP deficient. The brain growth, however, generally cannot be denied, and it will grow transversely with an accommodating sagittal suture. The head becomes wide or brachycephalic. The interplay here is between the forces of brain growth and suture response.

In the long bones, there are cartilaginous structures, the epiphyseal plates that are pacemakers of growth. These are programmed and responsive to circulating growth factors. They ultimately are timed to shutdown and fuse. The closest analogous structures in the craniofacial skeleton are skull-based synchondroses and the nasal septum. It appears though that these structures do not work as directly as the long bone growth plates. Craniofacial growth is rather unique in the body.

Three lines of control of craniofacial growth can be considered [18]:

1. There can be an intrinsic bone pattern within the bony structure itself. The mandible, for example, will be a certain size because of genetic controls within the bone or perhaps in the adjacent soft tissue.
2. There can be cartilaginous pacemakers, such as in the long bones. For example, it has long been held that cartilage septal surgery on the nose of a growing child can affect future growth.
3. There can be soft tissue and functional epigenetic forces on the craniofacial structures. This is seen with great frequency. A tongue that is unilaterally enlarged with lymphatic malformation will affect the growth of the maxilla and mandible on the affected side. A fetus that has deformational forces applied to the chin in utero (such as abutting the pelvic rim) will have a micrognathia at birth. Presumably, this is secondary to functional forces and not to intrinsic problems in the bony structure itself.

Moss proposed the importance of functional forces in control of craniofacial growth. This has become known as the Functional Matrix Theory and it accounts for much, but certainly not all, of the observed craniofacial growth patterns [19]. The Robin Sequence illustrates the issues regarding facial growth and the various theories.

In Robin Sequence, the mandible is small, the tongue is ptotic (retropositioned) secondary to the small mandible, and as a result the tongue position prevents the palatal shelves from achieving a horizontal position and fusing. The infant is born with micrognathia, glossoptosis, and a cleft palate. The Robin Sequence can be seen in syndromic and nonsyndromic situations alike. An example of a nonsyndromic pattern involves a fetus with an abnormal in utero lie, such as a chin tucked against the pelvis (as noted earlier). The mandible does not grow because of this deformational force, the tongue cannot position itself anteriorly because of the force, and in turn the tongue results in obstructive forces on the developing palatal shelves so that they cannot close.

This is completely a cascade (or sequence) of deformational forces resulting in an airway that is small and tenuous.

Conversely, a fetus with the Treacher-Collins Syndrome can have a similar outcome but with a different incitement. The mandible is intrinsically small in Treacher-Collins syndrome [20]. This is not because of extrinsic deformational forces, but because of a genetic effect on the bone and/or surrounding soft tissues. The glossoptosis and lack of fusion of the palatal shelves, however, are most likely secondary to deformational forces from the small mandible. Even this is not clear, because there is pharyngeal hypoplasia in the syndrome and this may predispose to a more significant glossoptosis and palatal obstruction. In this syndrome, genetics result in the Robin Sequence [21].

The arguments and conclusions regarding the interplay of bony morphology and functional forces can become almost circular—a true chicken or egg dilemma. Mouth breathing and the so-called adenoidal facies illustrate this point. Orthodontists see a pattern of narrow maxilla pinched nares and anterior open bite. This is associated with difficulty in nasal breathing and a pattern of open mouth breathing. It is assumed, with some justification, that nasal obstruction such as enlarged adenoids or enlarged nasal structures from allergy result in the mouth breathing and the skeletal changes. This is a clear-cut Functional Matrix argument. Alternatively, one can argue that the craniofacial structures are intrinsically narrow, and this gives the characteristic shape and mouth-breathing pattern. The structure causes the abnormal function. It is most probable that both explanations can apply in varying degrees. Research bears out the complexity and multifactorial nature of these growth patterns [22–24].

Craniofacial Patterns and OSAS

The narrow, obstructed, or high-resistance airway is seen in many craniofacial growth patterns. At times, the structures are so abnormal that there is little doubt as to the relationship with sleep-disordered breathing. An infant with a severe micrognathia and marked encroachment of the tongue on the pharynx is such an example. Other times, the abnormality may be minor and its ultimate impact on OSAS can be debated. A child with a mild retrognathia of the mandible with only a slightly narrowed airway space can fall into this category. This is a good time to recall confounding and compounding factors that must be considered. Such factors include a significant muscle tone problem, the child's weight, and other aspects of body habitus such as neck shape, waist size, intermittent swelling in the airway secondary to allergies, and gastroesophageal reflux [18,22,25,26].

A vivid example of this interplay is provided by a case by the Children's Hospital Craniofacial group. A 12-year-old with Crouzon Syndrome had a midface advancement. Afterward, the mother noted signs of OSAS at home with snoring and gasping. At the sleep lab, in 2 separate studies, only mild OSA was present. A videotape that she provided clearly revealed a sleep pattern at home that was more severe than noted in the lab. Detective work revealed that this small house was heated with wood, and the wood smoke was causing an allergic response in this patient. This is a patient with known anatomic reasons for OSAS. He had midface deficiency that was corrected but with some residual OSAS. The pattern at home was markedly worse because of wood fume–induced allergy. This illustrates the importance of maintaining an expansive view of the clinical presentation.

The ideal study to observe points of obstruction in the upper airway is a noninvasive, dynamic, 3-dimensional study in real time that would allow natural sleep in all positions. Such gated scans are routinely performed for cardiac diagnoses but are not widely available in upper airway analysis, especially in pediatric patients who may lack full cooperation. The orthodontic radiograph, the lateral cephalogram, is inexpensive, widely available, and requires some, but only momentary, cooperation [27–30]. Even though it is done standing and awake, it has produced some patterns and measurements that do correlate with OSAS. This together with clinical observation provides a good initial assessment [27]. Three-dimensional computed tomography scans of the airway somnofluoroscopy and, if needed, upper airway endoscopy provide additional important information [25,28–34].

The craniofacial patterns in the cephalogram that have correlated with OSA are provided in the list below and a line tracing of a

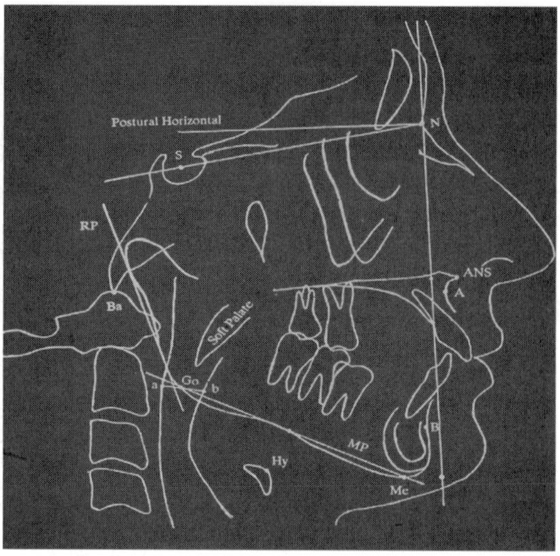

Figure 23.3 Lateral cephalogram. See text for discussion of landmarks.

normal cephalogram is provided as a reference [35–38] (Figure 23.3).

1. SNA (sella-nasion A point) is an angle that measures maxillary retrusion. The more acute the angle, the more retrusion is noted. It is in common usage but there are many exceptions to its predictability.
2. SNB (sella-nasion B point) is an angle that measures mandibular retrusion. The statements about SNA apply to SNB.
3. NSBa (nasion-sella-basion) is an angle of the anterior cranial base. The less obtuse the angle, the shorter the anterior cranial base. NS (or SN) is a linear measurement of anterior cranial base.
4. The PAS (posterior airway space) is a linear measurement of the radiolucent airway column made along a line from B point through gonial angle (Go).
5. MP to Hy is a linear measurement of the perpendicular from the mandibular plane (roughly the plane of the mandibular inferior border to a tangent at the most superior point of the body of the hyoid).
6. PNS = posterior nasal spine; P = tip of soft palate. PNS-P: linear measurement of the soft palate.
7. Mandibular angle is formed from intersection of MP and SN. The steeper the mandible, the less acute the angle. Steep mandibular angle correlates with OSA.

Some normal cephalometric values in children:

- Maxillary AP deficiency (decreased SNA) (nl = 82 degrees)
- Mandibular deficiency (decreased SNB) (nl = 79 degrees)
- Short anterior cranial base (decreased SN) (nl = 71 mm)
- Less obtuse basicranial flexure angle (decreased NSBa) (nl = 137 degrees)
- Short mandibular body (decreased pogonion-gonion; Pg-Go < 88 mm men, 79 mm women)
- Steep mandibular plane (less acute SN to MP angle; nl = 37 degrees)
- Long soft palate (PNS-P)
- Decreased sagittal posterior airway space (decreased PAS; nl ≥ 11 mm)
- Increased distance of the hyoid bone from the mandibular inferior border (decreased MP-H) (nl ≤ 15 mm)

Note: normal measurements are provided as an approximate guide because variability can be great

Adenoidal tissue may also be seen on the lateral cephalogram. A recent study reviewed past studies to evaluate and quantify the usefulness of the lateral cephalogram in visualizing adenoidal tissue. The conclusion reached is that the cephalogram view of adenoidal tissue correlates quite well with the adenoidal size. The cephalogram was less suited for estimating the nasopharyngeal airway space [39].

Abnormal Patterns of Craniofacial Growth in OSAS

The patterns of abnormal growth of the craniofacial skeleton are rarely confined to one anatomic site. There is often a major site of obstruction and several associated sites. For clarity of discussion, however, the major patterns will be discussed in groups and overlaps will be noted. Tonsils and adenoids have already been covered. The major patterns are as follows:

1. Midface deficiency in all 3 dimensions involving cranial base, the nose, nasopharynx, maxilla, hard palate, and soft palate.
2. Maxillary deficiency involving the upper jaw, parts of the nasal skeleton, hard and soft palates, and some of the nasopharynx.
3. Nasal obstructions involving the nasal passages, the anterior choanae, the posterior

choanae, the turbinates, the septum, and the nasopharynx.

4. Mandibular deficiency with retropositioning of the tongue, the floor of mouth, the suprahyoid muscles and soft tissue, and the hypopharynx.
5. Enlargements or masses that can obstruct the airway. These include both malformations and neoplasms. Examples include malformations or masses such as lymphatic malformations and neurofibroma of the nose, nasopharynx, palate, tongue, and floor of mouth. Tongue enlargement can be seen in the mucopolysaccharidoses, in Beckwith-Widemann syndrome and trisomy 21.
6. Neuromuscular disorders and metabolic disorders that have anatomic repercussions.

1. The midface deficiency syndromes are generally associated with fibroblast growth factor receptor defects, craniosynostoses, brachycephaly, and anteroposterior/vertical deficiencies of the midface. The orbits are small with exophthalmos, constricted nasal passages, zygoma hypoplasia, retrusion of the maxilla, underbite, and thickened palate. There is a "pseudo-mandibular prognathism"; the mandible is very rarely large in an absolute sense. It is usually small to normal, but it looks larger in relationship to the retruded maxilla. There can be posterior choanal atresia and cleft palate (Figures 23.4 and 23.5).

   Such a constellation of findings results in a short anterior cranial base and nasopharynx. The palate can be very close to the posterior pharyngeal wall, the nasal passages are exceedingly crowded, the maxilla can be narrow, and the tongue encroaches on the soft palate [35–38]. All these characteristics can predispose to a very compromised airway. Added to this are enlarged turbinates, significant nasal mucus, adenotonsillar hypertrophy, and possible central apnea from Chiari malformation and poor CPAP mask fit because of facial deformity. Clearly, the clinical problem can become severe, complex, and multifactorial. Crouzon, Pfeiffer, Apert, and Saethre Chotzen syndromes are the common presentations. There can be lesser degrees of developmental midface deficiency without clear-cut etiology [35,40].
2. Maxillary deficiency without full midface deficiency is also associated with OSAS. The zygomas, orbits, anterior cranial base, and much of the superior nasopharynx can be normal. The soft palate, however, is retropositioned and the tongue base, the soft palate,

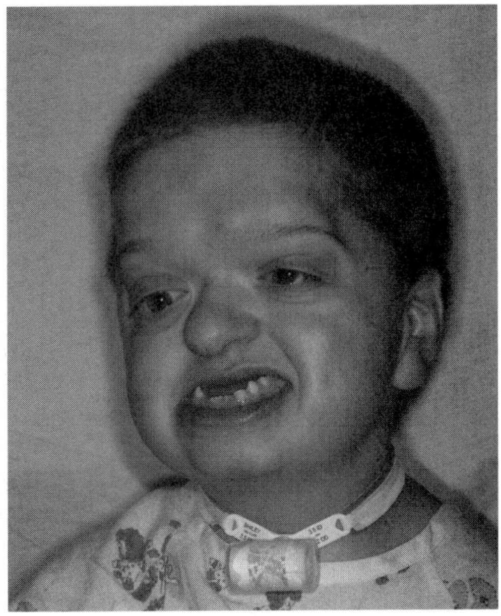

Figure 23.4 Syndromic midface deficiency in Crouzon syndrome. Note exopthalmos, maxillary hypoplasia, short nose, and open mouth.

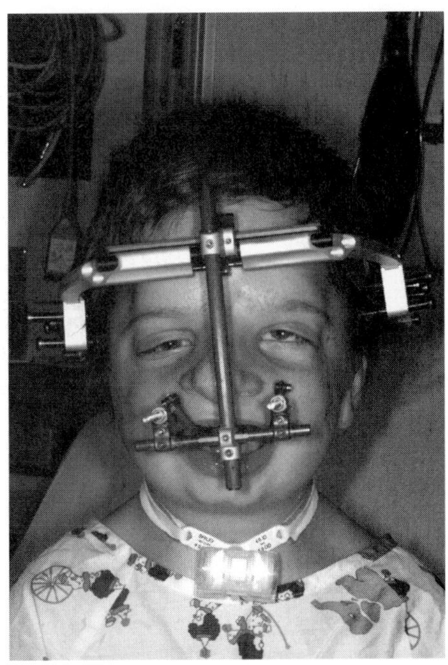

Figure 23.5 Midface distraction device in place for midface advancement.

and the posterior pharyngeal wall can form a zone of obstruction. The maxillary teeth are in an underbite. Patients with cleft lip/palate deformities form a significant portion of this group [41–46]. Midface deficiency can also be seen in families or without clear-cut etiology. Binders syndrome results in patients with naso-maxillary hypoplasia without full midface deficiency. Another anatomical abnormality is the maxilla that is transversely narrow, affecting the nasal airway and contributing to increased upper airway resistance [47].

3. Isolated nasal and/or nasopharyngeal deficiency exists. It can be congenital, developmental, or acquired. A patient with a nasal encephalocele may have nasal obstruction at presentation and after resection may have scarring of the nasal airway. A hypoplastic growth pattern may be noted in severe septal trauma. Nasopharyngeal stenosis after surgery has also been reported. The pharyngeal flap that is placed to partially occlude the passage from nasal pharynx to oral pharynx treats velopharyngeal insufficiency. Such flaps can result in snoring and sometimes in OSAS.
4. Mandibular deficiency in children exists with a wide spectrum of etiologies. The end result of mandibular deficiency is a retropositioned tongue, shortened floor of mouth, and possibly constricted hypopharynx. It is reasonable to recognize 4 groups of patients with mandibular deficiency. Some have already been discussed above (Figures 23.6, 23.7, and 23.8).
   a. Infants with deformational forces in utero that result in a micrognathia. When the deformational forces are removed, there can be complete or partial "catch-up" growth.
   b. Syndromic micrognathia does not exhibit "catch-up" growth. The more common of these disorders include Treacher Collins Syndrome, Bilateral Facial Microsomia, other first and second branchial arch disorders, Nager Syndrome, and Agnathia-Aglossia Syndrome. The Robin Sequence can be part of these syndromes [21,48,49].
   c. Acquired disorders can also result in micrognathia during the growing years. These include autoimmune disorders (such as juvenile rheumatoid arthritis),

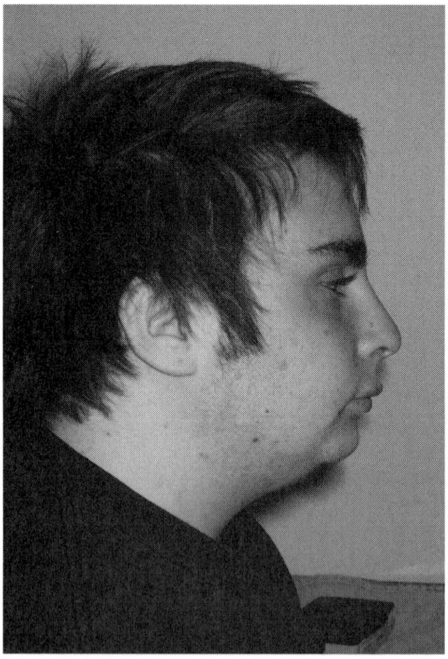

Figure 23.6 Mandibular deficiency in deformational Robin Sequence with Klippel-Feil syndrome.

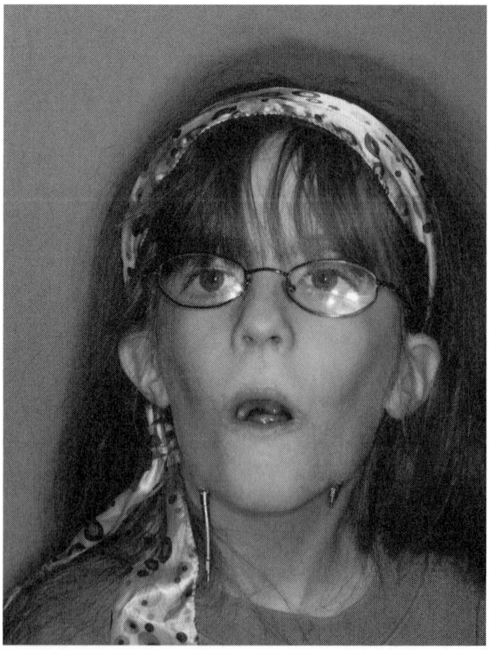

Figure 23.7 Mandibular distractors in place for mandibular advancement. Parents use special screw-drivers to turn the distractors. One distractor has an extension for ease of use.

mandibular condylar fractures with or without ankylosis, and the peculiar condition of idiopathic mandibular condylolysis [50–53].

d. Varying degrees of mandibular deficiency are also quite commonly seen in the population. It is a common problem seen by orthodontists. There may be a familial tendency, but no clear-cut cause. This may be the largest group of mandibular deficient patients with OSA tendencies. A recent study draws a relationship between small mandible and apparent life-threatening events [54].

5. Masses or enlargements in the upper airway can be congenital or develop after birth. Lymphatic malformations (previously discussed) are a well-known cause of upper airway compromise. Cervicofacial lymphatic malformation (which was previously known as cystic hygroma) is a well-known cause of upper airway compromise. Hemangiomas can develop after birth and might be in strategically unfortunate locations in the airway (such as in the larynx). Macroglossia is observed in a number of conditions (as noted above), but tongue elevation can also be seen with midline cysts and neoplasms such as foregut cysts, dermoids, teratomas, ectopic thyroid, and other floor of mouth and upper neck neoplasms.

   Intranasal, nasopharyngeal, and palatal masses must also be considered. By far, the most common enlargement resulting in upper airway compromise in children is adenotonsillar hypertrophy.

   Enlargements of the bony structures are also recognized. These bony expansions can result from a number of lesions including odontogenic masses, giant cell lesions, ossifying fibromas, fibrous dysplasia, and neurofibromas. One disorder, craniometaphyseal dysplasia, can be quite dramatic. The Children's Hospital experience includes a patient with severe OSAS as a result of craniometaphyseal dysplasia. There was resulting enlargement of the maxilla and encroachment on the nasopharyngeal airway. This was compounded by an anterior enlargement of the transverse process of C1, also encroaching on the airway.

   Finally, obesity must be considered. Although strictly not a mass or localized enlargement, deposition of fat in various locations in the upper airway is a well-known risk factor for OSA [55].

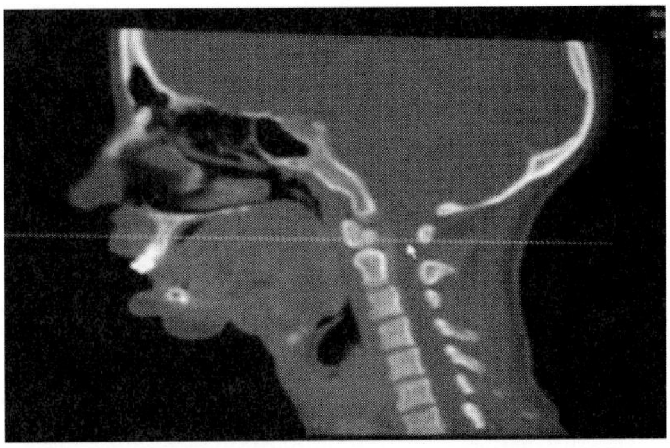

Figure 23.8 Midsagittal computed tomography view of airway occlusion with tongue against pharyngeal wall in severe micrognathia.

6. Much of this chapter involves the anatomic-neuromuscular relationship. Neuromuscular disorders that can affect the upper airway are numerous, though some are quite rare. Suffice to say that any neuromuscular disorder that affects muscle tone, strength, and posture can have an effect on the patency of the upper airway. These disorders can be genetic or acquired, congenital or postnatal, or progressive or static. They can range from muscular dystrophy to the aftermath of anoxic encephalopathy.

Conclusion

The message of this chapter is cautionary in regard to evaluation of upper airway patency in craniofacial disorders.

1. Anatomy and neurophysiology interact in ways that we are only beginning to understand.
2. An expansive view is needed in making diagnoses. Discount nothing until it has been duly considered.
3. Interdisciplinary cooperation and creativity are needed for the best treatment outcomes.
4. Always consider the fourth dimension, time, in diagnosis and treatment. The process is dynamic; therefore, the follow-up should be equally dynamic. Regular reassessment is the rule.

References

1. Marcus CL, Lutz J, Hamer A, Smith PL, Schwartz A. Developmental changes in response to subatmospheric pressure loading of the upper airway. *J Appl Physiol.* 1999;87(2):626–633.
2. Marcus CL, Fernandes Do Prado LB, Lutz J, et al. Developmental changes in upper airway dynamics. *J Appl Physiol.* 2004;97(1):98–108.
3. Arens R, Marcus Cl. Pathophysiology of upper airway obstruction: a developmental perspective. *Sleep.* 2004;27(5):997–1019.
4. Katz ES, Marcus CL, White DP. Influence of airway pressure on genioglossus activity during sleep in normal children. *Am J Respir Crit Care Med.* 2006;173(8):902–909.
5. Hudgel DW, Suratt PM. The human airway during sleep. In: Saunders NA, Sullivan CE, eds, *Sleep and Breathing.* 2nd ed. New York, NY: Marcel Dekker; 1994:191–208.
6. Castro Barbosa R, Aloe F, Tavares S, Baptista Silva A, et al. Mandibular-lingual repositioning device–MLRD: preliminary results of 8 patients with obstructive sleep apnea syndrome–OSAS. *Sao Paulo Med J.* 1995;113(3):888–894.
7. Schmidt-Nowara W, Lowe A, Weigand L, Cartwright R, Perez-Guerra F, Menn S. Oral appliances for the treatment of snoring and obstructive sleep apnea: a review. *Sleep.* 1995;18(6):501–510.
8. Schmitz JP, Bitonti DA, Lemke RR. Hyoid myotomy and suspension for obstructive sleep apnea syndrome. *J Oral Maxillofac Surg.* 1996;54: 1339–1345.
9. Riley RW, Powell NB, Guilleminault C. Currant surgical concepts for treating obstructive sleep apnea syndrome. *J Oral Maxillofac Surg.* 1987; 45:149–157.
10. Lin SY, Halbower AC, Tunkel DE, Vanderkolk C. Relief of upper airway obstruction with mandibular distraction surgery: long term quantitative results in young children. *Arch Otolaryngol Head Neck Surg.* 2006;132(4):437–441.
11. Steinbacher DM, Kaban LB, Troulis MJ. Mandibular advancement by distraction osteogenesis for tracheostomy-dependent children with severe micrognathia. *J Oral Maxillofac Surg.* 2005; 63(8):1072–1079.
12. Sorin A, McCarthy JG, Bernstein JM. Predicting decannulation outcomes after distraction osteogenesis for syndromic micrognathia. *Laryngoscope.* 2004;114(10):1815–1821.
13. Mixter RC, David DJ, Perloff WH, Green CG, Pauli RM, Popic PM. Obstructive sleep apnea in Apert's and Pfeiffer syndromes: more than a craniofacial abnormality. *Plast Reconstr Surg.* 1990;86(3):457–463.
14. Edwards PD, Rahbar R, Ferraro NF, Burrows PE, Mulliken JB. Lymphatic malformation of the lingual base and oral floor. *Plast Reconstr Surg.* 2005;115(7):1906–1915.
15. Wilkinson DJ, Baikie G, Berkowitz RG, Reddihough DS. Awake upper airway obstruction in children with spastic quadriplegic cerebral palsy. *J Paediatr Child Health.* 2006;42(1–2):44–48.
16. Sudo A, Fukumizu M, Sugai K, et al. Improvement of obstructive sleep apnea by uvulopalatopharyngoplasty and tonsillectomy in a case of Duchenne muscular dystrophy. Abstract. *No To Hattatsu.* 2000;32(4):352–357.
17. Preciado DA, Sidman JD, Sampson DE, Rimell FL. Mandibular distraction to relieve airway obstruction in children with cerebral palsy. *Arch Otolaryngol Head Neck Surg.* 2004;130(6);741–745.
18. Enlow DH. *Facial Growth.* 3rd ed. Philadelphia, PA: Saunders; 1990.
19. Moss ML, Salentijn L. The primary role of functional matrices in facial growth. *Am J Orthod.* 1969;55:566.
20. Anderson PJ, Netherway DJ, Abbott A, Moore M, David DJ. Mandibular lengthening by distraction for airway obstruction in Treacher-Collins syndrome: the long-term results. *J Craniofac Surg.* 2004;15(1):47–50.
21. Shprintzen RJ, Croft C, Berkman MD, Rakoff SJ. Pharyngeal hypoplasia in Treacher Collins syndrome. *Arch Otolaryngol.* 1979;105:127–131.
22. Cole P. *The Respiratory Role of the Upper Airways.* St Louis, MO: Mosby-Year Book, 1993.
23. Weider DJ, Baker GL, Salvatoreillo FW. Dental malocclusion and upper airway obstruction, an otolaryngologist's perspective. *Int J Otolaryngol.* 2003;67(4):323–331.
24. Shanker S, Vig KW, Beck FM, Allgair E Jr, Vig PS. Dentofacial morphology and upper respiratory function in 8-10-year old children. *Clin Orthod Res.* 1999;2(1):19–26.
25. Gibson SE, Myer CM III, Strife JL, O'Connor DM. Sleep fluoroscopy for localiz2ation of upper airway obstruction in children. *Ann Otol Rhinol Laryngol.* 1996;105(9):678–683.
26. Ward SL, Marcus CL. Obstructive sleep apnea in infants and young children. *J Clin Neurophysiol.* 1996;13(3):198–207.
27. Frohberg U, Naples RJ, Jones DL. Cephalometric comparison of characteristics in chronically snoring patients with and without sleep apnea syndrome. *Oral Surg Oral Med Oral Pathol.* 1995; 80(1):28–33.
28. Hochban W, Brandenburg U. Morphology of the viscerocranium in obstructive sleep apnea syndrome—cephalometric evaluation of 400 patients. *J Craniomaxillofac Surg.* 1994;22:205–213.
29. Lowe AA, Santamaria JD, Fleetham JA, Price C. Facial morphology and obstructive sleep apnea. *Am J Orthod Dentofacial Orthop.* 1986;90(6): 484–491.
30. Miles PG, Vig PS, Weyant RJ, et al. Craniofacial structure and obstructive sleep apnea syndrome-a qualitative analysis and meta analysis of the literature. *Am J Orthod Dentofacial Orthop.* 1996;109(2):163–172.
31. Riley RW, Powell NB, Guilleminault C. Obstructive sleep apnea and the hyoid: a revised surgical procedure. *Otolaryngol Head Neck Surg.* 1994; 111:717–721.
32. Trenouth MJ, Timms DJ. Relationship of the functional oropharynx to craniofacial morphology. *Angle Orthod.* 1999;69(5):419–423.

33. Aboudara CA, Hatcher D, Nielsen IL, Miller A. A three-dimensional evaluation of the upper airway in adolescents. *Orthod Craniofac Res.* 2003;6(suppl 1):173–175.
34. Arens R. McDonough JM, Corbin AM, et al. Linear dimensions of the upper airway structure during development: assessment by magnetic resonance imaging. *Am J Respir Crit Care Med.* 2002;165(1):117–122.
35. Donnelly LF, Surdulescu V, Chini BA, Casper KA, Poe SA, Amin RS. Upper airway motion depicted at cine MR imaging performed during sleep: comparison between young patients with and those without obstructive sleep apnea. *Radiology.* 2003;227(1):239–245.
36. Goldberg S, Shatz A, Picard E, et al. Endoscopic findings in children with obstructive sleep apnea: effects of age and hypotonia. *Pediatr Pulmonol.* 2005;40(3):205–210.
37. Myatt HM, Beckenham EJ. The use of diagnostic sleep nasendoscopy in the management of children with complex upper airway obstruction. *Clin Otolaryngol Allied Sci.* 2000;25(3):200–208.
38. Cistulli PA, Sullivan CE. Pathophysiology of sleep apnea. In: Saunders NA, Sullivan CE, eds. *Sleep and Breathing.* 2nd ed. New York, NY: Marcel Dekker; 1994:405–448.
39. Goldberg JS, Enlow DH, Whitaker LA, Zins JE, Kurihara S. Some anatomical characteristics in several craniofacial syndromes. *J Oral Surg.* 1981;39:489–498.
40. Jamieson A, Guilleminault C, Partinen M, Quera-Salva MA. Obstructive sleep apnea patients have craniomandibular abnormalities. *Sleep.* 1986;9: 469–477.
41. Peterson- Falzone SJ, Pruzansky S, Parris PJ, Laffer JL, et al. Nasopharyngeal dysmorphology in the syndromes of Apert and Crouzon. *Cleft Palate J.* 1981;18(4):237–250.
42. Steinberg B, Fraser B. The cranial base in obstructive sleep apnea. *J Oral Maxillofacial Surg.* 1995;53(10):1150–1154.
43. Major MP, Flores-Mir C, Major PW. Assessment of lateral cephalometric diagnosis of adenoid hypertrophy and posterior upper airway obstruction: a systematic review. *Am J Orthod Dentofacial Orthop.* 2006;130(6):700–708.
44. Ferraro NF. Dental and oral maxillofacial evaluations and treatment in Apert syndrome. In: Upton J, Zucker RM, eds. *Clinics in Plastic Surgery. Apert Syndrome.* Philadelphia, PA: Saunders. 1991: 291–307.
45. Josephson GD, Levine J, Cutting CB. Septoplasty for obstructive sleep apnea in infants after cleft lip repair. *Cleft Palate Craniofac J.* 1996;33(6): 473–476.
46. Chaisrisookumporn N, Stella JP, Epker BN. Cephalometric profile evaluations in patients with cleft lip and palate. *Oral Surg Oral Med Oral Pathol Oral Radiol Endod.* 1995;80(2):137–144.
47. DeLuke DM, Marchland A, Robles EC, Fox P. Facial growth and the need for orthognathic surgery after cleft palate repair: literature review and report of 28 cases. *J Oral Maxillofac Surg.* 1997;55:694–697.
48. Orr WC, Levine NS, Buchanan RT. Effect of cleft palate repair and pharyngeal flap surgery on upper airway obstruction during sleep. *Plast Reconstr Surg.* 1987;80(2):226–232.
49. Rose E, Staats R, Thissen U, Otten JE, Schmelzeisen R, Jonas I. Sleep-related obstructive disordered breathing in cleft palate patients after palatoplasty. *Plast Reconstr Surg.* 2002;110(2):392–396.
50. Mochidra M, Ono T, Saito K, Tsuiki S, Ohyama K. Effects of maxillary distraction osteogenesis on the upper airway size and nasal resistance in subjects with cleft lip and palate. *Orthod Craniofac Res.* 2004;7(4):189–197.
51. Cistulli PA, Richard GN, Palmisano RG, Unger G, Berthon-Jones M, Sullivan CE. Influence of maxillary constriction on nasal resistance and sleep apnea severity in patients with Marfan's syndrome. *Chest.* 1996;110(5):1184–1188.
52. Deegan PC, McGlone B, McNicolas WT. Treatment of Robin sequence with nasal CPAP. *J Laryngol Otol.* 1995;109(4):328–330.
53. James D, Ma L. Mandibular reconstruction in children with obstructive sleep apnea due to micrognathia. *Plast Reconstr Surg.* 1997;100(5): 1131–1138.
54. El-Sheikh MM, Medra AM, Warda MH. Bird face deformity secondary to bilateral temporomandibular joint ankylosis. *J Craniomaxillofac Surg.* 1996;24(3):96–103.
55. Ferguson KA, Ono T, Lowe AA, Ryan CF, Fleetham JA. The relationship obesity and craniofacial structure in obstructive sleep apnea. *Chest.* 1995;108(2):375–381.
56. Bettega G, Pepin JL, Levy P, et al. Surgical treatment of a patient with obstructive sleep apnea syndrome associated with temporomandibular joint destruction by rheumatoid arthritis. *Plast Reconstruct Surg.* 1998;101(4):1045–1050.
57. Perkins JA, Sie KCY, Milczuk H, Richardson MA. Airway management in children with craniofacial anomalies. *Cleft Palate Craniofac J.* 1997;34(2):135–139.
58. Sugahara T, Mori Y, Kawamoto T, Sakuda M. Obstructive sleep apnea associated with temporomandibular joint destruction by rheumatoid arthritis: report of case. *J Oral Maxillofac Surg.* 1994;52:876–880.
59. Horn MK, Kinnamon DD, Ferraro NF, Curley MA. Smaller mandibular size in infants with a history of an apparent life-threatening event. *J Pediatr.* 2006;149(4):499–504.

CHAPTER 24

Multidisciplinary Team Approach for the Evaluation of Children With Sleep Disorders

Umakanth A. Khatwa, Rachel Rosen, Eric H. Chiou, and Greg R. Licameli

Introduction

Important functions of the upper aerodigestive tract include respiration, deglutition, and phonation. Due to the complex embryology of this region, anomalies of upper aerodigestive tract development can lead to disorders of breathing, swallowing (risk for aspiration) and speech. This chapter highlights the usefulness of a combined multidisciplinary team approach when evaluating infants and children with breathing and swallowing problems in aerodigestive clinic. This includes children with complex upper airway difficulties (laryngomalacia, vocal cord paresis, laryngeal cleft, tracheoesophageal fistula (TEF), and tracheomalacia [TM]), chronic pulmonary diseases (aspiration-related lung disease, bronchiectasis, and primary ciliary dyskinesia), craniofacial anomalies (Pierre Robin sequence and Treacher Collins syndrome), dysphagia, gastroesophageal reflux (GER), and neuromuscular disorders. Table 24.1 lists the common presenting complaints in our aerodigestive center.

Traditionally, patients are seen by individual specialists for their symptoms. However, we know that diseases may not be specialty specific, and hence can have multisystem involvement and presentation. This is the rationale for the combined multidisciplinary approach where members from various specialties see patient as a team in a single setting. The members of a multidisciplinary aerodigestive team include physicians from otolaryngology, pulmonary medicine, gastroenterology, general surgery, sleep medicine, radiology, genetics, and speech and language pathology. The overall goal of this approach is to improve patient outcomes by coordinating clinical evaluations, diagnostic testing, and operative procedures in a timely and efficient manner. This is achieved by reducing waiting time for appointments and testing, limiting the number of individual clinic visits, facilitating better communication between providers, and improving parent satisfaction.

Table 24.1 Common presenting problems in the aerodigestive clinic

1. Persistent tachypnea
2. Recurrent croup
3. Chronic cough
4. Recurrent stridor
5. Infant apnea or apparent life threatening event
6. Atypical or difficult to control asthma
7. Recurrent pneumonia
8. Abnormal radiological examination
9. Cough or choking with feeding
10. Aspiration noted on swallow study
11. Persistent hypoxemia
12. Exercise induced dyspnea
13. GERD
14. Dysphagia
15. Nocturnal choking or "panic attack"

Otolaryngological Perspective

The upper airway is the air conducting pathway from the anterior nares to the carina. Various pediatric studies have reported that about 3% to 4% of the general pediatric population have upper airway anomalies. It is not uncommon for neonate or young infant to present with anomalies of upper airways at multiple levels, which can pose challenges for diagnosis and management.

Causes of upper airway obstruction include congenital anomalies (choanal stenosis or atresia, macroglossia, laryngomalacia, vocal cord paralysis, subglottic stenosis, and TM), inflammation of upper airways (reflux related injury), and infections (croup, laryngitis, and epiglottitis). Cranio-facial anomalies can also contribute to airway compromise and include retrognathia, (Pierre Robin sequence), micrognathia, and midfacial hypoplasia [1]. While adeno-tonsillar hypertrophy, nasal allergies, and obesity are the major causes of airway obstruction and obstructive sleep-disordered breathing (SDB) in older children, congenital anomalies of upper airways are the most common cause of SDB in neonates and infants. Any degree of airway narrowing can pose a risk for developing SDB. Three physical properties of upper airways increase the risk for airway obstruction. These include compliance or elasticity of the soft tissue, anatomical narrowing, position of the upper airway, and sleep-related changes in upper airway properties, which include reduction in the tone of the upper airway dilators with increased propensity of the upper airways to collapse.

Therefore, the approach to the patient with obstructed breathing will depend on the age of the patient and the historical data obtained from the caretakers [2].

Causes of Upper Airway Obstruction

It is useful to consider the anatomic levels of the airway separately concerning the pathology that may be present. Historical and clinical exam will dictate where the clinician's focus should be, but often a complete evaluation of the upper airway with various diagnostic modalities is undertaken.

Nasal Obstruction

The most common cause for obstruction of the nasopharynx is adenoid hypertrophy. However, based on the age and symptoms at presentation, other lesions such as angiofibromas and gliomas need to be entertained and can usually be diagnosed with nasal endoscopy in the office and imaging studies as needed. The adenoids are located in the nasopharynx and are often difficult to examine in a young child. The advent of thin, flexible fiberoptic telescopes allows the examiner a complete view of this region and is superior to a lateral neck x-ray. Due to the proximity of the adenoids to the Eustachian tube, the sinuses and the soft palate, the examiner should elicit in the history for otitis media, chronic nasal obstruction and discharge, or postnasal drainage. Hypertrophy of the adenoids classically presents with obligate mouth breathing and snoring while asleep, and hyponasal speech when awake. However, adenoid enlargement alone without palatine tonsillar enlargement less commonly may lead to a frank obstructive apnea. In the presence of markedly enlarged adenoids, its removal is usually effective in improving breathing, particularly in the younger population. Care must be taken in attempting removal of the adenoids in any child with a palatal abnormality as velopharyngeal insufficiency can occur.

The most common congenital abnormality of the nose is choanal atresia. The lesion is often associated with other craniofacial anomalies and is usually suspected by the inability to pass a flexible catheter through the nares into the nasopharynx. Confirmation with flexible endoscopy leads to performing computerized tomography to characterize the anatomic abnormalities for surgical planning. Bilateral atresia will require very urgent intervention and presents with symptoms of respiratory distress and feeding difficulties present at birth; whereas, unilateral obstruction may present with only chronic unilateral nasal discharge diagnosed later in childhood [3].

Oropharyngeal Obstruction

The most common cause of obstruction at this level is tonsillar hypertrophy (Figure 24.1). The adenoids and palatine tonsils, although commonly considered as a single disease process, should be evaluated individually for their contributions to any upper airway obstruction [4]. Palatine tonsillar enlargement, like adenoid enlargement, may be related to recurrent or chronic infection causing lymphoid hyperplasia. Enlargement of

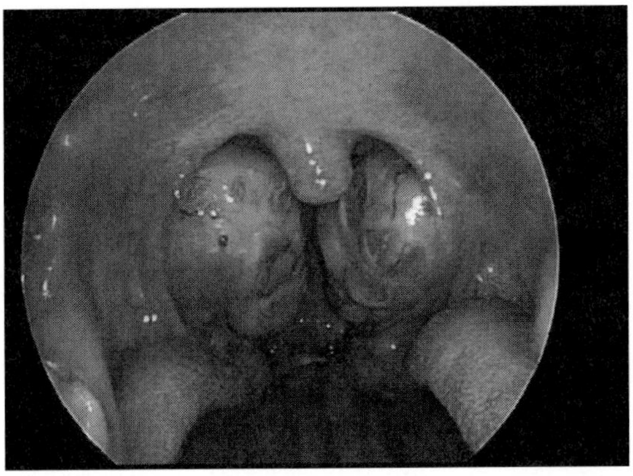

Figure 24.1 This picture reveals significantly hypertrophied palatine tonsils leading to airway obstruction.

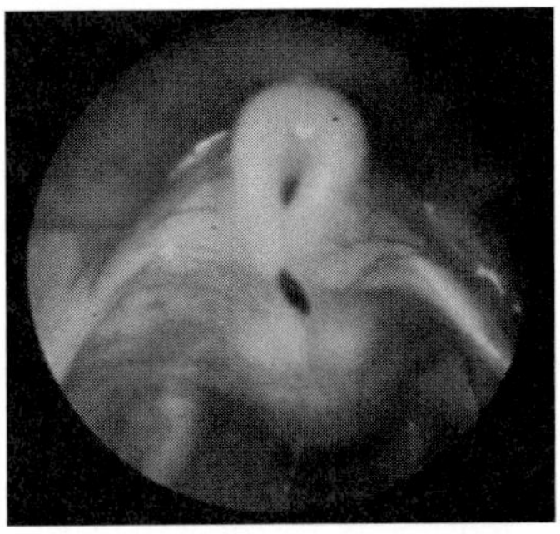

Figure 24.2 This is a picture of laryngomalacia. Note inspiratory collapse of the immature soft supra laryngeal tissues like epiglottis and aryepiglottic folds into the laryngeal inlets resulting in airway obstruction during inspiration.

the tonsils may cause apnea, feeding difficulties manifest by choking on solid food, and "muffling" of the voice. After an acute infection, the tonsils can take weeks to months to return to their baseline size. Although many children present with hypertrophy with no specific history of infection and indeed, on pathologic analysis of the tonsil, normal airway flora is often present. Tonsils that are significantly enlarged (occupying $\geq$ 50% of the oropharyngeal airway) have a higher likelihood of contributing to obstructive sleep apnea (OSA); however, in children with hypotonia (Trisomy 21 or cerebral palsy) or with craniofacial abnormalities, tonsils deemed small to average size may also be contributing to respiratory distress in combination with other anatomic issues such as macroglossia or retrongathia and neuromuscular dysfunction with increased tendency to airway collapse. In the older patient with findings of small adenoids and palatine tonsils, occult hypertrophy of the lingual tonsils, which reside at the base of the tongue, should also be considered.

Glottic Obstruction

Laryngomalacia: It is the most common laryngeal anomaly and the most common cause of stridor in children, usually presenting at birth. Stridor and upper airway obstruction results from the inspiratory collapse of the immature soft supra laryngeal tissues including the aryepiglottic folds (Figure 24.2) while crying, with agitation, or during feeding. Gastroesophageal reflux is felt to aggravate this condition due to local mucosal irritation. The majority of cases are mild and self-resolve in 12 months. Surgical intervention is relegated to the patient with severe respiratory distress, usually manifest by nasal flaring and chest/neck retractions or with feeding difficulties leading to failure to thrive. The majority of patients can be diagnosed with flexible nasopharyngoscopy in the office setting. For children who present with primarily noisy breathing, this often suffices. However, in the patient with associated clinical findings, such as feeding difficulties, a more thorough evaluation is required [5]. Laryngotracheobronchoscopy under general anesthesia is performed with attention to the supraglottic, glottic regions, and tracheal anatomy. Visual inspection and palpation are used to rule out laryngeal clefts, cysts, webs, or other associated lesions, which can be present in conjunction with laryngomalacia. Other associated comorbidities include hypotonia, developmental delay, cardiac malformation, and vascular rings compressing airways. In severe cases, life-threatening OSA, failure to thrive, and cor pulmonale can develop as complications. Hence, timely evaluation and treatment are of utmost importance.

In patients with laryngomalacia usually presenting with stridor rather than snoring, associated OSA needs to be ruled out via performing a sleep study, if the degree of laryngomalacia is moderate to severe. If the degree of OSA is mild, positional therapy (sleeping in nonsupine position) and optimization of gastroesophageal reflux disease (GERD) treatment (anti-reflux medication, thickening of feeds, and promotility agents) would be sufficient, as in most cases laryngomalacia resolves within 1 to 2 years. If laryngomalacia is accompanied with severe OSA, then surgical repair of laryngomalacia by supraglottoplasty is indicated. In extremely severe cases, tracheostomy has been performed. In a retrospective case series of 10 patients with laryngomalacia and OSA, Zafereo et al reported that 70% of the patients had significant improvement, 20% complete resolution, and 10% had mild improvement in stridor and snoring after supraglottoplasty. In addition, they also reported significant improvement in apnea hypopnea index (AHI), respiratory disturbance index, and oxygen nadir after supraglottoplasty [6].

Vocal Cord Paralysis

Vocal cord paralysis, either unilateral or bilateral, may result in airway compromise. The unilateral vocal cord usually presents with hoarseness of voice and risk for aspiration. Rarely airway obstruction can occur, leading to SDB. If there is no obvious cause such as cardiac surgery, repeated intubation, and trauma, then central nervous system causes like Arnold–Chiari malformation, hydrocephalus, neurofibromatosis, and hypoxic brain injury should be ruled out. Bilateral vocal cord paralysis can result in severe airway compromise and may require tracheostomy in some cases. Over 50% of these patients may achieve decannulation within 1 to 2 years due to spontaneous improvement in the vocal cord function [7].

Subglottic/Tracheal Obstruction

Narrowing of the subglottis presenting with inspiratory stridor in the first 6 months of life is often due to a subglottic hemangioma. Suspicion is raised when skin hemangiomas also coexist, and asymmetry of the subglottis is seen on plain film x-rays. Croup also causes inspiratory stridor, but with symmetric subglottic narrowing radiographically and in conjunction with an episodic barking cough. Anomalies of the trachea are classified as intrinsic from primary malacia of the cartilaginous rings, or secondary to extrinsic compression of the airway from vascular rings or slings, which are very common. Symptoms include stridor, respiratory distress, and feeding difficulties. Magnetic resonance imaging (MRI) in conjunction with rigid airway endoscopy aids the surgical management.

Otolaryngologic Evaluation

Two forms of airway endoscopy exist for the evaluation of the airway: rigid and flexible and are considered complementary to each other. Rigid endoscopy remains the primary method for evaluation as it allows not only in the diagnosis, but also for tissue biopsy. The rigid bronchoscope also serves to protect the airway by allowing mechanical ventilation of the patient during the procedure. It also acts as a conduit for optical forceps, is used for foreign body removal or tissue biopsy, and for balloon dilatation of the airway with catheters. It also allows the use of fixed beam or fiberoptic laser surgery to be performed. Disadvantages to the use of the rigid bronchoscope in children include the need to perform the procedure under general anesthesia, the inability to evaluate the distal airways, and the potential inability to use it in patients with craniofacial anomalies or cervical spine fixation.

Flexible endoscopy of the nasal passages up to the glottis typically is performed in the wake patient with topical anesthesia of the nasal mucosa in the office setting. Endoscopy below the glottis should be performed in a monitored setting as local anesthesia of the glottis along with intravenous sedation is used. Flexible endoscopy is advantageous in the evaluation of dynamic processes of the upper airway, such as stridor or hoarseness. Flexible endoscopy is often performed before rigid endoscopy to help ensure that administration of anesthesia can be performed safely.

Pulmonary Perspective

Many disorders of the aerodigestive tract may present with pulmonary symptoms like chronic cough, wheezing, and recurrent respiratory tract infections. At times, different comorbidities like cystic fibrosis, primary ciliary dyskinesia, and immune deficiency can coexist, and these conditions need to be identified and treated appropriately. Aspiration is the most common clinical problem in this group of children; however, symptoms can be atypical and are often misdiagnosed. It is crucial to differentiate between structural or functional defects leading to aspiration as management depends on the etiology. Abnormalities of the upper airway may present with recurrent croup and stridor, which is described elsewhere; however, it can also present with chronic cough, wheezing, upper airway obstruction, and increased risk for SDB. In this chapter, we will focus on the common pulmonary problems encountered in this clinic and the common pulmonary complications seen in children with neurological disorders (Table 24.2).

Tracheomalacia

Tracheomalacia (TM) refers to weakness of the trachea either because of reduction in muscular fibers or cartilaginous integrity leading to softer airway, which is more susceptible to collapse leading to prolonged expiration or coughing. TM may be localized to the trachea alone or may be associated with laryngomalacia or bronchomalacia [8]. TM is the most common congenital tracheal anomaly and is commonly seen in preterm infants [9,10]. Some of the common disorders associated with TM include Tracheo-esophageal fistula (TEF), CHARGE syndrome, VATER syndrome, DiGeorge syndrome, Trisomy 21, and Pierre Robin syndrome [8]. Secondary or acquired TM may be a complication of prolonged intubation, tracheostomy, recurrent severe tracheobronchitis, vascular rings or slings compressing trachea, kyphoscoliosis, and after trauma [8]. The most common clinical presentation includes stridor, croup-like attacks, chronic barking cough, recurrent respiratory distress, wheezing, recurrent respiratory tract infections, apneic spells, and reflex apnea. TM can be diagnosed by multidetector CT (MDCT) scanning of chest and techniques with two- and three-dimensional processing of MDCT data with appropriate image interpretations. This can be done during both inspiration and expiration to assess the degree of airway collapse [11]. Magnetic resonance angiography may be more useful in identifying vascular lesions compressing the trachea [11]. However, even with recent advances in the imaging technology, the main limitation includes inadequate assessment of airways with dynamic maneuvers, particularly in young children. Hence, many experts suggest upper airway evaluation using direct airway endoscopy during spontaneous breathing under general inhalation anesthesia, thus avoiding paralytics and intubation [12].

Table 24.2 Pulmonary complications of neurological diseases in children

1. Aspiration related pulmonary problems
   - Chronic cough and wheezing
   - Recurrent pulmonary infection
   - Parenchymal lung disease
   - Reactive airway disease
   - Obstructive lung defect
   - GER related lung disease
   - Bronchiectasis
   - Bronchiolitis obliterans
2. Restrictive lung disease
   - Scoliosis and khyphosis
3. Poor airway secretion clearance–respiratory muscle weakness
   - Recurrent atelectasis
   - Chest congestion
4. Sleep-disordered breathing
   - Hypoxemia
   - Hypoventilation
   - Obstructive sleep apnea
   - Central sleep apnea

Chronic Cough

Cough is one of the most common clinical problems encountered in pediatric practice. Pediatric chronic cough (ie, cough in children aged younger than 15 years) is defined as a daily cough lasting for more than 4 weeks. This time frame was chosen based on the natural history of upper respiratory tract infections (URTIs) in children and differs from the definition of chronic cough in adults [13]. According to one study, 9% of children between 7 to 11 years of age reported chronic cough [14]. It could be due to various causes, and at times, diagnosis could be challenging. Various etiologies of chronic cough are listed in Table 24.3. Nocturnal cough is a common clinical presentation in children with asthma, GER, post-nasal drip, pertussis, aspiration, or untreated obstructive SDB. Children with neurological disorder can also present with nocturnal cough. Symptoms of asthma typically worsen during the night and early morning hours. The exacerbation of asthma during the night represents the changing status of biological functioning due to circadian rhythms in bronchial patency in relation to plasma cortisol, epinephrine, histamine,

Table 24.3 Common causes of chronic cough in children

1. Asthma
2. Protracted bacterial bronchitis
3. Cystic fibrosis
4. Primary ciliary dyskinesia
5. GERD
6. Post-nasal drip cough syndrome
7. Aspiration
8. Bronchiectasis
9. Chronic tonsillitis
10. Tracheomalacia (TM)
11. Pertussis
12. Tuberculosis
13. Bronchiolitis obliterans
14. Habit cough
15. Allergies
16. OSA

and cyclic AMP. It has been shown in healthy adults that endogenous circadian rhythms contribute to nocturnal decline in pulmonary function, with the FEV_1 nadir coinciding with the nadir of cortisol around midnight [15]. Certain chronic pulmonary disorders like cystic fibrosis and primary ciliary dyskinesia can be potentially misdiagnosed as asthma. Certain structural anomalies of airways like TM or bronchomalacia can also be confused with asthma.

Cough and Sleep

Sleep disruption is common in patients with chronic nocturnal cough. Normally, sleep suppresses cough reflex, particularly so during REM sleep [16]. There have been reports that unexplained nocturnal chronic cough may be the presenting symptom of OSA [17,18]. Most of the guidelines for evaluation and treatment of chronic cough focus on diagnosis of asthma, GER, cystic fibrosis, and bacterial bronchitis and do not give any recommendation regarding evaluation of OSA. In a recent study, children who presented with isolated undiagnosed chronic cough evaluated by polysomnography (PSG) were found to have OSA in 44%, and 93% of these patients had improvement in their cough after treatment of the OSA [18]. Hence, if there is no obvious cause of chronic cough identified, PSG should be considered to rule out OSA.

Evaluation of Chronic Cough

Detailed history including response to medications is very important in the diagnosis of chronic cough. The common etiologies for cough in children are different from those in adults. The adult-based diagnostic approach like treating asthma first followed by reflux and post-nasal drip cough may lead to misdiagnosis and diagnostic delays [19]. According to one study that evaluated etiologies of chronic cough, the final diagnosis was reached in about 91% of their patient population. The most common pre-evaluation diagnoses in their cohort were asthma (50%), no diagnosis (31%), and bronchitis (2%). The common diagnoses after extensive evaluation included protracted bronchitis (40%) with normal resolution (22%) and other minor causes included asthma, GERD, post-nasal drip cough, aspiration, bronchiectasis, OSA, and habitual cough [19]. Although a detailed discussion of evaluation of chronic cough is beyond the scope of this textbook, the various diagnostic modalities for evaluation of aerodigestive disorders including chronic cough are listed in Table 24.4.

Exercise Induced Dyspnea

The common causes of exercise induced dyspnea or shortness of breath include asthma, cardiac disease, vocal cord dysfunction (VCD), anxiety, GER, and hyperventilation [20]. VCD is a functional disorder of the vocal cords rather than a structural abnormality. The presentation can be acute with severe dyspnea, "wheezing", and/or throat closure. Patients are usually misdiagnosed as asthma [21], but their pulmonary function tests are usually normal, and they fail to respond adequately to bronchodilators and/or steroids. They typically resolve spontaneously with a period of rest. Diagnosis involves direct visualization of vocal cord using a flexible laryngoscope following exercise challenge to look for vocal cord adduction that persists during both inspiration and expiration. Treatment involves involvement of a speech-language pathologist (SLP) who can teach patients to take control of vocal cord motions voluntarily. Use of ipratropium bromide aerosol inhaler before exercise may help prevent the symptoms, suggesting that this disorder may be vagally mediated [22].

Table 24.4 Various tests for evaluation of aerodigestive disorders

Test	Diagnosis
1. Sweat test	Cystic fibrosis
2. Immune work up	Immune deficiency
3. Chest x-ray (CXR)	Hyperinflation, pneumonia, atelecteasis, and follow-up
4. Chest CT scan/MDCT	Bronchiectasis and interstitial lung disease/airway malacia
5. Pulmonary function tests	Obstructive and restrictive lung defect
6. Exercise and cold air challenge tests	Asthma
7. Triple endoscopy	
▶ Rigid upper airway endoscopy	▶ Laryngomalacia, laryngeal cleft, and subglottic stenosis
▶ Flexible pulmonary bronchoscopy	▶ Airway inflammation, pulmonary toileting, TM, and obtain BAL
▶ Upper GI endoscopy and biopsy	▶ Esophagitis and celiac disease
8. Flexible nasopharyngoscopy	Adenoidal hypertrophy, VCD, FEES, and laryngeal irritation
9. Allergy work up (RAST and skin test)	Environmental and food allergies
10. Sinus CT	Chronic sinusitis
11. Modified swallow study	Aspiration from above
12. Radionuclide salivogram	Salivary aspiration
13. Upper GI study	TEF, malrotation of intestine, and vascular rings
14. pH probe/impedance	GER
15. Esophageal manometry	Esophageal dysmotility and cricopharyngeal achalasia
16. Radionucleotide gastric emptying scan	Delayed gastric emptying
17. Naso-ciliary biopsy	Primary ciliary dyskinesia (PCD)
18. Genetic testing	
▶ CF testing (eg., Delta F508)	▶ Cystic fibrosis
▶ PCD testing (eg., DNAI1, DNAH5)	▶ Primary ciliary dyskinesia
19. Polysomnogram	Sleep-disordered breathing
20. MRI brain	Arnold–Chiari malformation (vocal cord paresis)

Aspiration Related Lung Disease

Chronic pulmonary aspiration is defined as repeated passages of food material, gastric refluxate, and/or saliva into the subglottic airways in a manner sufficient to cause chronic or recurrent respiratory symptoms [23]. Aspiration can occur at multiple levels; it can occur at upper level due to swallowing dysfunction (due to anatomical defects such as laryngeal cleft or neuromuscular dysco-ordination), mid level as in TEF, and at lower level as in GER. The common manifestations of chronic pulmonary aspiration include chronic cough, recurrent wheezing, recurrent pneumonia, choking and coughing with feeds, tachypnea, and apparent life-threatening event (ALTE). Long standing pulmonary aspiration can potentially result in lung injury. There is currently no gold standard test for diagnosing chronic pulmonary aspiration; hence, a multidisciplinary approach in evaluation and identifying the cause of aspiration is much needed.

Evaluation of Chronic Aspiration in Children

The following tests are commonly used for evaluation of aspiration in children.

Videofluroscopic Swallow Study or Modified Barium Swallow Study (MBS)

This can evaluate both oral and pharyngeal phases of swallowing. An SLP and a radiologist are the integral part of the evaluation team. This test can evaluate premature spillage, velopharyngeal insufficiency, penetration, aspiration in to trachea, residue after swallow, and subsequent clearance of the residue. This test is generally effective in evaluating swallowing, assesses risk for aspiration, and makes feeding recommendations [24]. The limitation of this test is high false negative rate, subsequent risk for aspiration pneumonia [25], poor inter- and intra-observers reliability, and the associated risk of radiation exposure. As aspiration can occur intermittently, this can be completely missed on the MBS. Hence, a completely normal MBS does not rule out aspiration.

Fiberoptic Endoscopic Evaluation of Swallowing

This study involves an otolaryngologist and an SLP working together. It evaluates all phases of swallowing including the functional anatomy. This involves direct visualization of the swallowing of the food bolus. It can be done at the bedside, and there is no risk for radiation and/or sedation. A nasopharygyngoscope is placed just below the soft palate and above the epiglottis, and multiple swallows using different consistencies are directly visualized by the otolaryngologist and SLP on the video monitor. It can assess premature spillage, penetration, aspiration, post swallow residue, and attempts to clear the residue. Fiberoptic Endoscopic Evaluation of Swallowing (FEES) in children should be used as a complimentary test to MBS. Although there is a general agreement between the results obtained from MBS and FEES, FEES can provide independent information, which can help in accurately diagnosing swallowing abnormalities in certain situations [26].

Salivary Aspiration

Chronic salivary aspiration is one of the least commonly recognized forms of aspiration and is usually diagnosed late. These children are at risk for recurrent aspiration pneumonia, reactive airway disease, and lung abscess. Most of these children are neurologically challenged and have difficulty with handling salivary secretions due to abnormal neuromuscular swallowing mechanisms. Other causes of salivary aspiration include laryngo-tracheo-esophageal clefts, vocal cord paralysis, CHARGE syndrome, and other craniofacial defects [23]. Radioactive tracer is placed in the mouth and serial images are recorded to assess radioactivity in the trachea or lungs to confirm aspiration. This test can be used in children who are not fed orally; therefore, no oral challenge is necessary.

Gastroesophageal Reflux and Extraesophageal Manifestation

In addition to the common gastrointestinal complaints of reflux, there are several extraesophageal symptoms of GER including chronic cough, laryngitis, hoarseness of voice, wheezing, chest pain, recurrent sinus or ear infections, sleep disturbances, SDB, and aspiration related parenchymal lung injury [27, 28]. The evaluation of GER is described elsewhere.

Pulmonary Function Tests

These tests include spirometry, lung volumes, exercise or cold air challenge testing, flow-volume loops, diffusing capacity of carbon monoxide (DLCO), and maximal respiratory pressure. Spirometry can be performed in children 6 years of age or older; it can be performed before and after administration of bronchodilators to assess reversibility. Certain airway provocation testing like exercise, cold air and methacholine challenge can be used to induce bronchospasm in patients with normal baseline spirometry, which can help in the diagnosis of asthma. Flow-volume loops can be obtained before and after the challenge to evaluate any extrathoracic, intrathoracic, or fixed airway obstruction. It can also be helpful in the evaluation of vocal cord dysfunction. DLCO helps to assess interstitial lung disease in conditions such as idiopathic interstitial pneumonitis and post infectious bronchiolitis obliterans. Maximal respiratory pressure helps to assess respiratory muscle weakness such as in children with Duchenne's muscular dystrophy. The symptoms of hypoventilation in patients' neuromuscular disorders include headache, lethargy, anorexia, and poor growth. In patients with neuromuscular disorders, pulmonary function tests can predict presence of hypoventilation. In adults, REM hypoventilation ensues when inspiratory vital capacity (IVC) less than 60% predicted and maximal inspiratory pressures (MIP) less than 45 cm H2O, continuous nocturnal hypoventilation occurs when IVC $<$ 40% predicted and MIP $<$ 40 cm H2O, and daytime hypoventilation ensues when IVC $<$ 35% predicted and MIP $<$ 35 cm H2O. Hence, annual screening pulmonary functions should be considered in patients with neuromuscular disorders who are older than 6 years and/or when there are symptoms of hypoventilation described previously to predict onset of respiratory muscle weakness.

Fiberoptic Flexible Bronchoscopy

Fiberoptic flexible bronchoscopy (FFB) allows one to visualize the upper airways, trachea, and gives access to more distal tracheobronchial tree to assess airway anatomy, airway inflammation, airway compression, foreign body, endobronchial lesions, characteristic of airway secretion, as well as dynamic movements to assess tracheobronchomalacia. It can also help to obtain samples of airway secretions via bronchoalveolar lavage (BAL). It can be performed through the nose, using a laryngeal mask airway (LMA) or through an endotracheal tube. Different size scopes can be used based on the age of the child. It can be done under conscious sedation or general anesthesia. The BAL is performed using bacteriostatic normal saline to assess end organ damage. BAL samples can be sent for cytology and microbiological testing. Neutrophils and lipid laden macrophage index (LLMI) in BAL can act as surrogate markers of lung inflammation.

Sleep Evaluation in Children With Aerodigestive Disorders

Although there is no data looking into the incidence of sleep-related problems in children with aerodigestive disorders, our experience suggests that sleep disturbances and sleep-related breathing disorders are common. Sleep symptoms are often under-reported by the parents as the main focus of their visit relates to the underlying pulmonary or gastrointestinal problems. As sleep can be affected by multiple factors like chronic nocturnal cough, medication effect on sleep, and GER. In fact these children may present with significant sleep disruption. As a result of chronic sleep fragmentation due to various aforementioned causes, they may present with daytime somnolence, learning difficulties, adverse cardiovascular findings, and/or neurocognitive impairment. Laryngomalacia, TM, chronic cough, GER, associated craniofacial malformations, and neuromuscular disorders along with adenotonsillar hypertrophy are the common causes of OSA in this population. We recommend a careful sleep history in all children referred to the aerodigestive disorder clinic to determine whether a sleep study is indicated.

Common Abnormalities Noted on Polysomnography

In our anecdotal experience, the common PSG findings observed in children with aerodigestive disorders include frequent disruption of sleep architecture and sleep fragmentation due to frequent arousals caused by the various conditions mentioned previously. In addition, respiratory abnormalities noted during sleep include a wide spectrum of obstructive SDB, hypoxemia, and hypoventilation particularly during REM sleep. Patient with brain stem abnormalities (Chiari malformation) and certain neuromuscular disorders can also present with central sleep apnea and central hypoventilation [29]. SDB can be potentially worse in supine position in patients with laryngomalacia, obesity, neuromuscular disorders, and GER.

Pulmonary Disease and Severity of Sleep Disordered Breathing

Nocturnal hypoxemia can be a sign of underlying parenchymal lung disease and/or hypoventilation. Long-standing hypoxemia may reset the central ventilatory chemoreceptors to accommodate chronic hypercapnia and can tolerate longer period of hypoxemia, which then becomes the predominant drive for respiration in these situations. However, sleep-related hypoxemia can result in dramatic desaturation, even with milder obstructive events, as well as with brief central pauses; hence, the degree of SDB may be potentially overestimated. With persistent nocturnal hypoxemia, even mild degree of obstructive events can result in dramatic desaturation. Hence, recognizing the cause of persistent nocturnal hypoxemia is very important as appropriate treatment is based on diagnosis, such as bi-level ventilation for hypoventilation and oxygen therapy for parenchymal lung disease.

Gastroenterological Perspective

There is a complex interaction between the gastrointestinal tract and the lungs, which has necessitated a multidisciplinary approach to the patient with chronic lung disease. The primary role of the gastroenterologist is threefold: to rule out anatomic abnormalities that may be contributing to the lung disease, to evaluate for the presence and causes of GER, and to evaluate for allergic gastrointestinal diseases such as eosinophilic esophagitis. Extensive testing may suggest an association between the lung and gastrointestinal disease but proving causality is often difficult. This is especially true of GER which has been associated with many diseases including asthma, chronic cough, OSA, and hoarseness. Treatment of these conditions with antireflux therapy has produced inconsistent results, suggesting that while pathologic reflux may be present, its role in disease causality is not clear [30].

In particular, GER is common in patients with sleep disorders. More than 12% of patients with sleep disorders have symptoms of reflux [31]. Conversely, in patients with GER, the rates of sleep disorders are three times higher than in patients without reflux [32]. To explain the pathophysiology of reflux and sleep disorders, multiple different testing modalities including esophageal pH monitoring and esophageal motility testing have been employed. During episodes of airway obstruction, intraesophageal pressures fall accompanied by a concurrent rise in lower esophageal sphincter and upper esophageal sphincter pressures [33]. While the reduction in esophageal body pressures should, in theory, create a favorable environment for reflux, the rise in sphincter pressure effectively prevents reflux to such an extent that reflux only occurs in up to one quarter of all obstructive events, and when it does occur, it occurs during transient lower esophageal sphincter relaxations [34].

When reflux does occur during sleep, it tends to occur during times when sleep is the lightest, during N1 and N2 phases [33]. The presence of acid in the esophagus produces arousals in both patients with GERD and in healthy controls [35]. Examination of the overall nocturnal reflux burden, however, has shown that although the number of reflux events is reduced during sleep, clearance of reflux is often delayed because of reductions in swallowing, particularly during the deep sleep stages [36]. The reduction in swallows combined with decrease sensation at night results in more proximal reflux events, which can have a direct impact on the airway [37]. Reflux effects may be further potentiated by the reduction in the salivary bicarbonate as well as total saliva volume at night, which results in more esophageal and airway acid exposure [38].

There are two primary mechanisms by which reflux might affect the airway: a direct effect from aspiration or a neurally-mediated effect. There are studies in both animals and adults which suggest that acid instillation into the trachea results in increased lung resistance and decreased sensitivity of the larynx, which leads to a predisposition for further aspiration of acidic contents [39,40]. Recently, there has been an increasing body of literature on the damaging effects of bile, another component of gastric refluxate, on the lung. The mechanism by which this damage occurs is unknown, but one hypothesis is that bile depletes or inactivates the surfactant stores or has a direct proinflammatory effect [41,42]. Bile may have clinical ramifications as well; the presence of bile in the lungs of transplant patients is associated with an increased risk of bronchiolitis obliterans in the transplanted lungs and changes in lung flora [43].

The second pathway, that of neurally-mediated damage, stems from animal and human studies which show that airway resistance increases with distal esophageal acid infusion [44,45]. Interestingly, apart from the impact on resistance, there is animal data to suggest that the stimulation of the distal esophagus with acid results in release of inflammatory mediators in the lung [46]; whether this occurs in humans is unknown. There is only one pediatric study which looked at the impact of distal acid infusion on pulmonary function in 9 children with a history of nocturnal asthma; patients who experienced heartburn with distal HCl acid infusion also had evidence of concomitant bronchoconstriction and overt wheezing [47].

Relationship Between Reflux and Sleep Disturbances

The complex relationship between GER, pulmonary manifestations, and sleep disorders has been the topic of several studies but understanding remains incomplete. Sleep-related GER is associated with poor sleep quality, arousals from sleep, and daytime fatigue in adults [48]. It is unclear whether these findings simply reflect common risk factors or truly indicate a cause-and-effect relationship. The concept of a causal connection is supported by recent studies that demonstrated improvements in both subjective and objective measures of sleep function following treatment of GER with acid-suppression medications [49–51].

The clinical consequences and impact of nighttime GER on sleep quality may be unique compared to GER experienced during the daytime. In addition to typical manifestations such as heartburn and acid regurgitation, GER has been linked to pediatric SDB, with conditions ranging from apnea in infants, to upper airway resistance syndrome (UARS) and OSA syndrome (OSAS) in older children. SDB is believed to occur in 1% to 3% of children [52], but pediatric data examining the clinical connection between GER and SDB is limited.

The majority of pediatric research has focused on the relationship between GER and respiratory abnormalities in infants, though not necessarily limited to sleep. While several studies demonstrated a positive association between episodes of GER with apnea [53–55], others showed a poor temporal correlation [56–58]. There is also debate whether the link between reflux and certain sleep disorders may be bidirectional. OSA has been hypothesized to cause more negative intraesophageal pressures, which could increase the predisposition to GER [59]. One study found that although GER appeared to be overall more frequent in children with OSAS, reflux parameters did not correlate to OSAS severity, and a temporal relationship between GER and apnea-hypopnea events was not observed [60].

Further studies are needed to corroborate findings in adults, which have suggested a stronger link between GER and OSAS. Not only have adults with OSAS been found to experience more sleep-related reflux than healthy controls [61], treatment of OSA with continuous positive airway pressure (CPAP) reduced GER [62–64], and treatment of GER with acid-suppression improved OSAS parameters [65,66]; while these findings are suggestive, they also highlight the incomplete understanding of the nature and direction of the relationship between OSAS and GERD. Whether a cause-and-effect relationship between GER and sleep disturbances exists is not conclusive, and it may depend on the specific age and clinical manifestation of interest.

Diagnostic Testing

Multiple different tools have been used to evaluate reflux in children and adults.

Barium Contrast Radiography

Barium contrast studies of the esophagus are neither sensitive nor specific for the diagnosis of GERD. Compared to esophageal pH monitoring, the sensitivity of the upper GI (UGI) series ranges from 30% to 70% [67,68]. The UGI series may be helpful to rule out anatomic abnormalities such as esophageal stricture, achalasia, TEF or intestinal malrotation, which can present similarly to GERD. Because the UGI series provides only a snapshot in time however, there is a risk of false-negative results for the detection of reflux. On the other hand, presence of reflux episodes during an examination does not necessarily indicate pathologic reflux either. Radiographic studies, therefore, are not primarily useful to diagnose reflux or GERD.

Nuclear scintigraphy: Evidence of GER and aspiration can be documented using gastroesophageal scintigraphy in which patients ingest food or formula labeled with 99-technetium followed by scanning of the stomach, esophagus, and lungs to detect the distribution of the isotope. Potential advantages compared to esophageal pH monitoring are the ability to demonstrate the reflux of nonacidic gastric contents and assessment of the rate of gastric emptying, which may be delayed in children with GERD. Sensitivity for the detection of acid reflux was only 79% when compared to 24-hour esophageal pH monitoring [69]. As a result, nuclear scintigraphy is not recommended in the routine diagnosis and management of GERD in infants and children.

Esophageal pH monitoring: Esophageal pH monitoring, which quantifies the frequency and duration of acid reflux episodes, can be used to confirm abnormal esophageal acid exposure and/or correlate symptoms with acid reflux episodes. Most tests are performed using a transnasal catheter with a pH sensor located in the distal esophagus, typically for 24 hours. Episodes of acid reflux are conventionally identified by a drop in intraesophageal pH less than 4. The reflux index, which is the percentage of the entire monitoring period with pH less than 4, is generally considered the single most important variable in clinical practice with well-established normative cutoffs for infants and children [70]. The estimated sensitivity of pH monitoring for reflux esophagitis ranges from 83% to 100% [71], but the sensitivity of pH monitoring for GERD, which includes both erosive and nonerosive disease, has been difficult to ascertain.

Proximal or pharyngeal pH monitoring: The addition of a second pH sensor in the proximal esophagus or pharynx has been used to enhance the evaluation of supraesophageal manifestations of GERD, such as cough, wheezing, or laryngitis (Figure 24.3). Current limitations of proximal pH monitoring, however, include a lack of consensus on the best anatomic location for proximal probe placement and ongoing debate regarding the optimal pH criteria for the detection of a clinically significant proximal reflux event. Studies employing proximal pH monitoring in children have had mixed results in terms of sensitivity and specificity for supraesophageal manifestations of reflux as well as intra-subject reproducibility [72,73]. Although new devices for the monitoring of proximal esophageal and pharyngeal pH have been introduced, the clinical advantage of these diagnostic tests is not yet clearly proven.

Multi-channel intraluminal impedance with pH (pH-MII): pH-MII is a pH-independent method of measuring reflux. The catheter that has 7 impedance sensors and 1 distal pH sensor offers advantages over the standard pH probe, because the catheter can (1) differentiate the direction of flow (swallows versus reflux), (2) identify the height of the refluxate at 6 different heights, and (3) detect both acid and nonacid reflux (Figure 24.4). In the pediatric population, who have significantly more nonacid reflux particularly in the postprandial period, this technology offers significant advantages. In the realm of sleep disorders, the catheter is able to detect full column reflux, which may predispose patients to obstructive events, if aspirated. In the pediatric population, the sensitivity of pH-MII in patients who were not taking acid suppression therapy was 76 ± 13 compared to the pH probe whose sensitivity was 80 ± 18. When patients taking acid suppression were studied, the sensitivity of the pH probe dropped to 47 ± 36, whereas the sensitivity of pH-MII in treated patients was 80 ± 21 [74]. In untreated infants, the sensitivity of pH-MII to detect acid reflux events was 54% compared to the pH probe [75].

Esophageal manometry: Esophageal manometry is used to evaluate the motor function of the esophagus and can determine the efficacy of the upper and lower esophageal sphincter relaxations and esophageal peristalsis. Standard manometry catheters have a pressure sleeve and 4 to 8 sensors at different spacings depending on the size patient being studied. During sleep studies, manometry has been used to document the mechanisms of reflux (relaxations of the sphincter) relative to obstructive sleep events, and to clarify the airway protective mechanisms of the sphincters. In the last several years, high resolution manometry, which uses 36 pressure sensors, has been used to evaluate the esophagus; it offers the advantage of having more data on multiple different esophageal heights simultaneously such that both upper and lower sphincters as well as the esophageal body can be studied without needing to pull the sensors through the esophagus to capture the different esophageal regions. While manometry has been found to be extremely sensitive in detecting reflux events, manometry is not used routinely in the evaluation of GER because of the time-consuming nature of interpretation, its inability to detect the type (acid versus nonacid), and duration of reflux events [76].

Utility of esophageal pH, impedance and pressure monitoring during polysomnography: Although there is data to support the association of GER with sleep disturbances in general, the diagnosis of SDB secondary to GER in a given individual is not always clear. PSG can show an abnormal pattern of breathing, but the pathologic mechanisms may not be evident. On the other hand, separate establishment of pathologic GER by esophageal pH monitoring in a patient with an abnormal PSG does not necessarily confirm that GER is the cause of the breathing disorder either. Simultaneous recording of PSG variables and esophageal pH has the potential to reveal a cause-and-effect relationship between GER and SDB, and ultimately offer guidance in treating the underlying mechanism.

In studies of infants with unexplained SDB who were examined with simultaneous PSG and esophageal pH monitoring, GER and apnea were both relatively common findings, but they were temporally related in only 1% to 7% of patients [77,78]. One possible explanation for the lack of a strong relationship between changes in esophageal pH and apnea in infants may be due to a failure to account for nonacidic episodes of reflux. The addition of multichannel intraluminal impedance-pH (MII-pH) monitoring in conjunction with PSG in infants with a history of breathing irregularities was shown to increase the percentage of apnea episodes related to reflux from 6% with pH monitoring alone to 30% with MII-pH [79].

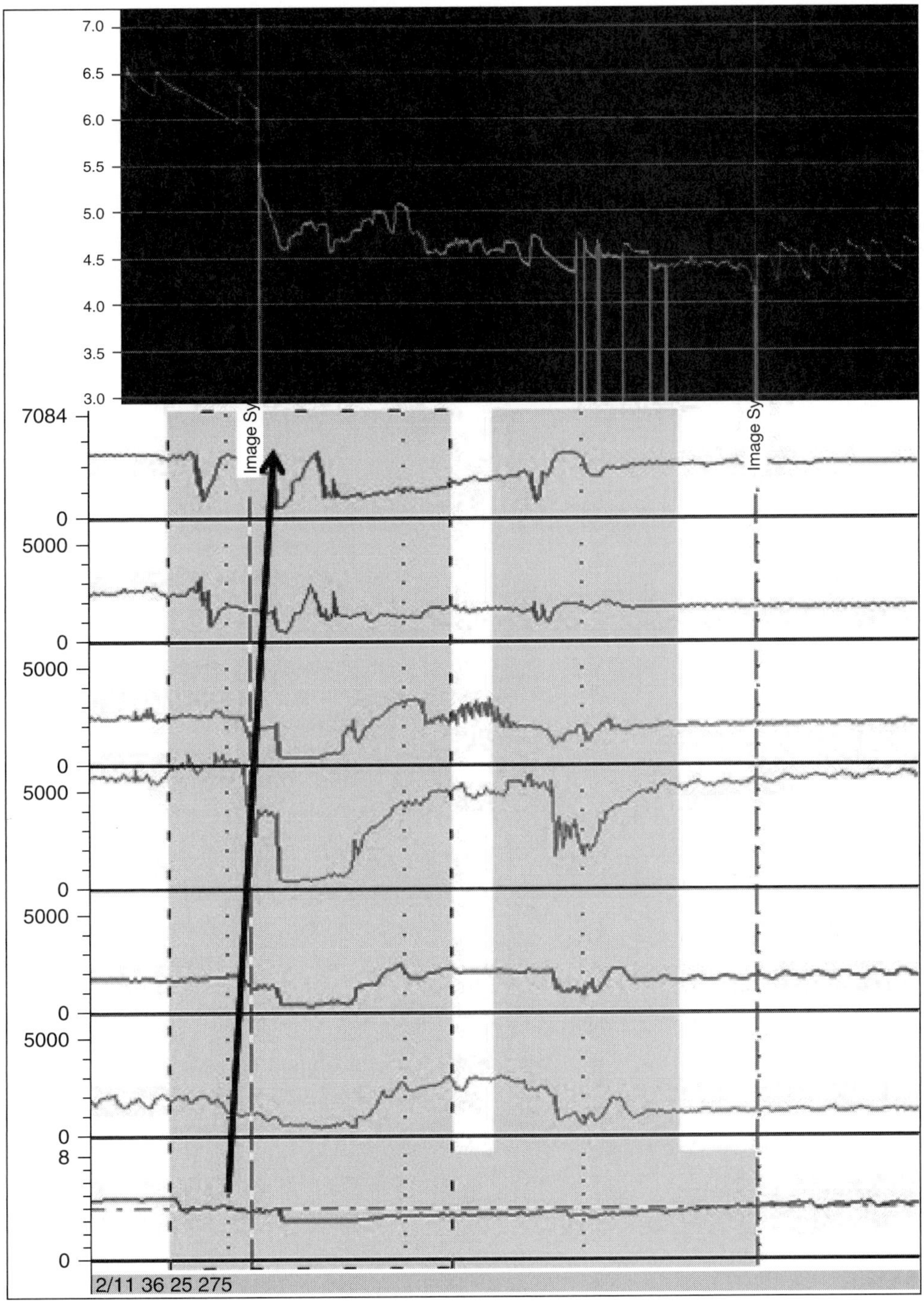

Figure 24.3 This combined diagram shows simultaneous recording of a reflux event with pharyngeal pH (top tracing) and esophageal MII-pH monitoring (bottom tracing with 6 impedance channels and distal pH). The acute drop in pharyngeal pH is preceded by a drop in distal esophageal pH as well as evidence of retrograde liquid reflux (arrow) on esophageal impedance monitoring.

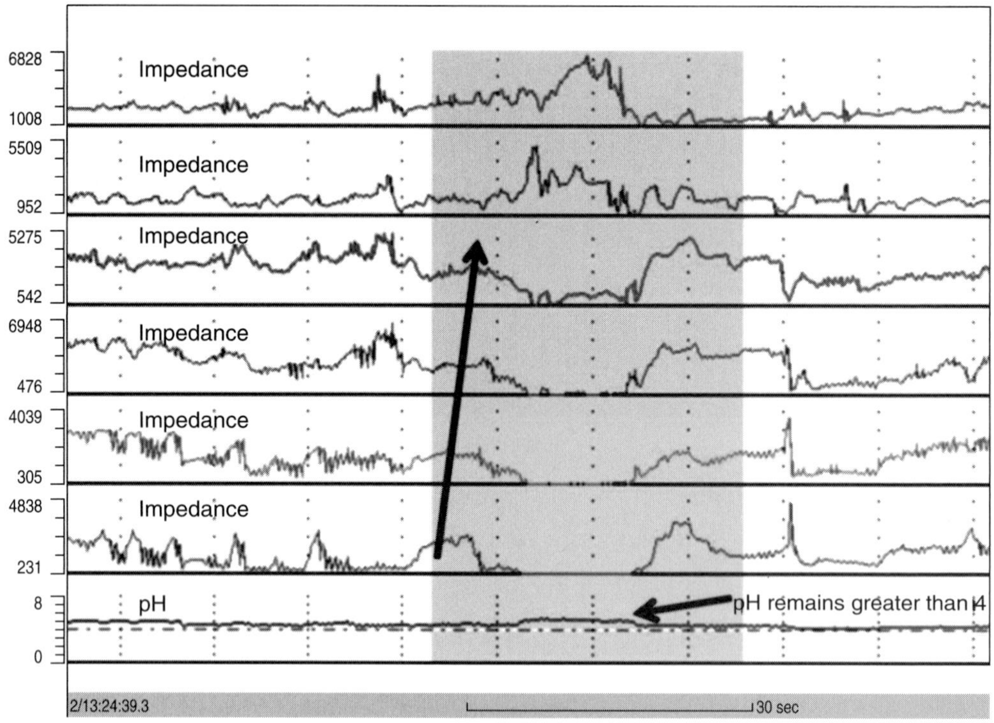

Figure 24.4 An example of a nonacid reflux episode. There is a drop in impedance that progresses from the distal esophagus proximally (long arrow). The lack of an associated drop in pH to less than 4 categorizes this as a nonacid reflux episode.

On the other hand, a more recent study using MII-pH found that less than 3% of cardiorespiratory events were preceded by either acid or nonacid reflux in preterm infants [80]. Therefore, because the relationship between GER and SDB remains controversial, there is currently insufficient evidence to support the routine use of simultaneous pH monitoring with PSG in infants with apnea. The addition of MII-pH may increase the yield of testing, but further studies are needed to establish whether nonacid reflux is clinically significant in the development of SDB in children.

The addition of esophageal pressure monitoring (EPM) to PSG has not been customarily used to improve the diagnosis of GER, but it is considered the gold standard for detection of increasing upper airway resistance that leads to arousals and for differentiation between obstructive and central apneas [81]. The use of EPM in the evaluation of SDB in children is now routine in some clinical centers [82]. From a research perspective, EPM may also ultimately help to elucidate the relationship between GER and OSAS by shedding light on changes in intraesophageal and esophageal sphincter pressures relative to both events [33].

Conclusion

In summary, children with aerodigestive disorders present with multisystem involvement along with atypical symptoms which can be challenging for appropriate diagnosis. Multiple medical as well as surgical problems coexist; hence, assessment should include a careful history along with coordinated evaluation and communication with other specialist. Therefore, a multidisciplinary team approach is optimal for comprehensive evaluation and time efficient management for these complex disorders. In addition, sleep problems are also common in aerodigestive disorders in children; hence, screening for sleep-related problems helps with their early diagnosis and appropriate treatment, which will ultimately prevent its long-term adverse cardiovascular and neurodevelopment outcomes.

References

1. Sculerati N, Gottlieb MD, Zimbler MS, Chibbaro PD, McCarthy JG. Airway management in children with major craniofacial anomalies. *Laryngoscope*. 1998;108(12):1806–1812.
2. Rutter MJ. Evaluation and management of upper airway disorders in children. *Semin Pediatr Surg*. 2006;15(2):116–123.
3. Ramsden JD, Campisi P, Forte V. Choanal atresia and choanal stenosis. *Otolaryngol Clin North Am*. 2009;42(2):339–352, x.
4. Darrow DH, Siemens C. Indications for tonsillectomy and adenoidectomy. *Laryngoscope*. 2002: 112(8, pt 2)(suppl 100):6–10.
5. Zoumalan R, Maddalozzo J, Holinger LD. Etiology of stridor in infants. *Ann Otol Rhinol Laryngol*. 2007;116(5):329–334.
6. Zafereo ME, Taylor RJ, Pereira KD. Supraglottoplasty for laryngomalacia with obstructive sleep apnea. *Laryngoscope*. 2008;118(10):1873–1877.
7. Miyamoto RC, Parikh SR, Gellad W, Licameli GR. Bilateral congenital vocal cord paralysis: a 16-year institutional review. *Otolaryngol Head Neck Surg*. 2005;133(2):241–245.
8. Carden KA, Boiselle PM, Waltz DA, Ernst A. Tracheomalacia and tracheobronchomalacia in children and adults: an in-depth review. *Chest*. 2005;127(3):984–1005.
9. Holinger LD. Etiology of stridor in the neonate, infant and child. *Ann Otol Rhinol Laryngol*. 1980;89(5, pt 1):397–400.
10. Jacobs IN, Wetmore RF, Tom LW, Handler SD, Potsic WP. Tracheobronchomalacia in children. *Arch Otolaryngol Head Neck Surg*. 1994; 120(2): 154–158.
11. Lee EY, Boiselle PM. Tracheobronchomalacia in infants and children: multidetector CT evaluation. *Radiology*. 2009;252(1):7–22.
12. Benjamin B. Tracheomalacia in infants and children. *Ann Otol Rhinol Laryngol*. 1984;93(5, pt 1): 438–442.
13. Chang AB, Glomb WB. Guidelines for evaluating chronic cough in pediatrics: ACCP evidence-based clinical practice guidelines. *Chest*. 2006;129(1) (suppl):260S-283S.
14. Leonardi GS, Houthuijs D, Nikiforov B, et al. Respiratory symptoms, bronchitis and asthma in children of Central and Eastern Europe. *Eur Respir J*. 2002;20(4):890–898.
15. Spengler CM, Shea SA. Endogenous circadian rhythm of pulmonary function in healthy humans. *Am J Respir Crit Care Med*. 2000;162(3, pt 1): 1038–1046.
16. Lee KK, Birring SS. Cough and sleep. *Lung*. 2010;188(suppl 1):S91–S94.
17. Chan KK, Ing AJ, Laks L, Cossa G, Rogers P, Birring SS. Chronic cough in patients with sleep-disordered breathing. *Eur Respir J*. 2010;35(2): 368–372.
18. Sundar KM, Daly SE, Pearce MJ, Alward WT. Chronic cough and obstructive sleep apnea in a community-based pulmonary practice. *Cough*. 2010;6(1):2.
19. Marchant JM, Masters IB, Taylor SM, Cox NC, Seymour GJ, Chang AB. Evaluation and outcome of young children with chronic cough. *Chest*. 2006;129(5):1132–1141.
20. Weinberger M, Abu-Hasan M. Pseudo-asthma: when cough, wheezing, and dyspnea are not asthma. *Pediatrics*. 2007;120(4):855–864.
21. Christopher KL, Wood RP II, Eckert RC, Blager FB, Raney RA, Souhrada JF. Vocal-cord dysfunction presenting as asthma. *N Engl J Med*. 1983; 308(26):1566–1570.
22. Ayres JG, Gabbott PL. Vocal cord dysfunction and laryngeal hyperresponsiveness: a function of altered autonomic balance? *Thorax*. 2002;57(4): 284–285.
23. Boesch RP, Daines C, Willging JP, et al. Advances in the diagnosis and management of chronic pulmonary aspiration in children. *Eur Respir J*. 2006;28(4):847–861.
24. Martin-Harris B, Logemann JA, McMahon S, Schleicher M, Sandidge J. Clinical utility of the modified barium swallow. *Dysphagia*. 2000;15(3): 136–141.
25. Croghan JE, Burke EM, Caplan S, Denman S. Pilot study of 12-month outcomes of nursing home patients with aspiration on videofluoroscopy. *Dysphagia*. 1994;9(3):141–146.
26. Leder SB, Karas DE. Fiberoptic endoscopic evaluation of swallowing in the pediatric population. *Laryngoscope*. 2000;110(7):1132–1136.
27. Malfertheiner MV, Kandulski A, Malfertheiner P, Schreiber J. [Bronchopulmonary manifestations of gastroesophageal reflux disease]. *Internist (Berl)*. 2010;51(suppl 1):246–254.
28. Moore JM, Vaezi MF. Extraesophageal manifestations of gastroesophageal reflux disease: real or imagined? *Curr Opin Gastroenterol*. 2010;26(4): 389–394.
29. Seddon PC, Khan Y. Respiratory problems in children with neurological impairment. *Arch Dis Child*. 2003;88(1):75–78.
30. Kahrilas PJ, Shaheen NJ, Vaezi MF, et al. American Gastroenterological Association Institute technical review on the management of gastroesophageal reflux disease. *Gastroenterology*. 2008;135(4): 1392–1413, 1413, e1–e5.
31. Guda N, Partington S, Shaw MJ, Leo G, Vakil N. Unrecognized GERD symptoms are associated with excessive daytime sleepiness in patients undergoing sleep studies. *Dig Dis Sci*. 2007; 52(10):2873–2876.
32. Jansson C, Nordenstedt H, Wallander MA, et al. A population-based study showing an association between gastroesophageal reflux disease and sleep problems. *Clin Gastroenterol Hepatol*. 2009;7(9):960–965.
33. Kuribayashi S, Kusano M, Kawamura O, et al. Mechanism of gastroesophageal reflux in patients with obstructive sleep apnea syndrome. *Neurogastroenterol Motil*. 2010; Jun;22(6):611–e172.
34. Kuribayashi S, Massey BT, Hafeezullah M, et al. Upper esophageal sphincter and gastroesophageal junction pressure changes act to prevent gastroesophageal and esophagopharyngeal reflux during

apneic episodes in patients with obstructive sleep apnea. *Chest*. 2010;137(4):769–776.
35. Orr WC, Johnson LF, Robinson MG. Effect of sleep on swallowing, esophageal peristalsis, and acid clearance. *Gastroenterology*. 1984;86(5, pt 1): 814–819.
36. Kahrilas PJ, Dodds WJ, Dent J, Haeberle B, Hogan WJ, Arndorfer RC. Effect of sleep, spontaneous gastroesophageal reflux, and a meal on upper esophageal sphincter pressure in normal human volunteers. *Gastroenterology*. 1987;92(2): 466–471.
37. Orr WC, Elsenbruch S, Harnish MJ, Johnson LF. Proximal migration of esophageal acid perfusions during waking and sleep. *Am J Gastroenterol*. 2000;95(1):37–42.
38. Schneyer LH, Pigman W, Hanahan L, Gilmore RW. Rate of flow of human parotid, sublingual, and submaxillary secretions during sleep. *J Dent Res*. 1956;35(1):109–114.
39. Sant'Ambrogio FB, G. Sant'Ambrogio, Chung K. Effects of HCl-pepsin laryngeal instillations on upper airway patency-maintaining mechanisms. *J Appl Physiol*. 1998;84(4):1299–1304.
40. Allen GB, Leclair TR, von Reyn J, et al. Acid aspiration-induced airways hyperresponsiveness in mice. *J Appl Physiol*. 2009;107(6):1763–1770.
41. D'Ovidio F, Mura M, Ridsdale R, et al. The effect of reflux and bile acid aspiration on the lung allograft and its surfactant and innate immunity molecules SP-A and SP-D. *Am J Transplant*. 2006;6(8):1930–1938.
42. Zecca E, De Luca D, Baroni S, Vento G, Tiberi E, Romagnoli C. Bile acid-induced lung injury in newborn infants: a bronchoalveolar lavage fluid study. *Pediatrics*. 2008;121(1):e146–e149.
43. Blondeau K, Mertens V, Vanaudenaerde BA, et al. Gastro-oesophageal reflux and gastric aspiration in lung transplant patients with or without chronic rejection. *Eur Respir J*. 2008;31(4): 707–713.
44. Schan CA, Harding SM, Haile JM, Bradley LA, Richter JE. Gastroesophageal reflux-induced bronchoconstriction. An intraesophageal acid infusion study using state-of-the-art technology. *Chest*. 1994;106(3):731–737.
45. Harding SM, Schan CA, Guzzo MR, Alexander RW, Bradley LA, Richter JE. Gastroesophageal reflux-induced bronchoconstriction. Is microaspiration a factor? *Chest*. 1995;108(5):1220–1227.
46. Hamamoto J, Kohrogi H, Kawano O, et al. Esophageal stimulation by hydrochloric acid causes neurogenic inflammation in the airways in guinea pigs. *J Appl Physiol*. 1997;82(3):738–745.
47. Davis RS, Larsen GL, Grunstein MM. Respiratory response to intraesophageal acid infusion in asthmatic children during sleep. *J Allergy Clin Immunol*. 1983;72(4):393–398.
48. Dubois RW, Aguilar D, Fass R, et al. Consequences of frequent nocturnal gastro-oesophageal reflux disease among employed adults: symptom severity, quality of life and work productivity. *Aliment Pharmacol Ther*. 2007;25(4):487–500.
49. Johnson DA, Orr WC, Crawley JA, et al. Effect of esomeprazole on nighttime heartburn and sleep quality in patients with GERD: a randomized, placebo-controlled trial. *Am J Gastroenterol*. 2005;100(9):1914–1922.
50. Orr WC, Goodrich S, Robert J. The effect of acid suppression on sleep patterns and sleep-related gastro-oesophageal reflux. *Aliment Pharmacol Ther*. 2005;21(2): 103–108.
51. Dimarino Jr AJ, Banwait KS, Eschinger E, et al. The effect of gastro-oesophageal reflux and omeprazole on key sleep parameters. *Aliment Pharmacol Ther*. 2005;22(4): 325–329.
52. Redline S, Tishler PV, Schluchter M, Aylor J, Clark K, Graham G. Risk factors for sleep-disordered breathing in children. Associations with obesity, race, and respiratory problems. *Am J Respir Crit Care Med*. 1999;159(5, pt 1):1527–1532.
53. Menon AP, Schefft GL, Thach BT. Apnea associated with regurgitation in infants. *J Pediatr*. 1985;106(4):625–629.
54. Sacre L, Vandenplas Y. Gastroesophageal reflux associated with respiratory abnormalities during sleep. *J Pediatr Gastroenterol Nutr*. 1989;9(1): 28–33.
55. Corvaglia L, Zama D, Gualdi S, Ferlini M, Aceti A, Faldella G. Gastro-oesophageal reflux increases the number of apnoeas in very preterm infants. *Arch Dis Child Fetal Neonatal Ed*. 2009;94(3):F188-F192.
56. Paton JY, Macfadyen U, Williams A, Simpson H. Gastro-oesophageal reflux and apnoeic pauses during sleep in infancy—no direct relation. *Eur J Pediatr*. 1990;149(10):680–686.
57. Peter CS, Sprodowski N, Bohnhorst B, Silny J, Poets CF. Gastroesophageal reflux and apnea of prematurity: no temporal relationship. *Pediatrics*. 2002;109(1):8–11.
58. Di Fiore JM, Arko M, Whitehouse M, Kimball A, Martin RJ. Apnea is not prolonged by acid gastroesophageal reflux in preterm infants. *Pediatrics*. 2005;116(5):1059–1063.
59. Arad-Cohen N, Cohen A, Tirosh E. The relationship between gastroesophageal reflux and apnea in infants. *J Pediatr*. 2000;137(3):321–326.
60. Noronha AC, de Bruin VM, Nobre e Souza MA, et al. Gastroesophageal reflux and obstructive sleep apnea in childhood. *Int J Pediatr Otorhinolaryngol*. 2009;73(3):383–389.
61. Ing AJ, Ngu MC, Breslin AB, Obstructive sleep apnea and gastroesophageal reflux. *Am J Med*. 2000;108(suppl 4a):120S–125S.
62. Kerr P, Shoenut JP, Millar T, Buckle P, Kryger MH. Nasal CPAP reduces gastroesophageal reflux in obstructive sleep apnea syndrome. *Chest*. 1992;101(6):1539–1544.
63. Green BT, Broughton WA, O'Connor JB. Marked improvement in nocturnal gastroesophageal reflux in a large cohort of patients with obstructive sleep apnea treated with continuous positive airway pressure. *Arch Intern Med*. 2003;163(1):41–45.
64. Tawk M, Goodrich S, Kinasewitz G, Orr W. The effect of 1 week of continuous positive airway

pressure treatment in obstructive sleep apnea patients with concomitant gastroesophageal reflux. *Chest*. 2006;130(4):1003–1008.

65. Bortolotti M, Gentilini L, Morselli C, Giovannini M. Obstructive sleep apnoea is improved by a prolonged treatment of gastrooesophageal reflux with omeprazole. *Dig Liver Dis*. 2006;38(2):78–81.
66. Senior BA, Khan M, Schwimmer C, Rosenthal L, Benninger M. Gastroesophageal reflux and obstructive sleep apnea. *Laryngoscope*. 2001; 111(12):2144–2146.
67. Chen MY, Ott DJ, Sinclair JW, Wu WC, Gelfand DW. Gastroesophageal reflux disease: correlation of esophageal pH testing and radiographic findings. *Radiology*. 1992;185(2):483–486.
68. Thompson JK, Koehler RE, Richter JE. Detection of gastroesophageal reflux: value of barium studies compared with 24-hr pH monitoring. *AJR Am J Roentgenol*. 1994;162(3):621–626.
69. Seibert JJ, Byrne WJ, Euler AR, Latture T, Leach M, Campbell M. Gastroesophageal reflux—the acid test: scintigraphy or the pH probe? *AJR Am J Roentgenol*. 1983;140(6):1087–1090.
70. Vandenplas Y, Rudolph CD, Di Lorenzo C, et al. Pediatric gastroesophageal reflux clinical practice guidelines: joint recommendations of the North American Society for Pediatric Gastroenterology, Hepatology, and Nutrition (NASPGHAN) and the European Society for Pediatric Gastroenterology, Hepatology, and Nutrition (ESPGHAN). *J Pediatr Gastroenterol Nutr*. 2009;49(4): 498–547.
71. Rudolph CD, Mazur LJ, Liptak GS, et al; North American Society for Pediatric Gastroenterology and Nutrition. Guidelines for evaluation and treatment of gastroesophageal reflux in infants and children: recommendations of the North American Society for Pediatric Gastroenterology and Nutrition. *J Pediatr Gastroenterol Nutr*. 2001;32(suppl 2):S1-S31.
72. Arana A, Bagucka B, Hauser B, et al. PH monitoring in the distal and proximal esophagus in symptomatic infants. *J Pediatr Gastroenterol Nutr*. 2001;32(3):259–264.
73. Cucchiara S, Santamaria F, Minella R, et al. Simultaneous prolonged recordings of proximal and distal intraesophageal pH in children with gastroesophageal reflux disease and respiratory symptoms. *Am J Gastroenterol*. 1995;90(10): 1791–1796.
74. Rosen R, Lord C, Nurko S. The sensitivity of multichannel intraluminal impedance (MII)compared to pH probe in the detection of gastroesophgeal reflux in children. *Clinical Gastroenterology and Hepatology*. 2006;4(2):167–172.
75. Wenzl TG, Moroder C, Trachterna M, et al. Esophageal pH monitoring and impedance measurement: a comparison of two diagnostic tests for gastroesophageal reflux. *J Pediatr Gastroenterol Nutr*. 2002;34(5):519–523.
76. Shay S, Richter J. Direct comparison of impedance, manometry, and pH Probe in detecting reflux before and after a meal. *Dig Dis Sci*. 2005;50(9): 1584–1590.
77. Greenfeld M, Tauman R, Sivan Y. The yield of esophageal pH monitoring during polysomnography in infants with sleep-disordered breathing. *Clin Pediatr (Phila)*. 2004;43(7):653–658.
78. Harris P, Muñoz C, Mobarec S, Brockmann P, Mesa T, Sánchez I. Relevance of the pH probe in sleep study analysis in infants. *Child Care Health Dev*. 2004;30(4):337–344.
79. Wenzl TG, Schenke S, Peschgens T, Silny J, Heimann G, Skopnik H. Association of apnea and nonacid gastroesophageal reflux in infants: investigations with the intraluminal impedance technique. *Pediatr Pulmonol*. 2001;31(2):144–149.
80. Di Fiore J, Arko M, Herynk B, Martin R, Hibbs AM. Characterization of cardiorespiratory events following gastroesophageal reflux in preterm infants. *J Perinatol*. 2010; Oct; 30(10):683–687.
81. Sleep-related breathing disorders in adults: recommendations for syndrome definition and measurement techniques in clinical research. The Report of an American Academy of Sleep Medicine Task Force. *Sleep*. 1999;22(5):667–689.
82. Kushida CA, Giacomini A, Lee MK, Guilleminault C, Dement WC. Technical protocol for the use of esophageal manometry in the diagnosis of sleep-related breathing disorders. *Sleep Med*. 2002;3(2):163–173.

CHAPTER 25

Drug Development for Pediatric Sleep Disorders: Opportunities and Challenges

O'Neill D'Cruz and Virinder Nohria

Introduction

Sleep disorders in children account for several million office visits each year, with 75% to 80% of children with pediatric insomnia receiving off-label prescriptions for various medications, including antihistamines, alpha-2 agonists, and hypnotics approved for use in adult insomnia [1,2]. Despite the high prevalence of pediatric sleep disorders, there are no Food and Drug Administration (FDA)—approved medications for pediatric sleep disorders. This chapter summarizes the clinical, regulatory, and pharmaceutical industry (sponsor) considerations in drug development for pediatric sleep disorders.

Clinical Background

The National Sleep Foundation—sponsored conference on "Pharmacological Management of Insomnia in Children and Adolescents" defined pediatric insomnia as repeated difficulty with sleep initiation, duration, consolidation, or quality that occurs despite age-appropriate time and opportunity for sleep and results in daytime functional impairment for the child and/or family [3]. Patients with pervasive developmental disorders and attention deficit hyperactivity disorder who had comorbid insomnia were among the suggested subpopulations suitable for clinical trials of sleep-promoting agents due to well-defined diagnostic criteria, high prevalence of both the primary disorder and comorbid insomnia, and high likelihood of use of off-label medications. In contrast, circadian rhythm disorders, medical disorders with comorbid insomnia, idiopathic and psychophysiologic insomnia were not considered suitable for early pediatric clinical trials. Primary sleep disorders (including sleep-related breathing disorders, restless legs syndrome (RLS), and periodic limb movement disorder) and comorbid psychiatric disorders (conduct disorder, major depressive disorder, oppositional defiant disorder, and anxiety disorder) were endorsed as relevant exclusions for pediatric insomnia trials.

Controlled trials for pediatric insomnia have not been successful so far. The TIRED study was terminated early after diphenhydramine failed to show a benefit over placebo in infants with frequent nighttime awakenings [4]. Similarly, zolpidem did not significantly decrease latency to persistent sleep compared with placebo in a pediatric trial [5]. Both diphenhydramine and zolpidem were reported to have higher incidence of adverse events (AEs) compared with placebo.

Consensus diagnostic criteria for pediatric RLS and periodic limb movement disorder were recently published by the International Restless Legs Study Group [6]. In children, clinical description of RLS symptoms may be supported by sleep disturbances, periodic sleep movements in sleep on polysomnography (PSG), and family history of RLS. Iron supplementation may be helpful in children with evidence of low serum ferritin or iron levels [7], but practice parameters for dopaminergic treatment of RLS and PLMD exclude children [8]. Trials of dopaminergic agents and other treatments in pediatric RLS require demonstration of significant unmet clinical need, as well as development and validation of an RLS scale for children.

Evaluations during trials include subjective and objective assessments. Sleep diaries and questionnaires, which are used for assessing eligibility and treatment effects, in either paper or electronic format, have not been validated in the pediatric population. Caregivers often have to complete the subjective assessments in pediatric trials, and validation requires special considerations for caregiver assessments. Objective evaluations using PSG and actigraphy are appropriate and complementary tools. Standardized and validated, age-specific normative data and ranges for the assessment tools need to be defined in the trial subpopulations before conducting randomized, controlled trials.

Besides off-label medications, pediatric sleep disorders are treated with behavioral therapy and environmental modifications. These interventions are often quite effective in behavioral insomnia. Although age-appropriate sleep hygiene practices are acceptable during clinical trials, the types and duration of behavioral interventions must be clearly outlined and controls for confounding effects established before enrolling subjects in clinical trials.

Regulatory Aspects

General Regulatory Principles for Drug Development in Infants and Children

Many of the general principles of both clinical and nonclinical pediatric drug development have been published by International Conference on Harmonization of Technical Requirements for Registration of Pharmaceuticals for Human Use (ICH) [9,10]. There are many factors that should be taken in to consideration before undertaking a pediatric development program for a product. These may include some or all of the following:

- The seriousness of the condition to be treated.
- The prevalence of the condition to be treated in the pediatric population.
- The availability and suitability of alternative treatments for the condition in the pediatric population, including the efficacy and the AE profile (including any unique pediatric safety issues) of those treatments.
- The nature and the pharmacology of the medicinal product—is it novel or one of a class of compounds with known properties and are there unique pediatric indications for the product.
- The need for the development of pediatric-specific end points.
- The age ranges of pediatric patients likely to be treated with the medicinal product.
- Any unique pediatric (developmental) safety concerns with the medicinal product, including any nonclinical safety issues such as those observed in repeat dose toxicity, genotoxicity, reproductive toxicity, or juvenile animal toxicity studies. In addition, it is important to note that the most relevant safety data for pediatric studies ordinarily come from adult human exposure.
- The potential need for pediatric formulation development.

Over the last 10 to 15 years, the FDA in the United States and European Medicines Agency (EMA) developed regulations and legislation addressing the development of drugs for use in children. These are summarized in Table 25.1.

According to ICH, the pediatric population has been classified into 5 categories, the basis of possible developmental biology and pharmacology, although these categories may vary depending on the disease and the medicinal product. In the categories below, ages are defined in completed days, months, or years.

- preterm newborn infants
- term newborn infants (0–27 days)
- infants and toddlers (28 days to 23 months)
- children (2–11 years)
- adolescents (12–16–18 years [dependent on region])

Pediatric studies should not be undertaken until the safety and efficacy in adults have been established and unless the product is going to be developed only for pediatric use. The regulatory authorities have mechanisms for providing a waiver or deferral from the requirements for pediatric studies in any or all age ranges, and justification for seeking such waiver/deferral needs to be provided by the sponsor of the pediatric program.

The FDA uses a clinical decision tree to guide the pediatric development plan after adult data are available. The tree is based on the disease condition,

Table 25.1 Summary of regulatory regulations for pediatric drug development

Agency	Initiative	Key features
FDA	Pediatric Rule, 1994	Data on PK/safety/efficacy of medication used in children
	FDA Modernization Act (FDAMA), 1997	6-month patent extension (pediatric exclusivity) for FDA-requested pediatric trials
	Best Pharmaceuticals for Children Act (BPCA), 2002	Pediatric exclusivity, NIH studies for off-patent drugs
	Pediatric Research Equity Act (PREA), 2003	Pediatric exclusivity, FDA authority to require pediatric studies
	FDA Amendment Act (FDAAA), 2007	6 month of full exclusivity (adult and pediatric) for pediatric studies, and FDA can mandate studies if condition with adult indication exists in children-Pediatric Plan
EMA	Pediatric Regulation 1901/2006, 2007	Pediatric Committee to assess and approve Pediatric Investigation Plans (PIP) for products in development before submission of marketing authorization approval (MAA) in adults
		Pediatric Use Marketing Authorization (PUMA) granted if PIP provisions completed for products without patent or data exclusivity

Abbreviations: EMA, European Medicines Agency; FDA, Food and Drug Administration; NIH, National Institutes of Health.

response to intervention, concentration-response relationship between adults and pediatrics populations, the availability of pharmacokinetic and pharmacodynamic data, and the need for safety data in the pediatric population. The decision tree is outlined in Figure 25.1.

Regulatory Guidance for Development of Drugs for Pediatric Sleep Disorders

The only guidelines that have been published by the FDA for sleep disorders make no reference to development of hypnotics in the pediatric population [11]. Over the last 15 years, there have been a number of drugs that have been approved in the United States for the treatment of insomnia in adult patients. These include zolpidem (Ambien), zolpidem CR (Ambien CR), eszopiclone (Lunesta), zaleplon (Sonata), and ramelteon (Rozerem). None of these products have an indication for treatment of insomnia in infants and children. However, the product label for zolpidem (Ambien) includes a pediatric randomized, controlled trial that was conducted after a written request from the FDA under the Pediatric Research Equity Act (PREA), 2003. Despite evidence that zolpidem may be ineffective in pediatric populations, an additional 6-month exclusivity was granted. Based on the evidence that Ambien was ineffective or may be unsafe in all pediatric ages, Ambien CR was granted a waiver from the requirements of PREA. It is advisable to discuss the details and obtain agreement from the FDA before commencing a pediatric drug development program.

The EMA has published draft guidelines for the development of medicinal products for the treatment of insomnia [12]. In this draft document, the EMA has provided extensive guidance as to the nature and design of studies necessary for development of products in adults and children. Specifics of any proposed programs are submitted as Pediatric Investigation Plans (PIP) and discussed and agreed with the Pediatric Committee and subsequently validated by the EMA.

Because sleep disorders such as insomnia in children may be a comorbidity of another disorder, it is important that proof of concept should be established in a homogenous patient group, such as patients with autism/learning difficulties, ensuring that patients are age matched, matched for cognitive level, and not treated with concomitant drugs that may interfere with sleep.

Pivotal efficacy trials should establish dose-response in specific pediatric subgroups

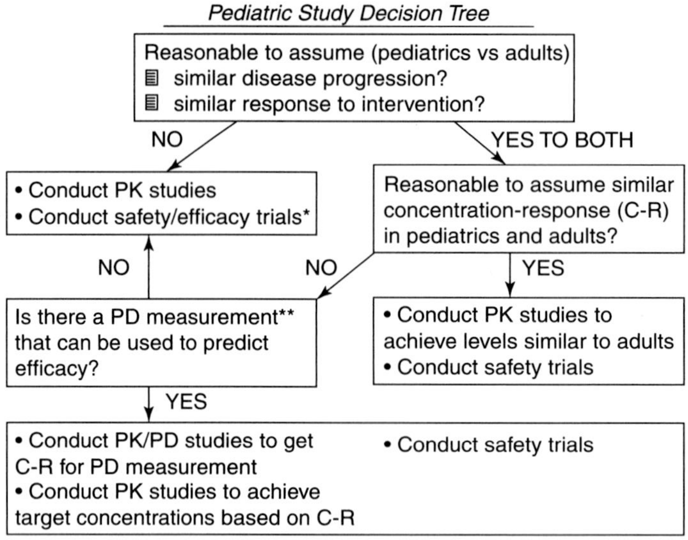

Figure 25.1 Food and drug administration pediatric study decision tree. PK, pharmacokinetic; PD, pharmacodynamic.

(as described under general principles above) compared with placebo; however, 3-arm studies including placebo and an active comparator are preferred. Because of the general ethical principle that children should only be subjected to clinical trials if they are likely to benefit from the intervention, the trials should include a run-in period with standardized behavioral interventions. Only patients nonresponsive to an adequate period of standardized behavioral interventions should be randomized to treatment. In general, clinical outcome measures as primary end point are preferred in the pediatric population as well. However, based on expert recommendation, results might be more reliable with the use of objective primary outcome measure criteria such as actigraphy or PSG, in this population. In such cases, next-day performance or school performance should be explored as a coprimary end point. The duration of efficacy trials should be as for the adult population and should be at least 2 to 4 weeks duration for agents that are intended for short-term use and up to 6 months duration for agents that are intended for long-term use. A follow-up period should be included to assess withdrawal/rebound reactions and AEs emergent after treatment discontinuation.

Secondary end points should be clearly defined and should include the effect of the medication on neurocognitive/neurobehavioural parameters. Assessment of functioning at school (concentration and academic performance) and of mood and general well-being should be performed using validated methods. Effects on quality of life for the caregiver, impulsivity, attention, vigilance, learning and memory, verbal fluency, complex/divergent/creative thinking, functioning at home, and behavioral problems are also of interest and should be sondiered for assessment using appropriate validated age-appropriate scales.

As sleep disturbances in children may adversely affect the pulsatile growth hormone release, effects of treatment on height, weight, and pubertal status should be assessed. Rather than relying on spontaneous AE reporting, potential treatment-emergent AEs such as somnolence, affective symptoms such as suicidality, depression, and so on should be clearly defined and actively monitored for. Validated questionnaires/scales should be used for monitoring AEs. The duration of long-term safety trials should be adequate to assess any effects on sexual development or growth.

The EMA publishes reviews of its opinions, including PIPs for medicinal products being developed for treatment of pediatric insomnia. Of the 2 published opinions, the sponsor for melatonin (Circadin) was required to resubmit the PIP after denial of a waiver request. The product eplivanserin was granted waiver in preterm newborn infants, term newborn infants, and infants and toddlers from 0 to less than 2 years for film-coated tablet and oral use. The approved PIP for eplivanserin in children from 2 to less than 12 years and adolescents from 12 to less than 18 years is summarized in Table 25.2 [13]. This summary outlines the type and amount of information required for obtaining an indication in the pediatric population.

Pharmaceutical Industry (Sponsor) Perspective

Sponsors assess the clinical needs and regulatory guidance and precedence for a therapeutic area and formulate a development program if there is a good match with the firm's strategy, areas of expertise, capabilities, and resources. The considerations that influence the feasibility of a successful drug development program for pediatric sleep disorders include the following.

- *Ethics:* Minimizing risk to vulnerable populations is a core ethical consideration for pediatric trials, and there are specific safeguards for research involving children, as laid out in the Code of Federal Regulations [14]. Hence, pediatric studies are typically deferred till data regarding safety and efficacy are available for adults. Specific guidelines for informed consent, sparse sampling with physiologically based pharmacokinetic modeling, and the use of data safety–monitoring boards are among the ethical safeguards to minimize risk and discomfort in pediatric clinical trials.
- *Science:* Protocols of clinical trials must be developed and substantiated by scientifically relevant information and principles. Protocol objectives vary based on the phase of clinical development and trial design. The study hypothesis must be clearly formulated, population selected by appropriate inclusion/exclusion criteria, and study end points assessed by appropriate trial design and valid statistical analysis.
- *Operations:* Type of clinical trial (placebo vs active comparator as control arm), selection of a homogenous study population after screening by appropriate inclusion/exclusion criteria, availability of validated assessments (including age-, language-, and culture-specific scales), identification of adequate number of suitable

Table 25.2 Approved pediatric investigation plan for Eplivanserin

Area	Subarea	Number	Description
Quality	Pharmaceutical Form	1	Development of a film-coated tablet formulation for the pediatric population from 6 to less than 18 years.
Quality	Pharmaceutical Form	1	Development of an age-appropriate formulation for the pediatric population from 2 to less than 6 years.
Nonclinical	Juvenile animal study	1	Dose-ranging safety study in juventile rats.
Nonclinical	Juvenile animal study	1	Definitive oral safety study in juventile rats.
Clinical	Pharmacokinetics, efficacy	1	Open-label with sequential single ascending dose administration of three doses in children aged from 6 to less than 18 years with insomnia.
Clinical	Pharmacokinetics, efficacy	1	Open-label with sequential single ascending dose administration of three doses in children aged from 2 to less than 6 years with insomnia.
Clinical	Efficacy, safety	1	8-week, randomized, double-blind, placebo-controlled "proof-of-concept" trial of eplivanserin hemifumarate for insomnia associated with attention deficit disorder in patients aged from 6 to less than 18 years.
Clinical	Efficacy, safety	1	8-week, randomized, double-blind, placebo-controlled trial of eplivanserin hemifumarate for insomnia associated with attention deficit disorder and/or pervasive developmental disorder and/or blindness in patients from 2 to less than 18 years including 4 months of open-label extension and 12 months of long-term follow-up.

sites and trained investigators capable of performing study assessments, duration of studies, feasibility of age-appropriate formulations, and other operational factors need to be considered.

- *Statistics:* Variability of baseline characteristics and response rates, knowledge of effect size, and onset and duration of effect influence the validity of trials and chances of achieving statistically significant outcomes on primary end points. The FDA's guidance document E9 summarizes principles of trial design and conduct, data analyses, evaluation of safety and tolerability, and reporting of clinical trial results [15].
- *Pharmacoeconomics:* A target product profile is developed for commercial assessment of clinical usage and takes into account the minimal, expected, and best-case outcomes that would support commercial viability of a product. Commercial assessments also include the type of indication (orphan, first-in-class, etc.) and availability of other therapeutic options that may compete or complement the product or device under consideration. Outside the United States, price and distribution of approved drugs must often be negotiated with payers to obtain a Marketing Authorization Holder license.

If a potential therapeutic drug meets the sponsor's criteria for proceeding with a clinical development program, a standard sequence of development phases is outlined in Table 25.3.

The course of clinical development typically lasts up to a decade and is fraught with several uncertainties. If the compound fails to meet objectives and end points at any phase, further development is delayed, or in many cases, halted entirely. If early phases show promise of both statistically significant and clinically relevant effects, phase III studies are undertaken and must be replicated before submission for approval. Regulators formulate a benefit-risk analysis and grant approval if a favorable analysis is supported by data in the new drug application submitted by the sponsor. Further safety and clinical trials or additional studies may be required by regulators, either in the form of requirements (especially for safety concerns) or commitments (for further assessment of clinical relevance) at approval. Phase IV studies and pharmacovigilance assessments continue for several years after initial approval.

Because of withdrawal of several marketed agents, pharmacovigilance assessments have evolved from passive collection of AEs and periodic reporting to various types of risk evaluation and mitigation strategies (REMS). The Xyrem Success Program is part of the extensive REMS for sodium oxybate that includes education, controlled prescribing and dispensing, and periodic recertification of prescribers. FDA's Sentinel Initiative and other pharmacovigilance programs and algorithms are beyond the scope of this chapter [16].

Many of the ongoing clinical trials for pediatric sleep disorders are conducted on marketed agents, diet supplements, devices, and behavioral therapies [17]. Currently, there are several sponsor commitments for investigational use in pediatric sleep disorders (see Table 25.4). Depending on the duration and outcome of these studies, we may expect to add safe and effective medications

Table 25.3 Drug development phases and features

	Trial design	Subjects	Typical end point(s)
Phase I	Open-label	Healthy Volunteers, 10–50 per trial	ADME, drug interaction
Phase II	Open-label, placebo-crossover	Patients, <100 per trial	PKPD, dose-response
Phase III	Randomized, DBPC or active-comparator	Patients, 100 to >300 per trial	Efficacy, tolerability, and safety
Phase IV (postapproval)	Open-label, varying doses or subpopulations	Patients, >100 per trial	Safety, efficacy, specific clinical subpopulation/ indication

ADME, absorption, distribution, metabolism, excretion; PKPD, pharmacokinetic, pharmacodynamic; DBPC, double-blind, placebo-controlled.

Table 25.4 Pediatric sleep disorders—drugs in clinical development (studies recruiting subjects)

Candidate agent	Indication	Phase	Sponsor
Eszopiclone	Insomnia in ADHD	III	Sepracor
Donepezil	Sleep in autism	II	NIMH
Zolpidem	Insomnia	IV	Astellas Pharma
Bupropion	Sleep and depression	IV	NIMH
Ramelteon	Insomnia	I	Takeda
Atomoxetine	Insomnia in ADHD	IV	Eli Lilly

Abbreviations: ADHD, attention deficit hyperactivity disorder; NIMH, National Institute of Mental Health.

to the therapeutic options for the treatment of childhood sleep disorders.

References

1. Stojanovski SD, Rasu RS, Balkrishnan R, et al. Trends in medication prescribing for pediatric sleep disorders in US outpatient settings. *Sleep*. 2007;30:1013–1017.
2. Owens J, Rosen C, Mindell J. Medication use in the treatment of pediatric insomnia: results of a survey of community-based pediatricians. *Pediatrics*. 2003;111:e628–e635.
3. Mindell J, Emslie G, Blumer J, et al. Pharmacologic management of insomnia in children and adolescents: consensus statement. *Pediatrics*. 2006;117:e1223–e1232.
4. Merenstein D, Diener-West M, Halbower AC, et al. The trial of infant response to diphenhydramine: the TIRED study—a randomized, controlled, patient-oriented trial. *Arch Pediatr Adolesc Med*. 2006;160:707–712.
5. Zolpidem [package insert]. Sanofi-aventis U.S. LLC Bridgewater, NJ Label Approved 2008. http://www.accessdata.fda.gov/drugsatfda_docs/label/2008/019908s027lbl.pdf.
6. Allen RP, Picchietti D, Hening WA, et al. Restless legs syndrome: diagnostic criteria, special considerations and epidemiology. *Sleep Med*. 2003;4:101–119.
7. Simakajornboon N, Kheirandish-Gozal L, Gozal D. Diagnosis and management of restless legs syndrome in children. *Sleep Med Rev*. 2009;13(2):149–156.
8. Littner MR, Kushida C, Anderson WM, et al. Practice parameters for the dopaminergic treatment of restless legs syndrome and periodic limb movement disorder. *Sleep*. 2004;27(3):557–559.
9. Guidance on nonclinical safety studies for the conductofhumanclinicaltrialsandmarketingauthorization for pharmaceuticals, 2009. http://www.ich.org/LOB/media/MEDIA5544.pdf. Accessed March 26, 2010.
10. Clinical investigation of medicinal products in the paediatric population, 2001. http://www.ema.europa.eu/pdfs/human/ich/271199en.pdf. Guidance is from 2009, accessed March 26, 2010.
11. Guidelines for the clinical evaluation of hypnotic drugs. FDA, 1977. http://www.fda.gov/downloads/Drugs/GuidanceComplianceRegulatoryInformation/Guidances/ucm071711.pdf. Accessed March 26, 2010.
12. Guidelines on medicinal products for the treatment of insomnia, Guidence is from 2009. http://www.ema.europa.eu/pdfs/human/ewp/1627409en.pdf. Accessed March 26, 2010.
13. European Medicines Agency Division on Application for agreement of a pediatric investigation plan for eplivanserin hemifumarate. http://www.ema.europa.eu/pdfs/human/paediatrics/000114-PIP01-07.pdf. Accessed March 26, 2010.
14. Code of Federal Regulations, Subpart D: Additional protections for children involved as subjects in research, Effective, July, 2009. www.hhs.gov/ohrp/humansubjects/guidance/45cfr46.htm#subpartd. Accessed March 26, 2010.
15. Guidance for Industry E9 Statistical Principles for Clinical Trials, September, 2009. www.fda.gov/downloads/Drugs/GuidanceComplianceRegulatoryInformation/Guidances/ucm073137.pdf. Accessed March 26, 2010.
16. FDA-Sentinel Initiative. www.fda.gov/Safety/FDAsSentinelInitiative/default.htm. Accessed March 26, 2010.
17. Clinicaltrials.gov, search performed. www.clinicaltrials.gov. Accessed March 26, 2010.

Index

Note: Page numbers followed by *f* and *t* refer to figures and tables, respectively.

2-process model, 246, 246*f*
6-hydroxymelatonin, 145
6-sulfatoxymelatonin, 248
20/24 to 20/33 genotypes, 315, 334, 342*t*
180-degree reversal of sleep phase, 18
α-Amino-3-hydroxy-5-methylisoxazole-4-propionic acid receptors, 368
ε4 genotype, 372
Γ-Aminobutyric acid (GABA) transmission, 11

AASM Manual for the Scoring of Sleep and Associated Events, 2007, 354
Acetylmelatonin methyltransferase (ASMT), 148–149
Achondroplasia (AC), 288
  treatment strategies for, 290
  varying combinations of SDB in, 289–290
Actigraphic studies
  in depressive disorders, 175
  in pediatric bipolar disorder (PBD), 177
Actigraphy, 37, 142, 196, 250–251
  for sleep and headache, 421–422, 424*t*
  for sleep fragmentation, 356
Active sleep, 6
Addendum–paraneoplastic syndromes, 203–205
Adenoid hypertrophy, 450
Adenosine (AD), 11, 87
  hypothesis, 108
  and sleep, treatment of, 172
Adenosine kinase (ADK), 87
Adenotonsillar hypertrophy (ATH), 151
Adenotonsillectomy (AT), 276, 285
  for OSA, 310, 311, 312, 313, 319, 320
ADHD-C symptoms, 48
ADHD-PHI, 48
Adiponectin, 362
Adolescents, insomnia in, 395–396
Advance sleep phase disorder (ASPD), 249
Adverse events (AEs), 469, 473
Aerodigestive disorders. *See* Multidisciplinary aerodigestive team approach
Agnathia-Aglossia syndrome, 444
Airway endoscopy, 452–453
Akathisia, 32
Alzheimer disease, 7
Ambien CR, 471
American Academy of Sleep Medicine, 251
American Sleep Disorders Association (ASDA), 1992, 354
American Thoracic Society (ATS) Statement on CCHS, 332
Amitriptyline, 425
Amphetamine, 202, 225, 224, 224*t*
Amphibians, sleep behavior in, 1
Angelman syndrome (AS), 160
  types of sleep problems in, 161
Anorexia, 178
Antiepileptic drugs (AEDs), 80, 92–93, 93*t*, 148
Antihypertensive agent clonidine, 391
Antipsychotic drugs, 181–182
Anti-voltage gated potassium channel (VGKC), 204
Anxiety, 51
Anxiety disorder, 170–171
  AD and sleep, treatment of, 172
  anxiety disorders, polysomnographic studies in, 171–172
  obsessive compulsive disorders, 171
  posttraumatic stress disorder, 171
Apert syndrome, 440, 444
Apnea hypopnea index (AHI), 144, 404, 405, 452
Apnea index (AI), 201
Apolipoprotein ε4 genotype, 372
Apparent life-threatening event (ALTE), 456
Architecture and cycling, of sleep, 4, 5*f*
  maturation of sleep, 6–7
Aripiprazole, 401
Armodafinil, 226, 403

Arnold-chiari malformation and syringobulbia, 375
Arousal mechanisms, 7, 8, 8*f*
Arousal parasomnias, 407–408
Arousals, 354
Arylalkylamine N-acetyltransferase (AANAT), 144, 145
Aspiration related lung disease, 455–458. *See also* Chronic pulmonary aspiration
Aspiration related pulmonary problems, 453
Aspirin, 147
Atomoxetine, 404, 475*t*
Atonia, 10
Atonic drop attacks, 222
Attention deficit hyperactivity disorder (ADHD), 45, 163, 222, 374, 399
  comorbidities, 48
  medications and daytime and nighttime behaviors, 54–55
  and sleep-phenotypes, 49
    ADHD comorbidities, 50
    ADHD per se, 49–50
    anxiety, 51
    learning, 51
    mood, 50–51
    oppositional defiant disorder (ODD) and conduct disorder (CD), 50
    substance abuse, 52
    Tourette syndrome/Tic disorder, 51
  sleeping child and its ADHD phenotypes, 52
    daytime sleepiness, 53
    restless legs syndrome (RLS) and periodic limb movements in sleep, 54
    sleep disorder, 53
    sleep per se, 52–53
    sleep-disordered breathing, 53–54
  sleep problems in children with, 48*t*
  umbrella, 47–48, 50
Augmentation, 72–73
Autism spectrum disorders (ASD), 157–160, 399
Autoimmune hypothesis, 214–215
Autonomic nervous system (ANS), 331
  overview of, 332*f*
Autonomic nervous system dysregulation (ANSD) symptoms, in congenital central hypoventilation syndrome, 337, 337*f*
Autosomal-dominant nocturnal frontal lobe epilepsy (ADNFLE), 82
Awakening, 29

Barium contrast radiography, 460–463
Basal forebrain (BF), 7
Beckwith-Wiedmann syndrome, 438, 439*f*, 443
Behavioral sleep, 1
Benign epilepsy of childhood with occipital paroxysms (BECOP), 85
Benign epilepsy with centro-temporal spikes (BECT), 84
Benign focal epilepsy of childhood (BFEC) variants, 118
Benign sleep myoclonus of infancy, 99
Benzodiazepines, 229, 406, 407–408, 425
Benzodiazepines hypnotics, 400
Best Pharmaceuticals for Children Act, 2002, 471*t*
Bilateral abductor vocal cord paralysis, 291–294
  diagnostic approach to evaluating sleep breathing disorders in children with, 291–292
Bilateral facial microsomia, 444
BiLevel positive airway pressure, 277
Bipolar disorder (BPD) and ADHD, 50
Birds and REM sleep, 2
Bradypnea, 433
Brain-derived neurotrophic factor (BDNF), 372
Brain injury
  potential mediators, in sleep disorders, 369–370
Brain physiology and sleep, 16–17
Brain temperature, 6
Brainstem aminergic nuclei, 420–421
Breathing disorders, in epilepsy patients, 91–92. *See also* Sleep-disordered breathing (SDB)
  central sleep apnea (CSA), 91–92
  obstructive sleep apnea (OSA), 91
Bright light exposure, 254
Bromocriptine, 163
Bronchoalveolar lavage (BAL), 457
Bruxism, 99, 418
BTBD9 allele, 64
BTBD9 homeobox gene complex, 132
Bupropion, 73, 181, 475*t*

C-reactive protein, 362
Caffeine, 223
Calmodulin kinase II, 368
Cancer, clinical problems of children with, 199–202
Cancer/brain tumors, in children, 191–194
Cancer-related fatigue, 196–197
Carbidopa, 405–406
Cardiac asystoles, 337
Cardiorespiratory management
  in Duchenne muscular dystrophy, 295–297
Cardiovascular changes in sleep, 17
Caregivers, 470
"Cataplectic facies", 217
Cataplexy, 32, 100, 209, 216–217, 222
  treatment of, 228, 403–404
    sodium oxybate, 229
    tricyclic antidepressants, 228–229
Catathrenia, 98
Central apneas, in Prader-Willi syndrome, 278, 279, 280*f*
Central Brain Tumor Registry of the United States (CBTRUS), 192
Central hypersomnia, in PWS, 282
Central pattern generators (CPGs), 125

Central sleep apnea (CSA), 197–198, 434
Cerebral blood flow (CBF), 6
Cerebral palsy (CP), 266–267, 319–320
  SDB in children with, 285–286
Cerebrospinal fluid (CSF) hypocretin, 196
Cervicofacial lymphatic malformations, 438, 439*f*, 445
Cervicomedullary compression in children with CM1, symptoms and signs of, 291
CHARGE syndrome, 453, 456
Chest wall deformities (CWD), 309. *See also* Sleep-disordered breathing
Chiari malformations (CM), 318–319
Chiari 1 malformations
  cervicomedullary compression and, 291
  sleep-disordered breathing and, 291–293
Childhood onset-schizophrenia (COS), 179
Children
  with aerodigestive disorders. *See* Multidisciplinary aerodigestive team approach
  with epilepsy, 286–287
  with intellectual disabilities (ID)/cerebral palsy (CP), 285–286
  sleep-disordered breathing in. *See* Sleep-disordered breathing
Children's Sleep Habits Questionnaire (CSHQ), 36
Chloral hydrate (CH), 397
  benzodiazepines hypnotics, 400
  clonidine, 400
  melatonin, 398–399
  neuroleptics, 401–402
  nonbenzodiazepine hypnotics, 400–401
Chlorpromazine, 181
Choanal atresia, 450
Chronic cough, 454–455
  causes in children, 454*t*
  evaluation of, 454–455
  sleep disruption, 454
  tests for evaluating aerodigestive disorders, 455*t*
Chronic fatigue syndrome, 417
Chronic migraine, 417–418
Chronic paroxysmal hemicrania (CPH), 418, 419
Chronic pulmonary aspiration, 455–458
  fibreoptic endoscopic evaluation of swallowing, 456
  fibreoptic flexible bronchoscopy (FFB), 457
  gastroesophageal reflux and extraesophageal manifestation, 456
  polysomnography, common abnormalities noted on, 457–458
  pulmonary disease and sleep disordered breathing severity, 458
  pulmonary function tests, 457
  salivary aspiration, 456
  sleep evaluation with aerodigestive disorders, 457
  videofluroscopic swallow study, 456
Chronic sleep deprivation with erratic sleep-wake schedule, 221
Chronic tension-type headache, 417–418
Chronotherapy, 254
Chronotype, assessment of, 249–250
Circadian clock in Smith-Magenis Syndrome, 150–151
Circadian integrator pathway of brain, 19*f*
Circadian period, 249
Circadian rhythm disorders, 245, 375
  advance sleep phase disorder, 256
  circadian rhythm sleep disorders (CRSD), 249, 251
    actigraphy, 250–251
    chronotype, assessment of, 249–250
    sleep diaries, 250
  delayed sleep phase disorder (DSPD), 252–254, 253*f*
  free-running disorder (FRD), 254–256, 255*f*
  irregular sleep-wake rhythm (ISWR), 256
  sleep and circadian rhythms
    intrinsic processes, 246–247
    light and measuring circadian timing system, 247–249
  sleep regulatory process across adolescence, 251–252
Circadian rhythm sleep disorders (CRSD), 249, 251
  actigraphy, 250–251
  chronotype, assessment of, 249–250
  sleep diaries, 250
Circadian rhythms and sleep
  circadian timing system, light and measuring, 247–249
  intrinsic processes, 246–247
    2-process model, 246, 246*f*
    circadian timing system, 247
    sleep homeostatic system, 247
Circadian sleep regulation, 15–16
Circadian timing system, 247
  measuring, 247–249
Cleveland adolescent sleepiness questionnaire, 36
Clomipramine, 224*t*, 228, 403
Clonazepam, 72, 127, 229, 400, 407–408
Clonidine, 72, 391, 400
Clotiapine, 181
Clozapine, 181
Cluster headache (CH), 418, 419
Cognitive behavioral therapy (CBT), 130, 172
Cognitive-behavioral therapy for insomnia (CBT-I), 425
Comorbid ADHD, 73
Comorbid depression/anxiety, 73
Comorbid epilepsy, 265
Comorbid psychiatric disorders, 469
Comorbidity, 70–71
Confusional arousals, 96, 127–128
Congenital anomalies, 450

Congenital Central Hypoventilation Syndrome (CCHS), 374–375
  autonomic nervous system dysregulation (ANSD) symptoms, 337, 337*f*
  cardiac asystoles, 337
  clinical evaluation, 341–343
  continuous ventilatory dependence, 335
  dermatoglyphics, 338
  diagnosis, 341
  facial dysmorphology, 337–338
  Hirschsprung disease (HSCR), 336
  later-onset CCHS, 338–339
  long-term prognosis, 344
  mosaicism in subset of parents with, 339–340
  neural crest origin, tumors of, 336
  non-polyalanine repeat expansion mutations (NPARM), 338
  PHOX2B, 333–334, 335*f*, 340–341
  ROHHAD, 339
  sleep-disordered breathing treatment in, 315
    respiratory abnormalities in, 315–317
  ventilatory management, 343–344
Continuous positive airway pressure (CPAP), 38, 91, 162, 201, 277, 310, 311, 437
Continuous spikes and waves during sleep (CSWS), 109
  clinical presentation, 109
  epidemiology and definitions, 109
  history, 109
  vs. Landau-Kleffner syndrome (LKS), 117*t*
  neuroimaging and EEG findings, 109–112, 110–111*f*
  neuropsychological manifestations, 112
  treatment, 112
COPS3 gene, 150
Core body temperature (CBT) rhythm, 247
Cortisol, 108
Cough, chronic, 454–455
Cranial radiation and brain tumors, 196
Cranial radiation therapy (CRT), 196
Cranio-facial anomalies, 449, 450
Craniocervical junction disorders (CCJ), 287
  achondroplasia, 288
    treatment strategies for, 290
    varying combinations of SDB in, 289–290
  chiari malformations, spina bifida, and meningomyelocele, 291–294
    cervicomedullary compression in CM1, symptoms and signs of, 291
    diagnostic approach, 292–293
    SDB in, 291–292, 293–294
  clinical symptoms of, 287*t*
Craniofacial anomalies
  micrognathia, 322–323
  midface hypoplasia, 323
Craniofacial disorders and sleep
  obstructive sleep apnea syndrome (OSAS)
    abnormal growth patterns of craniofacial skeleton in, 443–446
    craniofacial patterns and, 441–443
    principles of craniofacial growth, 440
    upper airway patency, anatomic and physiologic relationships in, 437–439
Craniopharyngiomas, 194
Creb binding protein (CREB), 145
Croup, 452
Crouzon syndrome, 323, 440, 441, 443*f*, 444
CSF Hcrt-1 analysis, 220–221
Cyclic alternating pattern (CAP), 85, 354, 354*f*, 357
Cyproheptadine, 425
Cystic hygroma, 438, 439*f*

D-amphetamine, 224
D-isomer of amphetamine, 224
Daytime sleepiness, 53, 223–228, 431, 433
  armodafinil, 226
  modafinil, 226
  pemoline, 227–228
  psychostimulants, 224–225
  reboxetine, 227
  ritanserin, 227
  selegiline hydrochloride, 225–226
  sodium oxybate, 226–227
  treatment, 403
Definite RLS, 66–67
Delayed sleep phase disorder (DSPD), 249, 252–254, 253*f*
Delayed sleep phase syndrome, 395–396
Dental therapy
  in children with OSA, 312
Depression, 473
Depression and sleep, effects of treatment of, 175–176
Depressive disorders
  actigraphic studies in, 175
  depression and sleep, effects of treatment of, 175–176
  EEG spectral analysis studies in, 174–175
  polysomnographic studies in, 173–174
Dermatoglyphics, in CCHS, 338
Desipramine, 147, 224*t*, 228
Dextroamphetamine, 224, 224*t*
Diabetes, 371
Diffusing capacity of carbon monoxide (DLCO), 457
DiGeorge syndrome, 453
Dim light melatonin onset (DLMO), 145, 248
Dimlight melatonin offset (DLMOff), 145–146
Diphenhydramine, 469
Diphenhydramine hydrochloride,2-(diphenylmethoxy)-N,N-dimethylethylamine hydrochloride, 396–397
Disturbed night sleep, 29
Donepezil, 475*t*

Dopamine, 405
Dopaminergics, 72–73
Dorsal and median raphe nucleus (DR/MR), 7
Dorsomedial nucleus of the hypothalamus (DMH), 16
Down syndrome (DS), 268, 275–277, 320, 321*f*
DQB1*0602 haplotype, 210
DRB1*1501 haplotype, 210
Dreaming, 6, 10–11
  distinctive features of, 10
  function of, 10–11
Droperidol, 181
Drosophila melanogaster, 1
Duchenne muscular dystrophy (DMD), 295–297, 321–322
Dysexecutive syndrome, 47
Dysphagia, 449

Early onset Hunter syndrome (MPS IIa), 282–283
Eating disorders, sleep in, 178
EEG spectral analysis studies in depressive disorders, 174–175
Electrical status epilepticus in slow wave sleep (ESES), 84, 108
Electroencephalogram (EEG), 1, 80
Elongator Protein Complex 4 gene (ELP4), 115
Endocrine function in sleep, 18
Energy conservation theory, of sleep, 3
Enzyme replacement therapy (ERT), for MPS I, II and VI, 284
Eosinophilic esophagitis, 458
Epilepsy, 79, 265
  effect of, on sleep, 88
    breathing disorders, 91–92
    epilepsy treatment, effect of, 92–93
    polysomnographic findings, 89–91
    potential causes of sleep disruption, 88–89
    prevalence of sleep complaints, 88
  effect of sleep on, 80
    different sleep stages on seizures and IEDs, 85
    sleep and epilepsy, 86–88
    sleep deprivation on epilepsy and IEDs, 85–86
    sleep-related epilepsy, 80–85
  factors inherent to, 91
  polysomnographic findings in children with, 90*t*
  SDB in children with, 286–287
  sleep phenomena mimicking seizures, 93
    daytime episodes, 100
    disorders and REM sleep, 98
    parasomnias and NREM sleep, 96–98
    paroxysmal events, 99–100
    rhythmic movement disorders, 99
    sleep-related movement disorders, 98–99
Epileptogenesis, 108
Episodic nocturnal wanderings (ENW), 82
Eplivanserin, 473
Epworth Sleepiness Scale (ESS), 32, 35, 211, 219, 361
Esophageal manometry, for gastroenterology, 462–463
Esophageal pH monitoring, 460
  for gastroenterology, 460
Esophageal pressure monitoring, 39
Eszolpiclone, 400, 401, 471, 475*t*
Ethanolamines, 398
Ethics, for pediatric trials, 473–474
European Medicines Agency (EMA), 470, 471*t*, 471–472
Excessive daytime sleepiness (EDS), 80, 162, 192, 209, 215–216, 402, 403
  in PWS, 317–318
Exercise induced dyspnea, 455
Exogenous melatonin, daily timed administration of, 256
Expiratory positive airway pressure (EPAP), 314
Extraesophageal manifestation and gastroesophageal reflux, 456

Facial dysmorphology, in CCHS, 337–338
Familial advance sleep phase disorder (FASPD), 256
FDA Amendment Act (FDAAA), 2007, 471*t*
FDA Modernization Act (FDAMA), 1997, 471*t*
FGFR3 protein, 288
Fibreoptic Endoscopic Evaluation of Swallowing (FEES), 456
Fibreoptic flexible bronchoscopy (FFB), 457
Fibromyalgia, 417
"First-night effect", 357
Fixed sleep-wake schedules, 256
Flexible endoscopy, 452–453
"Flip-flop switch", 12, 13*f*
Flow-volume loops, 457
Fluoxetine, 181, 224*t*, 228
Fluticasone, 404
Fluvoxamine, 147
Focal epilepsy with centrotemporal spikes (BECTS), 112
  clinical presentation and seizure semiology, 112–113
  epidemiology, 112
  genetics and pathophysiology, 115
  management and prognosis, 115
  neuroimaging and EEG, 113, 114*f*
  neuropsychological manifestations, 113–115
Folliclestimulating hormone (FSH), 18
Food and Drug Administration (FDA), 469, 470, 471, 471*t*, 472*f*
"Forced desynchrony", 249
Fragile X Mental Retardation 1 (*FMR1*) gene, 267
Fragile X Mental Retardation Protein (FMRP), 267
Fragile X Syndrome (FXS), 267–268, 399
Free-running disorder (FRD), 254–256, 255*f*
Frontal lobe epilepsy (FLE), 80

Function of sleep, 2
energy conservation theory, 3
learning and memory theory, 3–4
restorative theory, 2–3
Functional Matrix Theory, 441
GABAergic neurons, 11
Gabapentin, 72
Gamma hydroxybutyrate (GHB), 226, 402–403
Gastaut syndrome
clinical presentation and seizure semiology, 115
EEG findings, 115
epidemiology, 115
management and prognosis, 115
neuropsychological manifestations, 115
pathophysiology and genetics, 115
Gastroenterological perspective, 458
barium contrast radiography, 460–463
esophageal manometry, 462–463
esophageal pH monitoring, 460
impedance and pressure monitoring during polysomnography and esophageal pH, 463
multi-channel intraluminal impedance with pH (pH-MII), 460, 462, 462*f*
nuclear scintigraphy, 460
proximal/pharyngeal pH monitoring, 460, 461*f*
diagnostic testing, 460
reflux and sleep disturbances, relationship between, 459–460
Gastroesophageal reflux (GER), 100, 449, 456, 458
Gastroesophageal reflux disease (GERD), 18
treatment, 452
Gastrointestinal physiology in sleep, 18
Gene-environment interactions, 372
Ghrelin, 18
Gliomas, 194
Glottic obstruction, 451–452
laryngomalacia, 451, 451*f*
vocal cord paralysis, 452
Glycogen synthase kinase 3 beta, 368
"Growing pains", 68
Growth hormone (GH) in children with PWS, 280–281
Growth hormone (GH) therapy, 162
in PWS, 318
Guanine–cytosine (GC)-rich polyalanine region, 333

Haloperidol, 181
Hcrt-deficient mouse models, 230
Hcrt pathway, 212–214
Head trauma, sleep disorders following, 431–434
Headache disorders
diagnostic tools
actigraphy studies, 421–422, 424*t*
polysomnography, 422
sleep logs and sleep questionnaire studies, 421
future research, 425–426
pathophysiology
brain stem aminergic nuclei, 420–421
hypothalamic regulation, 420
SCN-Pineal-Melatonin Axis role, 421
secondary to sleep disturbances
in periodic limb movement of sleep, 417
in sleep disordered breathing, 415–417
relating to insomnia and chronic disorders, 417
and sleep disorders in pediatric population, 424*t*
and sleep disturbances
chronic migraine and chronic tension-type headache, 417–418
and sleep physiology
chronic paroxysmal hemicrania, 419
cluster headache, 419
hypnic headache, 419–420
migraine, 418–419
treatment strategies, 422–425
Headbanging, 99
Heart disease, 65
Heart rate
and beat-to-beat variability, on sleep fragmentation, 359
in REM sleep, 17
Hemangiomas, 445
Hemodynamic function, 371
Highest human leukocyte antigens (HLA) association, 210
Hirschsprung disease (HSCR), 333, 336
Histamine 3 (H3) receptors, 230
Histocompatibility, 221
History, of sleep, 29
daytime history, 29–32
nighttime history, 32–34
Homeostatic regulation, of sleep, 15
Hunter syndrome, 282–283
Hurler syndrome, 282, 283
Hydroxyindole-O-Methyl transferase (HIOMT), 145
Hyperactivity, 47
Hypercapnea, 313
Hypercapnia, 17
Hypernycthemeral syndrome, 254
Hypersomnia, 172, 433–434. *See also* Central hypersomnia, in PWS
recurrent, 221–222
Hypertension, 65
Hypnagogic, 100
Hypnagogic/hypnopompic hallucinations, 217–218
Hypnic headache (HH), 418, 419–420
Hypnic jerks. *See* Sleep starts
Hypnopompic hallucinations, 100
Hypnotic medications, 229
Hypocretin. *See* Orexin
Hypocretin (Hcrt) neurons, 212–213
Hypocretin-1 (Hcrt-1) neurons, 212, 282
Hypocretin-1 levels in CSF, 432
Hypotension, 72

Hypothalamic regulation, of sleep and headache, 420
Hypothalamus, 420
Hypoventilation, 39
  symptoms of, 457
Hypoxemia, 313, 458
Hypoxia, 369–370, 371
Ictal hypoxemia, 91
Idiopathic CNS hypersomnia, 221
IEDs and epilepsy, sleep deprivation on, 85–86
IEDs and seizures, different sleep stages on, 85
Imaging modalities in pediatric sleep medicine
  arnold-chiari malformation and syringobulbia, 375
  circadian rhythm disorders, 375
  congenital central hypoventilation syndrome, 374–375
  functional neuroimaging, 373–374
  Kleine-Levin syndrome, 374
  narcolepsy, 374
  sleep apnea, 374
  sleep deprivation and fragmentation effects, 370
    gene-environment interactions, 372
    hemodynamic function, 371
    inflammation, 371
    metabolic function, 371
    neurogenesis, 371
    vascular function, 371
  sleep disorders, 367–369
    hypoxia, 369–370
    potential mediators of brain injury in, 369–370
    vulnerability of pediatric brain in, 368–369
  structural neuroimaging, 372–373
Imipramine, 224*t*, 228, 403
Impulsivity, 47
Inattention, 47
Infantile spasms, 85
Inflammation, 371
Insomnia, 170, 431, 434, 471, 472
  headaches relating to, 417
  in infants, 395
  pharmacological treatment of
    in adolescents, 395–396
    in infants, 395
    in toddlers, 395
  symptoms of, 160–161
Inspiratory positive airway pressure (IPAP), 314
Intellectual disabilities (ID)/cerebral palsy (CP)
  sleep problems in children with, 285–286
Interleukin 6, 362
International Classification of Sleep Disorders, 406
International Conference on Harmonization (ICH), 470
International RLS Study Group (IRLSSG), 66, 469–470
Intracranial pressure (ICP), 17
Intrinsically photosensitive retinal ganglion cells (ipRGCs), 248
Ipratropium bromide aerosol inhaler, 455
Iron deficiency in pathophysiology of RLS, 64–65
Iron metabolism with RLS, 405
Iron supplementation, 72
Irregular sleep-wake rhythm (ISWR), 256
Isolated sleep paralysis (ISP), 126
Jactatio capitis, 99
Juvenile myoclonic epilepsy (JME), 84
Juvenile rheumatoid arthritis (JRA), 357

K-complexes, 5
Karolinska sleepiness scale, 35
Ketogenic Diet (KD), 93
Killer whale, 2
Kleine-Levin syndrome, 32, 38, 221–222, 374
Klippel-Feil syndrome, 445*f*
Kyphoscoliosis, 34

Landau-Kleffner syndrome (LKS), 84, 116–118
  vs. continuous spikes and waves during sleep (CSWS), 117*t*
Laryngeal mask airway (LMA), 457
Laryngo-tracheo-esophageal clefts, 456
Laryngomalacia, 451, 451*f*
Laryngotracheobronchoscopy, 451–452
Late Onset Central Hypoventilation Syndrome with Hypothalamic Dysfunction, 339
Late-onset Hunter syndrome (MPS IIb), 283
Later-onset CCHS, 338–339
Lateral cephalogram, 442, 442*f*, 443
Lateral hypothalamus (LHA), 7
Laterodorsal pontine tegmentum (LPT), 9
Laterodorsal tegmental (LDT) nucleus, 7
Learning, 51
Learning and memory theory, of sleep, 3–4
Leptin, 18, 362
Leutenizing hormone (LH), 18
Levodopa, 405–406
Light and measuring circadian timing system, 247–249
Limp man syndrome, 217
Lipid laden macrophage index (LLMI), 457
Lithium, 181
Locus coeruleus (LC), 7
Long-term potentiation (LTP) process, 4
Loxapine, 181
Lymphatic malformations, 438, 439*f*, 445

Macroglossia, 445
Maintenance of Wakefulness Test (MWT), 41, 220, 360–361
Major depressive disorders (MDD), 170
Mammalian sleep, 1–2
Mandibular deficiency, 443, 444, 445*f*

Marine mammals and REM sleep, 2
Maturation of sleep, 6–7
from childhood to adult period, 7*f*
Maxillary deficiency, 443, 444
Mean sleep latency (MSL), 39
Mechanistic target of rapamycin (mTOR), 268
MECP2 gene, 163
Medication side effects, drug/alcohol abuse, 222
Medications and daytime and nighttime behaviors, 54–55
Medications for children with cancer, 199
Medulloblastomas, 194
Melanin-concentrating hormone (MHC), 7
Melatonin, 14, 87, 108, 146, 147, 163, 248, 254, 398–399, 423
and AUT, 148–149
and sleep, 144
Melatonin synthesis offset, 145
Meningomyelocele (MM), 291–294
diagnostic approach to evaluating sleep breathing disorders in children with, 291–292
sleep-disordered breathing in, 291–292
Mental retardation (MR), 263. *See also* Sleep and circadian dysfunction
cerebral palsy (CP), 266–267
comorbid epilepsy, 265
Fragile X Syndrome (FXS), 267–268
septooptic dysplasia (SOD), 268–269
Trisomy 21 (Down syndrome), 268
tuberous sclerosis complex (TSC), 268
Mentally/physically disabled child, clinical approach to sleep in, 263–264
Mesoridazine, 181
Messenger RNA (mRNA), 267
Metabolic disorders, 443
Metabolic function, 371
Methamphetamine, 224, 224*t*, 225
Methyl-CpG binding protein 2 (MECP2) gene, 163
Methylphenidate, 202, 224*t*, 225, 434
Micrognathia, 322–323
Midface deficiency, 443
Midface deficiency syndromes, 443–444, 443*f*, 444*f*
Midface hypoplasia, 323
Migraine, 70, 417–419, 423*t*
and narcolepsy, 218
Mirtazapine, 181, 425
Modafanil, 202, 224*t*, 226, 230, 282, 318, 403, 434
Modified barium swallow study (MBS), 456
Monoamine oxidase (MAO), 181, 224
Montelukast, 404, 405
Mood, 50–51
Mood disorders, 172, 417, 418
Morbid obesity, 192
Morning awakening time, 29
Morningness-Eveningness Questionnaire (MEQ), 249
Mouth breathing, 150, 441
Mucopolysaccharidoses (MPSs), 282–285
obstructive sleep apnea in children with, 284–285
Multi-channel intraluminal impedance with pH (pH-MII)
for gastroenterology, 460, 462, 462*f*
Multidisciplinary aerodigestive team approach for children, 449–463
common presenting complaints in aerodigestive center, 449*t*
gastroenterological perspective, 458
barium contrast radiography, 460–463
diagnostic testing, 460
reflux and sleep disturbances, relationship between, 459–460
otolaryngological perspective, 450
evaluation, 452–453
glottic obstruction, 451–452
nasal obstruction, 450–451
oropharyngeal obstruction, 451
subglottic/tracheal obstruction, 452
upper airway obstruction causes, 450
pulmonary perspective
aspiration related lung disease, 455–458
chronic cough, 454–455
exercise induced dyspnea, 455
tracheomalacia, 453–454
tests for evaluating aerodigestive disorders, 455*t*
Multiple sleep latency, age-specific normal values for, 40*t*
Multiple sleep latency test (MSLT), 39–40, 49, 112, 144, 162, 200, 282, 360–361, 403

N-acetyl aspartate, 369
N-acetyl-5-methoxytryptamine, 398
N-acetyltransferase, 150
Nager syndrome, 444
Naltrexone, 163
Napping, 30–31
Narcolepsy, 100, 209
behavioral approaches, 223
cataplexy treatment, 403–404
clinical features of, 215
cataplexy, 216–217
CSF Hcrt-1 analysis, 220–221
excessive daytime sleepiness, 215–216
hypnagogic/hypnopompic hallucinations, 217–218
laboratory findings, 219–220
sleep paralysis, 217–218
symptoms, 218–219
diagnostic criteria for, 215
sodium oxybate, 229
differential diagnosis, 221
atonic drop attacks, 222
chronic sleep deprivation with erratic sleep-wake schedule, 221

idiopathic CNS hypersomnia, 221
medication side effects, drug/alcohol abuse, 222
primary sleep disorders, 222
psychiatric disorder/depression, 222
recurrent hypersomnia/Kleine-Levin syndrome, 221–222
secondary narcolepsy, 222–223
treatment, 223
daytime sleepiness treatment, 403
epidemiology, 209
age of onset, 210
gender differences, 210
genetic factors, 210–211
gamma hydroxybutyrate/sodium oxybate, 402–403
pathophysiology, 211
autoimmune hypothesis, 214–215
Hcrt pathway, 212–214
neurotransmitter dysfunction, 211
pharmacological treatment, 223
of cataplexy, 228
daytime sleepiness, 223–228
hypnotic medications, 229
pharmacology of, 224*t*
secondary, 222–223
Nasal obstruction, 443, 450–451
Nasal steroids, role in treatment of children with OSA, 404
Nasopharyngeal deficiency, 444
National Ambulatory Medical Care Survey (NAMCS), 392
National Cancer Institute's, Surveillance, Epidemiology and End Results program, 192
National Sleep Foundation, 469
Nefazodone, 181
Neoplasms, 203
Neuroblastomas, in CCHS, 336
Neurogenesis, 371
Neuroleptics, 148, 401–402
Neurological disorders
sleep-disordered breathing in children with. *See* Sleep-disordered breathing (SDB)
Neuromuscular disease (NMD)
and sleep-related breathing disorders, 294–298
Neuromuscular disorders, 443, 446, 449, 457
Neurotransmitter dysfunction, 211
Neutrophils, 457
Night terrors, 127
Nightmares, 98, 130
Nocturnal bruxism (teeth grinding), 131
Nocturnal cough, 454
Nocturnal frontal lobe epilepsy (NFLE), 80–82, 82*t*, 128
Nocturnal groaning, 98
Nocturnal hypoxemia, 458
Nocturnal nasal intermittent positive pressure ventilation (NIPPV), 297
Nocturnal panic attacks (NPAs), 99, 129
Nocturnal paroxysmal dystonia (NPD), 82
clinical features of, 83*t*
Nocturnal polysomnogram and MSLT, 219–220
Nocturnal polysomnography (NPSG), 35, 38–39
Nocturnal psychogenic nonepileptic seizures (PNES), 99
Nocturnal temporal lobe epilepsy (NTLE), 82–83
and nocturnal frontal lobe epilepsy, 83*t*
Nocturnal urinary–free cortisol (NUFC), 173
Non-24-hour sleep-wake syndrome, 254
Nonbenzodiazepine hypnotics, 400–401
Noninvasive nocturnal ventilation (NIV), 297–298
Noninvasive positive pressure ventilation (NIPPV)
overview, 313–314
side effects of, 315*t*
technical aspects and outcomes, 314–315
Non-polyalanine repeat expansion mutations (NPARM), 333
Non-rapid eye movement (NREM) sleep, 1, 34, 355, 370
Nonsteroidal anti-inflammatory drugs (NSAIDs), 147
Norepinephrine, 145, 179
Normal sleep, 4
NREM sleep, parasomnias of, 127
confusional arousals, 127–128
management of, 128
night terrors, 127
nocturnal frontal lobe epilepsy (NFLE), 128
nocturnal panic attacks (NPAs), 129
NREM arousal sleep parasomnias, 128
sleepwalking, 127
Nuclear scintigraphy, 460
for gastroenterology, 460

Obesity and narcolepsy, 219, 223
Obsessive compulsive disorders, 171
Obstructive sleep apnea (OSA), 29, 32, 34, 80, 99, 197, 268, 404–405, 415, 416, 434
in children with mucopolysaccharidoses, 284–285
in children with NMD
dental therapy, 312
pharmacologic therapy, 310–311
positive pressure/oxygen therapy, 311
surgical therapy, 311–312
weight loss, 312–313
Obstructive sleep apnea (OSA) syndrome, 368, 437, 459
Obstructive sleep apnea syndrome (OSAS), 438
abnormal growth patterns of craniofacial skeleton in, 443–446
craniofacial patterns and, 441–443
Olanzapine, 181, 401
Oppositional deviant disorder (ODD) and conduct disorder (CD), 50
Orexin neurons, 7, 8, 14

Ornicus orca, 2
Otolaryngological perspective
  evaluation, 452–453
  glottic obstruction, 451–452
  nasal obstruction, 450–451
  oropharyngeal obstruction, 451
  subglottic/tracheal obstruction, 452
  upper airway obstruction causes, 450
Overlap parasomnia, 98, 131–132
Overnight oximetry analysis, 37–38
Oximetry, 38
Oxygen desaturation, 91
Oxygen therapy
  in children with OSA, 311

Pace maker, 107
Pain in children with cancer, 198–199
Paired-like homeobox 2B (PHOX2B) gene, 333–334, 374, 375
  schematic of, 335*f*
Palatine tonsils, 451, 451*f*
Paliperidone, 181
Panayiotopoulos syndrome, 85
  epidemiology and definition, 116
  management and prognosis, 116
  neuroimaging and EEG findings, 116
  neuropsychological manifestations, 116
  pathophysiology and genetics, 116
  seizure semiology and clinical presentation, 116
Parasomnias, 95, 125, 406
  benzodiazepines and arousal parasomnias, 407–408
  classification of, 126, 126*t*
  epidemiology, 125
  nocturnal bruxism (teeth grinding), 131
  and NREM sleep, 96–98, 127
    confusional arousals, 127–128
    management of, 128
    night terrors, 127
    nocturnal frontal lobe epilepsy (NFLE), 128
    nocturnal panic attacks (NPAs), 129
    NREM arousal sleep parasomnias, 128
    sleepwalking, 127
  overlap parasomnia, 131–132
  pathophysiology, 125–126
  of REM sleep, 126
    behavior disorder, 130–131
    nightmares, 130
  sleep enuresis, 131
  sleep-wake transition parasomnias, 126
    isolated sleep paralysis (ISP), 126
    rhythmic movement disorder, 126
    sleep starts, 126
  status dissociatus, 131
  with migraine headaches, 418–419
Paroxysmal arousals, 82
Paroxysmal events, 99–100
Pediatric bipolar disorder (PBD), 176
  polysomnographic and actigraphic studies in, 177
  subjective reports of sleep in, 176–177
  treatment of, 177
Pediatric chronic cough, 454
Pediatric Daytime Sleepiness Scale (PDSS), 32, 219
Pediatric drug development, in infants and children, 470–471
Pediatric Investigation Plans (PIP), 472
Pediatric Quality of Life Inventory (PedsQL), 269, 297
Pediatric Regulation 1901/2006, 2007, 471*t*
Pediatric Research Equity Act (PREA), 2003, 471, 471*t*
Pediatric RLS diagnostic criteria
  definite RLS, 66–67
  research criteria, 67–68
  supportive criteria, 67
Pediatric Rule (1994), 471*t*
Pediatric sleep disorders
  clinical background, 469–470
  drug development for, 469–475, 471*t*
  drugs in clinical development, 475*t*
  investigation plan for eplivanserin, 473*f*
  pharmaceutical industry (sponsor) perspective, 473–475
  phases and features, 474*t*
  regulatory aspects, 470–473
Pediatric sleep history, 34*t*
Pediatric sleep medicine, imaging modalities in. *See* Imaging modalities in pediatric sleep medicine
Pediatric sleep pharmacology
  chloral hydrate, 397
    benzodiazepines, 400
    clonidine, 400
    melatonin, 398–399
    neuroleptics, 401–402
    nonbenzodiazepine hypnotics, 400–401
  diphenhydramine, 396–397
  general principles of pharmacology for, 391
    dosage and timing, 393–394
    other roadblocks, 392–393
    parental expectations, 392
    sedation and sleep, 393
    social environment, 394
  insomnia, 394
    adolescents, 395–396
    infants, 395
    toddlers, 395
  narcolepsy, 402
    cataplexy treatment, 403–404
    daytime sleepiness treatment, 403
    gamma hydroxybutyrate/sodium oxybate, 402–403
  obstructive sleep apnea, 404–405

parasomnias, 406
benzodiazepines and arousal parasomnias, 407–408
restless legs syndrome/periodic limb movements in sleep, 405
carbidopa/levodopa, 405–406
selective dopamine agonist, 406
Pediatric sleep questionnaire, 36–37
Pediatric study decision tree, 472*f*
PedsQL 4.0 Generic Core Scale, 269
Pedunculopontine tegmental (PPT) nucleus, 7
Pemoline, 225, 227–228
Penile erections, 6
PER1 gene, 150
Pergolide, 406
Periodic limb movement disorder, 49, 53, 65, 68, 80, 98, 150. *See also* Restless legs syndrome/periodic limb movements in sleep (RLS/PLMS)
criteria for diagnosis of, 68*t*
headaches in, 415, 417
Peripheral arterial tonometry (PAT), on sleep fragmentation, 359–360
Pfeiffer syndrome, 444
PGO (ponto-geniculo-occipital waves), 6, 9, 10
Pharmaceutical industry (sponsor) perspective, 473–475
Pharmacologic therapy
in children with OSA, 310–311
Pharmacological Management of Insomnia in Children and Adolescents, 469
Pharyngeal hypotonia, 150
Phase angle, 249
Phase response curve (PRC), 248, 248*f*
Phasic REM sleep events, 6
Phenothiazines, 398
Phenyethylamine, 434
Phototherapy, 254
PHOX2B gene, 333–334
Phylogeny of sleep, 1–2
Pierre Robin syndrome, 453
Pittsburgh sleep quality index, 35–36
PLM index, 218
Polyalanine repeat expansion mutations (PARMs), 333, 334
Polysomnogram (PSG), 49, 200
in children with neuromuscular diseases, 295
Polysomnographic studies
in anxiety disorders, 171–172
in depressive disorders, 173–174
in pediatric bipolar disorder (PBD), 177
Polysomnography (PSG), 38, 67, 89, 219, 249, 454
common abnormalities noted on, 457–458
impedance and pressure monitoring during, 463
for sleep and headache, 422
for sleep fragmentation, 356–359
in sleep-related disorders, 433
Positive pressure/oxygen therapy
in children with OSA, 311
"Possible RLS", 67
Postconceptional age (PCA), 6
Posttraumatic stress disorder, 171
Prader-Willi syndrome (PWS), 161, 277–282, 317
central hypersomnia common in, 282
clinical features of, 278*t*
excessive daytime sleepiness (EDS) in, 162, 317–318
growth hormone (GH) therapy in, 280–281, 318
sleep-disordered breathing in, 162, 280, 318
sudden death in, 281–282
treatment of sleep disturbances in, 162
Pramipexole, 72, 406
Primary sleep disorders, 222, 469
Primitive neuroectodermal tumors (PNET), 194
"Probable RLS", 67
Process C, 14
Process S, 14
Prolactin, 18
Promazine, 181
Protriptiline, 224*t*
Protriptyline (PROT), 404, 425, 228
Proximal/pharyngeal pH monitoring, for gastroenterology, 460, 461*f*
Pseudo-mandibular prognathism, 443
Psychiatric disorders and sleep, 169
anxiety disorder, 170–171
AD and sleep, treatment of, 172
anxiety disorders, polysomnographic studies in, 171–172
obsessive compulsive disorders, 171
posttraumatic stress disorder, 171
depressive disorders
actigraphic studies in, 175
depression and sleep, effects of treatment of, 175–176
EEG spectral analysis studies in, 174–175
polysomnographic studies in, 173–174
drugs for, 179
antipsychotic drugs, 181–182
bupropion, 181
lithium, 181
mirtazapine, 181
monoamine oxidase (MAO), 181
nefazodone, 181
selective serotonin reuptake inhibitors, 179–181
trazodone, 181
tricyclic antidepressants, 179
eating disorders, sleep in, 178
mood disorders, 172
pediatric bipolar disorder (PBD), 176
polysomnographic and actigraphic studies in, 177
subjective reports of sleep in, 176–177
treatment of, 177

Psychiatric disorders (*Continued*)
  psychosis, sleep in, 179
  sleep disturbances and suicide, 178
  sleep problems as predictors of, 170
Psychiatric disorder/depression, 222
Psychosis, sleep in, 179
Psychostimulants, 224–225
Pulmonary disease
  and sleep disordered breathing severity, 458
Pulmonary function tests, 457
Pulmonary perspective, aerodigestive tract with
  aspiration related lung disease, 455–458
  chronic cough, 454–455
  complications of neurological diseases in children, 453*t*
  exercise induced dyspnea, 455
  tracheomalacia, 453–454
Pulse transit time (PTT), on sleep fragmentation, 359, 360*f*
Pulse wave amplitude, on sleep fragmentation, 360

Quetiapine, 181
Quiet sleep, 6

R-modafinil, 226
Ramelteon, 396, 425, 471, 475*t*
Rapid eye movement (REM) sleep, 1, 9–10, 9*f*, 112, 205, 247, 313*f*, 354, 416, 433
Rapid Eye Movement sleep behaviour disorder (RBD), 406
Rapid maxillary expansion, 312, 320
Rapid-onset obesity with hypothalamic dysfunction, hypoventilation, and autonomic dysregulation (ROHHAD), 339
Rats, sleep in, 2
Rebound insomnia, 396, 401
Reboxetine, 227
Rechtschaffen, Allan, 1
Reflux and sleep disturbances, relationship between, 459–460
"REM-off" neurons, 9
  discharge rates of, 9
"REM on" cholinergic neurons, 9
REM sleep, parasomnias of, 126
  behavior disorder, 130–131
  nightmares, 130
REM sleep behavior disorder (RBD), 98, 130, 218
REM sleep without atonia (RSWA), 98
Reptiles, sleep behavior in, 1
Resistin, 362
Respiratory abnormalities in CCHS, 315–317
Respiratory cycle–related EEG changes (RCREC), 354, 358
Respiratory insufficiency, during sleep
  noninvasive positive pressure ventilation (NIPPV), 313–315
Respiratory physiology in sleep, 17–18
Restless legs augmentation, 406
Restless legs syndrome (RLS), 32, 53, 63, 152
  clinical course, 65–66
  comorbidity, 70–71
  diagnostic criteria, 66
    pediatric RLS, 66–68
    periodic limb movement disorder (PLMD), 68
  diagnostic interview, 70
  differential diagnosis, 68–70, 69*t*
  epidemiology, 63
  future research, directions for, 73
  impact, 65
  pathophysiology, 64
    genetics, 64
    heart disease, 65
    hypertension, 65
    iron, 64–65
    neuroanatomy, 64
    neurotransmitter dysfunction, 64
    stroke, 65
  and PLMS, 54, 405
    carbidopa/levodopa, 405–406
    selective dopamine agonist, 406
  potential exacerbating factors for, 71*t*
  severity assessment, 70
  treatment, 71
    iron supplementation, 72
    lifestyle changes, 71
    medication, 72–73
Restorative theory, of sleep, 2–3
Rett syndrome (RS), 163–164, 317
Rhythmic movement disorders, 99, 126
Rigid endoscopy, 452
Risk evaluation and mitigation strategies (REMS), 474
Risperidone, 181, 401
Ritanserin, 181, 227
RLS-like syndrome, 67
"RLS with PLMS", 67, 68
Robin sequence, 322, 441, 444
Ropinirole, 72, 406

S-modafinil, 226
Saccadic eye movements, 7
Saethre Chotzen syndrome, 444
Salivary aspiration, 456
Sandifer syndrome, 100
Sanfilippo syndrome (MPS III), 282, 283–284
SCN-Pineal-Melatonin Axis role
  in sleep and headache, 421
Seizures, sleep phenomena mimicking, 93, 94*t*
  daytime episodes, 100
  disorders and REM sleep, 98

parasomnias and NREM sleep, 96–98
paroxysmal events, 99–100
rhythmic movement disorders, 99
sleep-related movement disorders, 98–99
Seizures and IEDs, different sleep stages on, 85
Selective dopamine agonist, 406
Selective serotonin reuptake inhibitors (SSRIs), 98, 147, 172, 222
Selegiline, 224*t*, 225
Selegiline hydrochloride, 225–226
Septooptic dysplasia (SOD), 268–269
Serotonin, 108, 179–181, 211–212
Serotonin n-acetyltransferase, 144
Shortness of breath, 455
Sleep and circadian dysfunction
cerebral palsy
clinical approach in disabled child, 263–264
comorbid epilepsy, 265
Fragile X Syndrome, 267–268
in mental retardation/cerebral palsy, 263–269
septooptic dysplasia, 268–269
trisomy 21, 268
tuberous sclerosis complex, 268
Sleep and headaches. *See* Headache disorders
Sleep and wakefulness, neuroanatomy of, 195
addendum–paraneoplastic syndromes, 203–205
cancer-related fatigue (CRF), 196–197
central sleep apnea (CSA), 197–198
clinical problems of children with cancer, 199–202
cranial radiation and brain tumors, 196
medications, 199
pain, 198–199
psychiatric/behavioral, 198
sleep-disordered breathing, 197
sleep problems, evaluation and treatment of, 203
terminal phase, sleep during, 199
Sleep apnea, 374
Sleep deprivation and fragmentation effects, 370
gene-environment interactions, 372
hemodynamic function, 371
inflammation, 371
metabolic function, 371
neurogenesis, 371
vascular function, 371
Sleep diaries, 35, 250
Sleep disorder, 53
Sleep-disordered breathing (SDB), 50, 53–54, 80, 150, 264, 197, 201, 415–417, 450, 453*t*, 458, 459
cerebral palsy, 319–320
chiari malformations, 318–319
in children with epilepsy, 286–287
in children with intellectual disabilities/cerebral palsy, 285–286
in children with neurological disorders, 275–298
in children with neuromuscular disease, 309–323
congenital central hypoventilation syndrome (CCHS), 315
respiratory abnormalities in, 315–317
craniocervical junction disorders, 287
achondroplasia, 288–290
chiari malformations, spina bifida, and, meningomyelocele, 291–294
clinical symptoms of, 287*t*
craniofacial anomalies
micrognathia, 322–323
midface hypoplasia, 323
diagnostic and treatment paradigm, 309–310
Down syndrome, 320, 321*f*
duchenne muscular dystrophy, 321–322
and genetic type, 162
neurodevelopmental disorders
Down syndrome, 275–277
mucopolysaccharidoses, 282–285
Prader-Willi syndrome, 277–282
neuromuscular disorders
cardiorespiratory management in Duchenne muscular dystrophy, 295–297
noninvasive nocturnal ventilation in, 297–298
polysomnographic findings in children with, 295, 295*t*
predicting in children with, 294–295
obstructive sleep apnea (OSA)
dental therapy, 312
pharmacologic therapy, 310–311
positive pressure/oxygen therapy, 311
surgical therapy, 311–312
weight loss, 312–313
Prader-Willi syndrome, 317
excessive daytime sleepiness in, 317–318
growth hormone (GH) therapy in, 318
sleep-disordered breathing in, 318
respiratory insufficiency during sleep
noninvasive positive pressure ventilation (NIPPV), 313–315
Rett syndrome, 317
spinal muscular atrophy, 322
treatment of, 315–323
Sleep disruption, 454
Sleep disturbances and suicide, 178
Sleep drunkenness, 96
Sleep enuresis, 100, 131
Sleep evaluation
in children with aerodigestive disorders, 457
Sleep fragmentation
clinical utility, 355
defining, 353–355
in research and clinical settings
actigraphy, 356
animal studies, 355
heart rate variability, 359
human studies, 355–356
peripheral arterial tonometry, 359–360
polysomnography, 356–359
pulse transit time, 359, 360*f*

Sleep fragmentation (*Continued*)
pulse wave amplitude, 360
objective and subjective consequences
MSLT, MWT, and sleepiness scales, 360–361
neurocognitive, behavioral, and hormonal outcomes, 361–362
recovery from, 362
Sleep habits questionnaire, 36
Sleep Habits Survey (SHS), 36
Sleep homeostatic system, 247
Sleep-induced hypoxemia, 294
Sleep-inducing neurons, 11
Sleep laboratory diagnostic tests, 37
actigraphy, 37
Multiple Sleep Latency Test (MSLT), 39–40
nocturnal polysomnography (NPSG), 38–39
overnight oximetry analysis, 37–38
wakefulness test, maintenance of, 40–41
Sleep logs, 219
and questionnaires
screening tools for sleep and headache problems, 421
Sleep loss, 91
Sleep-onset REM period (SOREMP), 38, 40, 282
Sleep paralysis, 100, 217–218
Sleep per se, 52–53
Sleep pharmacology, *See* Pediatric sleep pharmacology
Sleep phase disorder, 256
Sleep-potentiated spiking, mechanisms of, 107–109
adenosine hypothesis, 108
cortisol, 108
epileptogenesis, 108
melatonin, 108
serotonin, 108
suprachiasmatic nuclei (SCN) and "pace maker", 107
thalamus, role of, 107–108
Sleep pressure score (SPS), 359
Sleep problems, evaluation and treatment of, 203
Sleep process matrix, 203
Sleep regulatory process across adolescence, 251–252
Sleep-related breathing disorder, 99
Sleep-related breathing disturbance (SRBD), 36–37
Sleep-related disorders
clinical presentation, 431–432
diagnostic evaluation and assessment, 433
evaluation, 433
in traumatic brain injury in children, 431–434
pathophysiology, 432–433
prognosis, 434
treatment, 433–434
Sleep-related epilepsy, 80–85
Sleep-related hypoventilation, in PWS, 278, 279*f*
Sleep-related movement disorders, 98–99
Sleep-related problems (SRPs), 170
Sleep starts, 99, 126
Sleep talking, 99
Sleep terrors, 96
Sleep-wake problems, 29
history, 29
daytime, 29–32
nighttime, 32–34
sleep laboratory diagnostic tests, 37
actigraphy, 37
Multiple Sleep Latency Test (MSLT), 39–40
nocturnal polysomnography (NPSG), 38–39
overnight oximetry analysis, 37–38
wakefulness test, maintenance of, 40–41
sleep-related examination, 34–35
survey tools for assessing, 35
Children's Sleep Habits Questionnaire, 36
Cleveland Adolescent Sleepiness Questionnaire, 36
Epworth Sleepiness Scale (ESS), 35
Karolinska Sleepiness Scale, 35
Pediatric Sleep Questionnaire, 36–37
Pittsburgh Sleep Quality Index, 35–36
sleep diary, 35
sleep habits survey, 36
Sleep-wake transition parasomnias, 126
isolated sleep paralysis (ISP), 126
rhythmic movement disorder, 126
sleep starts, 126
Sleep/wake transitions, 11–14
Sleepiness, 29. *See also* Daytime sleepiness
scales for assessing, 33*t*
"Sleeping" brain-behavior relationships of ADHD, 48
Sleeping child and its ADHD phenotypes, 52
daytime sleepiness, 53
restless legs syndrome (RLS) and PLMS, 54
sleep disorder, 53
sleep per se, 52–53
sleep-disordered breathing, 53–54
Sleeplessness, problem of, 431, 432, 434
Sleepwalking, 96, 127, 406
Slow-wave activity (SWA), 178, 247
Slow-wave sleep (SWS), 3, 6, 172, 247
Slow-wave/delta power analysis, 370
Smith-Magenis Syndrome (SMS), 137
genes implicated in circadian clock in, 150–151
melatonin and AUT, 148–149
melatonin and sleep, 144
phenotype, 138
sleep in, 138–142
studying sleep in children with, 142–144
treatment of sleep disorders in, 148
unrecognized epilepsy and sleep disturbance, 151–152
Sodium oxybate, 224*t*, 226–227, 229, 230. *See also* Gamma hydroxybutyrate (GHB)
Somatic mosaicism for PARM, 339–340
Somnambulism, 96, 418–419
Somniloquy, 99

Somnolence, 473
Spectral analysis, EEG, 358
Speech-language pathologist (SLP), 455
Spike wave (SW), 84
Spina bifida (SB), 291–294
  sleep-disordered breathing in, 291–292
Spinal muscular atrophy (SMA), 322
Spirometry, 457
Stanford Sleepiness Scale (SSS), 219
"Status cataplecticus", 216
Status dissociatus, 131
Stroke, 65
Subglottic/tracheal obstruction, 452
Subparaventricular zone (SPZ), 16
Substance abuse, 52
Sudden death
  in Prader-Willi syndrome (PWS), 281–282
Sudden unexpected death in epilepsy population (SUDEP), 92
Suicidal ideation, 178
Suicidality, 473
Suprachiasmatic nuclei (SCN), 14, 144, 194, 247, 420
  and "pace maker", 107
Supratentorial PNETs (sPNET), 194
Surgical therapy
  in children with OSA, 311–312
Sympathovagal imbalances, 17
Syndromic micrognathia, 444
Syringomyelia, 291
  diagnostic approach to evaluating sleep breathing disorders in children with, 291–292
  sleep-disordered breathing in, 291–292

Tanner sleep stage–specific reference values, 39
Taylor's type focal cortical dysplasia (TFCD), 83
"Tellectual disability" (ID), 263
Terminal phase, sleep during, 199
Thalamo-cortical circuits, 107
Thalamus, role of, 107–108
Thioridazine, 181
Thyroid-stimulating hormone (TSH), 18
Thyrotrophin-releasing hormone (TRH), 230
Tic disorder, 51
Time spent awake and moving (TSPAM), 175
Timed light exposure, 256
TIRED study, 469
Toddlers, insomnia in, 395
Tonsillar hypertrophy, 451, 451*f*
Topiramate, 422
Tourette syndrome/Tic disorder, 51
Tracheoesophageal fistula (TEF), 453
Tracheomalacia (TM), 453–454
Traumatic brain injury in children, sleep in. *See* Sleep-related disorders
Trazodone, 181
Treacher-Collins syndrome, 441, 444
Trial of Infant Response to Diphenhydramine (TIRED study), 397
Triazolam, 396, 401
Trichloroethanol (TCE), 397
Tricyclic antidepressants (TCAs), 179, 222, 228–229, 403
Triptans, 420
Trisomy 21 (Down syndrome), 275, 268, 443, 453
Tuberous sclerosis complex (TSC), 268
Two-process model of sleep, 14, 15*f*
  circadian sleep regulation, 15–16
  homeostatic regulation, 15
Typically developing children (TYP), 142–143

Unrecognized epilepsy and sleep disturbance, 151–152
Upper airway obstruction causes, 450
Upper airway resistance syndrome (UARS), 459
Upper GI (UGI), 460
Upper respiratory tract infections (URTIs), 454

Vagal nerve stimulation (VNS), 93, 286–287
Vascular function, 371
VATER syndrome, 453
Venlafaxine, 404
Ventro-lateral preoptic (VPLO) nucleus, 420
Ventrolateral periaquaductal gray matter (vLPAG), 9
Ventrolateral preoptic nucleus (VLPO), 11–12
  targets of, 12*f*
Videofluroscopic swallow study, 456
Videosomnography, 142
Vocal cord dysfunction (VCD), 455
Vocal cord paralysis, 452, 456
Voluntary sleep deprivation, 2

Wake-time after sleep onset (WASO), 142
Wakefulness, 7–8. *See also* Sleep and wakefulness, neuroanatomy of
Wakefulness test, maintenance of, 40–41
"Waking" brainbehavior relationships of ADHD, 48
Weight loss, in children with OSA, 312–313
Williams syndrome (WS), 162–163

Xyrem® Success Program, 474

Zaleplon, 229, 396, 400, 401, 471
Zeitgeber, 265
Ziprasidone, 181
Zolpidem, 229, 400–401, 469, 471, 475*t*
  conrolled release, 471
Zolpidem CR, 471
Zopiclone, 229